Occupational Therapy and Mental Health
Principles, Skills and Practice

Occupational Therapy and Mental Health

Principles, Skills and Practice

Edited by

Jennifer Creek DipCOT
Senior Occupational Therapist
Tameside and Glossop Health Authority

CHURCHILL LIVINGSTONE
EDINBURGH LONDON MELBOURNE AND NEW YORK 1990

CHURCHILL LIVINGSTONE
Medical Division of Longman Group UK Limited

Distributed in the United States of America by Churchill
Livingstone Inc., 1560 Broadway, New York, N.Y. 10036,
and by associated companies, branches and representatives
throughout the world.

First published 1990

ISBN 0-443-03758-2

British Library Cataloguing in Publication Data
Occupational therapy and mental health: principles, skills
    and practice.
    1. Man. Mental disorders. Occupational therapy
    I. Creek, Jennifer
    616.89165

Library of Congress Cataloging in Publication Data
Occupational therapy and mental health: principles, skills,
    and practice/edited by Jennifer Creek.
        p. cm.
    1. Occupational therapy.   2. Mentally
    ill—Rehabilitation.
    I. Creek, Jeniffer.
    [DNLM: 1. Occupational Therapy. WM 450.5.02 0145]
    RC487.024   1990
    615.8'515—dc20

Produced by Longman Singapore Publishers (Pte) Ltd.
Printed in Singapore

Preface

The profession of occupational therapy grew out of a strong belief in people's capacity to influence their own health through what they do. This belief gave the profession a clear identity and direction, and the confidence to proclaim its own worth. And yet the unique attributes of occupational therapy, along with a working knowledge of the beliefs and theories that underpin it and give it its strength, are not always communicated successfully to students and practitioners.

This is regrettable because occupational therapy is a potent and uniquely valuable approach to health care that enables people to take control of their own lives and overcome their own disabilities. The tools and methods that we use are commonplace but the aims of occupational therapy remain original and exciting. After nearly 20 years of practice, I still feel a sense of discovery in my work almost every day.

My experience over the past 20 years has taught me the necessity of infusing practice with a thorough appreciation of underlying philosophy and theory. Without this knowledge, skills become mere tools that are applied haphazardly. However, as a student and in my early years as a therapist, I was not so fortunate as to be provided with a clear and coherent account of the nature of my chosen profession. Like many of my contemporaries, I learned about the roots of occupational therapy piecemeal, mainly by chance.

In the early 1970s I had the good fortune to work at the Royal Edinburgh Hospital, and I am indebted to Henry Walton, whose ward I was at-tached to, and to my then colleagues—Hester Monteath, Sheena Blair and the late Irene Affleck—for setting a standard of care that I have tried to live up to ever since and for making explicit the theories underlying that care. I then went into teaching and became fascinated by the richness of occupational therapy's theory and philosophy. I had always enjoyed being a practising therapist but my exploration of the occupational therapy literature meant that my work was now enhanced by a clearer understanding of what I was doing and a new ability to explain my work to others.

My primary intention in compiling this textbook has been to communicate to students and professionals the enormous potential of occupational therapy, and to give them a clear picture of the scope of the profession. By providing a thorough and carefully structured introduction to the history of the profession, and the philosophy and theory on which it is founded, followed by an account of key client groups and clinical skills in the area of mental health, I hope to give a firm grounding that will allow them to enter the profession with confidence and build on this knowledge as they gain experience.

The opportunity to edit this new textbook, which includes the work of some of the profession's most experienced and valuable members, has given me the chance to bring together systematically much of what I have absorbed through years of study and clinical experience. It has also given me the experience of becoming better acquainted with the work of some of the profession's most knowledgeable practitioners. I would like to pay tribute here to their labours.

The book's overall structure

The book is divided into two main parts: Part 1 looks at the theory of occupational therapy but also includes history and philosophy. This part pertains to occupational therapy as a whole and is not specifically related to mental health.

Part 2 covers clinical and managerial aspects of practice, specifically within the context of mental health. These two parts have been written to show the links between theory and practice.

Part 1

The first section of Part 1 explores the history and progression of the profession of occupational therapy. It is difficult to understand our present state of development and position in the field of health care without this temporal perspective.

Section 2 begins with a review of the knowledge base of occupational therapy. It then attempts to bring together the components of an overall paradigm that will take occupational therapy into the 21st century with the same vigour and sense of purpose that brought it into being at the beginning of this century. These components are: the beliefs and values at the core of the profession, the theories that have been collected to support those beliefs, the goals and scope of occupational therapy practice, the content of practice and the occupational therapy process. A structure is suggested to show the relationships between all these parts of the profession.

Section 3 first has a chapter on frequently used models. It then takes the reader through the occupational therapy process in detail, with chapters on assessment, treatment planning and implementation and evaluation (quality assurance). This is the process that is used in all the chapters on different areas of practice in other parts of the book.

Section 4 looks at the context in which occupational therapy exists today: the physical settings where therapists practise and the social context of therapy, including the many different roles taken on by practitioners. The chapter on 'Ethics' is the only chapter in the book not written by an occupational therapist. It is intended to give the reader a new perspective on the profession and perhaps to provoke thinking about aspects that we tend to take for granted.

Part 2

Section 5 is the first section of Part 2, where the book moves into the clinical area. It covers some of the media and techniques that occupational therapists use in implementing treatment. It is impossible to include all possible techniques for a profession that will use almost any activity that benefits the client. The selection given here is a range of commonly used techniques for developing skills in all areas of function: physical, cognitive, intrapersonal and interpersonal.

Section 6 covers the main fields where therapists work with clients with mental health problems. This section highlights the trend towards large institutions being closed and people's being cared for in the community. It also includes a chapter on transcultural issues in mental health.

The final section of the book discusses the infrastructure of a therapy service, without which it would be impossible to practise. This includes management, budgeting and record keeping. It also includes a chapter on clinical supervision of occupational therapy students, which is relevant for most clinical therapists. The final chapter is on research, highlighting methods and topics that all therapists should consider taking up.

The profession of occupational therapy can be endlessly fresh and exciting for its practitioners. Many therapists adopt a developmental approach to working with clients and should, perhaps, use the same approach for themselves. There are always opportunities to explore new ideas or learn new techniques. Inspiration may come from attending a course or conference, talking to a colleague or reading a journal article. Most readers of this text will find some or all of the chapters useful and I hope they may come across a number that challenge them to think about their work in a new way. But the book will ultimately be successful if it inspires therapists, as I have been in-

spired, to value what they are doing and be true
to their beliefs; if it enhances for each reader a
sense of professional identity and satisfaction in
being a part of a living, growing profession.

Jennifer Creek
Stockport
1990

Acknowledgements

Hester Monteath, who has always believed in my ability as an occupational therapist, and who suggested I write this book.

The late Professor Max Hamilton, without whose practical help, support and advice the book would not have been written.

My sister, Jane Steed, who was always willing to childmind, giving me time to write.

Belinda Thompson and Adrienne Payne, who supplied much of the material for Chapter 23, Mental Handicap.

Irene Paterson for reading and commenting on the occupational therapy process, Chapters 4 to 7.

Ann Arnthal for reading and commenting on Chapter 21, The Elderly.

Kit Sinclair and Pauline Jenks, who put me on the trail of occupational therapy philosophy and supplied me with references.

Joyce Hamilton, Wendy Jabri and Ann Hodges, who typed large parts of the manuscript.

Dorset House School of Occupational Therapy and the American Occupational Therapy Association for supplying references.

Jennifer Creek
1990

Dr Pat Barnet of the Open University and Dr David Dodwell of Manchester University for support in preparing Chapter 10; Dr Dominic Jackson also criticised parts of the chapter and all gave constructive advice.

Hazel Bracegirdle
1990

Contributors

Sheena E E Blair DipCOT MEd
Senior Lecturer
Queen Margaret College
Edinburgh

Hazel Bracegirdle BA DipCOT RDth
Community Paediatric Occupational Therapist
North Derbyshire Health Authority
Derby

Teresa Brown DipCOT Cert of Projective Techniques
Analytical & Associated Applications Group,
Institute of Human Relations
Senior Occupational Therapist
Psychotherapy Day Hospital, Southern General
Hospital, Glasgow

Jennifer Creek DipCOT
Senior Occupational Therapist
Tameside and Glossop Health Authority

Tessa Durham DipCOT SROT
Formerly Senior Occupational Therapist
Royal Dundee Liff Hospital
Dundee

Margaret Ellis FCOT
District Occupational Therapist
Tower Hamlets Health Authority
The London Hospital
Whitechapel

Linda Franklin
Formerly Head Occupational Therapist
Withington Hospital
Manchester

Sue Gore DipCOT
District Occupational Therapist
Stockport Health Authority

Clephane A Hume BA DipCOT Cert FE
Lecturer
Queen Margaret College
Edinburgh

Lily I H Jeffrey FCOT UCCAP
Unit Head Occupational Therapist
West Unit, Lothian Health Board
Formerly Head Occupational Therapist
and Honorary Occupational Therapy Tutor,
Newcastle University

Lesley Lougher BSc Soc DipCOT
Senior Occupational Therapist
Peterborough Family Consultation Service

Elizabeth Morrison
Formerly Head Occupational Therapist
Raigmore Hospital
Inverness

Lesley McCallion DipCOT
Senior Occupational Therapist
Tameside and Glossop Health Authority

Shaun McCallion DipCOT
Senior Occupational Therapist
Astley Hospital
Wigan Health Authority

Judith Reid DipCOT
Head Occupational Therapist
The Maudsley Hospital
London

Averil M Stewart BA FCOT TDip SROT
Head of Department of Occupational Therapy
Queen Margaret College
Edinburgh

Belinda Thompson SROT Cert IHSM
Head Occupational Therapist
High Peak Locality
North Derbyshire Health Authority

Ian E Thompson BA (Hons) PhD
Principal Professional Development Officer
Scottish Health Education Group
Edinburgh

Penny Wheeler MSc DipCOT
Occupational Therapy Practice Coordinator
Exeter Health Authority

Contents

Part 1

SECTION 1
Introduction

1

A history of the profession

Elizabeth Morrison

INTRODUCTION

'The importance of studying the history of medicine, or indeed, the history of any subject, lies in the fact that a mere summary of concepts and the results obtained therefrom without a knowledge of their evolution cannot give any true picture of the matter. Without being aware of the laborious foundations upon which an edifice is built we can gain but a superficial idea of the great superstructure.' (Lloyd 1968)

Occupational therapy has been described as 'an active method of treatment with a profound psychological justification' (Clark 1963). Today this statement may appear an oversimplification, but it remains a viable description of a method of treatment that has flexible limits and is adaptable in its use. The essence of occupational therapy lies in the use of activities of every description as treatment medium, with a minimum aim of improving the quality of life and a maximum aim of complete rehabilitation.

This brief survey of the evolution of occupational therapy as it is recognised and practised worldwide today will try to show something, not only of the 'laborious foundations' which underlie it, but also the inspiration which has continued the building of the profession, particularly since the early part of the 20th century.

THE EARLY USE OF OCCUPATION AS TREATMENT

The therapeutic use of activity and movement has been appreciated since the dawn of civilisation. As early as 2600 BC the Chinese taught that disease resulted from organic inactivity and used physical training for the promotion of health. They utilised a series of medical gymnastics called 'Cong Fu'. This, they felt, could not only prolong life but would also ensure the immortality of the soul (Levin 1938).

At around 2000 BC the Egyptians dedicated temples where 'melancholics resorted in great numbers in quest of relief.' Philip Pinel, a physician writing in Paris in 1803, described how games and recreations were instituted in the temples and all the patient's time 'was taken up by some pleasurable occupation' (Haworth & Macdonald 1940). The Persians used physical therapy at about 1000 BC in order to train their youth for military service. From the age of six the boys followed a systematic course of physical therapy into adulthood, becoming an army of physically fit, able-bodied fighting men.

ANCIENT GREECE AND ROME

The earliest written references to therapeutic activities appeared some time before 600 BC. Aesculapius, working at Epidaurus in Greece, is claimed to have soothed delirium with 'songs, farces and music' (Le Clerc 1699).

In the following period (600 BC to AD 200) Pythagoras, Thales and Orpheus all used music as a remedy. Hippocrates, who consistently emphasised the mind–body link in all treatment, recommended wrestling, riding and 'labour', which seems to have meant active, vigorous exercise, possibly an early form of aerobics.

Cornelius Celsus, a major contributor to the early study of anatomy and medicine, recommended the following for maintaining health; sailing, hunting, handling of arms, ball games, running and walking. He prescribed reading aloud for a weak stomach and wrote of 'several kinds of madness and their cures,' advising occupations that are suitable to the temper of each person (MacDonald 1976). He also seems to have used a method of application similar to modern behaviour therapy and laid stress on the *combined* use of treatment techniques (McDonald 1976).

At around 30 BC Seneca recommended employment for any kind of mental agitation, and in AD 17 Livy wrote 'toil and pleasure in their nature opposites are linked together in a kind of necessary connection.' The value of alternating work and play was equally stressed by Phædrus, also in the 1st century AD, 'the mind ought sometimes to be diverted that it may return the better to thinking' (quoted in Levin 1938).

RENAISSANCE EUROPE

During the Dark Ages (AD 200–1250) there appears to have been little development of the use of occupation as therapy. From AD 1100 onwards, however, the founding of a number of universities brought a revival in scientific study. A significant factor at this time was the introduction of examinations for would-be medical practitioners, and of state control over medical practice by licensing (MacDonald 1964).

After AD 1250 medical studies became more profound, with greater attention to detail. Anatomy and physiology, together with philosophy and psychology, became subjects for careful study. Hospitals were set up, though the care of the mentally ill remained basic.

Between AD 1250 and AD 1700 interest was directed to the analysis of movement, while Leonardo da Vinci, Descartes and Francis Bacon gave attention to industrial physiology, taking especial note of rhythm, posture and expenditure of energy. These studies were later followed up by Ramazzini, Professor of Practical Medicine at Padua, who stressed the importance of prevention rather than treatment and of observing the patient–worker in his workshop. He noted the value of weaving as exercise and referred to cobbling, tailoring and pottery, all contemporary trades.

At about the same time, Sanctorus Sanctorius developed his theories of metabolism, showing the influence of work by Descartes, Harvey and Galileo. Occupational exercises and recreation for increasing stamina and for enjoyment were recommended by physicians during this period, but there is little to suggest any consistency in experiment or systematised prescription.

18TH AND 19TH CENTURY WESTERN EUROPE

During the 18th and 19th centuries rapid developments took place in the fields of psychology, anatomy and physiology. With the increased understanding each new discovery brought, treatment became more refined and specialised. Very gradually the embryonic patterns of the specialisations of physiotherapy and occupational therapy appeared, although it was some time before they acquired recognisable form. The introduction of the use of electricity had a profound effect on the development of physiotherapy and the link of movement therapy with purposeful activity emerged largely as the realm of the occupational therapist.

Before this, in 1780, C. J. Tissot classified occupational exercise as active, passive and mixed, recommending activities such as sewing, playing the violin, sweeping, sawing, bell-ringing, hammering, chopping wood, riding and swimming. In 1786 Phillipe Pinel, in France, introduced work treatment in the Bicetre Asylum for the Insane, near Paris. In 1801 he prescribed physical exercise and manual occupation; following his insistence on freeing patients from the chains and other physical restraints popular as a means of handling the mentally ill at that time.

Around the same time William Tuke in York, England, founded 'The Retreat,' a hospital still used for psychiatric treatment today. Restraints here were also reduced to a minimum. Simultaneously, Johan Reil in Germany also reduced mechanical restraints, but he failed to offer this freedom in treatment conditions (MacDonald 1981).

In Britain from 1850 onwards, the supplementary treatment services began to emerge as identifiable professions, setting up training courses and establishing qualifications, recognised examinations and professional associations. Another relevant factor was the move for women to take up careers and become accepted in the professions. The Crimean War precipitated the establishment of nursing as a profession and the First World War that of physiotherapy. Although some occupational therapy was carried on earlier, it was in the Second World War that occupational therapy really came into its own (MacDonald 1976).

The emphasis in the early 19th century was in the psychological field, and by the end of the century occupational therapy was being practised, though in rather different forms, in the United Kingdom, Ireland, the USA, France, Germany, Switzerland, Austria, Norway, Portugal and Belgium (MacDonald 1976).

In England, the best known centres were the Retreat at York and Hanwell Asylum, now St. Bernard's Hospital, Southall. In Scotland, the use of occupation as treatment was to be found at Murray Royal Infirmary, Perth. Dr W. A. F. Browne (known as the father of occupational therapy in Scotland) had introduced such treatment in the late 1830s at Montrose, and later at Crichton Royal Hospital, Dumfries (Groundes-Peace 1957).

A notable scheme introduced in Scotland in 1898–9 was the Brabazon Scheme at Woodilee Asylum, Lenzie. This scheme, founded by the then Lady Brabazon, consisted of 'teaching infirm and crippled inmates of workhouses to employ their idle hands usefully.' The Scheme was managed by 12 ladies, each 'particularly gifted to teach some special subject.' So rugmaking, lampshade-making, macrame, drawn linen work, woodcarving, basket-making and wrought-iron work came to be taught in what were eventually known as the Brabazon Workshops (MacDonald 1976). This seems to have been a prototype for other establishments in both the mental health and physical fields. It has also been suggested that the inspiration for occupational therapy arose in America as a result of inspecting the Brabazon work (Groundes-Peace 1957), although none of the researched American records confirms this. History suggests that the profession of occupational therapy emerged as part of an upsurge in awareness of the value of occupations as treatment at the end of the 19th century.

THE BEGINNINGS OF THE MODERN PROFESSION

THE USA*

In 1752 the Pennsylvania Hospital, Philadelphia, was established in the USA, where the use of occupation as treatment for the mentally ill continued to develop until the Civil War in 1860. The war meant that treatment for the mentally sick was seen as relatively unimportant while there were great numbers of wounded to be treated (Hopkins 1983).

Towards the end of the 19th century, attention was once again focussed on work as a therapeutic agent, particularly for the mentally ill. In December 1892 Adolf Meyer, psychiatrist, reported that 'the proper use of time in some helpful and gratifying activity appeared to be a fundamental issue in the treatment of the neuro-psychiatric patient' (Meyer 1922). In 1895 Meyer's wife, a social worker, introduced a systematic type of activity into the wards of a state institution in Worcester, Massachusetts.

Meyer's philosophy of treatment and occupation was to have a marked impact on the development of the philosophy and history of occupational therapy in the USA. 'Our conception of man is that of an organism that maintains and balances itself in the world of reality and actuality by being in active life and active use . . . It is the use that we make of ourselves that gives the ultimate stamp to our every organ . . .' (Meyer 1922). Meyer saw mental illness as a problem of living, not merely as a disease of structure or function, or toxic in nature. He laid stress on the value of interpersonal relationships between patients, instructors and helpers.

In 1905 Susan E. Tracy, while training as a nurse, noted the benefits of occupation in relieving tension and making bedrest more tolerable for patients. She saw occupation as an important ad-junct to drug treatment, realised something of the value of instruction in self-help, and stressed the importance of interpersonal relationships. Tracy wrote the first book about the use of occupation in the treatment situation, *Studies in invalid occupations* (Hopkins 1983), containing compilations of her lectures as director of the Training School for Nurses at Adams Nervine Asylum, Boston, Massachussetts.

John Dewey wrote in 1910, 'The fundamental point of the psychology of an occupation is that it maintains a balance between the intellectual and the practical phases of experience' (Tracy 1910), a conclusion he reached while directing the Experiment Station for the Study of Invalid Occupations in Jamaica Plains, Massachussetts.

In 1904, Herbert J. Hall began prescribing occupation for patients in Concord, New Hampshire and in 1906 Harvard University became interested in his work, giving him a thousand dollars 'to assist in the study of the treatment of neurasthenia by progressive and graded manual occupation' (Hopkins 1983). He established a workshop at Marblehead, Massachussetts. Feeling, like Tracy, that nurses and social workers were the most suitable trainees, Hall began a training course for young women from these disciplines at Marblehead in 1908.

During the same year, a training course in occupations for hospital attendants was given in Chicago. Enrolled on this course was Eleanor Clarke Slagle, a social worker from Chicago. Her concern about the detrimental effects of idleness on mental patients in a local state hospital led her not only to complete her own course but to share her learning with other students in Newberry, Michigan. From there she went to the Johns Hopkins Hospital, Baltimore and worked under A. Meyer as his Director of Occupational Therapy. In 1915 Eleaner Clarke Slagle organised the first professional school for occupational therapists in Chicago. She became director in 1918 and held the post until 1922.

Concurrently William Rush Dunton Jr., known as the father of occupational therapy in the USA, was using occupation as treatment in Baltimore, where he worked as a psychiatrist. Inspired by Tracy's book on invalid occupations Dunton, in

---

* Helen S Willard and Clare S Spackman published the first edition of their comprehensive book 'Occupational Therapy' in 1947. A more recent edition is the source for this section.

1911, conducted a series of classes on the use of recreations and occupations for nurses at his own hospital. 1915 saw the publication of Dr Dunton's own book, 'Occupational Therapy—a Manual for Nurses', the first complete textbook on occupational therapy in the USA.

The evolution of the term 'occupational therapy'

In December 1914 architect George Edward Boston attended a meeting of hospital workers and the Massachussetts State Board of Insanity (Hopkins 1983). During his own recent illness he had received treatment through activities and, as a result of this, he coined the name 'occupational therapy'. During the ensuing years alternative terms have been suggested, since many therapists feel it is clumsy and carries unfortunate associations of occupation for occupation's sake, however, no substitute has yet been found that so aptly describes the art and science of 'not the making of an object, but the making of a man' (Dewey 1900).

The National Society for the Promotion of Occupational Therapy (1917)

At a meeting in March 1917 held at Consolidation House, Clifton Springs, New York, the National Society for the Promotion of Occupational Therapy was formed, incorporated and chartered under the laws of the District of Columbia. This body held its first AGM in September 1917 in New York City.

During the following years it quickly became apparent that organisations at a local level were needed for the exchange of ideas and concepts. William Dunton established the first in Maryland and a pattern of nationwide organisations affiliated with the national body were formed. This remains the basic pattern for the American Occupational Therapy Association (AOTA), as it has been known since 1923.

In 1922, the first journal, 'The Archives of Occupational Therapy' was published. This name became 'Occupational Therapy and Rehabilitation' in 1925, and changed again in 1947 to 'The American Journal of Occupational Therapy' when AOTA assumed total responsibility for its publication.

American involvement in the First World War gave a great boost to the expansion of occupational therapy in the USA as 'reconstruction aides', as they were called, were required to help rehabilitate the wounded. The emphasis was on physical disabilities.

After the war, the Boston School reopened in the autumn of 1919, followed closely by the Philadelphia and St Louis Schools (Hopkins 1983). Two of these still function; the Boston School as part of Tufts University and the St Louis School as part of Washington University. Sadly, the Philadelphia School, which trained the first occupational therapist for Scotland and the founder therapists for the first English training school, was phased out in 1981.

By 1928 there were six schools of occupational therapy in the USA, and in 1931 the National Registry of all qualified occupational therapists was established. In March 1931, AOTA requested the American Medical Association to undertake the inspection and approval of occupational therapy training schools. This process began in 1933 and a document called 'Essentials of an Acceptable School of Occupational Therapy' was produced. By 1938 13 schools had been evaluated, and 13% of hospitals approved by the American Medical Association had qualified occupational therapy staff. The majority of these were mental hospitals.

The first formal subjective registration examination had been developed by 1939. The Second World War (1941–5) meant that more occupational therapists were needed very quickly. Emergency courses were again organised so that occupational therapists could work as part of the re-conditioning programme in the Armed Forces. It was 1947 before the first national objective registration examinations were presented.

Occupational therapists in the USA have been working towards the establishment of an exact science of occupational therapy, while maintaining training standards. Notable among them are Mary

Reilly, who developed the occupational behaviour frame of reference, Clare S. Spackman and Helen Willard, Gail S. Fidler, and Anne Cronin Mosey. They have also been involved in the founding and development of a worldwide organisation for occupational therapists.

GREAT BRITAIN

The First World War

Sir Robert Jones, an orthopaedic surgeon, persuaded the War Office to set up Orthopaedic Centres. The first was opened at Shepherd's Bush Military Orthopaedic Hospital in March 1916 and its success led to the establishment of others, including centres in Edinburgh, Glasgow and Aberdeen (Watson 1934).

Occupational therapy for a modern psychiatric hospital was introduced into Scotland at Gartnavel Royal Mental Hospital in 1919 by Dr D. K. Henderson, later known as Professor Sir David Henderson (Groundes-Peace 1957).

In 1924 Dr Henderson read a paper on occupational therapy to a meeting of the Royal Medico–Psychological Society of Mental Science. Among the delegates was Dr Elizabeth Casson, the first woman doctor to graduate from Bristol University, who had chosen to specialise in psychiatry. This encounter was followed by a visit to the USA by Dr Casson in 1925–6, where she saw occupational therapy in practice at Bloomingdale Hospital, New York. Recognising its value she resolved to introduce it to her own nursing home in Clifton, Bristol.

1925 was a momentous year for occupational therapy in Scotland. The first qualified occupational therapist to be employed in Britain started work at the Royal Cornhill Hospital, Aberdeen. This was Margaret B. Fulton, who had received her training at the Philadelphia School. Fulton continued to work at Cornhill Hospital until her retirement, making a very considerable contribution to Scotland's occupational therapy, and to the profession worldwide.

It was to the same school in Philadelphia that Dr Casson arranged to send Constance Tebbit for training. Constance Tebbit returned to work in Dr Casson's Dorset House Psychiatric Nursing Home in Bristol, and set up an occupational therapy department (MacDonald 1981).

The first school of occupational therapy

It was at Dorset House that the first school of occupational therapy in the United Kingdom was founded in 1930 under Dr Casson's inspiration and with Miss Tebbit as its first principal. Within a few years other schools followed, in London, founded by Angela Rivett and Margaret Tarrant, and in Northampton and Exeter.

In 1936 Lt. Col. John Cunningham, the first medical superintendent at the Astley Ainslie Hospital in Edinburgh, enlisted the help of Canadian occupational therapists to found an occupational therapy department and a training centre. The first students qualified from here in 1939, becoming members of the Canadian Association because of the close ties between the centre and the University of Toronto, from which the founders had come.

Meanwhile, in addition to the psychiatric treatment at Dorset House, Dr Casson arranged for occupational treatment for physical cases at Bristol General Hospital and other centres. When Constance Tebbit left Bristol to work at a psychiatric hospital in Chester, two American, Philadelphia trained therapists ran the Dorset House School and treatment departments until 1938 (Macdonald 1981). It was in this year that E. Mary MacDonald, who had trained as an occupational therapist at Dorset House, became principal of the school, including the treatment departments. MacDonald was to remain in this post for over thirty years. In the same year, after a sponsored training visit to orthopaedic hospitals in the USA and Canada, she helped Dr Casson and her staff to set up the Allendale Curative Workshop, also in Bristol (MacDonald 1981).

The British Associations of Occupational Therapy

Scotland

1932 saw a meeting take place, attended by 11 occupational therapists working in Scotland, mostly from psychiatric hospitals. This group formed the first professional occupational therapy association in Great Britain. It had 30 members between that time and the outbreak of war in 1939. No meetings were held during wartime, and the Association was reformed in 1946 with 35 full members and three associate members. An Advisory Panel was set up on the advice of the President, Sir John Fraser (Hume & Lock 1982).

England

In 1935 a meeting took place at Dorset House School, under the chairmanship of Dr Casson. This was the first of a series which led to the formation of the Association of Occupational Therapists in March 1936.

By early 1937 Sir Hubert Bond had become President and an Advisory Board with 37 members had been set up (Hume & Locke 1982). The second Annual General Meeting was held in 1938, the year of the first final examination of the Association, and also the year the first Journal was published in August.

The Second World War

At the outbreak of the Second World War in 1939 the Council for AOT set up a War Executive Committee in case the Council was unable to meet. While the numbers of Diploma candidates continued to increase, they were still insufficient to meet the needs of the wartime situation. AOT therefore established a series of shorter courses:

- Occupational therapy auxiliaries: a modified course that could subsequently be upgraded to a full diploma.
- War Emergency Diploma: for those with previous qualifications, for example, teachers and nurses.
- The 1943 certificate: a partial qualification for mature people with useful training and experience (Hume & Locke 1982).

'Upgraders', as the occupational therapy auxiliaries were called in the immediate post-war years, became some of the most distinguished members of the profession.

These truncated courses were introduced to improve the input of qualified staff to the physical field in Emergency Service (EMS) Hospitals, established as a wartime measure. Very little new work took place in the psychiatric field during this period.

With the intensive bombing of Bristol following the fall of France in 1940 it became necessary to move Dorset House nursing home, school and workshop to safer areas. The nursing home went to Somerset while the school and workshop found accommodation in the EMS hospital attached to the Barnsley Hall Mental Hospital at Bromsgrove. The medical superintendent of this hospital, Dr Andrew Shepherd, was to prove an invaluable friend to the fast-developing profession. Dorset House School thus succeeded in remaining open throughout the war years.

In Scotland, meanwhile, the Department of Health opened occupational therapy departments in EMS hospitals. It was arranged, therefore, that eight qualified occupational therapists from Toronto, Canada, should be sent to Scotland to restart work there. Three of these therapists went to the Astley Ainslie Hospital and re-opened both the occupational therapy department and the training centre. Besides students attending for the normal course, 12 students were trained as assistant occupational therapists for the Department of Health, receiving a six-month course of instruction (Groundes-Peace 1957). Another Canadian went to Bangour Hospital and developed a large department, while yet another one went to Gleneagles, where a department was started for the new Rehabilitation Centre for Miners. This has now become the Bridge of Earn Rehabilitation Centre. Other departments were also developed under the EMS scheme in Scotland.

Post-war: the National Health Service

Following the end of the war in 1945 some EMS hospitals gradually closed down, but a great many continued to be used as general and specialist centres for the care of both civilians and troops. Barnsley Hall at Bromsgrove closed and Dorset House School found new premises at Churchill

Hospital, Oxford in 1947, moving finally to Headington in Oxford, where it is now.

In July 1948 the whole national approach to health care was revolutionised by the implementation of the National Health Act 1946 and the National Health Act (Scotland) 1947, which were largely based on the Beveridge report of 1942. The patient was to receive whatever care he needed free of charge, regardless of his ability to pay. Magnanimous and comprehensive in its aims, the service soon ran into financial problems which successive governments have tried to solve in a variety of ways, while still maintaining a growing and developing service using up-to-date methods.

This has meant periods of growth in occupational therapy departments when funds were available, and a stable situation regardless of clinical need when money was in short supply or, indeed, when claims for development in other areas gained priority. With the development of the NHS there has been overall growth and considerable development within the profession, particularly as areas of specialised interest have emerged.

The training schools established before and during the war, that is, Liverpool (by Constance Glyn-Owens, formerly Tebbit), Chertsey, Derby and York, were joined by schools at Glasgow, Cardiff and Dublin shortly afterwards. More recently, health-authority-based schools have been started in Belfast, Wolverhampton, Aberdeen and Colchester. Concurrently, courses have been established in Polytechnics at Salford, Belfast and Newcastle (MacDonald 1981). Some schools are hoping to change to degree courses, Edinburgh and Ulster being the first, while a new degree course is being introduced at Canterbury.

State Registration (1960)

The Professions Supplementary to Medicine Act 1960 gave official recognition to occupational therapy and allied professions (MacDonald 1976). Each Professional Board links state and professional interest and is responsible for 'promoting high standards of professional education and professional conduct' (HMSO 1960).

As a result of this Act, all occupational therapists practising in the National Health Service since 1962 have had to become State Registered. This regulation also applies to some other employing authorities.

Alongside this, the profession itself was developing. In 1943 the Association in England, including Wales and Northern Ireland, became incorporated. The Scottish Association was reconstituted in 1946, following the disruption of the war years. In 1951 the Association of Occupational Therapists in England held a first International Congress. At this, Jean Waterston, who had been responsible for starting the occupational therapy department in the Sick Children's Hospital in Edinburgh, gave an outline of occupational therapy in Scotland.

During the 1950s a Joint Council of Associations of Occupational Therapists in Great Britain was established and met regularly to consider matters common to AOT and SAOT, such as State Registration. A referendum conducted by this Joint Council in 1969 indicated that both AOT and SAOT were in favour of a merger to create one United Kingdom association. Working parties were set up to study all aspects of this. On 10 May 1974, at a ceremony in Newcastle upon Tyne, AOT and SAOT became united as the British Association of Occupational Therapists. The Right Honourable Lord Byers PC OBE became its first and deeply committed President, remaining so until his death. Since 1984 this post has been held by Lord David Ennals, a one-time Minister of Health.

In 1977 BAOT organised the first European Congress which was held in Edinburgh, the second taking place in London in 1985.

The climate of industrial relations in the 1970s led to BAOT becoming an independent certificated trade union on 4 December 1978. Educational and professional aspects of the Association's work were transferred to the College of Occupational Therapists, which was able to retain the charitable status previously enjoyed by the Association (Hume & Locke 1982).

THE WORLD FEDERATION OF OCCUPATIONAL THERAPISTS

FOUNDATION

In September 1951 a number of international representatives of occupational therapy attended the Congress of the International Society for the Welfare of Cripples held in Stockholm, Sweden, holding various meetings from which emerged a draft constitution for a World Federation of Occupational Therapists. This Federation was inaugurated on 7 April 1952. Margaret Fulton, the first trained occupational therapist in Scotland and first secretary of the SAOT was elected its first President, while Constance Glyn-Owens, (formerly Tebbit), a founder member of Dorset House School, became the first honorary secretary. 'Both the United Kingdom Associations faced the challenge of contributing to the growth of the profession in the international field' (Hume & Locke 1982).

The first World Congress was held in Edinburgh in 1954. It was attended by 400 delegates, representing 21 nations.

'The World Federation has linked the profession with the World Health Organization and has published data on the procedures and standards required for training courses in the many world countries so that they can be accepted and given official recognition' (MacDonald 1981).

FUNCTIONS

Since 1952 the Council of WFOT has met every 2 years and held congresses in different member countries at 4-yearly intervals. It works 'to further its original aims to promote the development of occupational therapy and to safeguard professional standards' (BAOT 1986).

In 1952 full member countries numbered 11. By 1986 this membership had risen to 28 countries, with five more in associate membership. The duties of member countries include 'the furtherance of effective practice of occupational therapy and to safeguard standards; to appoint delegates and instruct them properly; and to submit to the Federation an annual report. . . These reports represent the major item of communication between the secretariat and member organisations.' (BAOT 1986). It is from this information that data is extracted for the study of the state of the profession internationally. The annual report also provides facts which enable the Federation to publish accurate information for its members.

STRUCTURE

One delegate and two alternates are elected for each member country. The delegate and one alternate may attend the biennial Council Meeting. It is part of the role of delegates to promote understanding of the purpose and function of the World Federation within their own association, and

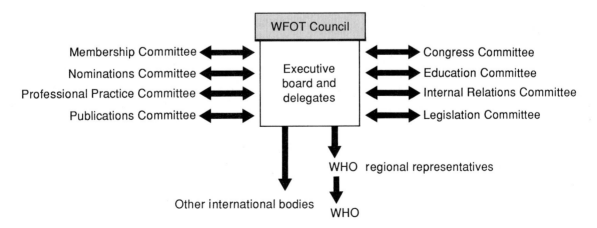

Fig. 1.1 The structure of the World Federation of Occupational Therapists. (Source: BAOT 1988)

to act as a link between the Federation and that organisation.

In order to make communication easier, WFOT has published a number of documents, such as 'Recommended Minimum Standards for the Education of Occupational Therapists,' as well as Proceedings of the International Congresses.

The functions of WFOT can be described as follows:

- 'To act as the official international organisation for the promotion of occupational therapy: to hold international congresses.
- To promote international co-operation amongst occupational therapy associations, occupational therapists and between them and other allied professional groups.
- To maintain the ethics of the profession and to advance the practice and standards of occupational therapy.
- To promote internationally recognised standards of education of occupational therapists.
- To facilitate the international exchange and placement of therapists and students.
- To facilitate the exchange of information and publications and to promote research.
- To be involved in matters where occupational therapy expertise can contribute to policy making in general preventative, curative and rehabilitative health matters.' (BAOT 1986)

MEMBER COUNTRIES

The 28 full member countries are: Argentina, Australia, Austria, Canada, Colombia, Chile, Denmark, Finland, France, Federal Republic of Germany, Hong Kong, India, Ireland, Israel, Japan, Kenya, Netherlands, New Zealand, Norway, Philippines, Portugal, South Africa, Spain, Sweden, Switzerland, United Kingdom, USA, Venezuela.
Associate members:
Iceland, Italy, Malaysia, Singapore, Zimbabwe. (BAOT 1986)

SUMMARY

In approximately three-quarters of a century occupational therapy has grown as an organised profession from the perception of its value among a few groups of dedicated people in different countries to a Federation maintaining professional standards and encouraging the exchange of information and experience throughout the world. From a virtually empirical beginning in clinical situations, it is now a largely research-based profession, as published documentation shows.

In the field of practice, from the simple use of craft activities, carefully analysed, the profession has moved through an emphasis on the Activities of Daily Living (ADL) and work-related activities to today's high technology. Whatever will improve the quality of life and, where appropriate, enhance rehabilitation remains the tool of the occupational therapist.

Occupational therapy began life in hospital wards and curative workshops. Today treatment is as likely to take place in the client's home as occupational therapy increasingly moves out into the community. Already, a growing practice in the Mental Health Service and changes in the provision of the Primary Care Services suggest that a developing role for the occupational therapist exists in this field (Walker 1986). This is over and above the excellent service provided through many social service and social work departments by the therapists who have chosen this field since the 1960s, particularly in the area of physical disability.

The future is bright for occupational therapy, the horizons unlimited. As the story of its development unfolds, it is seen to be well founded in dedicated and pioneering spirits who met every challenge and built upon each and every one. The resulting superstructure will become even more honourable if new challenges can be met with the same determination and vision.

REFERENCES

British Association of Occupational Therapists 1986 Occupational therapists' reference book. Parke Sutton, London

Clark D 1963 Psychiatry today, 2nd edn. Penguin, London

Dewey J, 1900 The school and society. University of Chicago Press, Chicago

Fidler G S, Fidler J W 1954 Introduction to Psychiatric Occupational Therapy. Macmillan, London

Groundes-Peace Z 1957 An outline of the development of occupational therapy in Scotland. Scottish Journal of Occupational Therapy 30

Haworth N A, MacDonald E M 1940 Theory of occupational therapy for students and nurses.

HMSO 1960 Professions Supplementary to Medicine Act. Bailliere Tindall, London

Hopkins H L 1983 An historical perspective on occupational therapy. In: Hopkins H L, Smith H D (eds) Willard and Spackman's Occupational Therapy, 6th edn. Lippincott, Philadelphia

Hume C A, Lock S J 1982 The golden jubilee 1932–1982. British Journal of Occupational Therapy 45(5): 151–153

Le Clerc D 1699 Translated: Drake, Baden The history of physick

Levin H 1938 Occupational and recreational therapy among the ancients. Occupational Therapy and Rehabilitation 17(5)

Lloyd W E B 1968 A hundred years of medicine, 2nd edn. Duckworth, London

MacDonald E M 1964 Occupational therapy in rehabilitation, 2nd edn. Bailliere Tindall, London

MacDonald E M (ed) 1976 Occupational therapy in rehabilitation. Bailliere Tindall, London

MacDonald E M 1981 Worldwide conquests of disabilities. Bailliere Tindall, London

Meyer A 1922 The philosophy of occupation therapy. The Archives of Occupational Therapy 1: 1–10. Reprinted 1977 in the American Journal of Occupational Therapy 31(10): 639–642

Rerek M D 1971 The depression years 1929–1941. American Journal of Occupational Therapy 25(5) 231–233

Walker J H 1986 The Casson Memorial Lecture: Out into the community. British Journal of Occupational Therapy 49(5): 144–146

Wallis M A 1987a Profession and professionalism and the emerging profession of occupational therapy, part 1. British Journal of Occupational Therapy 50(8): 264–265

Wallis M A 1987b Profession and professionalism and the emerging profession of occupational therapy: part 2. British Journal of Occupational Therapy 50(9): 300–302

Watson T 1934 (ed) The life of Sir Robert Jones. In: The cripple's journal. Quoted in MacDonald 1981.

Willard H S, Spackman C S (eds) 1963 Occupational therapy (3rd edn) Lippincott, Philadelphia

SECTION 2
The philosophical and theoretical basis of occupational therapy

2

The knowledge base of occupational therapy

Jennifer Creek

INTRODUCTION

In Chapter 1 we surveyed the ancient roots of occupational therapy and how it evolved into a
modern-day profession. Using this information as
a background, we can now look more closely at
the philosophical basis of occupational therapy,
the theories that have been explored in the past
and those that are being tested today. We will do
this by analysing the following:

● the three main phases of development of
 professional philosophy in the modern age
● the main areas of knowledge from which
 occupational therapy derives its theoretical
 base
● the relationship of the theoretical base and
 the practice of occupational therapy.

THE PHILOSOPHICAL DEVELOPMENT OF THE MODERN PROFESSION

As seen in Chapter 1, the profession of occupational therapy as we know it today dates from
approximately 1917. Since that time the profession
has undergone, and is still undergoing, changes in
its outlook and philosophy. Three main phases of
development can be distinguished and are discussed below under the following headings:

● the holistic era (early 19th century)

- the reductionist era (immediate post-war)
- the era of synthesis (the present).

In reality, the phases are not as distinct as these headings suggest; they merely help us to analyse general trends in the development of occupational therapy.

THE HOLISTIC ERA

During this first phase of occupational therapy, the profession operated with a holistic and humanistic view of human beings and occupation. Holism views people as whole entities who cannot be studied as a collection of discrete parts without losing sight of the interrelatedness of the parts which become something different if they are isolated (Smith 1983). People also change, according to this view, if they are separated from the environmental influences that have shaped them. They can only be understood as physical, intellectual, emotional and social beings operating in their natural environment.

Humanism views people as 'growing, developing, creating being(s), with the ability to take full self-responsibility' (Cracknell 1984). This includes taking responsibility for maintaining their own health and for making choices that determine what they become.

These beliefs in the mind–body–environment interrelationship and in the capacity of human beings to achieve health through what they do led occupational therapists to use broad and balanced programmes of occupation to treat mental health problems.

In 1922 Meyer wrote about the value of occupation in the management of psychiatric clients. Although Meyer did not attempt to define occupational therapy, he was aware that 'the proper use of time in some helpful and gratifying activity appeared to be a fundamental issue in the treatment of the neuropsychiatric patient.' He also outlined his philosophy as a recognition of:

'the need of adaptation and the value of work as a sovereign help in the problems of adaptation . . . .
Our conception of man is that of an organism that maintains and balances itself in the world of reality and actuality by being in active life and active use

. . . Our role (as occupational therapists) consists in giving opportunities rather than prescriptions . . .
Man learns to organise time and he does it in terms of doing things.'

Meyer described theories which we still recognise as being fundamental to our profession.

THE REDUCTIONIST ERA

Throughout the 1950s and 1960s occupational therapy gradually changed its philosophy under the influence of the reductionist model of science which was then being adopted by all the life sciences in an attempt to become scientifically respectable. Reductionism is based on the belief that the structure and function of the whole can best be understood from a detailed study of the parts by observation and experiment (Smith 1983). Reilly (1962) said that each person's need to be occupied should not be inferred from global generalisations but was being rigorously investigated under laboratory conditions. This comment sits uncomfortably within a talk which emphasises a holistic view of human beings, and demonstrates the confusion of identity that occupational therapists were experiencing at that time.

Shannon (1977) claims that occupational therapists not only lost sight of their holistic philosophy but adopted the medical model with 'its focus on pathology . . . and on the minute and measurable.' Medicine is concerned with acute illness, or with the acute phase of illness, whereas occupational therapy is traditionally and most usefully concerned with the needs of people with chronic health problems. Therapy began to focus on the techniques used rather than on the person, and became concerned with reducing symptoms without considering the quality of life that the client would have at the end of intervention.

With the increasing complexity of treatment and accompanying need for specialisation, the focus moved from health to illness, and responsibility for wellness moved from the client to the medical profession. Occupational therapy, in accepting this change, lost its humanistic perspective and began to prescribe activities for patients rather than giving them opportunities to influence their own health through occupation.

By adopting the reductionist model, occupational therapists were able to develop a great depth of expertise in various fields of practice, for example, many therapists became highly skilled in the use of projective media in analytic group psychotherapy, but the profession as a whole suffered from role diffusion and loss of identity (Kielhofner & Burke 1977).

THE ERA OF SYNTHESIS

During this period, which began in the 1970s and is still going on today, there has been a conscious effort on the part of occupational therapists to reassess the original philosophy of occupational therapy, which had become obscured during the 1950s and 1960s.

West (1984) suggests that society is moving from a mechanistic view of man and health to a systems view which is congruent with the holistic and humanistic perspective of occupational therapy. 'Health care of the future will consist of restoring and maintaining the dynamic balance of individuals, families, and social groups, and it will mean people taking care of their own health individually, as a society, and with the help of therapists.'

The profession is attempting to reassert the validity of occupational therapy traditions and values without losing the very real advances in theory and practice made during the reductionist era. The areas of belief which are being reassessed can be summarised as:

- concern with the whole person, who has a past, present and future, functioning within a physical and social environment
- belief in intrinsic motivation; an innate predisposition to explore and act on the environment
- acceptance of the social nature of people and the importance of social interaction in shaping what we become
- recognition of the importance of what we do in determining what we become; the primacy of function over structure
- view of health as a subjective experience of well-being, resulting from being able to achieve and maintain a sense of purpose and balance in life
- belief in the responsibility and capability of people to maintain their own health by what they do
- acceptance of the role of occupational therapists in serving the occupational needs of people in order to help them restore meaning and balance to their lives
- belief in the use of occupation as both the central organising concept of the profession and as the main treatment medium.

The current search for a clearer understanding of occupational therapy is not an academic exercise but a response to major changes both in society and within the profession. Occupational therapists, particularly in the USA, have been attempting to unite the profession within a commonly agreed paradigm. Although there has been a proliferation of models for practice, no one overall paradigm has been accepted.

'Occupational therapy theory into practice' on page 25 defines and explains paradigms, frames of reference and models but first we should briefly describe the areas of knowledge that occupational therapists have incorporated into their theoretical foundation.

AREAS OF KNOWLEDGE: THE THEORETICAL BASE OF OCCUPATIONAL THERAPY

Mosey (1981) states, 'the theoretical foundation of a profession is a statement of selected theories from various fields of inquiry.' The following list presents the main areas or fields of study on which occupational therapy is founded:

- theory of occupation
- biological sciences
- developmental theory
- physical medicine
- psychiatry
- psychology
- sociology
- the arts.

The wide-ranging nature of this list presents a problem in itself, as no-one can be fully informed on all these subjects, especially with the recent explosion of knowledge in all fields. It is important, therefore, to appreciate how these very varied subjects are of particular relevance to occupational therapy.

The following sections deal with each of the above areas of knowledge, concentrating on the aspects that are particularly relevant to the practice of psychosocial occupational therapy. Reference is also made to other chapters in this book where occupational therapy applications derived from these areas are explored in more detail.

THEORY OF OCCUPATION

The profession of occupational therapy was founded on the belief that people can influence their own health by being proficient in occupations which allow them to explore and interact with their environment in an adaptive way.

In order to understand this interaction and its effects, it is necessary to develop a theory of occupation, including:

- the role of occupation in human development
- the importance of occupation in maintaining physical and mental health
- the concept of occupational role
- the process of occupational choice
- balance of occupations
- concepts of motivation and volition.

Our knowledge of occupation has not yet been organised into a coherent and cohesive theory.

'Activity' and 'occupation' are often used synonymously, even by occupational therapists, but it is important to clarify the distinction. Reilly (1962) suggested that the very existence of occupational therapy depends on our knowledge of 'the difference between activity and occupation', and our capacity to 'act on the knowledge of this difference.' Activity has been defined as 'the state of being active; the exertion of energy.' 'Occupation' is defined as 'the being occupied with, or engaged in something.' To be engaged is to be attracted and held fast (Shorter Oxford Dictionary 1978). Thus, while occupation includes the use of activity it also implies involvement in what is being done.

Reed & Sanderson (1980) describe occupation as using the individual's resources of time and energy and being composed of skills and values.

Nelson (1988) divides occupation into two components:

- *occupational form* means the sociocultural and physical characteristics of an occupation that exist independent of the person engaging in the occupation, for example, the equipment, materials, context, rules and symbolism of a game make up its occupational form
- *occupational performance* is the actions of the individual elicited and guided by the occupational form, for example, playing a game.

In order to be able to apply occupation effectively as therapy it is necessary to have a sound understanding of the nature of occupation, the role of occupation in human development and the relationship between the individual and occupation. The theory of occupation is discussed in more detail in chapter 3, and activity analysis is described in chapter 6.

BIOLOGICAL SCIENCES

When working with people whose problem is emotional or behavioural it is essential to have a grounding in the biological sciences, since physical structures and systems underpin development in all other areas, and there are many physical abnormalities associated with psychosocial disorders. It is not within the scope of this book to cover the biological sciences in any detail but to review their importance to the knowledge base of occupational therapy.

Anatomy is the study of physical structures and systems. Physiology is the study of body functions. The understanding of certain disorders, such as dementia, depends on knowledge of anatomy and physiology, especially neuroanatomy and neurophysiology.

Some illnesses and handicaps are caused by chromosomal abnormalities, such as trisomy 21 (Down's syndrome), or genetic abnormalities, such as inherited microcephaly. Handicaps may also result from damage to the central nervous system of the foetus or young child by infection, toxins, anoxia or trauma. Effective intervention with such major handicaps depends on understanding the normal functioning of the nervous system and knowing where the focus of damage is. Other psychosocial problems arising from central nervous system malfunction include epilepsy, organic brain disease and the side effects of certain groups of drugs used in treatment.

Problems which may not have a physical cause but which have an important physical component in their presentation include eating disorders, addictions, anxiety neurosis, autism, catatonia, mania and depression.

Kinesiology is the study of the mechanics of movement, including range and coordination of movements and muscle strength. Movement and coordination are often affected in psychosocial disorders, for example, stereotyped movements in autism, or depressive stupor. A common feature of mental handicap is abnormal muscle tone, poor posture and unusual gait. Some methods of treatment can also affect the way a person looks and moves, for example, certain groups of drugs affect the central nervous system to produce Parkinsonian rigidity and tremor.

Any abnormality of appearance immediately marks a person as different and interferes with his acceptance by society, so effective treatment of movement patterns is essential in any resettlement programme.

The link between mind and body and the use of physical activity as treatment is covered in more detail in Chapter 7.

DEVELOPMENTAL THEORY

In order to understand and treat people with functional deficits it is necessary for the occupational therapist to have a basic understanding of normal structures, functions, and sequences of development. Development is the gradual evolution of an organism through a series of predictable stages to full growth. Maturation is the process of coming to full growth and development, mentally, physically and socially. Competent performance of age-appropriate skills depends on development and

maturation occurring in the appropriate sequence and at an appropriate pace.

Growth and development can be inhibited by internal or external factors so that maturation is seriously delayed or perhaps never completed. Disease or trauma can cause regression to an earlier stage of development. The theory of development is therefore central to occupational therapy and is not confined to the field of paediatrics.

Deficits due to developmental delay or regression can be physical, cognitive, intrapersonal or interpersonal, but problems in one area will affect the development of all the others. When assessing an adult with multiple handicaps it may be difficult to judge which was the area of primary deficit (see Case example 23.4).

Occupational therapy intervention usually follows the developmental sequence, as can be seen in the models outlined in Chapter 4 and in the paradigm described in Chapter 3.

PHYSICAL MEDICINE

In medicine, disease is classified according to aetiology or symptomatology. Care is taken to establish an accurate diagnosis so that the most appropriate treatment can be given. This may be to:

- remove the cause of the disease, for example, surgery to remove a tumour
- correct the pathology of the disease, for example, insulin for diabetes mellitus
- give symptom relief, for example, neuroleptics to control psychotic symptoms.

The occupational therapy student studies the classification, aetiology, presentation, treatment and prognosis of diseases affecting the cardiovascular, locomotor, respiratory, digestive, urogenital and endocrine systems. Emphasis is placed on neurology, including diseases and injuries affecting the nervous system such as brain, spinal cord and peripheral nerve injuries, cerebral palsy, poliomyelitis, chorea, multiple sclerosis and cerebral–vascular accidents.

A knowledge of basic medical theory is important to the occupational therapist because we work within a system which has a strong bias towards the medical model. This model helps us to understand some aspects of illness in depth but can be limiting, as it does not normally take account of the whole person functioning in his environment and in time (Lyons 1985).

PSYCHIATRY

Psychiatry uses a medical model, seeing mental disorder in terms of predisposing and precipitating factors (aetiology), signs and symptoms, course, treatment and prognosis. Diseases are usually classified by signs and symptoms. Treatment can be physical, for example, electroconvulsive therapy (ECT), or psychological, for example, psychotherapy.

Most psychiatrists take into account a range of factors affecting the client, such as pre-morbid personality, family history and environment, but these are grafted onto the medical model.

Occupational therapy students study the aetiology, presentation, classification and treatment of the more common psychiatric syndromes including psycho-neuroses, psychoses, organic states, drug addiction and alcoholism, personality disorders, psychiatric problems of children and developmental delay (mental handicap).

Like medicine, this model is useful for focusing on particular aspects of disease and for communicating with colleagues about those aspects, but it can be limiting with its focus on illness and its emphasis on treatment techniques rather than on people and social systems.

PSYCHOLOGY

Psychology is an important area of study throughout the three or four years of occupational therapy training. As well as providing theories to explain many aspects of human beings, such as personality and motivation, it has produced certain treatment techniques which have been widely adopted by occupational therapists, for example, some anxiety management techniques.

Areas of study include psychological development, which covers personality development, cognitive development and psychosocial development.

Perception, consciousness, memory, language and thinking are basic areas of study. Learning theory and conditioning are considered to be important to the occupational therapist, although some of the behavioural methods derived from these theories do not fit with the humanistic, client-centred approach. Humanistic psychology and psychoanalytic theory are studied in some depth and both give alternative insights into basic drives and motivation. Intelligence, creativity and methods of measuring these are studied, although occupational therapists are not usually expected to do formal testing. Knowledge of the effects of stress and methods used to cope with it are of particular importance to the occupational therapist. Finally, the technique of counselling is being given increasing emphasis.

Humanism and human development are two key concepts in occupational therapy that are discussed in more detail in Chapter 5. Theories of intelligence, learning theory, cognitive development and cognitive approaches to treatment are described in Chapter 12.

SOCIOLOGY

The body of knowledge in sociology has been expanding rapidly in recent years and has become increasingly useful to occupational therapists. The individual does not exist in isolation from other people and we do not assess or treat him in isolation, therefore an understanding of how society functions is crucial to the understanding of the individual.

Topics studied include social behaviour and socialisation, role theory, the family, group dynamics, deviance and stigma, work, organisations and social stratification.

Important concepts which will be expanded in other chapters include the family (Chapter 22) and stigma (Chapter 23).

THE ARTS

Occupational therapists use a wide variety of art media in every psychiatric setting. Only a limited number of techniques can be taught on the basic training course, but there are specialist postgraduate courses available in various media such as art, drama and music. Media commonly used include painting, printing, ceramics, music, poetry, literature, dance and drama. These all have the advantage of being very versatile and can be used on all levels from hobby to explorative psychotherapy. The arts have a symbolic and cultural value as well as having aesthetic, expressive and creative value for the individual.

The use of the arts in group psychotherapy is discussed in Chapter 13, giving examples of painting, poetry, music and clay modelling. Chapter 14 is about the use of drama.

The breadth of occupational therapy practice requires that the profession has this extensive knowledge base but different fields of practice will draw on different areas of knowledge. The ways in which the knowledge base is organised for use are covered in the next section, 'Occupational therapy theory into practice', and in Chapters 3 and 4.

OCCUPATIONAL THERAPY THEORY INTO PRACTICE

There is a need, within occupational therapy, for a coherent framework to encompass the philosophical, theoretical and applied aspects of the profession. The object is to establish a generally accepted structure that is sufficiently flexible to incorporate the values and beliefs of occupational therapists with the vast range of knowledge and practical skills available.

Such a structure would include an overall view of the nature of the profession, the different schools of thought coexisting within it, and the models used to translate theory into practice in different fields. These elements have come to be described by certain recognised terms:

- paradigm
- frame of reference
- model.

These terms, and the relationships between them, are defined here. Chapter 3 then looks in more

detail at the search for a universal paradigm and Chapter 4 presents four of the models commonly used in the mental-health field of occupational therapy.

DEFINITIONS OF TERMS

Paradigm

A paradigm is an agreed body of theory, explaining and rationalising professional unity and practice, that incorporates all the profession's concerns, concepts and expertise, and guides values and commitments. It reflects a profession's purpose, the nature and extent of its practice, the content of its educational curriculum and its research interests. (Alexander et al 1985, Kielhofner 1985, Shannon 1977).

Frame of reference

A frame of reference refers to the principles behind practice; the organisation of knowledge in a particular field to permit description of relationships between facts and concepts. For the purposes of this book, frames of reference are the different approaches used in occupational therapy that draw on particular areas of knowledge, for example, the occupational behaviour frame of reference. (Bruce & Borg 1987, Llorens 1984).

Model

A model is a simplified representation of the structure and content of a phenomenon or system. Its purpose is to describe or explain the complex relationships between concepts within the system and make it easier to think about them. Models are used to facilitate the translation of the occupational therapy paradigm into practice in particular fields. (Kielhofner 1985, Miller et al 1988, Mosey 1981).

The relationships between a paradigm, frames of reference and models

These three concepts operate at different levels. A

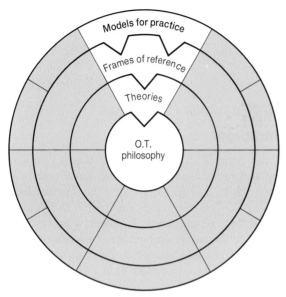

Fig. 2.1 A paradigm of occupational therapy.

paradigm is the overall structure of a profession that incorporates all the frames of reference and models (see Fig. 2.1).

Within the paradigm, the central unifying force is the professional philosophy. Theories are developed or collected to support professional philosophy. Some of these theories are compatible with each other, for example, neurodevelopmental theory and sensory integrative theory, while others are mutually incompatible, for example, behavioural theory and the theory of intrinsic motivation. Theories that are compatible and tend to be used together can be grouped into schools of thought called frames of reference.

Within a frame of reference one or more models may be used to translate theory and philosophy into practice. Each model will incorporate all the ethical and philosophical beliefs of the profession, but will only draw on particular areas of theory and technique. Models are designed to be used with specified client groups.

We have looked at some of the components of the occupational therapy profession: philosophy, theory and internal structures. We now look at a way of organising all this information into a rational whole.

GENERAL SYSTEMS THEORY

Reilly (1962) identified the need for a return to our roots and the organisation of our philosophies and knowledge into one unifying framework. The system she used to achieve this organisation, which is now being widely adopted, is general systems theory (GST) (Green 1977, Kielhofner & Burke 1977, 1980, Smith 1983, Lyons 1985).

Traditionally, scientific thinking has, to some extent, been either holistic or atomistic. Holism is the tendency to believe that it is best to study the whole unit because it is qualitatively different from, and more than, the sum of its parts. Atomism is the tendency to believe that the whole is made up of elementary units and that it can best be understood by studying these units separately before putting them together. Both these approaches are incomplete. Wholes and parts do not exist without each other: a part is always part of something and a whole is made up of parts.

General systems theory provides a way of thinking that is neither holistic nor atomistic but studies the interrelationship between parts and wholes. Each unit is both a combination of lesser parts and a part of a greater whole. This relationship can be described as a system. Systems have levels in which each unit is seen simultaneously as both a part and a whole.

Systems are hierarchical in nature, each level incorporating characteristics of all the lower levels. It has been suggested that all systems can be classified within eight levels of complexity, as shown in Figure 2.2 with frameworks being the lowest and social organisations being the highest (Smith 1983). The first three levels are called closed systems because they operate according to internal laws and structures. The higher levels are open systems which maintain themselves in equilibrium through interaction with the environment (Kielhofner 1978). An open system operates in a repetitive cycle of information intake, information processing, output and environmental feedback.

GST and occupational therapy

General systems theory has been described as a new paradigm of contemporary scientific thinking

Levels		
8	Organisations	Open systems
7	Man	
6	Animals	
5	Genetic – societal	
4	Open systems	
3	Cybernetics	Closed systems
2	Clockworks	
1	Frameworks	

Fig. 2.2 Boulding's classification of systems (adapted from Kielhofner 1978).

(Lazlo 1972). Its relevance to occupational therapy is within the context of a change in scientific thinking in general, a move away from the limitations of reductionism towards a view of the world in terms of relationships and basic principles of organisation.

Kielhofner and Burke (1977) suggest that the GST approach is relevant to occupational therapy because it:

- incorporates the advances made in knowledge during the reductionist era into a more holistic approach as conceptualised by our founders
- incorporates all our knowledge of man into one theoretical base so that man can be viewed as a whole, internally organised, growing, adapting, living system
- clarifies the relationship of man with his physical, temporal and symbolic world
- identifies the focus of concern of the profession, the goals of intervention and the methods used
- allows new knowledge to be incorporated into the theoretical base without having to create a new paradigm.

An example of a model based on general systems theory is the model of human occupation developed by Kielhofner and colleagues (Kielhofner & Burke 1980, Kielhofner 1980a, Kielhofner 1980b, Kielhofner, Burke & Igi 1980), which is outlined in Chapter 4.

SUMMARY

In this chapter we have looked at how the profession of occupational therapy has passed through various phases of philosophical development since its foundation in the early part of the 20th century.

The first phase was the era of holism, characterised by a strong belief in the humanistic and holistic ideals of the founders of the profession. The second phase was the era of reductionism when great gains were made in discrete areas of professional practice, with an accompanying loss of professional identity and universally accepted professional beliefs. The final, and current, phase of development is the era of synthesis, in which efforts are being made to reunite the profession under a new paradigm incorporating all the existing philosophical beliefs, theories and models for practice.

We then reviewed the areas of knowledge that occupational therapists have selected or developed to support the philosophical assumptions of the profession. These include the theory of occupation and selections from the biological sciences, social sciences, medicine and the arts.

Finally, we looked at general systems theory and the part it is playing in the move towards a new paradigm.

In Chapter 3 we look at the progress that has been made towards developing a paradigm, and in Chapter 4 we review four of the models that are being used in current practice in the field of mental health.

REFERENCES

Alexander L, French G, Graham J, King L, Timewell E 1985 Who needs a theory of occupational therapy? Do you? Australian Occupational Therapy Journal 32(3): 104–108

Bruce M A, Borg B 1987 Frames of reference in psychosocial occupational therapy. Slack, New Jersey

Cracknell E 1984 Humanistic psychology. In: Willson M (ed) Occupational therapy in short-term psychiatry. Churchill Livingstone, Edinburgh

Green M 1977 Development or oblivion? British Journal of Occupational Therapy Dec 1977

Kielhofner G 1978 General systems theory: implications for theory and action in occupational therapy. American Journal of Occupational Therapy 32(10)

Kielhofner G 1980a A model of human occupation, part 2. Ontogenesis from the perspective of temporal adaptation. American Journal of Occupational Therapy 34(10): 657–663

Kielhofner G 1980b A model of human occupation, part 3. Benign and vicious cycles. American Journal of Occupational Therapy 34(11): 731–737

Kielhofner G, Burke J P 1977 Occupational therapy after 60 years: an account of changing identity and knowledge. American Journal of Occupational Therapy 31(10)

Kielhofner G, Burke J P 1980 A model of human occupation, part 1. Conceptual framework and content. American Journal of Occupational Therapy 34(9): 572–581

Kielhofner G, Burke J P & Igi C H 1980 A model of human occupation, part 4. Assessment and intervention. American Journal of Occupational Therapy 34(12): 777–788

Kielhofner G (ed) 1985 A model of human occupation. Williams & Wilkins, Baltimore

Lazlo E 1972 The relevance of general systems theory. George Braziller, New York

Llorens L A 1984 Theoretical conceptualizations of occupational therapy: 1960–1982. Occupational Therapy in Mental Health 4(2): 1–14

Lyons M 1985 Paradise lost! . . . Paradise regained? Putting the promise of occupational therapy into practice. Australian Occupational Therapy Journal 32(2)

Meyer A 1922 The philosophy of occupation therapy. American Journal of Occupational Therapy 31(10) Reprinted from the Archives of Occupational Therapy 1: 1–10

Miller B R J, Sieg K W, Ludwig F M, Shortridge S D, Van Deusen J 1988 Six perspectives on theory for the practice of occupational therapy. Aspen, Maryland

Mosey A C 1981 Occupational therapy: configuration of a profession. Raven Press, New York

Nelson D L 1988 Occupation: form and performance. American Journal of Occupational Therapy 42(10): 633–641

Reed K L, Sanderson S R 1980 Concepts of occupational therapy. Williams & Wilkins, Baltimore

Reilly M 1962 Occupational therapy can be one of the great ideas of 20th century medicine. The Eleanor Clarke Slagle lecture. American Journal of Occupational Therapy 31(4)

Shannon P D 1977 The derailment of occupational therapy. American Journal of Occupational Therapy 31(4): 229–234

Smith A G 1983 Holistic philosophy and general systems theory: an overview for occupational therapy. Journal of the New Zealand Association of Occupational Therapists 34(1)

West W L 1984 A reaffirmed philosophy and practice of occupational therapy for the 1980s. American Journal of Occupational Therapy 38(1): 15–23

3

The development of a paradigm

Jennifer Creek

INTRODUCTION

The need for a systematic approach or framework to encompass the philosophical, theoretical and applied aspects of the profession was stressed in Chapter 2, which showed how general systems theory is being used to provide one such framework. In this chapter we will expand on this aspect by describing the philosophical assumptions of the profession, the key areas of the theoretical foundation, the content of practice, the occupational therapy process and the nature of the relationships between these different elements. The object is to move towards a generally accepted paradigm of occupational therapy which will organise the beliefs and knowledge of the profession in a way that both acts as a guide for practice and allows for further developments.

TOWARDS A NEW PARADIGM

Any attempt to condense all the knowledge and beliefs of the occupational therapy profession into one chapter, or even one book, would be unrealistic. The object of this chapter is not to include every detail of professional theory and practice but to provide a flexible framework that can be used to incorporate other areas of knowledge.

The starting point was the model outlined by Clark (1979b) and known by the title 'Human development through occupation.' After studying four of the major theoretical frameworks used by occupational therapists, Clark (1979a) identified the concepts common to all and used these to construct her model. They include:

- philosophical assumptions
- theoretical foundation
- content of practice
- sequence of practice (the occupational therapy process).

The material which it is proposed should be included in an occupational therapy paradigm is discussed under these headings in the sections that follow. The relationships between the different parts of the paradigm are discussed in the final section, and are illustrated in Figure 3.1.

The chapter draws on the work of many occupational therapy theorists, and acknowledgement is given in the text.

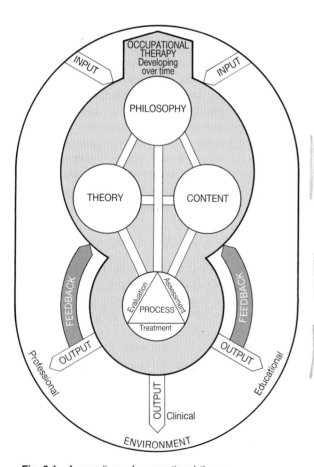

Fig. 3.1 A paradigm of occupational therapy.

PHILOSOPHICAL ASSUMPTIONS

Philosophical assumptions are the basic suppositions we share about the nature of living beings, the nature of the universe and the relationships between them upon which we build our knowledge. In occupational therapy we accept as true certain beliefs about people, society, the environment and the relationships between them, for example, that 'occupation is a central aspect of the human experience' (Kielhofner & Burke 1980). Without this assumption, we would not be convinced of the value of occupation as therapy. It is this sharing of fundamental beliefs that gives us a sense of identity as a profession (Mosey 1981). The three areas central to occupational therapy are beliefs about:

- the nature of human beings
- health and ill health
- the profession of occupational therapy.

VIEW OF HUMAN BEINGS

Occupational therapy is essentially client centred. The individual is seen 'not as an object or thing to be manipulated, controlled or made to conform but as a unique individual whose very humanness entitles him to choices in determining his own destiny' (Yerxa 1967). This belief in the right of the individual to be himself is made up of three separate beliefs:

- a concern with the whole person
- a belief in intrinsic motivation to be active
- an understanding of the social nature of people.

A holistic view is taken of people, and function and dysfunction can only be understood by seeing the relationships between mind, body and environment over time (Lyons 1985).

It is through the processes of growth, development and interaction with the environment throughout the life cycle that each individual reaches his own unique potential. Development can be studied by looking at different skill areas separately, but can only be understood by accepting that these areas are dynamically interrelated and interdependent (Daub 1983).

People as initiators of action

Western medical science is founded on the principle that human life should be preserved if possible. Occupational therapy takes the principle that human function should be preserved or restored where possible; it is the basic premise of our profession that being in a state of function is a desirable condition (Reilly 1962). It can be argued that life and function are the same thing; '. . . human reality does not exist first in order to act later; but for human reality, to be is to act, and to cease to act is to cease to be' (Sartre 1943). People have an intrinsic motivation to act on the environment in order to alter it for their own advantage. They do not wait for the environment to impinge on them before responding but are able to visualise the ends they wish to achieve and act to realise them. The drive to act is a basic human need and must be satisfied (Reilly 1962).

People as social animals

People are essentially social animals who develop and live in the context of a group. Human interaction stimulates biological, psychological, emotional and sociological development, and people deprived of company do not thrive. There is a long period of physical and emotional dependency in childhood, and it is normal to retain some emotional dependence on others once physical maturity is reached (Mosey 1980).

Social groupings take different forms in different cultures, for example, the village, the clan, the commune or the family. One social factor that people from all cultures find desirable is a small and stable social group. 'We enter the modern world with instincts and psyches which are those of a very intelligent omnivorous ape adjusted to family life within a small and intimate foraging group composed of individuals who know each other well' (Muir & Welfare 1983). When faced with a group that is too large for each person to know everyone else, such as a city, people use various rituals to limit and formalise their interactions with all but a small number of people.

VIEW OF HEALTH

Health is not merely the absence of disease. The Shorter Oxford Dictionary defines health as 'Soundness of body; that condition in which its functions are duly discharged.' The World Health Organization (1947, 1978) defines health as 'complete physical, mental and social well-being, and not merely the absence of disease.' Occupational therapists view health as the ability to function adequately in a balanced variety of roles, and achieve a sense of satisfaction from them. Each individual's needs, and the roles expected of him, change throughout the life cycle but a flexible balance of occupations is necessary to maintain health.

The individual is in a state of function when he has learned the skills necessary for successful participation in the range of roles he is expected to play throughout his life. These roles change throughout the life cycle and there may be times when existing skills lag behind new needs. Dysfunction occurs when the individual is unable to maintain himself within his environment because he does not have the skills necessary for coping with the current situation. Dysfunction is very individual. For a typist, the loss of a finger could be a major disability; for a singer, the same injury may be only a minor inconvenience.

The individual's ability to interact with his environment, achieve a workable balance, and direct his own life can be used as an indicator of health (Clark 1979b).

Why dysfunction occurs

Causes of dysfunction fall into four main groups:

- failure to develop and mature normally due to physical abnormality or environmental deprivation, for example, Down's syndrome
- environmental changes that the individual cannot cope with, such as bereavement
- new physiological or psychological needs, such as maternity, which cannot be met using existing skills
- pathology or trauma causing loss of skills, for example, head injury.

When the individual encounters a new situation

he uses his existing skills to try to master it. If these fail, he will try to learn effective new skills. Eventually, if the situation still remains outside his control, he will experience disequilibrium or crisis. The pace at which change occurs is important for maintaining equilibrium; too fast a pace means that new skills are not learned quickly enough, adaptation is disturbed, and a state of dysfunction may occur (Clark 1979b, Mosey 1968). The degree and pace of change that a person can manage without losing equilibrium is dependent on both internal factors, such as the ability to learn new skills quickly, and external factors, such as the amount of support available in the social environment.

Reilly (1962) also suggests that people have an innate drive to act and a need to use their muscular and intellectual tools, therefore psychological disorganisation will occur if they are deprived of occupation, irrespective of whether or not there are any other problems.

VIEW OF THE PROFESSION

The uniqueness of the occupational therapy approach to psychosocial dysfunction lies in the philosophy of human beings having the ability to influence their own health through occupation. Occupational therapy is concerned with treating the consequences of disease or injury as they affect a person's ability to function, rather than with the primary pathology. For example, the occupational therapist will try to slow down the process of senile dementia by involving the client in a balanced programme of activities to maintain physical and cognitive functioning, rather than by tackling the disease itself.

The aim of intervention is to develop each individual's highest level of competence, to enhance his quality of life and increase his satisfaction in daily living. The outcome of intervention should be that the client is able to enact a balanced range of occupations which will enable him to maintain physical and mental health.

The core of occupational therapy practice is activity analysis, synthesis and application. The outcome of occupational therapy intervention can be determined by the client's mastery of new tasks (Clark 1979b, Hopkins 1983, Mosey 1981, Reilly 1962).

THE THEORETICAL FOUNDATIONS OF OCCUPATIONAL THERAPY

Any profession must have special knowledge or skills. A coherent body of theory allows the therapist to make predictions about the outcome of intervention and so directs practice. Theories are also modified by practice and research.

One of the problems of occupational therapy has been that much of our knowledge is culled from other fields and many of our skills seem to be those of everyday living. This section describes in more detail three important areas of theory for the occupational therapist.

- occupation
- human development
- humanistic psychology.

OCCUPATION

Since the beginnings of occupational therapy it has been recognised that the concept of occupation is central to the profession, yet we have failed to develop a strong theory of occupation backed up by research. One reason is that the use of activity as therapy fell into disrepute during the 1960s and 1970s when therapists were trying to adapt their approach to fit into the medical model of dysfunction and treatment. In order to give occupational therapy the sound theoretical base it needs, we must extend our knowledge about occupation.

Occupation has been variously defined as:

- 'any activity which engages a person's resources of time and energy and is composed of skills and values' (Reed and Sanderson 1980)
- 'doing processes directed toward a planned or hypothesised end result' (Mosey 1981)
- 'the purposeful use of time by humans to fulfill their own internal urges toward exploring and mastering their environment that

at the same time fulfils the requirements of the social group to which they belong and personal needs for self-maintenance' (Kielhofner 1980b)

- 'the dominant activity of human beings that includes serious, productive pursuits and playful, creative, and festive behaviours' (Kielhofner 1983)
- 'any goal-directed activity meaningful to the individual and providing feedback to him about his worth and value as an individual and about his interrelatedness to others' (Johnson 1973).

For the occupational therapist, the key feature that differentiates occupation from activity is in having meaning and value for the individual. It is the quality of involvement, not the nature of the activity, that makes it an occupation.

Most occupations have both a real and a symbolic value, for example, cleaning the front doorstep has a realistic value in terms of safety and hygiene, but it also symbolises the respectability of the family.

Occupations can be divided into three areas:

- self-care
- play
- work

The amount of time devoted to each area of occupation is partly culturally determined and partly a matter of individual choice.

Self-care

Self-care is occupation that enables the individual to survive and that promotes and maintains health, including mental health. It includes:

- basic physical functions such as eating, sleeping, excreting, keeping clean and keeping warm
- survival functions such as cooking, dressing, shopping and maintaining one's living environment. Many of these functions have become specialised and have been delegated to members of society who have special skills, such as builders and bakers, but some remain with the individual.

The quality of self-care varies from person to person, although society tries to set minimum standards for certain aspects such as housing, clothing and income.

Play

Man is a very adaptable species. This adaptability has been achieved by developing flexible behaviour rather than specialised behaviour (Kielhofner 1980b). Play is the medium through which the child is able to learn and rehearse a wide range of skills that will enable him to respond appropriately and adaptively in different situations. Even in adult life, new skills are learned more thoroughly and integrated more successfully if the individual approaches learning in a playful and explorative manner.

Play also allows children to practise participating in their culture, and to learn its norms and values through the games and folk literature which are specific to that culture. For example, competitive games teach a child both society's rules and expectations about competition and his own position in the pecking order of a competitive society (Kielhofner 1980b).

In adult life play is usually called 'leisure' and is often used to satisfy individual needs that are not met by either self-care or work occupations. For example, playing squash can improve the physical well-being of a person who has a sedentary life-style, or provide social contacts for a housebound mother of small children, or give a sense of achievement to someone who has a low-level position at work.

Work

Work is any productive activity, whether paid or unpaid, that contributes to the maintenance or advancement of society as well as the individual. Work may help to maintain society, for example refuse collection, or contribute to its advance, for example theoretical physics.

The work in which a person spends most of his time usually becomes an important social role, giving him his position in society and a sense of his own value as a contributing member. Different jobs are given different social values, for example, a doctor is more highly valued in Western society than a housewife. In general, jobs which add to society's knowledge or cultural tradition are more highly valued than those which maintain its functioning (Kielhofner 1983).

Work serves many functions for the individual:

- it gives a major role in society and a social position
- it usually provides a means of livelihood
- it gives a structure to time around which other occupations can be planned
- it may give a sense of purpose and value to life
- it can be an important source of self-esteem
- it is a forum for meeting people who may become friends
- it can be an important interest and source of satisfaction.

Anyone who is unable to work misses all these benefits and is, in addition, usually given a low social position.

Balance of occupations

Self-care, work and play exist in a balance which changes throughout life. The healthy individual has his daily life activities organised into a satisfying pattern which is important to health and life satisfaction (Kielhofner 1980b).

For occupational therapists, the balanced use of time in daily living activities is an indicator of health.

HUMAN DEVELOPMENT

The Shorter Oxford Dictionary (1978) defines development as 'a gradual unfolding; a fuller working out of the details of anything.' In the case of human beings, this means the process of realising their genetic potential by passing through a series of stages of growth and maturation, in areas that are relatively independent of environmental influences. Psychological and social development are dependent on, but also influence, physical growth and maturation.

Conditions for development

Each person is born with genetic programming that determines his physical and psychological potential. However, in order to realise his potential, certain environmental factors must be present.

The growing child needs to have physiological needs, such as food, sleep, warmth, touch and physical handling, met. He needs to be protected from trauma by disease or injury, to be given loving attention and opportunities to explore his own potential and the environment. He interacts with his environment and reaches his potential through occupation; without occupation, development will not proceed normally.

Finally, the child needs a sense of security and belonging if he is to be able to move away from his existing situation towards greater independence (Hilgard et al 1979).

Physical development

Physical development follows a recognised sequence with certain skills always learned before others. For example, all children stand before they walk. Many skills are learned at the same time, especially in the first years of life, but not at the same rate. For example, some children are able to talk quite well before they can walk, while others learn to walk first. Various stages are passed through in learning new skills but not all children pass through all stages, for example, some children never learn to crawl before they walk.

Cognitive development

Swiss psychologist Jean Piaget suggested that children develop through a series of stages as their biological systems mature, psychological development being dependent on physical growth and maturation.

The four stages that Piaget postulated are:

- sensorimotor
- pre-operational
- concrete operational
- formal operational.

More details of Piaget's theories can be found in Chapter 12, p 183.

Cognitive development is not a passive process, the child actively seeks new information and generates and tests hypotheses about what he is perceiving.

Personality development

Each person is born with a genetic potential for personality, just as for physical characteristics. Individual differences are apparent from birth but personality is also shaped by experience. Some characteristics are influenced by the culture that the child grows up in, for example, aggression and competition are highly valued in some cultures but actively discouraged in others.

Although many people share a culture and have experiences in common with the other members of it, each person has unique experiences throughout life which shape his personality (Hilgard et al 1979). For example, the child of a diplomat may be widely travelled and have been to many schools by the time he leaves home. The child of a mill worker from the same town, by contrast, is likely to stay in the same house and at the same school until he starts work or further education. These two people will have very different views of the world and responses to events.

Psychosocial development

People are essentially social animals who develop and live in the context of a group. Human interaction stimulates biological, psychological, emotional and social development, and people deprived of human contact do not thrive.

The type of contact the developing child needs changes from the intense relationship with the mother, through various levels of group interaction, to adult intimacy and progressive emotional independence. Erik Erikson (1965) divided psychosocial development into eight stages, from birth to old age (Table 3.1).

He suggested that each stage involves a crisis that must be resolved if development is to continue normally.

Table 3.1 Erikson's stages of psychosocial development

Age	Psychosocial crisis	Key relationships
0–1	Trust v mistrust	Mother
2–3	Autonomy v shame and doubt	Parallel play
4–5	Initiative v guilt	Interactive play
6–puberty	Industry v inferiority	Idols
Adolescence	Identity v role confusion	Peer group
Early adulthood	Intimacy v isolation	Life partner
Middle adulthood	Generativity v self-absorption	Children
Late adulthood	Ego-integrity v despair	Self-sufficiency

HUMANISTIC PSYCHOLOGY

Occupational therapy can be said to have a traditionally humanistic base since many of our beliefs and values, and even our vocabulary, can be found in humanistic psychology.

Humanism, as well as being a theoretical approach, concentrates on the philosophical assumptions underlying therapy, with the basic belief that people can change themselves by their own efforts and have the responsibility to do so. It is concerned with what it means to become fully human.

Unlike an empirical approach to the study of human behaviour, based on observation and experiment, humanism accepts that subjective experience is valid and important. Two people might behave differently in response to the same situation because of their different perceptions of the situation. Humanism tries to include and understand variables such as feelings, spontaneity and involvement, as part of the whole person and his world.

The world of the humanist is made up of the physical self, the thinking and feeling self, the physical environment and the human environment, all interdependent and interacting (Briggs et al 1979, Corey 1977, Cracknell 1984, Willson 1983). The humanistic concepts that are most important to occupational therapists are described here.

Self-awareness

Human beings have a unique capacity for self-awareness that gives them the freedom to make choices. The greater the self-awareness a person has, the more realistic choices are open to him. Each person's perceptions of what he is and what he can do direct his behaviour, whether or not they coincide with reality. For example, someone in a hypomanic mood may spend huge amounts of money, without considering whether he can afford it, because he has a sense of being infinitely powerful.

Everyone also carries an image of what he would ideally like to be, the 'ideal self,' and usually tries to behave in a way that will bring him nearer to that ideal. Self-esteem is increased when the real self is perceived as being close to the ideal self, producing a feeling of harmony. Most people, if they have a realistic self-image, are aware that they fall short of their ideal and will work towards closing the gap.

Sometimes a discrepancy may arise between self-image and the feedback an individual receives about his behaviour from his environment. If the individual fails to alter either his behaviour or his self-image, this can lead to a separation from reality. In order to maintain an unrealistic self-image in the face of conflicting evidence, he must operate ego defence mechanisms, such as denial or projection, to block awareness of incongruity. As the gap between self-image and real behaviour becomes greater, so the individual operates more defence mechanisms and moves further out of touch with external reality.

In order to reverse this process the individual needs to become aware of and accept the more negative aspects of himself and to incorporate them into his self-image. A functioning person is able to change his self-image or his behaviour in order to maintain congruence within a changing environment (Cracknell 1984, Willson 1983).

Freedom and responsibility

Self-awareness gives human beings the freedom to choose and act within the limits imposed by external factors, that is, to be responsible for their own destiny. Acceptance of this responsibility brings 'existential anxiety'. Choices must often be made without being certain of the outcome, yet each person carries his own responsibility for the result. Avoiding making choices for oneself or failing to strive towards fulfilling one's own potential leads to guilt and depression.

Client-centred therapy

The humanistic approach to therapy is client centred, that is, the client is helped to become aware of his own potential and how he can work towards realising it. The therapist's main task is to understand the client, not to direct him, and any definition of function or dysfunction must be based on the client's own perception of himself. The client is not a passive recipient of treatment but must be active in developing his own goals and ways of achieving them. The final choices always rest with him.

The aim of therapy is to increase the client's self-awareness by creating a climate of acceptance and unconditional positive regard in which he may feel safe enough to drop some of his defence mechanisms and accept himself as he is (Briggs et al 1979, Corey 1977, Cracknell 1984).

CONTENT OF PRACTICE

A definition of the structure and scope of occupational therapy practice should derive from the philosophy and theoretical base of the profession, not from the constraints and demands of the service setting, although the way the service is applied will be influenced by such external factors. Practice can be defined as the actions taken by the therapist to serve the needs of the client (Agyris & Schon 1974). Only if these actions are based on a coherent philosophical and theoretical framework can the therapist make skilled predictions about outcome.

We will look at the content of occupational therapy practice under four headings:

● professional goals

- the population served
- the therapist's actions
- unique features of the service.

PROFESSIONAL GOALS

The major goal of occupational therapy is to enable the client to achieve a healthy balance of occupations through the development of skills that will allow him to function at a level satisfactory to himself and others. The desired outcome of intervention is the client's ability to meet his own needs throughout the life cycle so that his life is satisfying and productive.

Sub-goals which lead to the major goal are to:

- assess the client's needs in terms of the occupational roles required of him
- identify the skills needed to support those roles
- remove or minimise behaviours that interfere with occupational performance
- improve role performance
- assist the client to develop, relearn or maintain skills to a level of competence that will allow satisfactory performance of occupational roles
- help the client achieve an organised, purposeful and satisfactory use of time (Katz 1985)
- enable the client to perform outside the service setting at a level which will enable him to meet his needs in a way which is acceptable to himself and to society.

The focus of intervention is always the client rather than the problem or the method of treatment.

THE POPULATION SERVED

The premise that people can influence their own health by their actions can be applied to a wide range of problems once the appropriate specialist knowledge to support it has been acquired. The consumer is anyone who has problems of doing, whatever his age, sex or diagnostic category.

The consumer traditionally encountered occupational therapy in a medical setting, which predetermined, to some extent, the range of problems seen, the degree of dysfunction the client was experiencing and the amount of time the therapist could spend on treatment. As the service becomes more widely applied clients are also being encountered in other settings, such as social service agencies, educational settings, health centres, day centres, private homes, prisons, private practice and business.

In practice, referrals are often made by a doctor or other professional who makes the initial decision about who needs occupational therapy. The therapist selects clients from these referrals on the basis of information gained in her initial assessment (see Ch. 5). In some settings, such as long-stay wards, the therapist makes her own selection of clients from the entire ward population.

THE THERAPIST'S ACTIONS

The task of the therapist is to assess abilities and needs and to plan and implement effective programmes to meet those needs.

The relationship between therapist and client is an important part of the therapeutic process, from first meeting a newly referred client, through coping with transference and counter-transference relationships, to ending a treatment programme on a positive note. The therapist can use her interpersonal skills to deal with a whole range of needs, such as engaging the initial interest of an institutionalised client with a volitional disorder, supporting a bereaved client through the grieving process, helping someone release suppressed anger, making a client with chronic low self-esteem feel valued, and so on. This involves adopting a range of roles including:

- teacher, for example, in teaching a course of assertiveness skills
- counsellor, as in helping a client deal with the experience of sexual abuse
- listener, as when allowing a client to express painful or difficult feelings
- role model, for example, by expressing one's own feelings directly and appropriately
- friend, as when discussing clothes and make-up with a female client.

There are of course many other roles the therapist might adopt but some will feel more comfortable than others to the individual therapist.

In most settings it is appropriate for the therapist to use a version of the treatment process: selecting an appropriate model, assessment, treatment planning and implementation, and evaluation. These skills are discussed in more detail in Chapters 5, 6 and 7.

Activities are the means by which the client is able to have new experiences and learn new skills. The core of service delivery is therefore activity analysis, synthesis and application.

UNIQUE FEATURES OF THE SERVICE

The focus of intervention is human occupation in the context of the individual's total environment and over time.

The methods used by occupational therapists to achieve their treatment goals are usually commonplace and we find it tempting to dress our work up with fancy names or borrow more impressive techniques from other disciplines. However, the philosophy of occupational therapy is so comprehensive and great that we need not apologise for the simplicity of our tools. The unique concept of occupational therapy is that meaningful activity can be used by the individual to maintain or restore his functioning in daily life roles (Lyons 1985, Reilly 1962). Activities used may be from any area of human occupation: self-care, domestic, play or work.

Occupational therapy is essentially client orientated because an individual will only become engaged in activity which is appropriate to his age, sex, culture, interests, abilities and values. Occupational therapists have a unique appreciation of the dynamics between an individual and the activity he is performing (Westland 1986).

THE OCCUPATIONAL THERAPY PROCESS

Most writers agree that the occupational therapy process falls into three main stages:

- assessment
- treatment/intervention
- evaluation.

Selecting a model is also an integral step that must occur at the beginning of the process. Figure 3.2 illustrates this relationship, highlighting the three main stages in a triangle, but also giving prominence to the essential first stage of selecting a model.

The brief discussion which follows, and the chapters in Section 3, which examine the occupational therapy process in detail, relate to these four main stages:

- selecting a model
- assessment
- treatment/intervention
- evaluation.

SELECTING A MODEL

The occupational therapy process is a circular one, as shown in Figure 3.2. A model is selected to translate the occupational therapy paradigm into practice in a particular work setting or with an individual client. For example, an acute psychiatric setting might normally use a model of human occupation, but it may be more appropriate to use a psychodynamic model with certain clients.

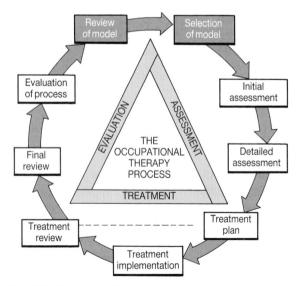

Fig. 3.2 The occupational therapy process.

Each stage of assessment and treatment is related to the chosen model, but its appropriateness can only be judged by evaluating the outcome of the process.

ASSESSMENT

Assessment is the basis for all intervention and must be both thorough and valid in order to ensure that treatment is appropriate. Assessment is in two stages:

1. initial assessment
2. detailed assessment.

Assessment begins from the moment a referral is received or, if specific referrals are not made in a particular setting, from the moment the therapist starts to identify those clients who could benefit from occupational therapy.

The initial assessment is a screening process to determine the main problem area of the client and whether or not occupational therapy can be of any value in this case. Factors influencing whether or not a client is accepted include:

- the needs of the client
- the facilities available
- the manpower available
- the expertise available
- the support available to the client outside treatment sessions
- the reason for referral.

Once the client is accepted for treatment a detailed assessment is carried out to determine his needs, assets, interests, and goals. Effective assessment will lead directly to setting long-term, intermediate and short-term goals and to choice of appropriate treatment methods.

Methods and content of assessment and screening will be discussed in chapter 5.

TREATMENT

There may be no clear division between assessment and treatment in occupational therapy, where clients are often assessed by being observed in activities. However, at some stage the therapist and client will establish goals and write a treatment plan. Treatment is in three stages which may

be repeated as necessary, depending on the client's progress:

1. formulation of treatment plan
2. treatment implementation
3. treatment review.

The preliminary treatment plan is formulated by the therapist and client together. The plan includes goals of treatment, methods to be used, an individual programme and a list of the people who need to be informed about the programme.

The treatment plan is put into practice and the client's progress is continuously monitored. Minor changes can be made without having to call a review or alter the plan. A close liaison is maintained with other disciplines involved so that any changes or problems observed in any setting can be shared. Regular reviews are held to evaluate the need for major programme changes. Records are kept to assist in the review process.

The treatment review serves several purposes:

- it gives the therapist and client an opportunity to review what progress has been made and to judge the success or otherwise of the programme
- it gives everyone involved in treatment a chance to get together and discuss progress
- it is an opportunity to set new short-term goals and to adjust intermediate and long-term goals.

After the review the treatment plan is updated, including the programme of activities. Other team members are informed of the new plan.

Treatment planning and implementation are discussed in more detail in Chapter 6.

EVALUATION

The circular process of occupational therapy is completed by the three stages of evaluation:

1. final treatment review
2. evaluation of process
3. review of model.

The final review of the client's progress is used to reach decisions about discharge or referral to other agencies. Major decisions are not usually made during one meeting but it is useful to meet to formalise decisions. The client and therapist can compare the present state of affairs with the position before intervention so that progress is obvious and termination of treatment is seen as positive.

Evaluation of the process should go on throughout the occupational therapy programme but formal evaluations of particular groups or of the process as a whole may be carried out at intervals. Programmes are not only judged for their effectiveness with particular clients but also for their congruence with the overall ethos of the department.

Evaluation may lead to changes in any part of the occupational therapy process. The most radical change likely to occur would be to modify or discard the model being used. Paradigm changes are unlikely to occur at this level.

Further discussion of evaluation and quality assurance methods can be found in Chapter 7.

THE STRUCTURE AND DEVELOPMENT OF A PARADIGM

In this chapter we have looked at some of the constituents that make up a paradigm for the profession of occupational therapy. In this section we will clarify the relationships between them and look at how changes take place.

THE RELATIONSHIPS BETWEEN PARTS OF THE PARADIGM

The internal structure of the occupational therapy profession is made up of philosophy, theory, content of practice and process, each influencing and being influenced by the others (Fig. 3.1). The nature of these relationships is examined here.

Philosophy, theory and content

The core of the occupational therapy profession is its shared beliefs, assumptions and values (philosophy). Theories are selected to support the professional philosophy; theories which do not

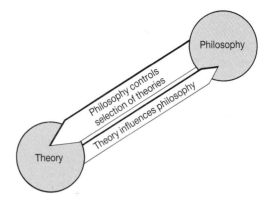

Fig. 3.3 The relationship between philosophy and theory.

support it are rejected. Philosophy therefore provides the profession with its sense of identity and exerts control over professional theory and practice. However, philosophy may be adjusted slightly over time as new theories are gradually absorbed, so control is not entirely in one direction (Fig. 3.3).

Philosophy and theory determine the content of practice. Beliefs and assumptions about man, health and how health can be maintained suggest goals of intervention. Theory produces methods of intervention to achieve the goals. Values lead to the formulation of ethical codes to control inter-

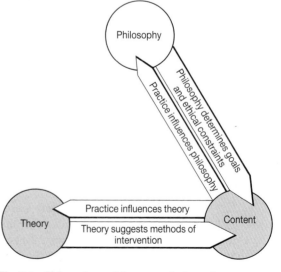

Fig. 3.4 Philosophy and theory control practice.

vention. Clinical practice also gives an opportunity to test theories and to modify them through experience, so that the content of practice influences theory development (Fig. 3.4).

The process

The occupational therapy process (see Fig. 3.2) is the means by which philosophy, theory and content are translated into practice. The process may vary slightly in different settings and with different clients, and some stages may be combined, such as assessment and treatment.

THE RELATIONSHIP BETWEEN THE PROFESSION AND THE ENVIRONMENT

The profession of occupational therapy is not static but changes gradually over time. Theories are continuously being added or discarded, as was shown in Chapter 2. Philosophies also change, though more slowly, under the influence of what is happening in the wider society.

Change is initiated both by changes in the social environment and by feedback about the results of professional practice (Fig. 3.5). The occupational therapy process can be seen as part of a loop through which the profession receives feedback about the outcomes of its practice. This feedback can lead to modifications of the process and of the philosophy, theory and content that initiated it.

External influences on the profession

There are few internally defined limits on the growth of occupational therapy as a profession, but external constraints determining growth include:

- new knowledge emerging
- the changing roles of other professions
- changing social values
- the national and international political climate
- economic pressures.

As was shown in Chapter 2, the great expansion of knowledge this century has changed how we see the human race and conceptualise health and dis-

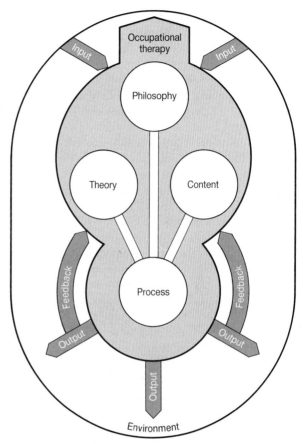

Fig. 3.5 The relationship between the profession and the environment.

ease. Vast areas of new knowledge have been incorporated into the theoretical base of the profession and will continue to be absorbed.

Occupational therapy is a relatively new profession and has not established clear boundaries to its field of practice. To some extent, the role of the profession is defined by the other professions that operate within similar areas. Some of the traditional roles of occupational therapists have been taken over by other professions, such as clinical psychologists and nurses, while our domain of concern has expanded into new fields (see Ch. 8).

Social values have changed since the beginning of the century when occupational therapy first took on a distinct identity, partly due to the experience of two world wars, partly to the technological revolution and partly to demographic changes. Modern health care and modern medicine have conquered many life-threatening diseases so that more and more people are living with disabilities that would have killed them in a previous age. For the first time in history, in some countries, old people outnumber children, posing new economic and moral dilemmas. Occupational therapy, with its commitment to achieving quality of life, has a major role in caring for the chronic sick in society, in carrying out social policies for elderly or disabled people and in influencing that social policy.

Social values are reflected in the political climate of a country, and health care policies are defined by politicians. At both the level of national government and at the level of institutional management, the degree of power and autonomy given to the different professions is a political decision.

Economic pressures also have an effect on the quality of health care in any country. When money is freely available there is an expansion of training and posts but when times are harder it is necessary to justify the existence of a profession in economic terms as well as social or humanistic ones.

All these external pressures are experienced by the profession and used to influence the way it develops. Other influences arise directly from the effects of our professional practice and are received as feedback.

Feedback from professional practice

Professional activity is in three main areas: clinical, education and professional (Fig. 3.6). Feedback from these three areas directs change within the profession.

Clinical

The type of feedback an occupational therapist receives in the clinical setting includes:

- results of intervention with individual clients, through evaluation
- effectiveness and efficiency of the service as a whole, through quality assurance measures and through research

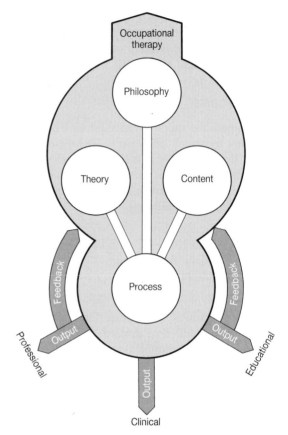

Fig. 3.6 Feedback from professional activity.

- the role and status accorded to the occupational therapist by her colleagues.

This feedback influences changes in:

- the method of service delivery in a particular setting
- the content of practice in a particular setting
- theories about function and dysfunction and the role of occupation in remediating dysfunction
- where occupational therapists choose to work, therefore their range of professional roles.

Education

The quality of education of occupational therapy students, together with the level of education, whether diploma or degree, has an influence on:

- standards of professional practice
- the quality and consistency of theories used
- the amount and quality of research carried out
- recruitment of students onto occupational therapy courses
- retention of staff in the profession
- the status of the profession, nationally and worldwide.

There are, therefore, continual moves to upgrade the level of the basic professional qualification and to create new higher qualifications.

Professional

Professional activity takes place at local, national and international levels. Occupational therapy changes over time, and the professional association is the body through which therapists can control and direct that change.

The functions of professional associations are to:

- establish a professional identity
- work towards reaching agreement on the parameters of the profession
- generate ideas
- produce a code of ethics
- set standards for education and practice
- monitor education and practice
- protect the interests of members
- facilitate intradisciplinary communication
- disseminate information
- facilitate interdisciplinary communication
- negotiate the role and status of the profession
- educate the public about occupational therapy.

It is part of the occupational therapy profession's domain of concern to help people to manage change, therefore clinical skills can be adapted to facilitate changes within the profession.

SUMMARY

This chapter summarised the elements that will go into a new paradigm of occupational therapy.

- Philosophical assumptions include beliefs about human beings, health and occupational therapy.
- The theoretical base of the profession is very broad but the three most important areas of knowledge are the theory of occupation, human development and humanistic psychology.
- The content of practice includes professional goals, population served, the actions taken by occupational therapists and the unique features of the profession.
- The occupational therapy process is in four main stages; selection of a model, assessment, treatment and evaluation.

The relationships between these elements were discussed and clarified. A diagram (Fig. 3.1) was used to illustrate how the elements relate to and influence each other. Finally, the process of change within the profession was discussed.

The next chapter looks at some of the models that are being used to translate aspects of this paradigm into practice.

REFERENCES

Agyris C, Schon D A 1974 Theory in practice: increasing professional effectiveness. Jossey-Bass, San Francisco

Briggs A K et al 1979 Case simulations in psychosocial occupational therapy. F A Davis, Philadelphia

Clark P N 1979a Human development through occupation: theoretical frameworks in contemporary occupational therapy practice, part 1. American Journal of Occupational Therapy 33(8)

Clark P N 1979b Human development through occupation; a philosophy and conceptual model for practice, part 2. American Journal of Occupational Therapy 33(9)

Corey G 1977 Theory and practice of counselling and psychotherapy. Brooks-Cole, Monterey

Cracknell E 1984 Humanistic psychology. In: Willson M (ed) Occupational therapy in short-term psychiatry. Churchill Livingstone, Edinburgh

Daub 1983 In: Hopkins H L, Smith H D (eds) Willard and Spackman's Occupational therapy, 6th edn. Lippincott, Philadelphia

Erikson E H 1965 Childhood and society. Triad Paladin, London

Hilgard E R, Atkinson P L, Atkinson R C 1979 Introduction to psychology, 7th edn. Harcourt Brace Jovanovich, New York

Hopkins 1983 In: Hopkins H L, Smith H D (eds) Willard and Spackman's Occupational therapy, 6th edn. Lippincott, Philadelphia

Johnson J A 1973 Occupational therapy: a model for the future. American Journal of Occupational Therapy 27(1)

Katz N 1985 Occupational therapy's domain of concern: reconsidered. American Journal of Occupational Therapy 39(8)

Kielhofner G, Burke J P 1980a A model of human occupation, part 1. Conceptual framework and content. American Journal of Occupational Therapy 34(9)

Kielhofner G 1980b A model of human occupation, part 2. Ontogenesis from the perspective of temporal adaptation. American Journal of Occupational Therapy 34(10)

Kielhofner G 1980c A model of human occupation, part 3. Benign and vicious cycles. American Journal of Occupational Therapy 34(11)

Kielhofner G 1983 Health through occupation: theory and practice in occupational therapy. F A Davies, Philadelphia

Lyons M 1985 Paradise lost! . . . paradise regained?: putting the promise of occupational therapy into pratice. Australian Occupational Therapy Journal 32(2): 45–53

Mosey A C 1968 Recapitulation of ontogenesis: a theory for the practice of occupational therapy. American Journal of Occupational Therapy 22(5)

Mosey A C 1980 A model for occupational therapy. Occupational Therapy in Mental Health 1(1)

Mosey A C 1981 Occupational therapy: configuration of a profession. Raven Press, New York

Muir R, Welfare H 1983 The National Trust Guide to prehistoric and Roman Britain. George Philip, London

Reed K L, Sanderson S R 1980 Concepts of occupational therapy. Williams & Wilkins, Baltimore

Reilly M 1962 Occupational therapy can be one of the great ideas of 20th century medicine. The Eleanor Clarke Slagle lecture. American Journal of Occupational Therapy 16(1)

Sartre J P 1943 Translated: Barnes H E 1966 Being and nothingness. Methuen, London

Westland G 1986 Letter to the editor. British Journal of Occupational Therapy 49(8): 269

World Health Organization 1947 Constitution of the World Health Organization. Chronicle of WHO 1(3)

World Health Organization 1978 Primary health care. Report of the international conference on primary health care. Alma Ata, USSR. WHO, Geneva

Willson M 1983 Occupational therapy in long-term psychiatry. Churchill Livingstone, Edinburgh

Yerxa E 1967 Eleanor Clarke Slagle lecture. Authentic occupational therapy. American Journal of Occupational Therapy 21: 3

As we stated in Chapter 3, most writers agree that the occupational therapy process falls into three main stages:

- assessment
- treatment/intervention
- evaluation.

However, selecting a model is also an integral step that must occur at the beginning of the process. The chapters in this section relate to these four stages:

- selecting a model
- assessment
- treatment/intervention
- evaluation.

Although evaluation is only one part of quality assurance, it seemed more beneficial to the student to include the larger topic.

SECTION 3
The occupational therapy process

4

Models for practice

Jennifer Creek

INTRODUCTION

In Chapter 2 it was shown that a profession needs a paradigm which incorporates the beliefs, values, knowledge and expertise of its members and serves as a unifying force. Chapter 3 suggested aspects of a paradigm for occupational therapy to take the profession into the 21st century.

Within this paradigm are various approaches, called frames of reference, that draw on particular theoretical systems and are appropriate to different areas of practice. The most commonly accepted frames of reference are listed here.

THE MAIN FRAMES OF REFERENCE

Various frames of reference have been developed over the years as new areas of knowledge have been incorporated into the theoretical base of occupational therapy. Some have wider application than others but all of those listed here are accepted and used within the mental health field.

In Britain there are four main frames of reference:

- the psychodynamic approach, which is derived mainly from psychanalytic theory
- the behavioural approach, based largely on learning theory
- the developmental approach, derived from theories of human development
- the humanistic approach, drawn from the philosophies and theories of the humanists (Finlay 1988).

A frame of reference drawing on the theory of human adaptation has also been proposed by Young (1984), based on the work of King.

In the USA, four main frames of reference have been identified:

- adaptive performance, developed by Fidler and Mosey
- biodevelopment, developed by Ayres, Wilbarger and others
- facilitating growth and development, developed by Llorens
- occupational behaviour, developed by Reilly and associates (Clark 1979)

A more recent approach is derived from cognitive theory (Allen 1985).

MODELS FOR PRACTICE

Within each frame of reference, one or more models has been developed to give more specific direction to practice in the various areas in which occupational therapists work. Some of these models have been extensively used, validated and reported, while others are still at an early stage of development. The four models described in this chapter are:

- activities therapy, from the adaptive performance frame of reference
- occupational therapy as a communication process, from the psychodynamic frame of reference
- facilitating growth and development, from the developmental frame of reference
- a model of human occupation, from the occupational behaviour frame of reference.

These four models have been selected because together they include most of the knowledge base of occupational therapy in mental health, each one has a wide application, and all are in common use. Humanism is seen as an aspect of occupational therapy philosophy that is incorporated into all models in contemporary practice, rather than as a separate model.

Each model example will include:

- a brief overview of the knowledge base
- how human beings are viewed

- how function and dysfunction are conceptualised
- the client group that the model was developed for
- the goals and processes of intervention
- the methods of intervention used
- a case example showing how the model is applied.

References have been given for the sources of the material presented here but later writings by the authors may have influenced the way the models were presented. For example, activities therapy was described by Mosey in 1973, but ideas from her later work have been incorporated into this presentation in order to bring it up to date and to do justice to Mosey's work. The same applies to each of the other approaches.

SELECTING A MODEL

Selection of an appropriate model is the first stage of the occupational therapy process. Many factors influence the choice of model used in a particular area of practice. These may include:

- the needs of the client, for example, it is appropriate to use a developmental model with a client who has developmental delay
- the skills and preference of the therapist
- the ethos of the work setting, for example, a psychodynamic model is appropriate in a psychotherapy unit.

More than one model may be used in a particular setting, or it may be possible to use only one, particularly if it is a model that has a wide application, such as activities therapy.

ACTIVITIES THERAPY*

This model, first presented by Mosey in the early 1970s, was one of the first attempts to bring together theories, goals of intervention and methods in a unifying framework. Although it has

---

* This model was developed and described by Mosey (1973, 1978) and this outline is taken from these two sources.

been further developed by Mosey to become more complex and comprehensive, the original model remains popular in occupational therapy practice.

THE KNOWLEDGE BASE

Activities therapy draws heavily on learning theory as a basis for practice, including the theory of operant conditioning and 'an integrated collection of various theories of learning.' It also draws on the theory of human occupation and on a knowledge of group dynamics (Fig. 4.1). Other theories used will depend on the area of practice. For example, when working with people who have a mental handicap it is also important to have some understanding of normal development, developmental abnormalities, genetics, deviance, labelling and stigma. Much learning takes place in groups, and a knowledge of group dynamics enables the therapist to see whether the group is assisting or hindering the learning process and to understand how she might make changes.

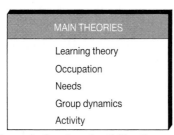

Fig. 4.1   The main theories of activities therapy.

It is impossible to make someone learn if he does not want to, therefore the therapist needs to know how to make the learning process easy and attractive to the client. The client needs to feel that it is worthwhile to learn how to carry out tasks effectively because this is the way to achieve satisfaction of needs. We know that learning has taken place when there is a permanent change in verbal or non-verbal behaviour.

VIEW OF HUMAN BEINGS

People are seen as self-motivated, feeling, thinking, acting, social beings made up of many different but interrelated facets (Fig. 4.2).

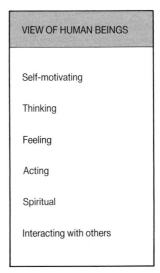

Fig. 4.2   Activities therapy: view of human beings.

People are self-motivated because they have a hierarchy of needs that they are always striving to gratify. These include physiological, safety, love and belonging, mastery, esteem and self-actualisation needs (Maslow 1973).

Feelings arise in response to how a person perceives his needs being met. If he has a sense of need satisfaction then he will feel positive emotion such as joy; if he feels deprived then he will experience negative emotion such as anger. Needs and emotions are inherent, not learned, but the skills needed to achieve need satisfaction and to express emotions appropriately have to be learned.

The thinking self is made up of factual knowledge, thinking processes and beliefs. Beliefs include what the individual thinks about himself: his appearance, personality, abilities and limitations. This is known as his self-concept. Each person also holds a set of beliefs about others; what they are like and how they might interact with him.

People are seen as being action-orientated. It is normal for the individual to be active during most of his waking hours, although he may have periods of passivity. The drive to act is inherent but competent action requires the use of learned skills.

People are also social beings who learn during normal development to relate to other people in a variety of ways. Social interaction occurs on different levels and may be one-to-one or in groups.

FUNCTION AND DYSFUNCTION

In order to function effectively in all these facets of his life, a person uses skills that are learned during normal development. A person is considered normal if he is able to do the things that other people of similar age and background can do.

A fully functioning person is one who is able to:

- *plan* and carry out a task
- *interact* comfortably in a group
- *identify and satisfy* personal needs
- *express* emotions in an acceptable manner
- *perceive* himself, other people and the non-human environment in a fairly accurate manner
- *function* within a value system that allows him to satisfy his own needs without infringing upon the rights of others
- carry out required *activities of daily living*
- *work* at a relatively satisfying job or participate in preparation for such a job
- *enjoy* avocational pursuits and recreational activities
- interact comfortably in *family and friendship* relationships
- perceive himself as a *member of a society*, nation, and world community
- attend to his *spiritual needs*.

When the developmental, process is disrupted or delayed, necessary skills are not learned at all or not learned to a sufficient level of competence. Psychosocial dysfunction, therefore, is the inability to carry out one or more of the above tasks so as to meet one's needs in a manner that is satisfying to oneself and not detrimental to others.

CLIENT GROUP

Activities therapy was developed for use in the area of psychosocial dysfunction or deficit, that is, with people suffering from mental disorder or developmental delay. It is applicable to various age groups, from young adulthood to old age, to the full range of social groups generally encountered in the mental health field and to a wide variety of psychosocial disorders.

GOALS AND PROCESSES OF INTERVENTION

The goal of activities therapy is to assist people to participate in the life of the community by minimising or eliminating deficits. In order to achieve this there are two parallel and interdependent goals:

- to help the client to identify faulty patterns of behaviour and the ideas, feelings and values that underlie them
- to help him to develop more effective ways of behaving.

This involves 'learning through doing,' using activities that emphasise present functioning. Exploration of the past is not relevant in this model.

Treatment is seen as a planned, collaborative interaction between the therapist, the client and the environment by which new skills can be learned. It is important that the relationship between the client and therapist is based on trust and mutual respect. The process of intervention is in seven stages.

1. Initial evaluation is done by observing what the client can and cannot do in a variety of situations over a period of time. When these observations have been interpreted and validated they become the starting point for planning treatment.

2. The client and therapist, together, decide on the immediate and long-term goals of treatment. If the client is unable to collaborate at this stage it may be necessary for the therapist to set the first goal and modify it as soon as the client is able to express his views. The immediate goal is the area of difficulty that the therapist and client decide to work on at a given time in treatment. Goals should be concrete and measureable so that it is easy to see when they have been reached.

3. A treatment plan is written, stating what is going to be done to try and achieve the goals.

4. The treatment plan is implemented as quickly as possible. Progress is monitored and the

plan is followed until the first evaluation, if satisfactory, or altered if not.

5. Monitoring should be frequent, formal and at regular intervals. Ideally, review meetings are attended by the client and all the staff involved in his treatment. The results show whether or not the programme is working and when goals have been reached.

6. When immediate goals have been reached further goals are set and the treatment programme is altered accordingly.

7. Monitoring also highlights when the client is ready to discontinue treatment.

The most basic skills to be learned are simple task performance and group participation. Other skill areas include self-care, domestic work, recreation, productive work and intimacy. The therapist can be only indirectly involved in this last area.

When trying to involve the client in an activity

there are three main points:

1. select an activity that interests, or has the potential to interest, him
2. start at the point the client is at and progress slowly or let him make the pace.
3. provide ample reinforcement for even small achievements.

METHODS OF INTERVENTION

This approach uses a wide range of activities including work-orientated, recreational and creative-expressive activities. Group or individual therapy is used, depending on the needs of the client, and the therapeutic relationship is seen as a significant factor in the learning process. It is emphasised that, while the therapist can set up learning experiences for clients, it is the individual who must do the learning and bring about change in himself.

CASE EXAMPLE 4.1

Mr Allison, a 38-year-old man with left spastic hemiparesis, was referred to the occupational therapist as an outpatient for clerical assessment and vocational counselling. He had done clerical work for many years but was given early retirement because he needed a series of operations on his foot. When he became mobile again, he went for vocational assessment and was employed to do clerical work in a sheltered workshop. Eventually, he was transferred to the shop floor where he did various light industrial tasks. He had been in this job for 8 years but was very unhappy with his situation and wanted to go back to clerical work. He had been seen as a psychiatric outpatient several times for anxiety and depression. However, he did not have the confidence to change jobs, especially as he had a mortgage and a wife and small child to support. His marriage was happy, and he saw work as his only problem.

At the initial interview, the therapist was struck by the high level of anxiety displayed by Mr Allison. His overall goal was to find a more satisfactory job, but he did not know how to go about this. The therapist arranged a second interview in order to give Mr Allison a chance to feel more relaxed with her before starting programme planning.

At the second meeting Mr Allison was still anxious, so the therapist decided that he would

need to be assessed in an informal, non-stressful environment, otherwise the anxiety might impair his performance. A short-term goal was agreed, that Mr Allison would have a series of individual sessions working with a technical instructor on a word processor in order to:

- see if he had any aptitude for this type of work
- build up his confidence in his capabilities
- see if he liked the work.

If this was successful, he would look for a word-processing course at one of the local colleges as a step towards changing jobs. The immediate goal would be reached when Mr Allison expressed readiness to try a college course.

The technical instructor allocated to work with Mr Allison was briefed to be very supportive and encouraging. She allowed him to work at his own pace and to feel confident about his skills at each stage before progressing to the next task. The therapist saw Mr Allison and the technical instructor regularly to discuss his progress and ensure that the programme was satisfactory.

He expressed interest in word processing from the first session and his anxiety gradually decreased as he mastered new skills. After seven sessions he decided to apply for an evening course in word processing at the local technical college and therapy was discontinued. Mr Allison did not feel he needed help to pursue his goals any further.

OCCUPATIONAL THERAPY AS A COMMUNICATION PROCESS*

This model was developed by Fidler and Fidler in the 1960s, when individual and group psychotherapy were being widely used for the treatment of all types of psychosocial dysfunction, and it is still the most comprehensive model of occupational therapy for use in this field. It is based on a psychodynamic view of human beings and their relationship to action and to others. Psychodynamics is the study of mental powers and processes (Greek—*psyche* mind, *dynamis* power—Butterworths Medical Dictionary 1978).

THE KNOWLEDGE BASE

The core of psychiatric occupational therapy is seen as the skilled use of activities, objects and relationships to assist the individual to explore and re-evaluate assumptions about himself and others and to gratify some of his frustrated basic drives in order to develop a more integrated self-identity (Fig. 4.3). It is mainly concerned with the use of action to express and communicate feelings and thoughts as a starting point for therapy. Purposeful action is the means by which man is able to:

● communicate with others
● express his feelings
● gain clearer understanding of his experiences
● achieve gratification of his basic drives
● test his perceptions and ideas about external reality.

In order to use activities as therapy, the therapist needs to have knowledge of psychiatry, psychoanalytic theory, non-analytic concepts of psychopathology, group dynamics, the nature and meaning of symbols and object relationships.

Object relationships is the term used to describe the relationship between the self and other human or non-human objects. The newborn child cannot

---

* This summary is taken from three sources: Fidler & Fidler (1963, 1968) and Clark (1979).

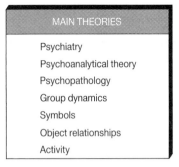

MAIN THEORIES
Psychiatry
Psychoanalytical theory
Psychopathology
Group dynamics
Symbols
Object relationships
Activity

Fig. 4.3 Occupational therapy as a communication process: main theories.

differentiate between himself and his environment, therefore he cannot have any conscious relationship. As he grows, he becomes aware of the mother as a separate, but vitally important, person because she is the source of satisfaction of his needs. The relationship is one of total dependence and the baby is 'in love' with the mother to the exclusion of everyone else. This type of dependent relationship is called an anaclitic relationship. Gradually the child realises that he can gratify some of his own needs and this leads to a narcissistic relationship with his own body. More mature object relationships are formed as the child grows and develops a stronger sense of identity, allowing him to relate to people and things in a variety of ways other than using them for immediate gratification.

VIEW OF HUMAN BEINGS

People are seen as having an innate drive to be active that is directed towards achieving gratification of basic drives and towards making satisfactory interpersonal relationships. Action is used to express and communicate feelings and thoughts. It arises from mental images, and feedback about the result of action allows these images to be modified to meet reality (Fig. 4.4).

The infant strives for competence in actions that will both meet his needs and increase his sense of personal identity and integrity. A sense of self-worth comes from the intrinsic gratification of doing well in the particular areas of life that he values. The more situations and actions the child

VIEW OF HUMAN BEINGS
Innate drive to be active
Action arises from mental images
Action is used to express and communicate
Feedback from action allows reality testing
Striving for competence in actions

Fig. 4.4 Occupational therapy as a communication process: view of human beings.

is able to experience, the greater will be his knowledge of his own potential and limitations, leading to greater adaptability. A knowledge of what patterns of action for survival and gratification are most useful and acceptable in a particular culture is learned through interaction with the social environment.

FUNCTION AND DYSFUNCTION

A functioning individual is one who has an integrated self-identity and a realistic concept of others, who continues to grow through exploration and experimentation throughout his life, who is able to satisfy his basic needs and who contributes to the needs and welfare of others. A well organised personality has a positive and realistic self-concept and good object-concepts.

Dysfunction is characterised by immature object relationships, which may be the result of a failure to develop realistic self- and object-concepts or may be due to regression and psychopathology. For example, a person experiencing psychological disorganisation in severe psychosis may have difficulty in recognising himself as separate from others, or may have anaclitic object relationships.

CLIENT GROUP

This psychodynamic model is appropriate for use with people of all ages and for treating a wide range of psychosocial disorders. It has been most widely used with adults with acute disorders but is also appropriate for long-stay clients and people with chronic psychosis. It requires that clients participate actively in the intervention process, therefore it is less appropriate for use with severely handicapped or very dependent clients.

GOALS AND PROCESSES OF INTERVENTION

The overall goal of therapy is to build a more healthy and integrated ego. Sub-goals are:

- to help the client express and deal with his needs and feelings
- to assist in the gratification of frustrated basic needs
- to strengthen ego defences
- to reverse psychopathology
- to facilitate personality integration
- to offer opportunities to explore and re-evaluate self-concepts and object-concepts
- to develop a more realistic view of the self in relation to action and others.

Activity analysis is in terms of the psychodynamics of activity, the real and symbolic components, interpersonal elements and cultural significance. For an activity to be of therapeutic value it should match the individual's developmental level and needs, both realistically and symbolically, and be socially and culturally appropriate.

METHODS OF INTERVENTION

The occupational therapy experience has three main aspects which are equally important and which, together, constitute the uniqueness of occupational therapy:

- the action which the client carries out
- the objects used in, or resulting from, the action
- the interpersonal relationships influencing and being influenced by the action.

The process of intervention begins with collection of relevant data about the client, including the team's views on appropriate general goals. Treatment programmes may be oriented towards exploration of unconscious material, support of existing ego defences or repression of problematic material.

Data analysis allows a tentative treatment plan to be made or a preliminary programme for the collection of more data to be set up. Close liaison with other team members is essential, especially with the client's psychotherapist if he has one. Treatment planning takes account of the amount of support and structure the client needs in his programme, the level and amount of social interaction that is appropriate and the type of activity to use. Treatment may be individual or in groups, but the group size should always be small enough to allow the individual to relate closely to everyone in it. Eight to 10 members is usually considered to be the optimum size.

Occupational therapy is seen as a part of a comprehensive treatment programme which involves all aspects of the treatment setting but the use of activities adds an extra dimension to the therapeutic experience. Therapists must be prepared to use a wide range of activities selected for their therapeutic value, including projective techniques (as described in Chapter 13) which have been developed to facilitate the expression and communication of painful feelings. The choice of which activities to use may be made by either client or therapist, depending on the needs of the client, but the client must be an active participant in the therapeutic process if it is to be of value to him.

In summary, it can be said that occupational therapy intervention consists of the relationships between the therapist, the client, the therapeutic environment and the activity.

CASE EXAMPLE 4.2

Case example 4.1 covers Mr Allison's case history.

The therapist discussed Mr Allison with his doctor and it was agreed that she would be the primary therapist. The doctor would continue to see him to monitor his medication and the therapist would make regular progress reports. The main goals of intervention would be to encourage Mr Allison to express his feelings about his disability and to reach a more satisfactory degree of adjustment to it. A secondary goal would be to help him explore his capabilities with a view to changing jobs.

At the first interview the therapist noted Mr Allison's high level of anxiety. He talked freely about how he perceived his problems but saw them all as caused directly by his physical disability and did not feel optimistic about making changes. The therapist decided to have further individual sessions to build up a good relationship with Mr Allison and to obtain more information.

As the therapeutic relationship developed, Mr Allison shared the experience of becoming disabled. He had been a bright boy who had gained a place at grammar school and had great expectations for his future. Four days after starting school he had a road traffic accident that left him with hemiparesis. He returned to school but dropped down from the A stream to the B stream and then to the C stream. He expressed the feelings of loss and despair that this had engendered.

It emerged that part of Mr Allison's dissatisfaction with his work was due to the gap between his earlier expectations about his future and the present reality. He believed that his brain still functioned as well as it had before the accident and that his low achievement was due to anxiety and depression. However, he had been reluctant to test this out by attempting demanding tasks.

It was agreed that Mr Allison would start weekly individual sessions with a technical instructor to learn to use a word processor. This would give him a chance to explore his capabilities and interests. In addition, it would arouse feelings about his performance that could be dealt with in psychotherapy sessions. The therapist suggested a small weekly group, rather than individual sessions, so that Mr Allison could receive more feedback about himself in relation to others. The group used various media, in addition to talking, thus providing additional opportunities for exploration of his capabilities. The therapist would see Mr Allison monthly for an individual session.

After 12 weeks in the group, Mr Allion felt confident enough to seek out a word-processing course at the local technical college. He had a much more realistic image of his abilities and weaknesses, and no longer needed to use his disability as an excuse for avoiding action. Treatment was terminated at this point.

FACILITATING GROWTH AND DEVELOPMENT*

Aspects of developmental theory are drawn on for most occupational therapy models but Llorens' model of facilitating growth and development is most explicit about the developmental nature of occupational therapy.

The model is based on 10 premises.

1. A person develops in parallel the areas of neurophysiological, physical, psychosocial and psychodynamic growth, social language, daily living and sociocultural skills.

2. All these areas continues to develop throughout the person's life.

3. Mastery of skills to an age-appropriate level in all areas of development is necessary to the achievement of satisfactory coping behaviour and adaptive relationships.

4. Such mastery is usually achieved naturally in the course of development.

5. Intrinsic factors and external stimulation received within the family environment interact to promote early growth and development.

6. The later influences of extended family, community, and social groups assist in the growth process.

7. Physical or psychological trauma can interrupt the growth and development process.

8. Such interruption will cause a gap in the developmental cycle resulting in a disparity between expected coping behaviour and the skills necessary to achieve it.

9. Occupational therapy can provide growth and developmental links to assist in closing the gap between expectation and ability through the skilled application of activities and relationships.

10. Occupational therapy can provide growth experiences to prevent the development of maladaptive behaviour and skills.

* This model has been developed by Llorens (1970, 1974, 1976) and this outline is taken from these three sources.

THE KNOWLEDGE BASE

This model is based on theories of human development (Fig. 4.5). It includes knowledge of the normal sequence of physiological, physical, cognitive, psychological, social and emotional growth and development. It draws on the biological, behavioural and social sciences and on medical knowledge. It also includes a knowledge of the properties of activities and the theory of human occupation.

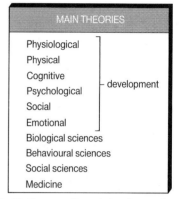

Fig. 4.5 Facilitating growth and development: main theories.

VIEW OF HUMAN BEINGS

People are seen as dynamic, changing, developing organisms whose life cycles go through stages of growth and decline that necessitate adaptation by the individual (Fig. 4.6). Early patterns of development become a part of the personality structure of the adult but developmental achievements are not necessarily permanent and regression to an earlier level can occur.

Development takes place in a sequence that is common to everyone, although the pace may vary widely. Each stage of development can only proceed normally if the developmental crises of the preceding stage have been successfully resolved. Age ranges can be suggested for particular skills to be mastered but these are not absolute and are mainly useful for checking if development in all areas is proceeding at the same pace. Growth and development continue into adulthood and middle age, especially in the areas of changing responsibility and relationships, and it can be

VIEW OF HUMAN BEINGS

Dynamic, changing, developing organisms

Life cycle goes through stages of growth and decline

Development takes place in a common sequence

Stress can cause regression to an earlier developmental stage

Development continues throughout the life cycle

Fig. 4.6 Facilitating growth and development: view of human beings.

assumed that some kind of development continues into old age, although not much is known about this.

FUNCTION AND DYSFUNCTION

A functioning individual is one who achieves satisfactory coping behaviour and adaptive relationships by developing appropriate skills, abilities and relationships at each stage of the life span. These adaptive behaviours allow the individual to adjust both to internal needs and to external demands.

Dysfunction occurs when the developmental level of the individual, in any aspect, is unequal to the age-related demands made on him. Trauma at any stage can interrupt the developmental process and inhibit the development of adaptive skills or cause regression to an earlier level of performance. Trauma may be due to disease, injury, environmental insufficiencies or intrapersonal vulnerability. A major disruption in any one area of development will affect all other areas and the longer the disruption is allowed to continue the more gaps there will be in the developmental process.

CLIENT GROUP

Occupational therapists are concerned with

promoting development at all ages, therefore this framework is applicable throughout the life span. It can be used with people suffering from any kind of chronic mental disorder, not just those with delay in physical or cognitive development.

GOALS AND PROCESSES OF INTERVENTION

The occupational therapist uses activities and relationships, applied with knowledge and skill, to facilitate growth and development. The overall goal is to increase skills in all areas, with emphasis being placed on the main area of deficit, so that the gap between expected coping behaviour and actual adaptive ability is closed or narrowed.

Occupational therapy is also concerned with maintaining health and preventing maladaptation through early detection of problems and early intervention. Intervention at an early stage will allow the individual to continue the growth process with a minimum of disruption.

The occupational therapy process includes:

- preliminary assessment to determine the need for occupational therapy intervention and to identify aspects that need further assessment
- formal assessment and analysis of developmental disruptions
- setting goals in relation to the individual's age, life role, sex, present developmental level and the skills and behaviours expected of him
- selection of activities on the basis of activity analysis
- application of activities selected to enhance remaining function and facilitate the learning of skills, working through of emotional conflicts and redevelopment of functions that have been lost
- continuous monitoring so that the client can move on to the next developmental level as soon as possible and treatment can be terminated when goals have been achieved.

METHODS OF INTERVENTION

Assessment methods include interviewing, testing, reviewing client records, projective techniques, developmental screening tests and clinical observation. Information gained is analysed to determine which areas of performance are affected and to assist in planning appropriate intervention.

Treatment techniques include activities and relationships. Activities are offered to the client to facilitate growth in areas of need. These may be sensory, physical, symbolic or interpersonal. Certain activities are known to be important for developing skills at particular developmental stages, for example, the young child needs access to a variety of objects for manipulating and sorting in order to learn classification skills. Developmentally appropriate activities are combined with a suitable level of interpersonal interaction to achieve the maximum benefit.

Continuous monitoring is an integral part of the therapy process so that the results of treatment can be determined.

CASE EXAMPLE 4.3

Case example 4.1 covers Mr Allison's case history.

The therapist was aware that Mr Allison had become disabled at the age of 11, following a road traffic accident. Prior to that he had been a bright, normal boy with an interest in sports. At the initial interview he displayed such a high level of anxiety that the therapist decided not to start programme planning until he felt more relaxed. She used the next two interviews to explore what he had done since the accident in the areas of physical activity, individual relationships, social activities, hobbies and work. His development appeared to have been normal in all areas except:

• cognitive development; following his accident he had dropped down from the A stream to the C stream at school, had left at the age of 16 and had taken an undemanding clerical job. His present job made no intellectual demands on him.

• psychodynamic development; he had a very poor self-image and saw himself as a failure, despite having a happy marriage, a car and a house.

The next task was to assess whether there was a primary cognitive deficit or whether his poor performance was due to low expectations. Mr Allison agreed to have weekly sessions on the word processor with a technical instructor, to see if he could master it. The therapist continued to see him weekly to evaluate his progress and offer emotional support.

After the first two sessions it became apparent that Mr Allison had no difficulty in understanding how to use the word processor and had an aptitude for technology. He had six further sessions, during which his confidence increased and his mood lifted until he felt ready to apply for a word-processing course at the local technical college. Treatment was terminated at this point.

A MODEL OF HUMAN OCCUPATION*

This model, first presented by Kielhofner, Burke and Igi in 1980, is based on three fundamental beliefs:

• humans cannot be healthy in the absence of meaningful occupation
• the occupations a person does can shape his health, therefore occupations can be used as a means to health
• occupational therapy must embody the characteristics of true human occupation; purposefulness, challenge, accomplishment and satisfaction.

THE KNOWLEDGE BASE

The model of human occupation has a broad knowledge base that includes general systems theory, theories of motivation and role theory (Fig. 4.7). Important concepts within the model are temporal adaptation, personal causation, habits and skills. The central concept is that of occupational behaviour, which is the developmental continuum of play, self-care and work, organised into a healthy balance throughout the life cycle.

Most adult roles can be divided into three types: family roles, personal-sexual roles and occupational roles. The occupational role, which is the main

---

* This outline is taken from a series of four articles (Kielhofner & Burke 1980, Kielhofner 1980a, 1980b, Kielhofner, Burke & Igi 1980); Kielhofner 1985 and the workbook from a workshop on the model of human occupation (Kielhofner 1988).

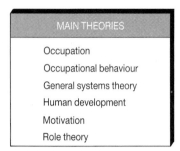

Fig. 4.7 A model of human occupation: main theories.

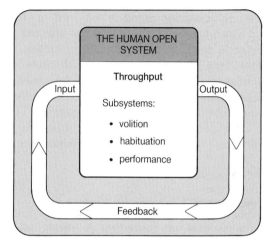

Fig. 4.9 A model of human occupation: subsystems within a human system. (Adapted from Kielhofner & Burke 1985)

focus of this model, is defined as the tasks a person performs for the greater part of his waking time plus the social position those tasks give him, for example, student, housewife or gardener.

VIEW OF HUMAN BEINGS

People are conceptualised as open systems, operating within and interacting with the environment (Fig. 4.8). Interaction takes place by a process of input, throughput and output. Input consists of information received from the environment, including feedback about the results of actions. Throughput is the organisation and reorganisation of available information in order to plan action and predict outcomes. Output is in the form of action; mental, physical or social. The whole process is one of continual adaptation to the environment through dynamic interaction with it. The system acts on the environment and changes in response to the input it receives.

The internal part of the system is described as three subsystems existing in a hierarchical relationship (Fig. 4.9):

- the volition subsystem is the highest subsystem, which controls the entire system and is activated by the urge to achieve mastery over one's own actions and interactions with the environment
- the habituation subsystem is the organising subsystem, which consists of internalised roles and habits
- the performance subsystem is the lowest subsystem, which is composed of skills and is most directly linked with the system's output.

The system's output is dependent on the range of skilled actions that the performance subsystem has generated. These skills are organised into habits appropriate to the individual's various social roles by the habituation subsystem. Roles are selected by the volition subsystem on the basis of personal values, interest and sense of efficacy. Each subsystem is dependent on the others, al-

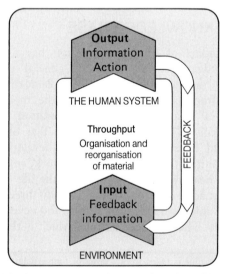

Fig. 4.8 A model of human occupation: view of human beings. (Adapted from Kielhofner & Burke 1980)

though the volition subsystem exerts overall control over how the system develops.

The system changes over time. Change is both internally motivated, by the urge towards mastery of one's own actions and interactions, and externally influenced by the demands of the environment. The process of change takes place as new knowledge is acquired, organised and reorganised and the person learns more about the environment and his effect on it. Actions become more refined as the individual learns how to use his skills effectively to achieve his own ends. The direction of change is towards increasing complexity.

FUNCTION AND DYSFUNCTION

A functioning individual is one who:

- adopts a balanced range of occupational roles
- has the skills and habits to support them
- is able to interact successfully with the environment.

Each action by the individual carries a chance of success or failure which he will try to gauge on the basis of previous experience. A successful outcome will confirm that the skills generated are useful, is likely to arouse interest in the action and will lead to a sense of competence. This, in turn, will make the individual more likely to act again so that he is in a benign spiral of increasing competence and self-confidence. A person who has a good balance of positive outcomes from his actions is able to adapt in a way that satisfies his own needs and the demands of the environment, and to develop a sense of himself as an active person.

Failure to achieve a good ratio of successes to failures may be due to physical or mental deficiency or to environmental factors. The individual learns to fear failure and holds back from action so that he does not have opportunities for learning new skills. He develops a sense of himself as incompetent and is less likely to initiate action, so that he is in a vicious, spiral of decreasing skill and confidence.

Cycles of interaction with the environment are initiated by the volition subsystem but problems of doing can be rooted in any of the three subsystems, volition, habituation or performance, or in the process of enacting occupation, or in the environment.

Examples of problems in the volitional subsystem include unrealistic personal goals, such as is seen in manic-depressive psychosis, and decreased personal causation, as seen in depression.

Disruption of habits and roles is frequently seen in psychosocial or organic disorders, such as acute anxiety or alcoholism.

Skills deficits may be caused by a failure to develop normally, due to environmental deprivation or organic damage, or may be lost later in life due to acute distress or organic illness.

CLIENT GROUP

This model has a wide application with people of all ages, from children to the elderly. Its focus is on occupational dysfunction, therefore it is appropriate for use with anyone suffering from either psychosocial or organic disorders, such as depression, anxiety, anorexia nervosa, schizophrenia and dementia.

GOALS AND PROCESSES OF INTERVENTION

This model is client centred and the client's own goals take precedence over what the therapist thinks should be attempted first. This is an acknowledgement of the importance of volition in determining what a person does.

Intervention follows a set format:

- identification of clinical questions to guide assessment
- data collection
- construction of an explanation of function or dysfunction
- identification of treatment options and decision about which ones to use
- treatment implementation with ongoing evaluation and adjustment.

METHODS OF INTERVENTION

Several assessment instruments have been developed for use within this model, such as in-

CASE EXAMPLE 4.4

Mr Allison's case history is covered in Case example 4.1.

At the initial interview the therapist observed that Mr Allison had a very high level of anxiety, so she used a structured interview format, the occupational role history, to help him feel more comfortable. This took two sessions as Mr Allison talked freely about his life. Analysis of the data produced showed that the primary area of dysfunction was occupational role; other life roles were normal and satisfactory. However, the present crisis seemed to have been precipitated by a reduction in social and physical activities since the birth of his son.

The hemiplegia had been caused by a road traffic accident when Mr Allison was 11 years old. Prior to that he had been a normal, lively boy. Following the accident he was unable to join in sports, and his academic performance deteriorated steadily. This triggered a loss of confidence, leading to withdrawal from activity, so that new skills were not learned and his confidence deteriorated further. This withdrawal had only been in the area of occupational performance, since he remained highly motivated to make social contacts and actively pursued relationships.

It was agreed that Mr Allison would have weekly sessions with a technical instructor to learn to use a word processor. This activity was chosen because he expressed an interest in it and because it might lead to a change of job. The activity would give him an opportunity to:

- learn new skills
- test his capabilities
- develop a new interest
- gain a realistic picture of his abilities
- explore a possible career option.

He was also included in an anxiety-management group and continued to see the therapist once a fortnight to assess his progress.

Mr Allison enjoyed word processing and was highly motivated to continue. His anxiety dropped to a level he could cope with, and he began to feel more in control of his life. After six weeks he felt confident enough to enrol at the local technical college for a word-processing course. Treatment was terminated at this point.

terest checklists (see Ch. 5), role checklists and questionnaires. Assessment data is analysed to construct an explanation of occupational function or dysfunction and to produce treatment options.

Activities used must be purposeful and have meaning and value for the client. Within this constraint, any activities may be used in treatment. However, the main focus of the model is on occupational roles and the minor roles that support them, therefore activities related to the client's major life role are seen as most relevant. For example, a housewife with agoraphobia, whose main aim was to be able to manage her household and care for her family, would be helped to engage in domestic chores and shopping. She may also be encouraged to take up new social interests to provide balance and variety in her life.

Therapy is conceptualised as an environment in which:

- the individual's curiosity is aroused so that he engages in explorative behaviour that generates skills
- he is presented with demands for performance so that routines of behaviour are established

and he gains competency in using patterns of skills
- the responses he makes bring positive feedback to the system that a sense of efficacy, interest and belief in the value of occupational roles are restored.

SUMMARY

In this chapter we have reviewed four models commonly used in occupational therapy practice in mental health. Activities therapy was described as an example of an adaptive performance approach, developed by Mosey in the USA. Occupational therapy as a communication process was described to illustrate the psychodynamic frame of reference, which is also described in Chapter 13. Facilitating growth and development was given as an example of a developmental approach. Finally, the model of human occupation was described, as an example of a model from the occupational behaviour frame of reference.

REFERENCES

Allen C 1985 Occupational therapy for psychiatric diseases: measurement and management of cognitive disabilities. Little Brown, Boston

Clark P N 1979 Human development through occupation: theoretical frameworks in contemporary occupational therapy practice, part 1. American Journal of Occupational Therapy 33(8): 505–514

Fidler G S, Fidler J W 1963 Occupational therapy: a communication process in psychiatry. Macmillan, New York

Fidler G S, Fidler J W 1968 Doing and becoming: purposeful action and self-actualization. American Journal of Occupational Therapy 32(5).

Finlay L 1988 Occupational therapy practice in psychiatry. Croom Helm, London

Kielhofner G 1980a A model of human occupation, part 2. Ontogenesis from the perspective of temporal adaptation. American Journal of Occupational Therapy 34(10): 657–663

Kielhofner G 1980b A model of human occupation, part 3. Benign and vicious cycles. American Journal of Occupational Therapy 34(11): 731–737

Kielhofner G, Burke J P 1977 Occupational therapy after 60 years: an account of changing identity and knowledge. American Journal of Occupational Therapy 31(10)

Kielhofner G, Burke J P 1980 A model of human occupation, part 1. Conceptual framework and content.

American Journal of Occupational Therapy 34(9): 572–581

Kielhofner G, Burke J P, Igi C H 1980 A model of human occupation, part 4. Assessment and intervention, American Journal of Occupational Therapy 34(12): 777–778

Kielhofner G (ed) 1985 A model of human occupation. William & Wilkins, Baltimore

Kielhofner G 1988 Workshop: The model of human occupation. York

Llorens L A 1970 Facilitating growth and development: the promise of occupational therapy. Eleanor Clarke Slagle lecture 1969. American Journal of Occupational Therapy 24(2)

Llorens L A 1974 The effects of stress on growth and development. American Journal of Occupational Therapy 28(2): 82–86

Llorens L A 1976 Application of a developmental theory for health and rehabilitation. American Occupational Therapy Association, Maryland

Maslow A H 1973 The further reaches of human nature. Penguin, Harmondsworth

Mosey A C 1973 Activities therapy. Raven Press, New York

Mosey A C 1978 Paper: Behavioural models in occupational therapy. The 7th International Congress of the World Federation of Occupational Therapists, Jerusalem

Young M 1984 Models of practice for occupational therapy. British Journal of Occupational Therapy 47(12): 381–382

5

Assessment

Jennifer Creek

INTRODUCTION

Assessment is an integral part of the occupational therapy process. An initial assessment is used to evaluate the client's problems, to determine whether or not occupational therapy intervention is appropriate and to establish a database prior to beginning programme planning. Ongoing assessments show any changes that have taken place during treatment and demonstrate when goals have been reached. Later assessments provide a picture of residual problems, which can be measured against the client's life demands in order to make recommendations about discharge and to plan follow-up.

Assessment is measurement of the quality or degree of the various factors in a situation or condition. In clinical practice it is used to measure the assets and deficits of the client that relate to his referral for therapy. The process of assessment is invoked when a client is referred to the occupational therapist because some change is judged to be necessary in his situation.

Assessment is not something that is done to the client. It involves his active cooperation both in providing information and in helping to interpret it.

This chapter will discuss what part assessment plays in the occupational therapy process, what is assessed, methods of assessment and how to determine the validity of results.

THE ASSESSMENT PROCESS

The process of assessment, as shown in Figure 5.1, relates to the occupational therapy process as a whole (see Ch. 3) and to the model being used in a particular treatment setting (Ch. 4).

A model defines the parameters of practice and the purpose of intervention. Information is only useful when it comes within those parameters and contributes to realising the therapeutic purpose (Fidler 1982), therefore the methods of assessment used and the type of data sought will be deter-

mined by the model used. This, in turn, is determined by the client group and treatment setting.

INITIAL ASSESSMENT

When a referral is received, the first step in the occupational therapy process is to collect and organise information about the client from a variety of sources in order to plan treatment effectively.

The initial assessment has three main functions:

1. it gives the therapist an opportunity to judge whether or not the client will benefit from occupational therapy intervention (screening)

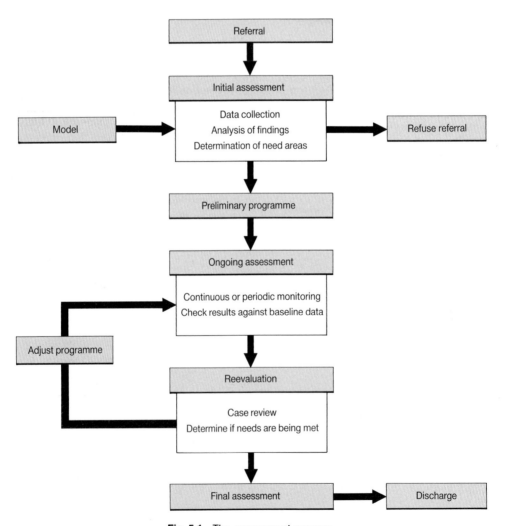

Fig. 5.1 The assessment process.

2. it provides an opportunity to begin to establish rapport and elicit the client's interest and cooperation
3. it produces a database.

The methods of data collection will be discussed in more detail in the section on methods of assessment.

Recording results of investigations not only provides a baseline from which to measure change but is also the starting point for interpretation. Methods of recording data are discussed in chapter 28. The process of organising information, which should be carried out as far as possible with the active cooperation of the client, is used to:

- produce a list of problems and strengths
- identify goals of treatment
- suggest activities to use.

This process is part of treatment planning and is described in more detail in Chapter 6.

Screening referrals

The outcome of an initial assessment may be a decision not to provide an occupational therapy programme. The main reasons why this decision might be taken are:

- the client's problem does not come within the domain of concern of the occupational therapist
- the client could not benefit from occupational therapy intervention at this particular time, for example, a person with alcoholism needs to acknowledge that he has a drink problem before he can benefit from intervention
- the resources of the department cannot meet the client's needs at this particular time.

Occupational therapy intervention only contributes directly to the treatment process when the programme is based on an assessment procedure that clearly indicates the need for such intervention (Gillette 1968). A programme that is not based on assessment results does not provide therapy but merely diversion. Occupational therapists are realising the need to provide high-quality treatment rather than large-scale diversion and are

learning to say 'No' (British Association of Occupational Therapists 1988).

Establishing rapport

Establishing rapport with the client in this initial meeting is important to the client–therapist relationship. It can take a great deal of courage for someone to admit he needs help and the experience of attending a hospital or clinic can be very traumatic, particularly if it is a first admission. Older clients may be distressed by having to share their difficulties with a young woman (or man) and may resent being asked to carry out activities if they cannot see their point. The therapist needs to appreciate these feelings and not feel personally threatened if a client is uncooperative at first.

The essential ingredients in establishing rapport with a client are as follows.

- *Respect* for the person, whatever his problems are. He is a person first and a client temporarily.
- *Empathy* It is not possible to like everyone we come into contact with but the therapist should be able to empathise with most problems she encounters. If there is a real personality clash that cannot be overcome with help from the supervisor then it may be advisable to pass the client to another therapist.
- *Honesty* about what occupational therapy is about and what it can offer. It may be tempting to promise great results or to try to sound mysterious and potent but, in the long run, the client's full cooperation can only be engaged if he understands the therapeutic process and feels in control.

Producing a database

Basic information such as the client's name, age, sex, marital status, etc. can usually be found in the case notes. Assessment must focus on the client's occupational performance so that therapy can help him to build on existing skills to improve his function (Moorhead 1969).

Florey and Michelman (1982) identify two major areas of information that are critical to occupational therapy assessment:

1. patterns of skills or patterns of dysfunction in past and current occupational roles
2. the degree of balance or imbalance between areas of occupation in the present.

Much of this information will emerge during the treatment process, the initial assessment being only a starting point from which the general direction of treatment is determined.

The database is used to:

- determine the need for occupational therapy intervention
- identify the client's needs and assets
- provide a baseline against which to measure the outcome of treatment
- identify which areas need further investigation
- produce a set of treatment objectives
- suggest methods of intervention.

When all the preliminary investigations have been completed, the database can be analysed to produce a list of problems and assets, which is the basis for programme planning.

ONGOING ASSESSMENT

Ongoing assessment is a part of the treatment process and is used to measure the client's progress, or lack of progress, so that the effectiveness of the treatment programme can be judged. In practice, it is very difficult to know whether it is occupational therapy or some other variable which is producing change. This problem is addressed in Chapters 7 and 30. However, if the clinician bases her practice on an accepted occupational therapy model, uses activities that have been analysed and chosen for their specific value and applies recognised and validated methods of assessment, she can assume for practical purposes that it is her intervention that is having an effect.

When the therapist and client have produced a set of treatment goals and considered how they may be achieved, a programme is planned and implemented immediately. It may be necessary to start with a temporary programme while further data is collected but this programme should be designed to help elicit the information required. This is shown in Case example 5.1.

CASE EXAMPLE 5.1

Jim Manson, a young man with a severe mental handicap, was referred for occupational therapy to find out whether any activities that would interest him could be found. The nursing staff felt that he had the potential to do more than wander around the home unit all day but they did not have time to work with him individually.

It was agreed that for his preliminary programme one therapist would see Jim individually twice a week and try various activities with him, using her judgement and skill to choose activities and to motivate Jim to stay in the sessions.

After a few weeks Jim's progress was reviewed. He had spent most of the time in his sessions either walking about, trying to leave or finger-flapping. His therapist noted two barriers to involvement in activity:

- Jim found it hard to tolerate one-to-one attention
- he could not concentrate on any one activity for more than a few minutes.

It was felt that Jim would do better in a parallel group where he would not receive the therapist's concentrated attention and where he could take time off from his own task to look at what other people were doing.

Jim continued to see his therapist once a week but they stayed in the occupational therapy workshop where many other people were also working and he was included in a small supportive psychotherapy group for people with severe communication and emotional disorders.

After a few weeks the staff involved noted that Jim seemed much more relaxed and made no efforts to leave either of these sessions. He was spending almost equal proportions of time involved in the activity, looking at other people and indulging in ritualistic behaviour, a great improvement on his performance in individual sessions.

The new programme was continued with 6-monthly reviews. The preliminary programme, while not successful in involving the client in therapy, gave staff the information they needed to design a more appropriate programme.

Assessing and reevaluating progress

During the treatment programme the therapist has many opportunities to observe the client's level of competence in the skills that it is designed to develop. Minor adjustments can be made at any time on the basis of observation and discussion with the client. For example, the therapist observes that a client's concentration span has increased so that he now has no difficulty in staying for a half-hour painting session. She points this out to him and suggests the length of the session be increased to three-quarters of an hour. He agrees to try, the relevant people are informed of the change and the new length of session is implemented.

More radical programme changes are usually discussed by all the people directly involved in the client's programme, if not by the whole team. A case review may be called by the therapist because she feels the client is ready for it, or the review may be routine. All clients should be reviewed regularly. In an acute setting this may take place weekly but in a long-stay setting 6-monthly may be adequate.

Programme
How often the client attends
What sessions or groups he attends
Whether or not his attendance is regular
Whether or not the client seems satisfied with his programme

Review
Brief recap of the last review
Clients performance in the areas of physical, cognitive, intrapersonal and interpersonal skills
Highlight any particular areas of interest or progress

Needs
A list of needs that the client and therapist have identified
Priorities for action
Suggestions about who might take action to meet each need
Suggested treatment for each need

Recommendations
A summary of treatment recommendations and who is responsible for ensuring that they are carried out

Fig. 5.2 A case review format.

The case review

In most departments a regular time each week is set aside for reviews so that all staff can attend, although an emergency review may be called at any time.

All staff members are invited to the review. It is important that as many people as possible attend because:

- the observations of everyone who sees the client are important
- a broad discussion may shed new light on the client's needs
- it may be necessary to ask new staff to become involved
- the review can serve as a teaching session.

Invitations may be sent to staff of other disciplines, such as nurses or social workers. The client should also be given the opportunity to attend for at least part of his review in order to give his views in person and to hear what other people think about his progress.

One person is responsible for preparing and presenting the review, usually the client's key worker. Her task is to collect all relevant information about the client from everyone involved and to organise it into a clear and comprehensible format. It is helpful to have a standard review format so that everyone knows how the material will be presented (see Fig. 5.2). This also ensures that no points are missed.

The review will cover the client's background and why he has been referred, his occupational therapy programme to date, his level of involvement in treatment, his progress and his current areas of deficit. By analysing this information, the team can determine what changes, if any, need to be made in his programme to meet those needs.

CASE EXAMPLE 5.2

A 6-monthly review meeting was called to discuss Mr Greg Hodges, a middle-aged man with a mild mental handicap living in a long-stay institution. He had been having occupational therapy for over a year, with the overall aims of intervention being to introduce him to new activities appropriate to his ability and age and to improve his social skills.

At the previous review, several recommendations had been made:

● Greg should continue with two structured individual sessions each week to work on specific skills
● he would be allowed to sit in the department every morning to read his newspaper and have a chat. He preferred to plan his own time without pressure from staff and was highly motivated to work on his own
● the advice of the speech therapist should be sought about helping him to control excessive salivation
● he should be given tactful encouragement to take more care of his appearance
● he would be invited to join in as many outings as possible to increase his social contacts.

The present review showed that Greg's performance continued to improve consistently in all areas. He enjoyed reading and his motivation to socialise had increased; his conversational skills were improving, although he sometimes did not listen and would interrupt other people; he had better control of salivation and his general appearance was much tidier. He was still a very messy eater and demanded staff attention at inappropriate times.

New recommendations were made to help with these problems:

● Greg could join a local library and go there every week, with a member of staff, to take out books
● staff would continue to remind him to swallow, especially in the afternoons when he tended to be tired and to forget
● he would continue to be encouraged to take an interest in his appearance
● Greg would be allowed to sit in one room in the mornings but would be asked to leave the department if he disrupted other people's sessions by making demands on staff
● he would be invited to join a small lunch cookery group to work on his eating habits.

This review shows how aspects of a programme that are still effective are continued at the same level, for example, reminding Greg to swallow, while other aspects are upgraded to take account of improvements, for example, joining the library rather than just continuing to read newspapers. Changes can also be made to deter unacceptable behaviour, such as asking Greg to leave if he is disruptive.

TERMINATION OF TREATMENT

The process of treatment, assessment, evaluation and replanning can take place as many times as is necessary for the client to reach his optimum level of functioning. Short-term goals are continually being met and updated and it may be necessary to change long-term goals in the light of new information acquired during therapy or if the client's progress does not match expectations.

At some stage it will become apparent that either the goals have been met or there are reasons why no further progress can be made at this time. The decision to terminate treatment is ideally taken by the therapist and client together but it may be a one-sided decision in some cases, for example, the therapist may feel that the client could benefit from further practice in the relatively protected environment of the department but he feels ready to take on his social responsibilities again and leaves.

Final assessment

Planned discharge is the ideal but many factors may intervene to cause treatment to be terminated before the client has attained maximum benefit. The occupational therapist does not make the final decision on how long a client remains in therapy, whether in the health or social services or in private practice.

If the discharge is planned, there will be time to do a final assessment with the client and write a discharge report. This can serve several purposes:

● it allows the client to see what changes he has made so that he can leave feeling positive about himself

- it gives the occupational therapist an opportunity to evaluate the effectiveness of her treatment programme
- a record of treatment goes into the case notes in the form of the discharge summary
- any gap between the client's existing level of skills and the skills he needs to carry out his expected roles and occupations is highlighted so that recommendations can be made for further treatment or advice given on where to find help.

WHAT IS ASSESSED?

As occupational therapy takes a holistic view of man, assessment is very broad. The therapist carries out a general assessment of the client's life roles and functions as follows:

- abilities and strengths, as well as areas of dysfunction
- the balance of activities in daily life and any major changes of roles or occupations that have taken place
- barriers to the development of competence and the individual's potential for change.

It is important to take a full occupational history as well as assessing present function in order to find out whether the client has had experience and developed competence in occupations that he has later lost, or whether he has never developed competence in certain areas.

It is not possible or necessary to learn everything there is to know about a client, therefore data is collected and organised in the context of the model being used. However, the broad areas that the occupational therapist is interested in include:

- volition (the will to act and the direction of action)
- performance (the skills that make up the action and the roles the individual acts out)
- environment (where the action takes place).

VOLITION

Man has a basic urge to act (intrinsic motivation)

but the type of action he takes is determined by the experiences he has throughout life. These experiences will influence his self-image, what he considers to be valuable and worth doing, the goals he sets out to achieve by action and what he enjoys or finds interesting.

The occupational therapist has traditionally taken an interest in motivation for the purpose of treatment, to assist in engaging clients in therapeutic activity. This aspect of motivation is discussed in more depth in Chapter 6 (page 97). However, an understanding of the theory of intrinsic motivation can also facilitate assessment of dysfunction.

Intrinsic motivation

Man has an innate urge to use his capacity to explore and interact successfully with his environment (Reilly 1962). The satisfaction in such action comes from the activity itself, not only from the external rewards that the action may bring. This intrinsic satisfaction is stimulated by novelty in the environment and is strong enough to sustain action even when the immediate consequences are not pleasant. Intrinsic motivation is discussed further in Chapter 6.

The occupational therapist looks for five factors in assessing a client's level of motivation (Burke 1977, Florey 1969, White 1971):

- level of stimulation in the environment
- satisfaction of basic needs
- opportunities to act on the environment
- experience of social disapproval (negative feedback) of actions
- sense of being able to achieve desired goals.

Direction of action

One important factor in how a person acts is his self-image (Kielhofner & Burke 1980). This is conceptualised in different ways depending on the model being used but all theorists agree that this factor influences how the individual performs.

Fidler and Fidler (1978) state that each person learns his own capacities by *doing*. Successful doing leads to a sense of satisfaction and a sense of competence. Persistent failure to succeed, due to lack of skill or lack of opportunity to do, leads to a sense of incompetence and lack of control.

The model of human occupation (Kielhofner & Burke 1980) also conceptualises self-image as arising from interactions of the human system with the environment during development. The balance of success to failure depends on how much the individual feels that events are within his control and how much they are outside it. This model suggests that three factors determine the actions a person takes:

- values
- goals
- interest.

Values

Values not only influence the actions of the individual but also influence how he interprets and reacts to other people's actions. It may therefore be important for the therapist to understand the values underlying the client's behaviour but this is not easy, particularly if the therapist and client are from different cultural backgrounds.

Goals

Goals are linked to values in that they are based on what the individual thinks is worth doing. In order to elicit the client's full cooperation the therapist must be able to elicit his personal goals through the assessment procedure. He will not strive to achieve the therapist's goals unless they coincide with his own.

Interest

Interest is the expectation of pleasure in an activity. It is aroused by a combination of experience and some degree of novelty. Experience tells the individual that he has enjoyed something similar in the past and novelty arouses the urge to try again. When we say a client is not interested in an activity we mean:

- that he has tried something similar before and not enjoyed it
- that he has tried something similar before and knows he cannot do it,

- that he has tried this activity before and there is no challenge in it
- that he has never tried this type of activity before and has no confidence in his ability to succeed at a new task.

The reason for not being interested has implications for suggesting alternative activities therefore it is important to assess a client's interests before planning intervention.

PERFORMANCE

Each person develops a repertoire of skills that are refined from the unskilled actions of the baby and young child. New skills are learned throughout the life cycle but they are not selected randomly. Skills are developed specifically to support the life roles that the individual undertakes and to carry out the occupations associated with those roles. The more skills a person has learned and the greater his competence in those skills, the more roles are open to him. A variety of roles will be adopted at any one period of life and these roles change throughout the life cycle.

Assessing competence in skills

To be competent means to be 'sufficient or adequate to meet the demands of a situation or task' (White 1971), therefore, skills must be developed to a level of competence if they are to enable the individual to function effectively in his occupational roles. When assessing clients, it should be taken into account that competence is not an absolute concept; norms for competence vary with age and are to some extent socially defined (Mocellin 1988).

For simplicity, function is divided into skill areas that are interdependent and interrelated but that can be looked at separately in the early stages of intervention. One example is Mosey's (1968) seven adaptive skills:

1. perceptual motor skill
2. cognitive skill
3. drive–object skill
4. dyadic interaction skill
5. primary-group interaction skill

6. self-identity skill
7. sexual identity skill

These adaptive skill areas can be broken down into hierarchies of sub-skills that are learned in a predictable sequence during normal development. Lower-level skills are normally learned before higher-level skills. Learning must progress at a similar pace for each skill area. A delay in learning one particular skill will affect the ability to learn other skills, for example, the ability to trust, a sub-skill of dyadic interaction skill, must be learned before a person can enter into a sustained heterosexual relationship, a sub-skill of sexual identity interaction skill.

The therapist can assess what level of sub-skills the client has attained in each adaptive skill area and compare it with:

- past performance
- expected performance for someone of the client's age, sex and cultural background; norms for comparison with people who have the same disability may also be available
- level of skills required for the client to fulfil his occupational roles.

In this way, the information can be used to set goals for intervention.

Assessing roles and occupations

Roles are patterns of behaviour associated with social position. They are defined by society and assigned to individuals on the basis of such attributes as age, sex, relationships, possessions, education, job, income and appearance. Each role carries expectations of performance, which the individual attempts to carry out if he accepts the role. A properly integrated role, supported by the skills and habits necessary for its performance, satisfies both society's expectations and the individual's needs. However, when a person is assigned a role that he is unable or unwilling to accept then dissonance occurs between society's expectations and his performance. This can lead to social rejection and stigma (Ch. 23, p. 394).

In order to support roles, skills are organised into the routines that are habitually used to carry out the individual's daily tasks, for example,

brushing one's teeth involves a sequence of actions that becomes habitual so that one does not have to think carefully about every stage of the operation. Habits mean that the individual can perform everyday tasks without having to consciously remember how to go about them. These routines are developed to suit the individual's needs at any one period of his life. New habits are learned and old ones discarded as circumstances change.

The therapist assesses how clients organise their time, that is, whether they have useful habits or have to expend a lot of time and energy in working out ways of performing. Habits may also have become too rigid to allow for necessary changes so that the client's behaviour no longer meets the needs of his situation. It is useful to take an occupational history to assess whether the individual's habits have been disrupted or whether he has never developed good habits. If possible, the therapist will want to identify the point at which habits broke down.

Roles exist in a balance that normally changes throughout the life cycle. A healthy balance is one that allows most of the individual's needs to be satisfied without causing him to be rejected by society. The balance can be disrupted by illness, disability or bereavement.

The therapist wants to know:

- if the client's needs are being met
- if he is able to carry out the roles expected of him
- any reduction in the expected number of roles he adopts
- any imbalance between work, personal and social roles
- his role history

ENVIRONMENT

Man is never independent of his environment but learns how to adapt to it, or adapt it to him, to satisfy his needs. Through acting on the environment and receiving feedback about the effect of his actions he learns how best to achieve his own aims. Skilled performance of actions is only developed through exploring the environment and acting on it. Failure to adapt to the environment leads to dysfunction.

Assessing opportunities for exploration and practice

Skills are learned through exploration of the environment and of one's own potential. Competence is developed through practising skills in a variety of situations. Some skills are learned by carrying them out in reality, such as learning to climb trees; competence in this can only be acquired by doing it. Other skills are learned by role-playing, for example, social roles are rehearsed through childhood play.

Lack of opportunity to practise skills and roles in childhood and adolescence prevents the individual from developing a realistic image of his capacities and from knowing what his interests and values really are.

Reasons for being unable to engage in exploration of the environment and to practise skills for coping with it include:

- physical disability
- impoverished environment
- lack of satisfaction of basic needs, for example, emotional insecurity
- overcontrolling or overprotective parental figures
- interruptions to normal development, such as injury or illness.

It should be remembered that the treatment situation itself may block engagement in occupation for several of the above reasons.

Once the problem has been identified, the therapist and client can plan intervention that will include new opportunities for exploration and skill generation with a high chance of success.

Assessing adaptation to the environment

Individuals have the ability to influence their own health through what they do. A healthy environment allows the individual to act in a way that will enable him to meet his needs.

Sometimes people find themselves in an environment that they cannot adjust to in a healthy way or that does not give them opportunities to make changes. Various constraints may exist, including:

- social expectations, such as the role expectations for young mothers
- physical factors, such as poor housing
- economic constraints, such as poverty or having to stay in an unsatisfactory job.

A person may become ill because of environmental factors and then discover that the illness allows him to meet his needs, either by removing him from the problem environment or by changing the attitudes and behaviour of people around him. The costs of being ill are outweighed by the benefits, which then act to maintain the illness behaviour.

METHODS OF ASSESSMENT

Occupational therapists use a wide range of assessment tools, from interviews to activity batteries. Some depend on the knowledge and skill of the tester, such as general observation, while others are standardised tests and can, in theory, be used objectively by anyone.

Several factors influence the methods of assessment chosen for a particular client:

- the model being used by the therapist
- the data required
- the level of ability of the client.

The first three assessment techniques described here, review of records, interview and home visits, are used by many professionals as well as by occupational therapists. Techniques more specific to occupational therapists are those involving activity or occupation. Described here are checklists, performance scales, occupational questionnaires and projective techniques.

REVIEW OF RECORDS

The therapist sometimes does not have easy access to case notes and other records, for example, if she works in the community. In this case, a well-designed referral form is essential to elicit the desired information before the client is seen.

It is sometimes suggested that the therapist should not read the client's records before seeing him as this may influence her perceptions of him. However, it is very frustrating for the client to have to give the same information to many people and if the therapist is aware of the danger of bias she can consciously try to avoid it.

Looking through medical and nursing records can be time-consuming, especially if the client has a long medical history but familiarity with the way case notes are organised (and with the handwriting of medical officers!) makes the search easier. Hemphill (1982) suggests that the therapist looks at:

- social history
- admission summary
- nurses' notes
- the psychologist's report
- the physicians' reports
- any other pertinent reports.

She recommends a checklist to use when reading case notes so that no relevant information is missed.

Information gained from the client's records can be used to plan the initial interview.

THE INTERVIEW

In most treatment settings the occupational therapist is in constant, informal communication with her clients. However, a formal interview can often be a useful additional method of communication and assessment.

Interviews can be structured or unstructured. No interview is truly unstructured if it is to be of use but there is a difference between knowing what you want to elicit and having a list of set questions to ask. The structured interview tends to be more popular with less-experienced therapists (Kielhofner 1988).

Unstructured interviews

Before the interview, the therapist collects any information she can about the client and decides what she wants to find out. Time need not be wasted during an interview in going over what the therapist already knows. The client is informed in advance about the time, place and purpose of the interview. The therapist may expect him to turn up on time or may collect him, depending on his needs.

The interview is carried out in an informal atmosphere without distractions or interruptions. Attention is paid to details such as height and positioning of chairs, in order to gain maximum rapport. Comfortable but straight-backed chairs, placed at an angle of 90° to each other, are probably ideal since both parties can then see each other without effort. Interruptions can usually be avoided if other staff are informed that the interview is taking place, where it is and how long it will take. It has been known for an entire ward staff to turn out to search for a missing client, only to find him being interviewed by a student who forgot to tell anyone that he was with her.

At the beginning of the interview the therapist calls the client by name and makes sure that he remembers her name and the purpose of the interview. She may take a more- or less-directing role in the interview, depending on the client's mental state and the purpose of the interview but a warm and accepting manner is usually most successful. The length of the interview may be set in advance, especially if there are many constraints on time, or it may be determined by the course of events. A confused person may not be able to tolerate a long interview whereas a client in acute distress may benefit from the therapist's undivided attention until he feels calmer.

Upon termination of the interview a brief summary of its main points by the therapist can help the client to continue thinking about it afterwards. The therapist then checks that the client knows where he is going and walks with him if it is appropriate. Notes are usually written up after the interview.

Structured interviews

The structured interview format may be designed for use in a particular treatment setting if the therapist finds it useful to collect the same information about each client. Alternatively, it may be designed as part of a particular model, for example, an occupational history is often taken to collect information about a client's performance in past and present occupational roles for use within the model of human occupation.

The structured interview consists of a series of questions designed to elicit the desired information. Such a series of questions could also be administered as a questionnaire if the therapist is confident that the client understands it fully but an interview is more personal and allows rapport to be developed (Florey & Michelman 1982). It is often acceptable to take brief notes during a structured interview.

An interview may also be semi-structured, that is, the therapist has a number of questions to ask but allows for digressions if they seem useful. Florey and Michelman (1982) suggest that, while the questionnaire or structured interview are effective for gathering a history of discrete events such as childhood illnesses, the semi-structured interview is useful for taking a history of more abstract events.

Many of the histories and checklists used by occupational therapists could be administered as interviews, self-assessment instruments or computer programs, depending on the needs and abilities of the client.

Content of the interview

During the interview the therapist can observe:

- the client's verbal and non-verbal communication skills
- any sensory deficits
- the quality of his self-care
- any mannerisms he may have
- his posture
- his facial expression.

By asking questions she can find out:

- his level of cognitive functioning
- his attitudes to his current situation, in general
- how he feels about being involved in therapy
- his mood
- what he expects from therapy.

Questions can be directed towards exploring a particular aspect of the client, such as his relationships with other people.

The interview is also an opportunity for giving the client information and feedback. At the initial interview, rules and expectations within the occupational therapy department can be explained, including how violations of the rules are dealt with. A discussion of the general function of the department and its potential value to the client helps him to make more informed decisions about becoming involved in treatment. Clients frequently complain that they do not see how occupational therapy can help them and a clear explanation can enhance the value of therapy.

During later interviews the client can be given feedback on his performance and on any changes that have been observed. He may also give feedback on how he feels about the programme. Modifications to the programme are discussed so that the client continues to be actively involved in his own treatment.

OBSERVATION

Observation involves noting and recording the type, frequency and duration of behaviours in the client and interpreting what is observed according to the model being used.

Mosey (1973) describes three steps in using observation as a method of assessment:

1. *Observation*: noting what the client does without ascribing meaning to it
2. *Interpretation*: using observed data to reach conclusions about the reasons for the client's behaviour
3. *Validation*: seeking to confirm the accuracy of interpretations by sharing them with the client or others who know him well.

There are three main types of observation:

- general observation of the client during activities
- observation of specified behaviours
- observation of performance of set tasks.

General observation

The range of activities provided by occupational therapy gives opportunities for observing clients under different circumstances so that a picture of their capabilities and deficits can be built up. However, clients' behaviour in the occupational therapy department is often very different from when they are in the ward, so staff also benefit from spending time out of the department to observe clients. In a small community, where clients are frequently encountered outside the treatment setting, the therapist also has opportunities to observe their social functioning in their normal environment.

Using a checklist to record behaviours observed can help to ensure accuracy and reduce subjectivity. Checklists make it possible to look at complicated areas of skills without becoming confused, although a description may also be needed to give additional information.

Much can be learned from the physical appearance of the client, his physique, posture, facial expression, mannerisms, gait, grooming and dress. Some diseases, such as severe depression, produce a characteristic stooped posture and flat expression. However, the use of certain drugs may mask symptoms of the underlying disorder with an array of side effects, for example, obesity or rigidity may be due to phenothiazine medication.

Form and content of speech provide clues to the client's inner life, including mood, insight, cognitive functioning and thought disorder. A good rapport with the client is helpful in that he will be more willing to share his thoughts in the context of a warm and trusting relationship.

The client's behaviour patterns can be observed in different situations to assess his energy level, diurnal variations in energy, interaction with others, willingness to cooperate, initiative and skills. He may respond in totally different ways to peers, junior staff, students and senior staff so that everyone in the treatment setting will have something to contribute to a total assessment.

Observation of specified behaviours

General observation tends to be descriptive and inevitably misses much of what happens. The occupational therapist is usually a participant observer, making it even more difficult to observe clients' performance. A more precise method of

observation is to specify what is to be observed and ignore all other behaviour. This method is commonly used by psychologists but can be useful for occupational therapists, particularly within a behavioural model. The process consists of:

- deciding what to observe
- selecting an observation technique
- making the observation
- recording the observation
- analysing the behaviour recorded.

The therapist may wish to observe the number of times a particular behaviour occurs (frequency) or the length of time the behaviour lasts (duration). The observation technique chosen will depend on what is to be observed but the three main methods are (Hogg & Raynes 1987, Felce & McBrien 1987)

- event counting
- time sampling
- duration recording.

Event counting and time sampling are used to count the frequency of behaviours that are brief, discrete and easily identified, such as head-banging. Duration recording is used for behaviours that last for longer periods, such as concentrating on a task.

Event counting

The therapist specifies the behaviour she wishes to observe, for example, the client makes eye contact with the therapist. The therapist then counts the total number of times the behaviour occurs either during the whole session or during a specified period of time. If the behaviour occurs infrequently then the whole session may be observed, for example, the client makes eye contact with the therapist twice during a half-hour session.

Interval recording and time sampling

If the behaviour to be observed occurs frequently it may be more appropriate to take samples than to record it continuously. This can be done by noting the number of times the behaviour occurs during brief, regularly spaced intervals of time, say, for 1 minute in every 10 (interval recording), or by making an observation at fixed intervals and noting if the behaviour is occurring at that moment (time sampling). The results can be noted on a record sheet that specifies the behaviour to be observed and only takes a moment to mark.

Duration recording

This method is used for behaviours that occur for longer periods or for variable periods of time. The easiest method is to use a cumulative stopwatch to record the total amount of time spent on the behaviour in a given period, for example, the amount of time a client concentrates on the task in hand during a 1-hour session.

Set tasks

When further information is required about a particular area of functioning, the client can be asked to participate in a task designed to measure that function, for example, cooking a meal or planning an outing. The task may demand practical skills, such as hand–eye coordination, or cognitive skills, such as problem solving. It may be a social task that requires interaction with others or it may be designed to highlight the client's attitudes by making unusual demands on him.

A careful and detailed analysis of the task ensures that it requires the skills that the therapist hopes to observe. A knowledge of 'normal' performance is also necessary so that the client's performance can be measured against it.

It is rarely possible to reproduce external conditions accurately within the treatment setting and it may be appropriate to visit the client's home or workplace to assess its particular demands or try out skills.

HOME VISITS

Home visits may be made at any stage of treatment for the purpose of assessment or treatment or both. Within a multidisciplinary team it is necessary to coordinate with other staff to limit the number of people who do home visits and to share information obtained. Doctors, nurses, social workers and therapists all commonly visit clients' homes but it may not be necessary for all of them to visit the same person.

Purpose

Home visits are an expensive use of staff time so it is important to establish the purpose clearly beforehand. The occupational therapist builds up a picture of the client's assets and needs from her assessment in the treatment setting, which she can use to determine what to assess in the home environment.

The home visit can be used to:

- gain a picture of the client's life demands and role expectations
- observe his level of functioning in his normal environment
- carry out specific assessments, such as using the kitchen
- observe the physical environment, including where the house is situated and what type of accommodation it is
- meet family and neighbours on their own territory.

The physical environment includes where the home is situated, whether it is convenient for transport, shops, libraries and open spaces, its distance from the workplace and the character of the neighbourhood. The home itself can be assessed for physical barriers to easy access, amount of space, opportunities for privacy, playing space outside for children, facilities, comfort and noise level.

The emotional environment is more difficult to assess in a single visit since the family dynamics will be changed by the presence of a stranger. However, the therapist may learn something about stresses and supports within the home by observing the number of family members and the amount of personal space each one has. More difficult to assess, but very useful to know, is how emotionally close to each other the family members are, what roles they take within the family, what methods of communication they use and their attitudes to the person who is receiving treatment. Neighbours' attitudes are also relevant, especially if the client lives alone.

Carrying out a home visit

A date and time for the visit are set to suit the therapist, the client and his family, taking into account transport. It will be easier to determine the length of the visit if the aims are very clear and specific. Uniform is not normally worn for home visits but the therapist can carry some form of identification for the benefit of the family.

The purpose of the visit is clearly explained to the family, especially if the therapist has not met them before. Many families like to offer a cup of tea to a visitor and this can provide an opportunity for getting to know them in a relaxed way. Further structuring of the visit depends on what the therapist wishes to assess.

After a home visit, the therapist can discuss with the other team members the client's level of functioning against his life demands. They can then help the client to decide if any adjustments can be made to the environment or whether he needs to make personal changes in order to cope. This visit resulted in a decision that affected Mrs Wilson's whole life. It was important that the therapist presented all her observations accurately and objectively to the team so that they could discuss the facts of the case, and not the occupational therapist's opinion, with Mrs Wilson.

CHECKLISTS, PERFORMANCE SCALES AND QUESTIONNAIRES

Occupational therapists have always used check-lists for assessing skills such as activities of daily living (ADL) and work skills but there has been an increase in the number of assessment procedures developed for use within particular models over the past 20 years. There has also been more interest in standardising assessments, although normative data has still to be collected for many tests that are in regular use.

Checklists can be used to make sure no skill area has been missed. The types of checklist commonly used by occupational therapists include:

- broad assessments, such as the Occupational Therapy Developmental Analysis, Evaluation and Intervention Schedule (DAEIS)
- assessments of specific skill areas, such as ADL checklists
- multidisciplinary assessments, such as the Personal Assessment Chart (PAC).

Some of the many areas of performance that can be assessed by the use of checklists or performance scales include adaptive skills, sensory integration, past and present life roles, balance of occupations, motivation, interests, locus of control and time structuring. Three of these will be described here: the Comprehensive Occupational Therapy Evaluation Scale (COTE), the Interest Checklist and the Occupational Questionnaire. Readers are recommended to follow up references at the end of the chapter for details of further methods.

CASE EXAMPLE 5.3

Mrs Wilson, an 83-year-old widow, had been admitted to hospital 6 weeks before in a confused state due to malnutrition. She had made a good recovery and was now very keen to return home but the team had some doubts about her ability to manage alone. The occupational therapist was asked to do a home visit with her to measure the home environment against her existing skills.

At first, Mrs Wilson refused to consider taking the therapist home with her, insisting that she could manage well. She changed her mind when the therapist, knowing that Mrs Wilson was a very sociable lady, suggested she cook lunch for them both and then call in at her local pub on the way back.

Mrs Wilson had some difficulty getting on a bus but managed her shopping without any problems. The flat was in an old house with many steps up to the front door, no bathroom, no hot running water and only old paraffin stoves for heating. From her observations, the therapist felt that Mrs Wilson would not be able to survive the winter in good health in that environment.

The visit to the pub was more successful, as Mrs Wilson was a popular regular and was bought many drinks before the therapist could persuade her to leave.

Using data provided by the occupational therapist's home visit, the team concluded that Mrs Wilson would do well in an old people's home where she would be well cared for and have company but would be able to go out to the pub when she wanted. She was at first reluctant to give up her home but quickly became very contented with her new life.

Comprehensive Occupational Therapy Evaluation Scale

This instrument was developed by occupational therapists working in an acute adult psychiatry unit in the USA to provide a broad but consistent range of information about clients for the purpose of coordinating occupational therapy programmes with the different approaches of other staff (Brayman & Kirby 1982). The four objectives of developing such an evaluation were specified as:

1. to identify behaviours relevant to the practice of occupational therapy
2. to define the identified behaviours in such a way that they can be reliably observed and rated
3. to record information in a way that can easily be read by the referring agent and that can provide a record of client progress
4. to provide an efficient method for data retrieval to assist in treatment planning and evaluation.

The evaluation scale is divided into three sections, general behaviour, interpersonal behaviour and task behaviour, each of which is subdivided into skills that are given a numerical rating from 0 to 4 (see Fig. 5.3). A total of 25 skills has been identified and clear definitions of the behaviour indicative of each skill are given on the back of the rating form. Performance in all the skills can be recorded for 16 days on a grid so that the results can be quickly recorded and compared.

Date																
1 GENERAL BEHAVIOUR	1	2	3	4	5	6	7	8	9	10	11	12	13	14	15	16
A Appearance																
B Non-productive behaviour																
C Activity level (a or b)																
D Expression																
E Responsibility																
F Punctuality																
G Reality orientation																

Scale   0 – normal 1 – minimal 2 – mild 3 – moderate 4 – severe

Fig. 5.3 A comprehensive occupational therapy evaluation scale. (Taken from: Hemphill B J 1982 *The evaluative process in psychiatric occupational therapy*. Slack, New Jersey. Reproduced by kind permission of Slack Inc.)

It has been found that the COTE shows up areas of competence and deficiency and is therefore useful for setting priorities in developing a treatment plan. However, some more extreme behaviours or more subtle changes are not reflected on the rating scale and it is recommended that a descriptive note is added in such cases.

The Interest Checklist

The interest checklist was developed by Matsutsuyu (1969) to assess clients' interests in order to facilitate the selection of therapeutic activities that would evoke and sustain interest throughout the treatment programme. It includes 80 items that the client can mark under the headings of 'casual interest', 'strong interest' or 'no interest'. These include activities such as cooking, gardening, solitaire, religion and swimming. There is space to add any other interests not included in the list and space for a written report on the client's interests from schooldays to the present.

Matsutsuyu suggested six propositions to describe the properties of the interest phenomenon:

1. interests are influenced by early experiences in the family
2. interests are affective in nature and evoke positive or negative emotional responses
3. making choices on the basis of interest leads to commitment to the roles chosen
4. interest leads the individual to engage in activities that teach him how to act effectively to achieve his goals
5. interest in a task can sustain action after the novelty of the task has worn off
6. interests reflect the image a person has of himself.

These six propositions became the theoretical basis for designing an interest checklist.

The data from this checklist can be classified by intensity of interest felt, ability to express personal preference, ability to discriminate type and intensity of interests and categories of interest. All the items on the list can be classified as manual skills, physical sports, social recreation, activities of daily living or cultural/educational.

From this information it should be possible to select activities that will maintain the client's commitment to treatment for the attainment of either short-term or long-term goals.

The Occupational Questionnaire

This questionnaire was developed for use within the model of human occupation (Kielhofner 1988). It consists of a daily timetable in half-hour blocks for the client to fill in to show his typical way of spending time on a working day or a non-working day (see Fig. 5.4). Each activity can then be rated by the client as being, in his perception:

- work
- a daily living task } habits
- recreation
- rest.

The client is also asked to rate each activity on a five-point scale for:

- how well he thinks he performs it—personal causation
- how important he thinks it is—values
- how much he likes it—interest.

The questionnaire is designed to provide data about the client's habits, balance of activities, feeling of competence, interests and values and to show up problems in any of these areas. Used in collaboration with the client, it can assist in setting therapeutic goals. The results can be displayed in various ways to give a visual picture that the client will understand, for example, a pie chart or a profile, since it is necessary for the client to be involved in interpreting the results.

The questionnaire can also be filled in for a time when the client feels he was functioning effectively, so that a comparison can be made with his present functioning.

Other versions of the questionnaire are now being developed to measure different aspects of the client, for example, one version highlights the amount of pain and fatigue the client is experiencing.

PROJECTIVE TECHNIQUES

Projective techniques were developed as a method of assessing emotions, motivations and values, all of which could not be measured with existing tools. Early techniques included the Rorschach Inkblot Test, Morgan and Murray's Thematic Apperception Test and Cattell's Sentence Completion Test. All these tests present the subject with ambiguous stimuli to which he is asked to give mean-

Time	Typical activities	Question 1 — I consider this activity to be:				Question 2 — I think that I do this:					Question 3 — For me this activity is:					Question 4 — How much do you enjoy this activity?				
		Work W	Daily living task D	Recreation R	Rest RT	Very well VW	Well W	About average AA	Poorly P	Very poorly VP	Extremely important EI	Important I	Take it or leave it TL	Rather not do it RN	Total waste of time TW	Like it very much LVM	Like it L	Neither like nor dislike it NLD	Dislike it D	Strongly dislike it SD
5.00 – 5.30 am		W	D	R	RT	VW	W	AA	P	VP	EI	I	TL	RN	TW	LVM	L	NLD	D	SD
5.30 – 6.00 am		W	D	R	RT	VW	W	AA	P	VP	EI	I	TL	RN	TW	LVM	L	NLD	D	SD
6.00 – 6.30 am		W	D	R	RT	VW	W	AA	P	VP	EI	I	TL	RN	TW	LVM	L	NLD	D	SD
6.30 – 7.00 am		W	D	R	RT	VW	W	AA	P	VP	EI	I	TL	RN	TW	LVM	L	NLD	D	SD
7.00 – 7.30 am		W	D	R	RT	VW	W	AA	P	VP	EI	I	TL	RN	TW	LVM	L	NLD	D	SD

Fig. 5.4 Sample worksheet from the Occupational Questionnaire. (*Source*: The relationship between volition, activity pattern and life satisfaction in the elderly (activity analysis, geriatrics, human occupation, personal satisfaction), by Smith, N. R., Kielhofner, G. and Watts, J. H. Copyright 1986 by the American Occupational Therapy Association, Inc. Reprinted with permission.)

ing. A projective test uses standard stimuli that allow the subject to make his own interpretations. The theory behind them is that the subject does not know what is expected of him, that is, what would constitute a good performance, therefore he performs spontaneously (Cutting 1968).

The material projected by the subject may be one of three types.

1. Projection was described by Freud as an ego-defence mechanism through which painful or unacceptable feelings are ascribed to someone else. This is an unconscious process.

2. Projection can also be a way of giving meaning to situations that are otherwise confusing by seeing them in terms of one's own motives and beliefs.

3. It may also be an unconscious method of wish fulfillment, for example, a woman who does not find it easy to attract men may think that all men have designs on her (Munn 1966).

All three aspects of projection are involved in projective techniques.

How projective tests are administered

Projective tests are presented in a standardised manner and order. The stimulus may be, for example, a sentence to be completed or a picture to be interpreted. The Rorschach Inkblot Test uses 10 standard inkblots which are shown to the subject one by one. He is asked what each blot might be. The test is scored on the number of items seen in each blot, whether the blot is perceived as a whole, the type of things perceived and the qualities perceived, such as form and movement. The tester must have experience in order to be able to interpret the results of the test.

In the Thematic Apperception Test the subject is shown a standard series of pictures and asked to build a story around each one. The themes of his stories are then analysed to discover his unconscious motivation. Again, the interpretation of results requires an experienced tester.

The assumption in all these techniques is that the subject projects his own perceptions, values and motivations onto the stimulus. The task of the tester is to relate what the subject says about the stimulus back to him and thus gain understanding of his motives and values. There is, of course, a danger that the inexperienced therapist might intrude her own unconscious feelings into the test.

Material projected in these tests will include that which falls within normal limits and that which relates to the client's problems. It is therefore necessary to standardise tests and testing procedures so that results show any deviations from the normal population.

The use of projective techniques by occupational therapists

Occupational therapists use projective techniques in two ways.

1. Creation of an object by the client, such as a painting, or presentation of a stimulus by the therapist, such as a poem, followed by a period of discussion in which the client is encouraged to express his feelings about the object freely. This is usually done in a group.

2. Presentation of a series of standard activities to the client with an assessment of how he copes with them.

Using projective techniques in groups

The distinguishing feature of occupational therapy as opposed to other therapies is the presence of objects that can be manipulated by the client. These objects may already be available or may be created by the client (Azima & Azima 1959). Thus, projective techniques are an appropriate method of assessment for occupational therapists because they involve doing as well as talking.

Most of the projective techniques used by occupational therapists involve a phase of creating, which can be structured or unstructured, and a phase of talking about the created object or free-associating about it (see Ch. 13, p 199). The technique is used as assessment and as a form of treatment simultaneously, in that the therapist helps the client to accept the projected material as his own and gain insight into how his own perceptions are formed.

The functions that are assessed by the use of projective techniques will vary according to the model being used, but may include:

- motor skills
- cognitive skills
- task skills
- interaction skills
- orientation
- motivation
- ego-organisation and control
- mood
- reality orientation
- level of activity
- self-image
- independence.

Projective tests developed by occupational therapists

Two types of projective tests developed by occupational therapists for individual use are the Azima Battery and the Goodman Battery.

The Azima Battery is a typical projective technique developed by an occupational therapist (Azima 1982). This utilises three tasks: a free pencil drawing, drawings of a person of each sex and a free clay model. These are presented to the client in a standard order and method. The client is given a set period of time to complete each task. During the 'doing' phase of the test the therapist records the time taken, the client's behaviour, any verbalisations and the techniques used. When the work is finished the client is asked to describe his productions.

An evaluation scale is used to interpret the results of the battery. This includes organisation of mood, organisation of drives and organisation of object relations, all of which are inferred from aspects of the client's observed behaviour and content of speech. Findings are analysed and presented as a summary to be used in differential diagnosis, treatment planning and prognosis (Azima 1982).

The Goodman Battery was developed from the Azima Battery and differs from it in that the tasks given are progressively less structured, thus making it possible to assess cognition and ego

functioning under decreasingly structured conditions. It was designed for use with young adults and adults suffering from psychiatric disorders.

The four tasks in the battery are: copying a mosaic tile, spontaneous drawing, figure drawing and free clay modelling. The tester assesses the client's ability to conceptualise, to organise and to plan procedures that will enable him to complete the tasks. The theory underlying this technique is that the individual's ability to carry out practical tasks will be affected by the presence of conflicts and defences that consume energy, and by weak ego boundaries. When ego boundaries are weak, performance may be expected to deteriorate as the external structure becomes looser.

A guide has been developed to help in the recording and interpretation of findings, and rating scales are used for the different aspects of performance. These include ability to organise, independence and self-esteem.

This battery is administered by a standardised procedure but the rating scales have not yet been standardised (Evaskus 1982).

VALIDATING RESULTS

An increasing number of assessment procedures that were originally developed by occupational therapists to meet the needs of their particular setting have now been made widely available. Some have been described in this chapter. Smith and Tiffany (1988) point out that there is still a lot of work to be done in establishing the legitimacy of many of these procedures and much research is still needed.

Procedures have been developed for use in particular settings but are not used anywhere else, and many of these have not been standardised or tested for reliability and validity. Occupational therapists tend to look at the individual and compare his current performance with past and desired performance, rather than looking at the norms for someone of his age, sex, social background, etc.

If treatment results in general seem satisfactory, then standardisation may not appear important to the therapist in the field who is working under pressure and simply wants to get through the work as efficiently as possible. However, we cannot justify our assessment results if the tests used will not stand up to scrutiny.

In developing new testing procedures, or looking at existing ones, there are seven main points to consider:

1. What aspects of the client does the therapist wish to assess?
2. Have these aspects been identified in such a way that they can be measured accurately? (Reliability.)
3. How can the desired function be elicited for assessment?
4. Does the proposed assessment procedure measure what it is intended to measure? (Validity.)
5. Is there a clearly defined way of administering the assessment? (Standardisation of administration.)
6. How are the results to be recorded and scored?
7. Can the results be compared with the normal results for a comparable population? (Standardisation of results.)

Most of these points have been covered in this chapter. The model being used determines what is to be assessed, how it is assessed and how the assessment results are interpreted. The method of recording is influenced by who is to read the results and what they will be used for. Reliability, validity and standardisation will be discussed here.

RELIABILITY AND VALIDITY

Vague and inaccurate assessment leads to vague and imprecise treatment. This is unacceptable for both ethical and practical reasons. The occupational therapist has a duty to use treatment that will benefit and not harm the client (see Ch. 9 p. 134), therefore intervention must be based on accurate knowledge of the client's needs and abilities. The two most important concepts in ensuring accuracy of assessment procedures are reliability and validity.

Reliability

The first concern in legitimising an assessment procedure is whether or not it reliably elicits accurate information. There are two main ways of determining reliability.

1. *Test-retest* The rater assesses the client and records the results. After a suitable interval to minimise the effect of practice, the test is given again and the results are compared. Obviously, results are more likely to be similar if the aspects being measured have been clearly defined and the testing procedure is standard (see p. 83).

2. *Inter-rater evaluation* The assessment procedure is carried out on the same client by two or more raters and their results compared. This method is appropriate for evaluating procedures that involve observation. If possible, the raters observe the client doing the same activity, perhaps by using a videotape. The results are more likely to be similar if the testing procedure is standard and the raters have been trained in its use.

Validity

Establishing the validity of an assessment procedure is more difficult than establishing reliability, so it is only carried out on procedures that are known to be accurate and therefore worth validating.

Validation involves checking that the procedure does measure what it is intended to measure. If we want to know whether a client is able to cook a meal on his gas cooker there is no point in assessing his performance on the department's electric cooker.

There are three main types of validity:

1. *content validity*: analysing the assessment procedure to see if it measures what it purports to measure
2. *criterion-related validity*: comparing the assessment results with an external criterion such as data collected from other sources
3. *construct validity*: looking at the accuracy of the assessment procedure in measuring the theories or hypotheses behind the intervention.

STANDARDISATION

If an assessment procedure is found to be both accurate and reliable then it may be appropriate and useful to standardise it for use in a particular way with the client group it was developed for. Establishing a clear and uniform procedure for applying the test is called standardisation of administration and establishing the performance of a similar group of people for comparison is called standardisation of results, or norming.

Standardisation of administration

This means that the procedure can be repeated in exactly the same way by different people, at different times and on different subjects. This involves defining the functions to be assessed very clearly and giving precise instructions about administering and scoring the test. Objective tests are easier to standardise than tests that require an observer to make a judgement. Observer bias must be minimised by training the rater (Garfield 1982).

Standardisation of results

This is a lengthy procedure and is most likely to be neglected when an assessment procedure is developed. It involves administering a reliable and valid assessment procedure to a large number of people who are matched for such factors as sex, age, cultural background and, possibly, disability. The results can be used to show the normal range of performance for that group, to use as a comparison with the scores of an individual.

SUMMARY

This chapter covered the assessment stages of the occupational therapy process, including initial assessment, ongoing assessment and final assessment. It looked at what is assessed by the occupational therapist; volition and motivation, performance, and relationship with the environment. Methods of assessment used by occupational therapists were reviewed, including review of client records, interviewing, observation, home visits, checklists, performance scales, questionnaires and projective techniques. Finally, there was a brief section on validating assessment results.

Chapter 6 covers the treatment planning and implementation stage of the occupational therapy process, which follows assessment.

REFERENCES

Azima F J C 1982 The Azima Battery: an overview. In: Hemphill B J (ed) The evaluative process in psychiatric occupational therapy. Slack, New Jersey

Azima H, Azima F 1959 Outline of a dynamic theory of occupational therapy. American Journal of Occupational Therapy 13: 1–7

British Association of Occupational Therapists Annual Conference 1988 Workshop: The District General Hospital and high turnover of beds. British Journal of Occupational Therapy 51(6): 201–202

Brayman S J, Kirby T 1982 The Comprehensive Occupational Therapy Evaluation. In: Hemphill B J (ed) The evaluative process in psychiatric occupational therapy. Slack, New Jersey

Burke J P 1977 A clinical perspective on motivation: pawn versus origin. American Journal of Occupational Therapy 31 (4): 254–258

Cutting D 1968 A review of projective techniques. American Occupational Therapy Association Regional Institute report. Unpublished

Evaskus M G 1982 The Goodman Battery. In: Hemphill B J (ed) The evaluative process in psychiatric occupational therapy. Slack, New Jersey

Felce D, McBrien J 1987 Workshop: Challenging behaviour in mental handicap. Stockport

Fidler G S, Fidler J W 1978 Doing and becoming: purposeful action and self-actualization. American Journal of Occupational Therapy 32 (5)

Fidler G S 1982 The activity laboratory: a structure for observing and assessing perceptual, integrative and behavioural strategies. In: Hemphill B J (ed) The evaluative process in psychiatric occupational therapy. Slack, New Jersey

Florey L L 1969 Intrinsic motivation: the dynamics of occupational therapy theory. 'Papers on research and development in occupational therapy' at Southern California

Florey L L, Michelman S M 1982 Occupational role history: a screening tool for psychiatric occupational therapy. American Journal of Occupational Therapy 36(5)

Garfield M 1982 The principles of developing assessment tools. In: Hemphill B J (ed) The evaluative process in psychiatric occupational therapy. Slack, New Jersey

Gillette N 1968 Principles of evaluation. From AOTA Regional Institute

Hemphill B J 1982 The evaluative process in psychiatric occupational therapy, Slack, New Jersey

Hogg J, Raynes N V 1987 Assessment in mental handicap: a guide to assessment, practices, tests and checklists. Croom Helm, London

Kielhofner G 1988 Workshop: The model of human occupation, York

Kielhofner G, Burke J P 1980 A model of human occupation, part 1. Conceptual framework and content. American Journal of Occupational Therapy 34(9)

Matsutsuyu J S 1969 The interest checklist. American Journal of Occupational Therapy 23(4): 323–328

Mocellin G 1988 A perspective on the principles and practice of occupational therapy. British Journal of Occupational Therapy 51(1)

Moorhead L 1969 The occupational history. American Journal of Occupational Therapy 23(4): 329–334

Mosey A C 1968 Recapitulation of ontogenesis: a theory for the practice of occupational therapy. American Journal of Occupational Therapy 22(5): 426–438

Mosey A C 1973 Meeting health needs. American Journal of Occupational Therapy 27(1): 14–17

Munn N L 1966 Psychology: the fundamentals of human adjustment (5th edn) Houghton Mifflin, Boston

Reilly M 1962 Occupational therapy can be one of the great ideas of twentieth century medicine. American Journal of Occupational Therapy 16(1): 1–9

Smith H D Tiffany E G 1988 Assessment and evaluation: an overview. In: Hopkins H L, Smith H D (eds). Willard and Spackman's occupational therapy (7th edn). Lippincott, Philadelphia

White R W 1971 The urge towards competence. American Journal of Occupational Therapy 25(6): 271–274

6

Treatment planning and implementation

Jennifer Creek

INTRODUCTION

In Chapter 5 we looked at the assessment stages of the occupational therapy process. This chapter looks in detail at the next stage, treatment planning and implementation, starting from the point where a database has been compiled and the therapist and client are ready to analyse it for the purpose of setting goals for intervention.

The chapter covers the process of analysing assessment data and setting long-term, or overall, goals that can then be broken down into intermediate and short-term goals. This process is illustrated with Case examples. Alternative methods of activity analysis and synthesis are described in detail, with an example of a generic activity analysis format and a sample activity analysis. Theories of motivation are discussed, highlighting their relevance to engaging clients in activity. The three factors of client goals, properties of activities and motivation determine the selection of activities for treatment which is described, together with a discussion of the four key elements of intervention: the client, the activity, the therapist and the environment. This section gives only an outline of the occupational therapy intervention process; Chapters 10 to 17 describe in detail the therapeutic use of activity.

TREATMENT PLANNING

Treatment planning is a collaboration between therapist and client in which assessment data are analysed and goals are set for intervention. As shown in the previous chapter, data collection is not random. The model being used determines what information is sought and provides an outline for analysing the information collected and for clarifying problem areas. The whole process should be made as simple as possible for the client so that he can be genuinely involved. Clients are more likely to become involved in treatment and to make changes if they are involved in setting their own goals and monitoring their own progress (Howell 1986).

Once the long-term goals of treatment have been agreed they can be broken down into short-term goals that lead, in smaller steps, to the achievement of the major goal. Long-term hospitalised clients may have difficulty accepting the overall goal of the treatment team, which usually involves major changes in their way of life, but they can move towards it in stages that they can accept (Drouet 1986).

The therapist uses her expertise in activity analysis and synthesis to identify appropriate activities for attaining goals but the client must feel that the activities are worth doing. The final decision as to whether to become involved in the activity rests with him. The treatment planning process is shown in Figure 6.1.

The treatment plan should be put in writing and copies given to the appropriate people, for example, the client, the doctor and the client's key worker. Formats for writing treatment plans are suggested in Chapter 28.

DATA ANALYSIS

Analysis of data obtained from the initial assessment produces three key areas of information:

1. the client's expected environment and occupational roles
2. areas of dysfunction that might interfere with the fulfillment of occupational roles

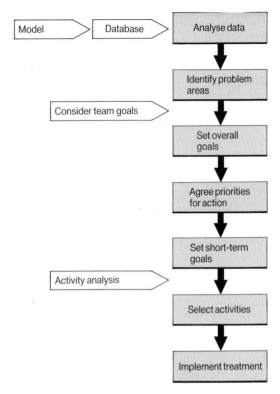

Fig. 6.1 The treatment planning process.

3. skills already available in the client's repertoire.

Environment and occupational roles

The client cannot be considered in isolation from his expected environment, since the skills he will require are determined by the demands of that environment and the roles he adopts within it. He may expect to return to his previous environment and previous level of functioning if the problem requiring intervention is an acute one. He may be moving from an institutional environment to the community, in which case there will be a lot of unknowns in his future. He may have a chronic disability that necessitates making changes in occupational roles.

The therapist needs to be clear about what the client expects to do in the future and what skills he will need in order to cope.

Areas of dysfunction

The client usually requires intervention because he is unable to meet the demands of his environment, either because the demands have changed, he has changed, or he has never coped adequately. The therapist's task is to identify areas of dysfunction where there is a gap between the skills the client needs and the skills he has. It may be a general deficit across several skill areas, as often occurs in mental handicap, for example, or it may be a specific deficit, such as inadequate social skills. Dysfunction can only be defined relative to the client's expected environment; there is no universal standard of achievement for all clients.

Skills in the client's repertoire

Skills must be learned in the developmental sequence so that higher-level skills are founded on lower-level skills, otherwise stress will cause regression to earlier modes of behaviour. The therapist tries to assess what level of skills the client has reached developmentally and starts her intervention from that point. Isolated skills will easily be lost.

As well as looking at the range of skills the client has, the therapist assesses whether or not he has achieved a sufficient level of competence to carry out his expected occupational roles and whether skills have been organised into habits that allow for efficient use of time and energy. This analysis highlights the skill areas that must be developed if the client is to fulfil his expected occupational roles and leads on to setting goals for achieving those skills.

SETTING GOALS

Goals are the targets that the client hopes to reach through involvement in occupational therapy. They define both the skills to be learned and the level of performance that is acceptable. Goals must be within the client's capabilities and he must adopt them as his own. When goals have been set the client should be absolutely clear about what is expected of him and how he is to achieve it. He and the therapist can easily see what progress has been made by looking at the goals that have been reached.

Levels of goals

Client goals are usually set on two or three levels:

1. long-term goals
2. intermediate goals (these will not be necessary in all cases)
3. short-term goals

as shown in Figure. 6.2

Long-term goals

These are the overall goals of the intervention process, the reasons why the client is being offered help and the expected outcome of intervention. They usually take account of:

- where the client might live after discharge
- the level of independence he might be expected to achieve
- the degree of support that is likely to be needed
- any necessary changes in life roles and the skills required to support them.

These can be described as occupational performance goals (Mosey 1986).

Intermediate goals

These may be clusters of skills to be developed or barriers to be overcome on the way to achieving the main goals of therapy. In a crisis intervention or other acute treatment it may not be necessary to use intermediate goals; the fluid nature of the problem and the short intervention time allow problems to be tackled rapidly.

Short-term goals

These are the small steps on the way to achieving major goals. They are organised into a hierarchy, with the most basic goal to be tackled first; they can be expressed in behavioural terms or subjective terms; and they are measurable. The short-

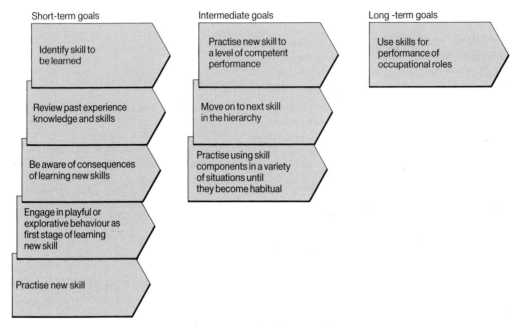

Fig. 6.2 The goals of intervention.

term goal is usually to learn a sub-skill or skill component of the adaptive skill that is needed for successful occupational performance (Mosey 1986).

Setting long-term goals

As discussed in the previous chapter, the occupational therapist will produce from her initial assessment a general picture of the client's occupational roles, balance of occupations, areas of skills deficit and future needs. These data, together with information from other team members, should suggest overall aims of intervention.

Whenever possible, the client's own perception of his needs is the guiding principle in setting aims, since he is the person who must achieve them. However, certain problems impair the ability to make rational decisions about the future. These may be temporary, as in severe depression, or permanent, as in dementia. In such cases the therapist may take a stronger lead in establishing

aims, while recognising that these are subject to review as the client changes during treatment and becomes able to express his opinions. If the therapist takes a strongly supportive role in the early stages of treatment it may be difficult to pass personal responsibility back to the client at a later stage, so one of the stated goals of intervention should be for the client to accept responsibility for his own progress.

In many cases the client will be expecting to return to his previous life roles, so treatment is designed to restore lost skills, teach additional skills or improve performance of existing skills in order to prevent recurrence of problems. In other cases the problem that caused the client to seek treatment is unlikely to be completely overcome, so that a change in life roles and the skills needed to support them can be anticipated.

The overall goals of the treatment team will also influence the occupational therapist's goals. Her programme is a part of the wider treatment programme and will play a greater or lesser part in achieving its aims.

CASE EXAMPLE 6.1

Lynn suffers from chronic anxiety of such severity that her performance of even simple tasks is seriously impaired. Most of her fear is focussed on magic and hypnotism; she is terrified of people being able to make her do things against her will. She also fears change, meeting new people, going out and failing in anything she attempts. These fears cause her to limit her sphere of activity to a few comforting rituals, such as overeating and bouncing a ball.

Lynn first received treatment for hyperactivity at the age of 18 months. Now, at the age of 32, she has experienced several admissions to hospital, various diagnoses and many different treatments. She lives at home and attends a day hospital 5 days a week, with occasional short admissions to give her parents a break. This situation is expected to continue for as long as her parents can keep her at home.

The team hopes to introduce Lynn gradually to a broader range of daytime activities without provoking further anxiety. She is expected to need long-term care eventually, preferably in a community setting such as a group home.

Lynn has insight into her present problems but is unrealistic about the future. She would like to marry, eventually, and to have children, or to look after her parents in their old age. She is able to give much more practical goals that she can start working towards now, which suggests that she recognises her long-term plans to be over-optimistic. She would like to start going out and meeting people, and doing the things other young adults do; to be helped to do more for herself so that she is less of a burden on her parents; to be able to visit the local shops, in company; and to have an interesting hobby such as cookery or sewing.

Taking all these factors into account, the long-term goals set by the occupational therapist in consultation with Lynn (see Fig. 6.3) are:

- to become independent in self-care
- to perform simple household tasks, such as making coffee, washing up, making beds
- to walk regularly to the local shops with a companion
- to learn simple embroidery

Achievement of these aims would satisfy Lynn, enable her to live at home longer, and help her to cope with life in a group home.

Setting intermediate goals

Long-term goals may not take a long time to reach, particularly in an acute treatment setting. However, in some cases they can take months or years to attain and may be modified to a greater or lesser extent during the treatment process. In the latter case, it may be difficult for the client to see himself ever attaining his ultimate goals and it can be useful to set intermediate goals, which can be seen as easier to reach. These are smaller goals that lead towards attainment of the long-term goals.

Certain disorders, such as dementia, interfere with client's ability to take a temporal perspective and therefore with their ability to plan for the long-term future. These clients will have difficulty in setting realistic long-term goals but may become involved in treatment planning by setting smaller goals. The acute phase of illness may also interfere with a person's perception of his own potential and make long-term goal setting impossible, although intermediate goals can still be discussed. For example, the therapist might feel that it is appropriate for a severely depressed client to aim to return home once the acute phase of the illness is over. During the acute phase, the client feels utterly hopeless about the possibility of ever leaving hospital, but is able to accept intermediate goals of attending a supportive psychotherapy group twice a week and a creative activities group once a week.

Three main factors determine what the intermediate goals should be:

1. any barriers to performance that need to be overcome, for example, fear of going out (agoraphobia)
2. the need to learn skills in a developmental sequence
3. the client's wishes.

CASE EXAMPLE 6.2

Lynn and the therapist spent some time discussing what skills would be needed to attain the long-term goals already agreed. They then decided which skills to tackle first. The factors taken into account in this process were:

- Lynn's fear of going out, which had to be overcome before she could go out to the local shops
- the need to build up Lynn's confidence by starting with goals that could be attained easily
- Lynn's strong interest in food and drink, which helped her to tolerate a certain amount of anxiety
- Lynn's request to be allowed to progress at her own pace in treatment.

It was decided to work towards all the long-term goals simultaneously, using small intermediate goals so that Lynn would develop a sense of achievement. These would be reviewed regularly but no pressure would be put on Lynn to perform any particular tasks in a set period of time. The first set of intermediate goals (see Fig. 6.3) was:

- to learn to tolerate a certain amount of anxiety while performing tasks
- to learn to comb her own hair
- to learn to make a cup of instant coffee independently
- to learn to wash up crockery independently
- to go to the local cafe with the therapist without being overwhelmed by anxiety
- to learn some simple embroidery stitches.

Setting short-term goals

When long-term and/or intermediate treatment goals have been agreed they can be broken down into a hierarchy of smaller steps. Each short-term goal needs to be realistically within the client's reach and a decision must be made about where to start. Each goal should also be measurable, so that client and therapist know when it has been reached.

Once short-term goals have been agreed, a programme of activities that will lead to their achievement is planned. The therapist's knowledge of activity analysis and synthesis enables her to identify or modify activities to incorporate all the skills, personal factors and environmental factors that will best bring about change.

CASE EXAMPLE 6.3

Lynn's first aim, to learn to tolerate a certain amount of anxiety while performing tasks, is broken down into steps that are given in the order in which they will be tackled. It is felt that Lynn would quickly learn to perform even the most complex task if not immobilised by anxiety. The aim is to enable her to perform despite her fears.

1. to feel at ease with the therapist
2. to identify occupations that she enjoys
3. to give each task its due importance and not take it too seriously
4. to remember to think through each task before beginning
5. to attempt simple tasks, such as combing her hair, with supervision
6. to stop and think about the task in hand if she starts to become anxious.

Some of the above stages are more easily measurable than others. Therapists may prefer to put all their goals into the form of measurable behavioural objectives to make evaluation of results easier. These six goals can be rewritten in objective format as follows.

At the end of treatment, Lynn will be able to:

1. remain in the company of the therapist for the duration of a treatment session without wanting to leave
2. state three activities that she has enjoyed in the past and would like to do again
3. state why she is carrying out each task
4. outline the stages involved in each task before beginning it
5. comb her hair, with verbal prompting
6. respond to anxiety by stopping what she is doing and reviewing the stages of the task in hand.

ACTIVITY ANALYSIS AND SYNTHESIS

Activity analysis is the process of identifying the various components of an activity. Activity synthesis is the process of designing an appropriate activity or adapting an existing activity by bringing together the desired components.

It is possible to identify all the components of an activity that come within the domain of the occupational therapist. Mosey (1986) calls this the generic approach and points out that there is no universally accepted conceptual framework for doing this.

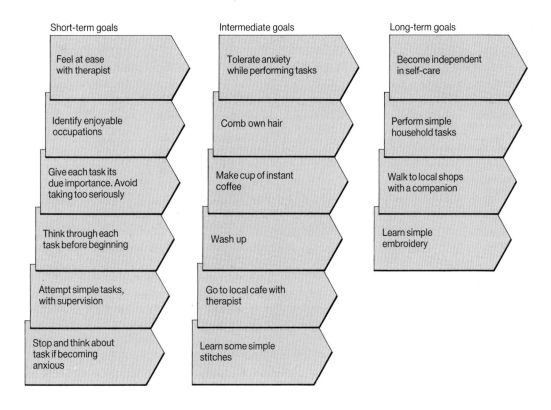

Short-term goals	Intermediate goals	Long-term goals
Feel at ease with therapist	Tolerate anxiety while performing tasks	Become independent in self-care
Identify enjoyable occupations	Comb own hair	Perform simple household tasks
Give each task its due importance. Avoid taking too seriously	Make cup of instant coffee	Walk to local shops with a companion
Think through each task before beginning	Wash up	Learn simple embroidery
Attempt simple tasks, with supervision	Go to local cafe with therapist	
Stop and think about task if becoming anxious	Learn some simple stitches	

An alternative approach is to study only components that are relevant to the model being used, for example, a psychodynamic model focusses on the psychological functions and psychosocial interactions involved in performing an activity (Katz 1985).

The format presented here is a generic one that was developed from several different frameworks (Mosey 1986, Fidler and Fidler 1963, Hopkins and Tiffany 1988, Llorens 1976).

Activity analysis

Activities are composed of many skills that can be divided for the purposes of analysis into:

- physical
- cognitive
- psychological
- interpersonal.

In order to understand the effect an activity will have on the client, the therapist needs to break it down into these skill areas and look at each one in detail.

Activity analysis also includes any potential for adapting the activity in order to allow for change in the client. This is called 'grading'. Grading allows the client to progress from exploration, through acquisition of skills, to attainment of goals. It also allows him to move on to the next stage once a skill has been learned. Grading may involve a gradual change in the nature of the activity by changing one or two components, or a complete change of activity.

Analysing an activity enables the therapist to:

- discover the skills required for its successful performance
- identify the sequence of sub-skills leading to the acquisition of mature skills and decide how they can best be presented

Name of activity
Timing/length of time/number of sessions
Environment
Brief description

Appropriateness for different ages and sexes
Social and cultural value
Preparation
Precautions

Requirements of activity

Physical

sensation
sensory integration
perception
spatial awareness
motor planning
gross motor
mobility
balance
fine motor
repetition
rhythm
coordination
strength
endurance
range of movement
posture
types of movement

Cognitive

attention
concentration
discrimination
generalisation
use of symbols
perceiving cause and effect
abstract thinking
reality testing
choice
language
following demonstration/directions
reading
writing
numbers
orientation
awareness of time
memory
range of knowledge
goal setting
planning
organisation
number of processes
speed
imagination
creativity
logic
problem solving

Psychological

expression of feelings
control of feelings
frustration tolerence
coping with pressure
expression of needs
gratification of needs
sublimation
playing/exploring
tolerating risk
trust
independence
passive or active
creativity
reality testing
ego-defence mechanisms encouraged or removed
exploration of feelings and motives
responsibility
involvement
sharing
interaction
self-image
body image
identification
sexual identity
end product
contrived or real experience

Interpersonal

individual or group/size of group
mixed or segregated sexes
communication
cooperation
competition
negotiation
compromise
leadership
structure
rules
interaction
isolation
variety of relationships
involvement
role opportunities

Potential for grading

Materials and equipment
Environment — human and non-human
Method
Related activities

Fig. 6.4 Activity analysis guidelines.

Name :   Guided fantasy
Duration :   Approximately 1 hour
Timing :   Participants need to be alert, so not after a meal
No. of sessions :   One, or a series
Environment :   Requires a quiet, comfortable room which can have the lights dimmed

Brief description:

Participants are taken through a relaxation process of about 20 minutes and asked to remain quiet and still during a fantasy lasting another 20 to 30 minutes. The therapist uses verbal directions to lead them on a fantasy journey. A few minutes rest is given, then everybody stretches and comes into a circle for discussion. Opportunity is given to share experiences and feelings in the group

Appropriateness:

Suitable for both sexes and any age above infancy

Social and cultural value:

Low social value is given to the use of imagination and expression of creative thought unless leading to financial reward. It is more highly valued in less industrialised cultures

Preparation:

Arrange mats or furniture in room. Try to ensure there will be no interruptions

Precautions:

Not appropriate for severely disturbed or restless people

Requirements of Activity

Physical:

Hearing verbal instructions
Sitting or lying still for about half an hour
Relaxing

Cognitive:

Attending to the therapist's voice
Concentrating for about half an hour
Following complex verbal instructions
Translating verbal instructions into mental images
Imagining a series of events cued by verbal instructions
Discriminating between fantasy and reality
Remembering and describing images

Psychological

Expression of feelings to therapist and group during discussion
Control of feelings for half an hour during fantasy
Allowing oneself to relax
Trusting the therapist enough to close eyes and relax
Allowing oneself to use imagination freely
Creating vivid mental images
Risking free use of imagination
Recognising that images are fantasy and not reality
Dropping defences to allow imagination to work
Exploring relevence of fantasy to oneself

Interpersonal:

Can be one-to-one or in a group
Requires cooperation in being quiet during fantasy
Not competitive
Therapist is group leader and the session is highly structured. Discussion may be less structured
Rule of silence during fantasy
No interaction during fantasy but requires verbal sharing and listening during discussion
Relationship to therapist as leader and peer participants
Some degree of involvement required in discussion
Opportunity to rehearse roles in imagination

Potential for Grading

Materials or equipment:

May be done lying on mats or sitting in chairs
Music could be used
Client could be given a tape to work alone

Environment:

Can be carried out one-to-one or in groups of various sizes

Method:

Different methods of relaxation
Instructions may be detailed or minimal
Fantasy may be simple or complex
Content of fantasy may be varied to change cognitive or psychological skills required
Rules may be implicit or stated
Participants could paint fantasy instead of talking
Participants could act out a fantasy
Discussion could be superficially descriptive or analytical and explorative or anywhere in between

Related activities:

Supportive psychotherapy
Explorative psychotherapy
Dream work
Drama

Fig. 6.5 A sample activity analysis.

- determine whether or not the activity is within a client's capacity
- assess what needs it might satisfy
- determine the extent to which it inhibits undesirable behaviour.

Figure 6.4 shows a generic activity analysis format and Figure 6.5 shows how it was used to analyse a particular activity, 'guided fantasy.'

Activity synthesis

When adapting or designing an activity it is useful to look at the different elements that have potential for change, that is:

- the materials and equipment used (media)
- the environment, including other people involved
- the method of carrying out the activity.

These three dimensions can be manipulated to achieve the desired therapeutic result.

Therapeutic media

Some activities, such as woodwork, centre on the materials and equipment used while in others, such as drama, these are of secondary importance. Certain skills can be more easily assessed and developed using activities that are materials/tools orientated, for example, to develop hand–eye coordination it would be more appropriate to use woodwork than drama. A variety of tools can be used to develop both physical and cognitive skills.

Materials can be selected for their power to evoke feelings, for example, wet clay may evoke the feelings of lack of control associated with the anal stage of development as described by Freud. Materials can also influence the outcome of the activity, for example, good-quality paints and paper will make it easier for a client to achieve a satisfactory painting than would poor-quality materials. Within a single activity, a whole range of skills can be upgraded by changing the materials or equipment used. Therapeutic media are discussed in more detail in chapters 10 to 17.

Therapeutic environment

The environment includes both human and non-human elements. The physical environment in which therapy is carried out is often the aspect of treatment least amenable to manipulation because of external constraints; the therapist works in the space she is given, rather than selecting an ideal environment for each activity. However, some environmental factors may be used to change the activity, such as being indoors or outdoors, working with groups or individuals, staying in the hospital or going out into the community, using public transport or the hospital bus. Smaller changes within the work setting can be brought about by using background music, altering the level of lighting, adjusting temperature or ventilation. Large or small alterations in the environment influence sensory stimulation, perception, concentration, work tolerance, enjoyment of the activity and social contact.

Other environmental factors are discussed in more detail under treatment implementation p. 100.

Therapeutic method

The method used to direct an activity is usually the simplest element for the therapist to manipulate. She can be directive or laissez-faire, supportive or demanding, involved or an onlooker. As a general rule, when starting a new activity the therapist will be more active herself, gradually taking less part as the group or individual develops and matures. Sensitivity and experience allow the therapist to make subtle adjustments to her approach as the need arises, without delay or preparation.

TREATMENT IMPLEMENTATION

Throughout the occupational therapy process described in Chapter 5 and earlier in this chapter, the therapist attempts to involve the client fully, to engage his interest, elicit his cooperation and earn his trust. If she succeeds, she will avoid problems in the implementation of treatment. However, some clients will come this far through the process and still not feel able to participate actively in treatment. It is therefore necessary to have an understanding of motivation in order to be able to select appropriate activities that will engage the client.

In this section we look at two theories of motivation:

1. intrinsic motivation
2. Maslow's hierarchy of needs

and how they can be applied in therapy. We then look at the four key elements of occupational therapy intervention:

- the client,
- the therapist
- the activity
- the environment

highlighting the relationships between them.

MOTIVATION

An understanding of the theory of motivation is necessary to successful treatment implementation because the success of occupational therapy intervention is dependent on the client being actively engaged in treatment, not passively receiving it from the therapist. There are many different theories of motivation but the most important one for occupational therapists is the theory of intrinsic motivation.

Intrinsic motivation

Intrinsic motivation is the urge to use one's capacity to have an effect on the environment, independent of any external reward. Every child is born with this urge but life experiences influence how it is used and developed.

What is intrinsic motivation?

Human beings have an inherent urge to be active and to explore the environment. In doing so they find out that they can have an effect on it and this, in turn, leads to an urge to influence the environment in a controlled way, to act competently to bring about desired changes. There is an inherent satisfaction in being able to act competently, independent of any extrinsic rewards action may bring. This satisfaction can be strong enough to sustain action even when the activity itself causes pain, for example, the marathon runner keeps going despite his physical exhaustion.

Exploration is prompted by something in the environment that is novel, different from usual in some aspect, puzzling or not understood for whatever reason; this arouses curiosity. The urge to try out one's capacities in new ways on the environment is so strong that people will seek or create puzzles to solve if there are none readily available. Intrinsic motivation prompts the individual to seek and master new skills throughout the life cycle.

Pawns and origins

When a child acts on the environment he receives feedback about the effect his action has had. If the result is satisfactory his self-respect is enhanced and he begins to build an image of himself as a competent performer. This increases the likelihood of him acting again to seek further satisfaction and proof of competence. A high proportion of satisfactory to unsatisfactory outcomes leads to the development of a positive image of the self as a 'doer'. Such a person's sense of competence is enhanced by his successes but he has the confidence to learn from his failures. The result is a benign spiral of action, feedback and satisfaction leading to more action (see Fig. 6.6).

If the child frequently experiences unsatisfactory outcomes when he acts, or fails to have any impact at all on the environment, his self-image will develop as an incompetent performer or passive observer of external events. Failure in action leads to a reduction of the urge to act, therefore the child receives less feedback and has reduced opportunities to build up a positive self-image. The process is a vicious spiral, as shown in Figure 6.7.

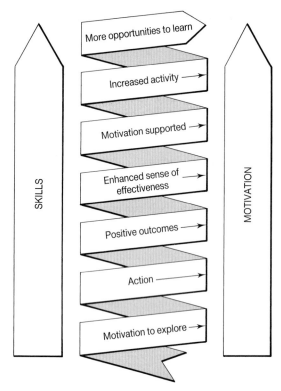

Fig. 6.6 A benign spiral of motivation.

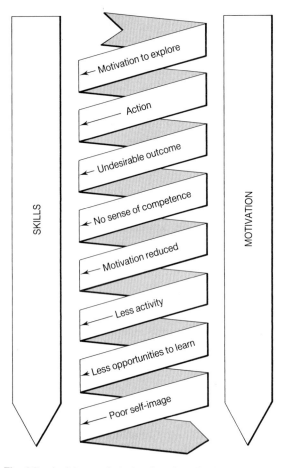

Fig. 6.7 A vicious spiral of reduced motivation.

People with a positive image of themselves as competent actors who can influence events in their environment are known as 'origins,' They have an internal locus of control, or belief that power to make changes lies with them.

People who have no sense of being able to control events are called 'pawns' and have an external locus of control. (Burke J. P. 1977, DeCharms R. 1968, Florey L. L. 1969, Robinson 1977, Smith 1974, White 1971.)

Maslow's hierarchy of needs

This is an example of a theory of external motivation, that is, it views people as acting to attain ends rather than gaining intrinsic satisfaction from action.

Maslow (1968) suggested that people are motivated by the drive to satisfy physical and psychological needs. Needs exist in a hierarchy, with physiological needs at the bottom and the drive to self-actualise at the top (see Fig. 6.8).

The lower needs, including physiological needs and safety needs, provide deficiency motives, that is, the individual acts to remove discomfort. For example, if someone is hungry he will take action to procure food. Only when the lower needs are largely satisfied will the person become concerned about satisfying higher needs.

Higher needs do not help the individual to survive, they are concerned with developing each person to his highest potential and are called growth motives. Each of these growth motives leads towards the ultimate goal of self-actualisation, which is the need to use one's capabilities and achieve one's unique potential. Maslow suggested

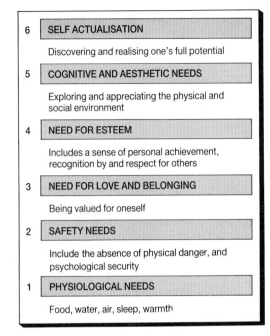

6	SELF ACTUALISATION
	Discovering and realising one's full potential
5	COGNITIVE AND AESTHETIC NEEDS
	Exploring and appreciating the physical and social environment
4	NEED FOR ESTEEM
	Includes a sense of personal achievement, recognition by and respect for others
3	NEED FOR LOVE AND BELONGING
	Being valued for oneself
2	SAFETY NEEDS
	Include the absence of physical danger, and psychological security
1	PHYSIOLOGICAL NEEDS
	Food, water, air, sleep, warmth

Fig. 6.8 Maslow's hierarchy of needs.

that very few people become self-actualised but that life satisfaction depends on striving towards that goal.

Motivation in therapy

Intervention necessitates motivating the client to voluntary action. Lack of motivation to act is rarely due to lack of interest in attaining valued personal or social goals; it is more likely to be a sense of hopelessness about the possibility of influencing whether or not they are attained. Every therapist has encountered clients who put their faith in drugs or electroconvulsive therapy (ECT) and see occupational therapy as a way of filling in time between treatment sessions.

There are various ways in which the therapist can increase the likelihood of a client being motivated to participate:

- provide a stimulating environment with objects for the individual to act on and people to interact with
- maintain enough novelty in the environment to arouse curiosity without causing fear

- provide opportunities for the environment to be explored and actions to be repeated
- ensure that competent role models are available, either peers or therapists
- help the client to build up a feeling of efficacy by starting with playful exploration, allowing time for skills to be learned thoroughly, and providing opportunities for skills to be used realistically
- select tasks that are appropriate to the individual's age, sex, cultural background, educational level, etc.
- ensure that lower-level needs are met before moving onto higher-level needs
- use activities the client sees as being personally or socially valuable
- allow people to use their particular talents
- ensure that there is a high probability of success in the activity by using activities that the individual is capable of completing and by providing the correct materials, equipment and instructions
- set tasks that offer some challenge but are not so difficult that they frustrate
- maintain motivation by grading activities as the client progresses
- consider the individual's interests when setting a task
- allow the individual to be responsible for the outcome of his actions
- ensure that feedback is available so that the individual knows when he has succeeded
- treat each person as someone who can attain valued goals
- show respect for the client as a person, believe in his potential for change, and listen to what he says.

In order to motivate a client successfully, the therapist must try to eliminate inhibiting factors as well as incorporating positive factors into her programme. Curiosity can be inhibited by:

- physical deprivation or stress, such as hunger, thirst, cold
- too much novelty or too many changes in the environment, which evoke fear rather than curiosity
- lack of stimulation or challenge in the environment.

By following these guidelines it should be possible to engage any client in therapy and to help him to develop a more positive self-image as an active and influential person. (Burke J. P. 1977, Florey L. L. 1969, Mocellin G. 1988, Robinson 1977, Smith 1974, Stewart 1975, White 1971)

KEY ELEMENTS OF INTERVENTION

The client, the therapist, the activity and the environment are the four elements available to the occupational therapist for assessing and motivating the client and for carrying out treatment programmes. Mosey (1986) calls these the 'legitimate tools' of occupational therapy.

Each of these elements is in a dynamic relationship with the others:

- the client's active participation in treatment, rather than his passive reception of it, is the factor that brings about change
- the quality of the relationship between the client and therapist is a crucial factor in motivating the client and engaging his active cooperation, thus determining the outcome of intervention
- the therapist's ability to analyse and understand activity allows her to select appropriately for individual clients' needs
- the context of treatment has a major influence on both process and outcome.

The client

Clients who receive occupational therapy for mental health problems can be of any age. They live in a variety of places and are seen in different settings. Each person has a unique problem or set of problems and each individual brings his own personality and experience to the therapeutic encounter.

When a client sees an occupational therapist for the first time, he will probably already have received psychiatric treatment, perhaps for many months or years. His expectations of the type of help he will receive and of the behaviour expected of him will be coloured by that experience. It may

take him a while to adjust to the different approach that occupational therapists use, with its emphasis on active involvement and on giving responsibility for health to the individual. Some people are unable to accept this type of treatment and prefer a more passive role while others are relieved to be allowed to take control of their own lives again.

Engaging the client in activity

If an activity is to be an occupation it must engage the client's resources and fit in with his value system, therefore an understanding of his existing skills and beliefs is essential to treatment planning. The client will not become engaged by an activity that does not match his needs, interests, values and abilities.

The initial assessment of the client includes those factors that influence the choice of therapeutic activity. These are:

- sex and sense of sexual identity
- chronological age
- any sensory deficits, perceptual problems or physical disability
- special aptitudes, such as musical talent
- stage of cognitive development
- any specific cognitive problems, such as short attention span
- educational level
- emotional needs
- stage of psychosocial development
- sense of personal and social identity
- personal values
- social skills and social preferences
- cultural and sub-cultural background
- communication and language skills
- any contraindications arising from specific problems or other treatment in progress.

In matching activity to client, the therapist needs to be aware of the relative importance of all these factors to the individual.

The therapist

The occupational therapist can be her own most powerful therapeutic tool. A knowledge of her own qualities, strengths and weaknesses allows her to function effectively and to have the satisfaction of knowing she is effective.

Personality

Personality is important. The therapist who chooses to specialise in psychotherapy is likely to be a very different person from the one who works contentedly in the long-term rehabilitation of institutionalised psychiatric patients, and they would not happily exchange positions. Personality also plays a part in determining her style of therapeutic interaction and the treatment techniques she selects to use. An understanding of her own needs, foibles and ways of relating to others will allow for more appropriate selection of roles in her relationship with the client.

Experience and skill

The experience and skill of the therapist also determine the treatment techniques she uses. Some techniques, such as psychodrama, require specialist postgraduate training. The basic occupational therapy training can only teach a limited number of activities, so the qualified therapist will add on new techniques to suit her interest and field of practice. Using a microcomputer to encourage a child with mental handicap to communicate, or helping a group of adults to explore causes of anxiety with projective art, is a long way from teaching basket weaving, although the same principles are used in selecting the treatment media.

Therapeutic relationship

There are many different kinds of therapeutic relationship, from a warm, mutual sharing of experience to a less personal relationship that allows the client to project feelings onto the therapist without fear of retaliation or rejection. The type of relationship developed will depend on

- *The therapeutic setting*, for example, it is usually considered inappropriate for staff to share personal information with clients in an analytical psychotherapy unit

- *The needs of the client:* these needs change as treatment progresses, so the therapist may start by being supportive and readily available but withdraw as the client becomes more independent
- *The age and experience of the therapist:* newly qualified staff may feel more comfortable with a sharing relationship. It takes experience and confidence to allow clients to project feelings, particularly negative feelings, without taking them personally.

The therapeutic relationship is a dynamic one, affecting the therapist as well as the client. In order to maintain objectivity and to avoid feeling threatened it is useful to have supervision from another occupational therapist. Even an experienced therapist can benefit from being able to discuss feelings and problems as they arise.

Staff availability

When planning treatment programmes to achieve both quantity and quality of treatment, the therapist takes account of several factors, including the number of staff available and their experience. Some activities cannot be used by a therapist working single-handed, either because of the nature of the activity, for example psychodrama, or because of the degree of disability or disturbance of the client. When working alone it may be necessary to reduce either the intensity of treatment or the number of clients in order to ensure safety.

The activity

Activity is at the core of occupational therapy practice. If the therapist cannot engage the client in activity that has meaning and value for him then there is no assessment and no treatment implementation. This is partly achieved by understanding the factors that will motivate the individual, as described on page 97, and partly by establishing an expectation that everyone attending the occupational therapy department will be active in his own treatment process.

The functions of activity for the individual have

been described in this chapter and elsewhere in the book and will only be summarised here.

Summary of activity functions

- Activity is essential for the normal development of the individual. Without activity no personal development can take place, and inability to perform activities competently leads to maladaptive development.
- People use activity to explore the environment and to test their own position in it.
- Activity is intrinsically satisfying.
- Activity is used to learn and practise skills that can be used for occupational role performance.
- The individual can gratify his needs through activity.
- Relationships with others can be made through shared activity.

The process of analysing activities into their component parts and synthesising therapeutic activities was described in the previous section. Details of how various activities are used can be found in chapters 10 to 17.

The environment

People cannot be considered in isolation from their environment and treatment cannot be considered separately from the environment in which it takes place. In this section we will look at the elements that make up the therapeutic environment and how they can be manipulated to achieve therapeutic goals.

What is the therapeutic environment?

The therapeutic environment consists of human and non-human elements that can, to a greater or lesser extent, be manipulated by the therapist to facilitate engagement in tasks and the achievement of goals. Some elements in the environment are physically or emotionally closer to the individual and some are further away.

The human environment consists of:

- the therapist

- other clients
- other staff
- relatives and friends
- neighbours
- peers.

The non-human environment consists of:

- the treatment setting (for example, hospital, community centre)
- the occupational therapy setting (for example, department, client's own home)
- the physical space where treatment occurs
- home
- workplace
- neighbourhood
- resources and facilities within the environment
- non-human objects within the environment, including aids to independent performance.

There are various ways of looking at both the human and non-human environment to assess the effect it might have on clients. One such system is PASS 3 (Programme Analysis of Service Systems), devised by Wolfensberger and Glenn (1975) to examine and rate 50 variables in the therapeutic environment. It was designed for use on services for people with mental handicap but the authors claim it can be applied to other settings without adaptation. Examples of some of the factors evaluated by this system are:

- physical resources
- age-appropriate facilities, environmental design and appointments
- staff development
- model coherency
- culture-appropriate labels and forms of address.

Many of these items are outside the control of the occupational therapist, such as location of the treatment centre, but other items are relevant, such as forms of address used with clients. The quality of the therapeutic environment gives the client a powerful message about how much he is valued as a person.

Manipulating the environment

The first task of the therapist is to ensure that the

therapeutic environment is so designed that it meets the needs of the client. As far as possible, the client is involved in this process. Dunning (1972) suggests that there are three environmental variables to be considered by the occupational therapist:

1. space
2. people
3. the task

and that the therapist should not neglect any one of them.

- Space can be arranged to promote stimulation.
- People can be organised to encourage social interaction.
- Tasks can be designed to develop skills.

It may be appropriate to teach people how to manipulate their own environments by:

- physically moving objects, such as moving the furniture around at home to give more privacy
- changing the function of rooms, for example, turning the spare bedroom into a study
- changing the way the house or workplace looks, for example, by decorating or buying house plants
- using space differently, for example, by going out more
- learning methods of communication and assertiveness
- learning new social skills
- going out to practise new skills in new social settings
- attending evening classes or community college to learn new skills.

SUMMARY

This chapter looked at the treatment planning stage of the occupational therapy process. This includes data analysis, goal setting, activity analysis and activity synthesis.

Data analysis includes looking at the client's environment and occupational roles, areas of dysfunction and available skills. Goal setting is in three stages, short-term, intermediate and long-term goals, which were illustrated by a case example.

Activity analysis can be generic, taking into account as many factors as possible, or specific to a particular model for practice. The format given here is for a generic activity analysis, and was illustrated by a sample activity, guided fantasy.

Activity synthesis involves manipulating the three elements of activity, media, environment and method, in order to achieve the desired therapeutic result.

The chapter also looked at the ways in which therapists can engage clients in treatment by evoking the intrinsic drive to be active and by ensuring that basic needs are met.

The four elements of intervention client, therapist, activity and environment, were discussed. The contribution that each element makes to the therapeutic process and the relationships between them were highlighted.

Therapeutic techniques used by occupational therapists are discussed in chapters 10 to 17, and treatment implementation with specific client groups is covered in chapters 18 to 25.

REFERENCES

Burke J P 1977 A clinical perpective on motivation: pawn versus origin. American Journal of Occupational Therapy 31 (4): 254–258

De Charms R 1968 Personal causation. Academic Press, New York

Drouet V M 1986 Individual behavioural programme planning with long-stay schizophrenic patients, part 1. British Journal of Occupational Therapy 49: 7

Dunning H 1972 Environmental occupational therapy. American Journal of Occupational Therapy 26 (2): 292–298

Fidler G S, Fidler J W 1963 Occupational therapy: a communication process in psychiatry. MacMillan, New York.

Florey L L 1969 Intrinsic motivation: the dynamics of occupational therapy theory. Papers: Research and development in occupational therapy, Southern California

Hopkins H L, Tiffany E G 1988 Assessment and evaluation: an overview. In: Hopkins H L, Smith H D (eds) Willard and Spackman's occupational therapy, 7th edn. Lippincott, Philadelphia

Howell C 1986 A controlled trial of goal setting for long-term community psychiatric patients. British Journal of Occupational Therapy 49 (8)

Katz N 1985 Occupational therapy's domain of concern: reconsidered. American Journal of Occupational Therapy 39 (8)

Llorens L A 1976 Application of a development theory for health and rehabilitation. American Occupational Therapy Association, Maryland

Maslow A H 1968 Towards a psychology of being. Van Nostrand, New York

Mocellin G 1988 A perspective on the principles and practice of occupational therapy. British Journal of Occupational Therapy 51 (1): 4–7

Mosey A C 1986 Psychosocial components of occupational therapy. Raven Press, New York

Robinson A L 1977 Play: the arena for acquisition of rules for competent behaviour. American Journal of Occupational Therapy 31 (4): 248–253

Smith M B 1974 Competence and adaptation. American Journal of Occupational Therapy 28 (1): 11–15

Stewart M C 1975 Motivation in old age. Physiotherapy 61 (6): 180–182

White R W 1971 The urge towards competence. American Journal of Occupational Therapy 25 (6): 271–274

Wolfensberger W, Glenn L 1975 PASS 3 Program Analysis of Service Systems. National Institute on Mental Retardation, sponsored by the Canadian Association for the Mentally Retarded, Toronto

7

Quality assurance

Margaret Ellis

INTRODUCTION

Much work has been done on quality assurance in other service areas. Quality assurance in the UK is now taking a more prominent position mainly due to the present political climate.

Occupational therapists should respond to the opportunities offered by quality assurance. For too long the role and tasks undertaken by the profession have lacked clarity and therefore understanding by others. By using the new quality-assurance standards described later in this chapter the services provided by occupational therapists will benefit, as will the disabled consumers using the service.

DEMAND FOR QUALITY ASSURANCE

In the UK the demand for assurance of quality developed in the 19th century when the traditional skills and experience required to achieve those skills started to be defined. Early in this century the government laid down systems of inspection for standards of goods. By the 1950s groups had started to create ideas for principles of quality assurance. Some of these helped formulate the system now known as British Standards, which applies quality controls in industry.

BS 5750 (British Standards Institution 1979) explains what is required in a quality system with emphasis on:

● understanding customers' needs

- designing a product or a service to meet these needs
- a guarantee of performance
- provision of clear instructions
- punctual delivery
- a back-up service
- a system of feedback of customer satisfaction.

A section of BS 5750 also explains the feasibility of independent assessment of services by a third party.

Although it is intended for the manufacturing industries, the general principles outlined in BS 5750 can also be applied to quality assurance in the area of health care.

QUALITY ASSURANCE IN HEALTH CARE

As general awareness increased about how quality might be assured, assessed and controlled, there was an appreciation that it could also be applied to health care, particularly where it was privately financed. The USA led the field in applying quality-assurance methods when comparing similar services. Private medical insurance companies set up their own systems of quality assurance, often making it a prerequisite for payment that the relevant assessment and treatment processes had been recorded in a particular format. Professional groups then began to develop their own policy and advisory networks to support individuals and help them to meet the growing quality-assurance standards.

Most of these developments were a response to economic pressures, spin-offs from social demands to have a reasonable service that gave value for money. In some countries, where the health-care system was state organised, there were also political pressures to develop quality-assurance systems, as a result of national policies. Other political influences came where one section of a private health-care organisation was seen to be in competition with another or with the state-run system. In applying quality assurance, the needs of four groups can be identified:

1. *consumers*: the people needing the health care

2. *professionals*: the people qualified to provide the health care
3. *managers*: the people with responsibility to plan and control the service, working frequently on the advice of financiers and statisticians
4. *organisations*: which may be the state providing a national scheme, or the employer or company providing the health care in a private system.

CONSUMERS

Consumers' views are increasingly based on better education, as newspapers, radio and television give rise to a better understanding of what range of health care is possible in a technical age.

Consumer groups, such as MIND in the UK, have been set up to help individuals with particular disabilities and illnesses. Such groups have heightened awareness of need and also of rights and eligibility for health care. Consumer groups have also produced pressure groups demanding that the consumer not only has a right to choose the health care being offered but also to choose to take risks in the decision-making process. The individual should have the right to decide whether or not an action should happen. Consumer groups occasionally support test cases to publicise the failure of the system to provide health care to an individual. Examples like this encourage others to use formal channels of complaint, such as Members of Parliament or the Health Service Ombudsman.

Representation of consumers on planning teams is important. This involvement must be to the benefit of the service provided and be encouraged. However, it is essential not to raise expectations without being able to meet them.

PROFESSIONALS

In addition to the basic professional qualification, the professional should have a desire to achieve high standards for the consumer. In many countries professional bodies for occupational therapists have developed quality assurance systems and policies encouraging their members to implement these. The systems have been created not only to encourage good practice but also to defend and support the professional workers in the day-to-day provision of health care.

Quality-assurance programmes have been most successful where there has been active involvement of the practising professionals (Holland and Bergen 1987). Therapists have welcomed the challenge of meeting standards and the opportunity for peer review. In some cases, particularly where systems have been imposed for financial benefit, workers have not reacted favourable to measures that may interfere or inhibit opportunity for the consumer or the profession as a whole to benefit.

MANAGERS

Quality assurance for the manager can be a simple procedure for identifying needs and matching services to need, the provision of the service being a simple equation of cost and manpower. Nevertheless, in times when profit from investment gains in importance the need for efficiency is increased. The need to compare like services, their cost and impact, necessitates creation of systems of measurement. Such systems were created in the Connecticut Mental Health Centre in the late 1960s (Siegel and Fischer 1981). There patient care, professional performance and utilisation of services were all reviewed regularly.

Inevitably, conflicts of interest have occurred, for example, meeting budgets can sometimes be perceived to be of greater importance than the standard of care. The need for the manager to meet health and safety regulations with the constraints these impose has to be balanced against the urge to allow greater freedom for the clients to experiment with independent living out of institutional care. Some local communities will have reservations about the mentally ill being housed outside institutions.

The manager should be encouraging coordination of work on quality assurance. He should be actively involved in a circle of activity with all the people providing the service (Fig. 7.1).

To maintain the balance of the circle each participant (the consumer, staff, manager, organis-

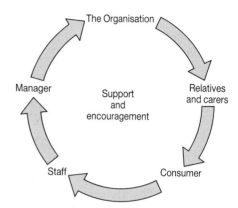

Fig. 7.1 The quality assurance circle of activity.

ation, and relatives and carers) must make an appropriate contribution. If the circle is not equally balanced then there will be difficulties for the consumer and the professional staff attempting to provide the service. The manager must wish to provide appropriate training for staff to develop techniques and have resources to meet the objectives of the service. Obviously skewing of the circle may occur because these values and priorities do not equate to budgeting allocations.

ORGANISATIONS

In this context the organisation in the UK is likely to be either the National Health Service (NHS), local government or a voluntary body. The organisation will probably seek to impose its views about quality assurance on its managers. In recent years the state's view of health care has been concern for overload: over demand, balanced by limited funding and facilities, and increasing opportunities with new technology. There is an emphasis on quantative measurement rather than concern for quality.

In some organisations *quality assurance* may take the form of *quality control* (Betts 1983). In the manufacturing industry, for example, random-sampling techniques may result in appropriate quality control. In health care, quality assurance is required for each individual. The Griffiths Management implementation in the NHS in the UK brought new views of health care. 'General management' as described by Griffiths, with presupposed management by non-professionals, removed some opportunities for consensus management whether that included the view of the multidisciplinary team of health-care workers or the consumer's view. 'Enterprise management,' which is directed towards income generation, also tends to ignore the voice of the consumer. However, the state now says it is welcoming the voice of the consumer. All governments wish to be seen to be contributing to good standards of policy, planning and provision for health care which should include quality assurance.

WHO RECOMMENDATIONS

The report of the World Health Organization's (WHO's) Working Group on the Principles of Quality Assurance (1983) remains one of the most useful sources of information on quality assurance. Seven major guidelines for working towards an effective approach to Quality Assurance were drawn up:

1. The methods employed should identify opportunities to improve health care and resolutions to problems with the physical, mental and social wellbeing of patients.

2. Quality assurance activities should consider efficiency, effectiveness and risk to achieve optimal results.

3. Programmes should consider emotional and social aspects as well as scientific and technical ones.

4. Quality assurance should be integrated into the total health-care system at all levels, with adequate resources provided.

5. All levels of the health-care system should be included.

6. The quality-assurance process must be allowed to evolve in a flexible way to meet the changing needs of the consumers.

7. Because health care is a rapidly changing field and health-care quality assurance methods are still in a period of experimentation and development, any quality assurance methods in member states should maintain the flexibility to change as quality assurance continues to evolve.

Advice on how to implement quality assurance in member states was also given.

In all of these summaries and overviews the real emphasis on quality-assurance programmes is that they must be seen as a whole and not as fragmented parts.

QUALITY ASSURANCE IN OCCUPATIONAL THERAPY

The King's Fund set up a review of the existing systems of health-care quality assurance in the UK in 1982. A small multidisciplinary team undertook this review and their work included visits to the USA to see the practice there.

Sadly, no paramedical member was part of the team but the nurse member was responsible for comparing findings with practice in the UK. The report was based on evidence of individuals and institutions, including the College of Occupational Therapists (COT). They also established an information system on activities related to and literature on quality assurance, and highlighted priorities for research and development. From this project many health-care organisations and professional bodies were encouraged to develop their own activities. Most of these were based on recommendations from the King's Fund Project (Shaw 1986) of literature searches, national and local observation of professional practice, consultation on views of practitioners, development of quality-assurance standards in combination with practitioners and then editing and regular review of these standards to ensure a practical format. In 1986 COT set up a Quality Assurance Working Party (COT 1987), which followed the King's Fund recommendations.

The initial literature search highlighted, in particular, the work already being done in Canada, Holland and the USA. In comparing work already undertaken here with that in other countries some area for urgent work were noted.

A national study day for a wide range of practitioners was held in 1986 and a group of therapists of varying backgrounds consulted. Special Interest Groups, such as Community Psychiatry, were involved.

A survey undertaken in 1987 (Ellis) of senior occupational therapist managers showed that only 28% were involved in quality-assurance assessment work whilst 70% were involved with quantity-of-service assessments. The majority of the 28% were projects that had been initiated by the occupational therapists themselves, rather than by other managers or by multidisciplinary team members. Respondents also stated why the were not involved in quality-assurance work; many responses reflected the national shortage of occupational therapists and the resulting pressure to treat clients rather than to assess need or satisfaction.

QUALITY-ASSURANCE MANUAL

COT in the UK is developing a quality-assurance manual (COT 1980), with eight sections on standards for care in mental health.

1. How the occupational therapist should accept the referral, whether medical or a self referral.
2. The assessment of need.
3. Preparation of a treatment programme in conjunction with other members of the multidisciplinary team, the consumer and their family as appropriate.
4. Implementation of the treatment programme and the need for reassessment.
5. The need to record progress and plan for discharge.
6. The need to reassess the chronically ill person.
7. The quality of care and outcomes of the services provided.
8. The need for follow through, research and planning for the future.

Other issues that occupational therapists should consider when planning and implementing their own quality-assurance programmes in psychiatry will depend on whether they work in a large institution or a more isolated setting in the community.

Most occupational therapists appreciate the need for more than a feeling of self-satisfaction in a job well done. There is a need to question the services we provide. We should all ask ourselves how we would feel as the consumer of the service we are providing.

THE QUALITY-ASSURANCE PROCESS

Quality assurance is part of the occupational therapy process at all stages, including assessment, planning, treatment and review. It should be noted that the consumer is involved in both planning and review, giving opportunities for assessing his satisfaction throughout the period of intervention.

The final stage of quality assurance involves evaluating the whole treatment process and the departmental structures and procedures that support it. Occupational therapists should use the COT Quality Assurance Manual of Standards and Policies when practising their profession.

THE QUALITY-ASSURANCE CYCLE

The quality-assurance process is a cyclical system of monitoring, assessment and improvement, as demonstrated in Figure 7.2.

Observing practice in occupational therapy may be the simplest assessment of treatment carried out. This can then be compared with the standard expected, findings are recorded, and accommodation for changing practice made. This cycle of quality assurance can then be reviewed at regular intervals.

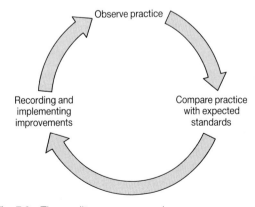

Fig. 7.2 The quality-assurance cycle.

QUALITY-ASSURANCE OBJECTIVES

The WHO (1985) defines quality assurance objectives as:

to assure that each patient receives such a mix of diagnostic and therapeutic health services as is most likely to produce the optimal achievable health care outcome for that patient, consistent with state of the art of medical science, and with biological factors such as the patient's age, illness, concomitant secondary diagnoses, compliance with the treatment regimen, and other related factors; with the minimal expenditure of resources necessary to accomplish this result; at the lowest achievable risk of additional injury or disability as a consequence of the treatment; and with maximal patient satisfaction with the process of care, his/her interaction with the health care system, and the results obtained.

Four components should be considered to meet this definition:

1. professional performance or technical quality
2. resource use or efficiency
3. risk management or risk of injury or illness associated with the services provided
4. client satisfaction with the services provided.

It is essential that any health service organisation consider all four and does not ignore one component in order to concentrate on the others.

Frequently, services have been assessed in terms of how many clients can be treated. The quality of treatment is seen as being of lesser importance and client satisfaction has been totally overlooked. This is particularly so in the UK where the public system of payment of health care is very remote from the service provided. There is little understanding by the service provider of how much the particular treatment costs and rarely any appreciation of the consequential costs of not providing treatment.

As the policy to transfer long-term mentally ill people from institutions to the community is being put into practice (Audit Commission 1981) then some Health Authorities are being forced to compare costs between these two types of service. This policy was adopted assuming that community-based services would be cheaper than those in larger institutions. Gradually, management are realising that this not correct. In planning, little or no account was given to client satisfaction, for ex-

ample, the theory that inmates of a large institution would wish to return to their place of birth may be real for only a minority.

This is an example of a government policy ideally conceived but not pursued on quality-assurance objectives. Only in recent times has the Office of Health Economics reported (Taylor 1976) on comparative costs of surgical procedures, such as joint replacements, against not providing such services.

QUALITY-ASSURANCE IMPLEMENTATION

Earlier in this chapter reference was made to the quality-assurance cycle: monitoring practice, comparing practice with expected standards and recording and implementing improvements. We can compare this cycle with the system of providing occupational therapy under three headings: structure, process and outcome (Maxwell et al 1983). Wherever we work we need:

- a structure in which to provide our service
- a process for providing the service
- a system of measuring outcomes that will define whether satisfaction has been achieved.

Structure

In any service there is a structure for provision, which includes an organisation to employ us and a room or department to undertake the service with relevant equipment and personnel.

Other publications (COT 1980) have already recommended minimum standards for staff, equipment, treatment space required, etc. for services for psychiatry. Compare your service structure with those recommendations as a base for defining whether it is feasible to provide reasonable care for mentally ill patients. It is essential to begin with that basic information because it may be that, for example, if you do not have physical space to provide a particular assessment or treatment or no secretarial support to provide reports for other members of the multidisciplinary team to read, then it will not be surprising if others are dissatisfied with your own contribution to the service.

Process

The process includes the methods of assessment whereby the consumers' needs are evaluated. In some services the methods of assessment are well documented and well established. Reference has been made to work in the USA (Siegel and Fischer 1981) in the Psychiatric Utilization and Review Evaluation Project (PURE). This project noted the need for occupational therapy as part of the rehabilitation programme. The variety of assessments used is enormous, and is dealt with in more detail in Chapter 5. Whatever the system adopted, all assessments must be recorded and be able to be repeated. Occupational therapists working in psychiatry should make detailed assessments, which may need to be repeated during the treatment process. Individual or group treatments may need to be assessed in order for the process to be comprehensive.

When considering the process of occupational therapy in quality assurance it is essential to consider the contributions to prevention and counselling as part of the whole.

Treatment usually follows assessment. The varying nature of the treatment has already been acknowledged. In some difficult cases the very fact that the client attends for treatment may be recorded as a success.

It is usual for a multidisciplinary team to be contributing to the process, which may make it difficult to assess whether one particular aspect of intervention has been the major contributor to the whole. However, it is important not to use this as an excuse not to make detailed records of the process. Importance will be placed on the consumer's contribution to the assessment process. This may be difficult for members of the team to accept because it may seem threatening or because the views of mentally ill people may seem unreliable. These issues also affect the third component of the quality-assurance service; outcome.

Outcome

Outcome is concerned with the improvement or restoration of good health, physically, mentally and socially, in consumer satisfaction and in the satisfaction of the organisation (employer or institution). Lack of documentation by occupational therapists means that there is little evidence to show they regularly use methods to record outcome. This is, of course, not unusual, as only in recent years have there been many examples to show outcome in health care, especially in psychiatry. This is born out in publications such as 'Consumer Feedback in the NHS' (Jones et al 1987) where, in over 200 references, only one specifically concentrates on work and the consumers' views on a psychiatric service.

As occupational therapists develop their own methods of assessment and recording they will also need to consider how these may be evaluated for the outcome of their service.

In some psychiatric services a system of peer review exists, through regular case conferences, where staff present feedback on their contribution to the treatment process. The development of outcome measures could be greatly assisted by this type of peer review if it were recorded and graded in some way. If no such system of multidisciplinary peer review exists it may be that peer review through an occupational therapy supervision system occurs. This can also be part of assessing outcome and be of great value. If neither form of peer review exists it is recommended that the occupational therapist should try to establish a regular system, either individually or in a group. This will assist in standard setting and measuring achievement.

Quality circles

Peer review may be provided by a formal quality circle set up for this specific purpose. A quality circle (Robson 1982) may be a group of four to 10 voluntary members working together with their manager to identify, analyse and solve their own work-related problems.

Such circles are more likely to be successful if:

- membership is voluntary
- there is a lack of bureaucracy
- the changes ensuing from the quality circle are at a pace suited to the members, not pressurised by management
- time is allocated so that developments

recommended by the quality circle members can occur
- the outcome is adequately documented.

In Ellis's (1987) survey of occupational therapy managers, 28% of the respondents reported that they had some kind of quality circle or staff group, to help develop change. Quality circles have proved of great value in encouraging change where management and workers have acknowledged their importance and supported their contribution.

In some organisations formal quality circles have been established but have not been successful. Some failures have been due to the lack of recognition by management that suggestions made by the quality circle should be implemented. The members of the quality circle have, in turn, become disillusioned about the usefulness of the circle and have withdrawn from it.

Checklists

A quality-assurance checklist is of help to all therapists. The checklist will follow the three sections of structure, process and outcome. Many articles advise of the need and the advantages of using guidelines in practice (Robson 1982, Chambers et al 1981, Lake and Modrow 1982, BAOT 1985, Management checklist 1985, Guidelines 1986) whether on documentation, the planning or the outcome of the service. You will need to create your own local checklist to follow your own standards, policies and procedures.

When creating your own checklist it will be essential to include headings covering the absence of any feature of the service as well as its presence. The process section of your checklist should record why a client did not attend treatment or occasions when the recommended treatment was not complied with by the client. If the process is terminated against the occupational therapist's advice, this should also be recorded. A doctor may discharge a client or the client discharge himself against the occupational therapist's advice. The checklist should also include a section on follow-up of care and reassess whether the original treatment aims were satisfactorily achieved or not. Where clients are referred and re-referred at regular intervals, the checklist should highlight

this so that an overview of care can demonstrate potentially unsatisfactory processes, especially if they occur regularly. Readmissions for treatment may result from the lack of community services in the locality.

Your checklist will require a method of communicating the quality assurance processes with other workers. Confidentiality, the need for unaltered records and the length of time the records should be kept are all essential procedures. You must also have some system of setting priorities for the service.

Record keeping

Good quality assurance requires good records (see Chapter 28). Good records will not necessarily result in good service but they are usually an indication of a good service. Written evidence of the treatment process may well be the only way the institution has of appreciating good practice. The emphasis on the need for better accountability to the mentally ill consumer in legislation such as the Mental Health Act predicates good records.

Occupational therapy departments increasingly use computers to maintain records (see Chapter 17). The Data Protection Act safeguards the consumer's rights to access to his own records, if they are computerised. If the content of the records is not well formulated they may not stand the testing of a court of law. Registration of the computerised systems will be essential.

SUMMARY

This chapter has reviewed quality assurance, its history and development. Comparisons of work in the UK and in other countries have been made. The particular need to relate quality-assurance principles and practice to the field of occupational therapy and psychiatry has been addressed. The need to develop the process in each service has been emphasised. The test of whether you have implemented some of the principles can be your own starting point. Would you want to be a client in your own service? A good base from which to proceed.

From that base, create a checklist of structure, process and outcome and decide how to establish the need for assessment, treatment and documentation systems. In the majority of cases outcome will probably be the area that requires greatest development, the consumer's viewpoint and that of the organisation being the most rarely measured. The occupational therapy profession will need to develop quality assurance systems but use will depend on the enthusiasm of local occupational therapists and on pressure by management.

Further research by practising occupational therapists standardising procedures in quality assurance at all levels will be needed.

At a time when the NHS is considering the development of greater awareness of enterprise management it will be essential for occupational therapists to be seen to accept responsibilities, not only for the actual treatment element of the process but also for helping to formulate the structure of documented process and outcome of care.

The future practice of quality assurance in occupational therapy and psychiatry is in your hands.

REFERENCES

American Occupational Therapy Association 1986 Reference manual of the official documents of the AOTA. AOTA, Rockville

Audit Commission 1981 Making a reality of community care. HMSO, London

Betts P L 1983 Supervisory studies. Pitman, London, ch 26

British Standards Institution. Getting to grips with quality. National Quality Campaign. Dept of Trade and Industry, London

British Standards Institution 1979 BS5750 Part I. Dept of Trade and Industry, London.

Canadian Occupational Therapy Association 1983 Guideline for client centered practice of occupational therapy. Minutes of National Health Welfare, Ontario.

Chambers L W et al 1981 Quality of care assessment. Clinics of Investigative Medicine. 4(1)

College of Occupational Therapists 1980 Recommended minimum standards for occupational therapy staff–patient ratios. COT, London

College of Occupational Therapists Quality Assurance Working Party 1976 Manual of official document (In press) COT & BAOT, London.

College of Occupational Therapists Quality Assurance Working Party 1987 British Journal of Occupational Therapists 50(7): 234–236

Ellis M 1987 Quality: who cares? British Journal of Occupational Therapy 50(6): 195–200.

Guidelines for occupational therapy documentation. 1986 American Journal of Occupational Therapists 40(12): 830–832

Holland S, Bergen B V 1987 Professional organisation of allied health disciplines assessments: A review from disciplines. Clinical Review, Australia, March, 36–40

Jones L et al 1987 Consumer feedback for the NHS. Kings Fund Centre, London

Luke R, Modrow R 1982 Professionalism, accountability and peer review, Health Services Research 1(17.2): 113–123

Management checklist for out-patient services, Appendix 2. 1985 Hospital and Health Services Review 277

Maxwell R J et al 1983 Seeking quality. Lancet 2: 45–48

Robson M 1982 Quality circles, Gower

Shaw C et al 1986 Quality assurance project. Kings Fund Centre, London

Siegel C and Fischer S K (eds) 1981 Psychiatric records in mental health care. Quality assurance.

Taylor D G 1976 The costs of arthritis and the benefits of joint replacement surgery. Office of Health Economics 192(11): 145–155

World Health Organization 1985 Report: The principles of quality measurement. WHO, Geneva

SECTION 4
The context of occupational therapy

8

Roles and settings

Belinda Thompson

INTRODUCTION

This chapter discusses the ways in which the work setting and working environment can affect the role of the occupational therapist. The work setting is the context of occupational therapy intervention, whether hospital, prison, community or elsewhere. Working environments include the place where the client receives occupational therapy and the occupational therapist's base or personal space where work materials and records are kept, where mail and telephone calls can be received and where visitors, colleagues and students can be met. The occupational therapist who is based in an institution or other residential setting will probably use the same area for both purpose. The community or peripatetic therapist may have an office but travel around to see clients. The working environment also includes other staff with whom the occupational therapist works and the way working relationships are structured.

In this chapter we first examine the settings in which occupational therapists work, ranging from a permanent base in one department to several different settings in any one week. We then look at the ways in which the working environment can affect work performance and therefore role. This is followed by a review of the concept of role. The roles we play are dependent on those around us, therefore it is necessary to examine how occupational therapists develop their role in relation to other members of the multidisciplinary team. The final section looks at team working and structure.

THE SETTINGS

The settings in which occupational therapists work are many and varied. Those relevant to the field of psychiatry include:

● acute wards
● long-stay wards
● hostels
● Secure Units
● Drug-Dependency Units
● Alcohol-Dependency Units
● ESMI (Elderly Severely Mentally Ill) Units
● Young People's Centre
● Travelling Day Hospital
● Psychiatric Day Hospital
● Psychiatric Work Assessment Unit
● Community Mental Health Teams, based both in hospital and in a community setting
● Community Mental Handicap Teams.

These include both residential settings and day services. A closer examination of their similarities and differences follows.

RESIDENTIAL SETTINGS

The occupational therapist working in a residential setting, such as a hospital or ESMI unit, may work on one type of ward or may find herself covering a variety of different wards with entirely different needs. Different types of residential establishment are described separately here but it should be borne in mind that there may be overlaps of function.

Acute admission wards

These are situated either within traditional psychiatric hospitals or alongside other acute services within District General Hospitals. A traditional ward contains male and female dormitories of about eight to 10 beds and a few single bedrooms. Some modern wards are divided into smaller bedrooms for two or four people. The ward will also have a lounge or dayroom, bathrooms, a kitchen, a dining room, a nurses' office, a treatment room and one or more small rooms for interviewing clients or holding ward rounds.

Admission wards take clients in the acute stage of illness, often in crisis. People are likely to display florid symptoms on admission and require intensive treatment, including drugs and other physical treatments. Some admission wards run community meetings, ward activities and therapeutic groups but others are just used to hold disturbed clients until their medication or other treatment takes effect. The length of stay of clients ranges from one night to a few months but a few weeks is most common.

The occupational therapist might work mainly on the wards, using lounges or side rooms for interviewing or group work, or she may see clients in a purpose-built occupational therapy department or a building that has been adapted for such use. Rooms need to be suitably equipped and furnished for individual and group work, with areas for specific activities such as art or domestic skills. The occupational therapist's personal base will be within the occupational therapy department.

Other staff working in the acute admission setting include nurses and psychiatrists, who both play a major role at this stage of intervention, social workers, psychologists and, possibly, a physiotherapist. There is the potential for much role overlap between professions, so teamwork and good communication are essential.

Long-stay wards

These are situated in large psychiatric hospitals and District General Hospitals. The old psychiatric hospitals were built to house many hundreds of people, with 20 or 30 sharing each ward. In recent years attempts have been made to improve sleeping arrangements by using wardrobes and screens between beds to provide some privacy.

As a result of the 'Care in the Community' policy, many large psychiatric hospitals are now closing. The people resident on long-stay wards are moving out, either into houses in their local communities or into medium/long-stay wards in District General Hospitals.

Wards in District General Hospitals are usually modern and like acute wards in their layout, with either small dormitories of between four and 10 people, or single or double rooms. There will also be at least one lounge, bathrooms, a kitchen, a dining area and rooms for staff to hold meetings and to store records and medication.

Many of the people who use medium/long-stay wards have been admitted from long-stay hospitals and require a longer time to adapt to living outside a hospital environment than do those on acute wards.

The other large group of people who live on long-stay wards are the elderly who have a dementing illness or who are totally dependent on others for their physical needs. Some of these long-stay wards are situated in small community hospitals, while others might be part of larger hospitals for the elderly.

Occupational therapists have an important role to play in helping people prepare to live out of hospital. They might, therefore, work in local community facilities as much as using the ward environment. When working with the elderly, community resources are used as much as possible, although the ward lounge or meeting room are used for groupwork or interviewing. Usually, occupational therapists working on these wards will have their base in the hospital psychiatric occupational therapy department, where facilities may also be used for work with clients.

Other team members working on these wards include nurses, social workers, doctors and psychologists, all of whom have the common aim of assisting people to adapt successfully to living out of hospital.

Hostels and group homes

The first people who moved out of long-stay hospitals moved into hostels or group homes, where between four and 20 people, male and female, live together. The buildings are therefore larger than average houses and have mostly single bedrooms and a few double bedrooms. The lounge, kitchen and dining areas are communal, although some bedrooms are large enough to be made into bedsits.

People who live in hostels and group homes are more likely to be able to take control of their own day-to-day lives than those who currently remain in long-stay hospitals.

Occupational therapists are not usually employed to work with residents in hostels or group homes on a full-time basis. An occupational therapist who works as part of a community team might work with a client who lives in a group with others and might, if appropriate, work with that person in their home, as they would with anyone else.

Other staff involved would include support workers, who assist clients with the running of the hostel or group home, and other members of a community team as and when necessary.

Specialist units

These might be based within the hospital setting or as part of the local community. They cater for people who are dependent on, for example, alcohol or drugs, or for people who have physical disabilities or illnesses that require specific treatments, such as AIDS. Because there are an increasing number of private specialist units, the standard of accommodation can vary greatly. Units that are run by the National Health Service provide accommodation for between 10 and 15 people in single and shared bedrooms, with other facilities including living rooms, kitchens, bathrooms and a dining area.

The people who use such units require an intensive and specific regime of treatment, which might consist of group work, psychotherapy and the responsibility of sharing the day-to-day running of the unit.

Specialist units vary considerably, according to the resources they have and the treatment approach used.

There are opportunities for occupational therapists to work in specialist units, where they would be part of a team consisting of psychiatrists, social workers, psychiatric nurses and sometimes psychotherapists. In some cases, the skills of drama therapists and art therapists are also used.

Units for the elderly mentally ill

Units for people who have a dementing (organic) or functional mental illness are frequently known as ESMI (elderly severely mentally ill), EPD (elderly psychiatrically disturbed), or EMI (elderly mentally ill) units.

They may comprise an acute admission/assessment ward, long-stay wards, a day centre, or any one of these. Such units are either purpose built or constitute part of a hospital. As the larger institutions close, services for this client group are developing in most health authorities into a speciality of their own.

There are many occupational therapists and occupational therapy staff working in this setting, either using the ward facilities for group work and individual interviewing, the day centre, or a separate occupational therapy department, where assessments and skill practice can take place.

Because the needs of the elderly people are varied, many members of the team are likely to be involved, and will include physiotherapists, nurses, social workers, doctors, psychologists and clients' relatives.

DAY SERVICES

Many occupational therapy departments treat people who are not resident on wards but attend daily or for specific therapy sessions. Other day services consist of day hospitals or day centres, either based in hospitals or in the local community.

Day hospitals

The purpose of day hospitals is to offer people a step between staying in hospital and staying at home. They can provide medical, nursing and other input on a daily basis and so avoid the need for an inpatient admission in many cases.

They are usually situated in hospitals and consist of a lounge/sitting area, a kitchen, a dining room, group work rooms, toilets and, sometimes, bathroom facilities.

Day hospitals for older people who have mental illness provide a monitoring and continual assessment service for people's physical, psychological and social functioning. In this way, people can remain in their own homes for longer before admission to a residential home or hospital might become necessary.

For people under the age of 65, attendance at a day hospital for between 1 and 7 days per week provides support and therapy appropriate to their needs. A person might attend a day hospital immediately following discharge from the acute admission ward so that he has continued support whilst in the home environment or day hospital attendance might be used as an alternative to hospitalisation.

Some people who have chronic mental illness and who experience difficulties in obtaining employment attend day hospitals and day centres for many months. In this situation, the day hospital team would be involved in helping that person to seek employment by helping him recognise his strengths, needs and skills and be channelling them appropriately and productively. This would be a primary role for the occupational therapist. She might work full-time at one day hospital, or work between an acute setting and the day hospital, providing an ongoing service to clients discharged from a ward to a day hospital.

Other team members working in this setting will include psychiatric nurses, community psychiatric nurses, doctors, physiotherapists, psychologists and social workers.

Day centres

These are based in the community and away from the hospital setting. They provide a focus for people living at home who require support either on a sessional or daily basis. People may also attend a day centre for specific activity or occupational therapy intervention, on an individual or group-work basis, away from their home setting.

Day centres usually consist of a large sitting area and perhaps a small number of separate rooms for group or individual work. There is usually a kitchen for making hot drinks and meals, and toilet facilities.

Occupational therapists are usually employed to work in one or more day centres on a sessional basis, rather than in one centre full-time. The occupational therapist who works on a community mental health team may provide input to a day centre as part of her job.

As in the day hospital, the occupational therapist's colleagues will include nurses or, where the centre is managed by Social Services, support workers and social workers. Psychologists, speech therapists, physiotherapists, doctors and creative therapists usually provide a service on a sessional basis when required. They, like the occupational therapist, are members of a community team.

Community settings

Community teams are normally based in office accommodation away from the hospital setting, in an attempt to remove the stigma that people still attach to a psychiatric hospital and also to facilitate access to the local community.

However, some community teams are based in hospitals, where communication with ward teams consultants and day hospitals is essential. An example of such a hospital-based team would be a team for the elderly who have mental illness.

Community-based teams use their office accommodation as a base for communication meetings and some teams use it for client contact. In those situations, in addition to office space, there will be rooms for individual and group work. In addition, a variety of different community settings will be used, according to the needs of the client. These could include the client's own home and local community resources, such as shops, cafes, leisure centres, etc. Indeed, as the demand for preventative care increases and the treatment of people who have mental health problems continues to be given out of the hospital environment, then those providing that care, including the occupational therapist, find themselves making extensive use of resources within the community.

Dasler (1987) says, 'for our professions, the price (of institutional security) is dilution of the ability to move patients towards meaningful activity by continuing to use the artificial environments of residential facilities for training. Like their patients, occupational therapists need to adapt their skills to fit the new 'outside' environment of the community. It is only in the community that the daily problems of living with a disability will become as clear to the therapist as it is for patients.'

The membership of community teams varies from team to team. However, there is a role for the occupational therapist to be a full member of the team. Other team members and their roles are discussed in the section on 'The multidisciplinary team', p. 123.

THE WORKING ENVIRONMENT

The concept of role and the different roles an occupational therapist might adopt are discussed in more detail later in the chapter. First, it is interesting to look at how the working environment affects performance and, therefore, the roles we play in contributing to the overall service given to the client. The working environment includes the therapist's personal office space, the place where clients are seen and the geographical location.

PERSONAL OFFICE SPACE

It is important for people in any work setting to have a place to write up notes and reports; read; use the telephone; meet visitors, colleagues and students; hang up their coats; and keep their personal belongings safe. Some occupational therapists have their own office; others share a desk or table with another member of staff.

Although the personal office space of an occupational therapist is not the main place for working with clients, it will nevertheless represent occupational therapy to colleagues, visitors and prospective new employees and students. It is worthwhile taking a few moments to step back from time to time and look around the space in which we work, checking whether any changes could be made to promote a better image of the service.

It is important to provide unqualified staff with office space so that they do not feel undervalued. For students, a space in the corner, or the use of the oldest desk, is a more welcoming gesture than to have no space at all.

WHERE CLIENTS ARE SEEN

The environment where the occupational therapist sees the client must be conducive to the work to be done and must be a place where clients feel comfortable. For example, for individual or group work such as anxiety management or relaxation sessions, the space used must be warm, with comfortable seating and curtains to block out sunlight. For an interview or individual work, the client must feel that the space being used is private and small. Facilities for hanging coats and making drinks make the setting welcoming to clients, as does an indication as to where toilets and washing facilities are.

GEOGRAPHICAL LOCATION

Looking finally at the working environment in its widest sense, the geographical location in which occupational therapists work can affect their role.

Occupational therapists who work in rural areas can become isolated from others who work in the same speciality. Local special-interest groups aim to create a forum for occupational therapists working in specialities to meet regularly, share ideas and give peer support. These can be very useful for occupational therapists working in rural areas who are likely to be few in number and to be attached to small local hospitals, or health centres and community teams.

Occupational therapists who work in cities or large towns have more opportunities for support from their peers. In such settings, there is usually a District General Hospital, which will contain acute and rehabilitation services employing many occupational therapists.

Most schools of occupational therapy are situated in large towns and cities, and this gives students opportunities to become familiar with the occupational therapy services in their locality. It is therefore more common to find students taking clinical placements, and their first position as trained therapists, in well-staffed departments in towns and cities, where they will have support and stimulation from experienced colleagues.

THE DIFFERENT ROLES OF THE OCCUPATIONAL THERAPIST

THE CONCEPT OF ROLE

All of us have several roles in our daily lives, some permanent, for example, male or female, and some changeable, for example, employee or student. At work we may also have several roles, therefore, since occupational therapists work with many different people, our roles must be clear to ourselves, our clients and our colleagues.

Problems in role identification

Many occupational therapists have difficulty replying to the question, 'What do occupational therapists do?' There are possibly three reasons for their difficulty:

1. The profession is still relatively new and small and is, therefore not widely understood, even by other health-care professionals.
2. Diversional activities, such as basket weaving, are still used in some settings and are sometimes called occupational therapy.
3. Occupational therapists are trained to use a philosophy and general approach that can be applied to a variety of problems in different situations. Specialisation in a particular field usually occurs after qualification. The breadth of the basic training may contribute to a sense of being less well qualified or well defined than other professionals.

However, occupational therapists can take advantage of the fact that their profession is new and developing, and is making use of new technology, such as computers, as clinical and administrative tools. Therapists also need to value the scope of the basic training and accept it as a starting point from which to develop a wide range of skills. Postgraduate specialisation is an option available, providing the opportunity to become expert in a particular field of interest. Furthermore, the broad range of skills an occupational therapist has makes it appropriate to transfer from one field of practice to another, giving enviable career options and opportunities.

Roles in team work

There is often no clearly defined role for each person within a health-care team and it becomes the responsibility of each team member to develop and identify her own role in relation to that of her colleagues. Members of an effective health-care team must share role expectations, that is, there must be agreement between how the individual views her own role and how it is viewed by her colleagues. Craik (1988) says that one of the many factors contributing to stress at work is role ambiguity. When a person is unclear about what is expected of her or receives conflicting expectations, then dissatisfaction and tension may result, leading to poor work performance. It is important, therefore, to establish clear roles in the work setting, but ensuring that they are sufficiently flexible to allow for change.

BALANCING DIFFERENT ROLES

There must be a balance between the different roles that one person takes. In addition to having a primary role as therapist to a client, the occupational therapist will find herself in several other roles throughout the working day, for example, that of a manager. It is important that role strain or pressure is prevented by balancing time spent in the various roles and by ensuring that colleagues also understand the therapist's commitments to the different roles.

The following examples show a typical working day for three occupational therapists working in widely different settings:

- an acute-service setting
- a day-hospital setting
- a community-service setting.

It is apparent that, in each setting, time is spent in roles additional to that of therapist, for example, student supervisor, manager of self and other occupational therapy staff, and consultant to colleagues.

The acute-service setting

8.30am   Arrive at work
          Check diary for today's appointments

Open mail, plan when to reply to correspondence, pass on relevant information to other staff, read documents/reports/articles received
Check student's timetable for the day

9.00am   Attend ward community meeting
9.30am   Attend ward round:

- report on clients being seen in occupational therapy
- collect two new referrals

11.00am   Write up details of new clients from case notes
          Talk to student about her caseload and about the new clients
12.00noon Occupational therapy staff meeting and sandwich lunch
1.00pm   Colleague asks to share ideas regarding occupational therapy for a new client
          Prepare for group
1.30pm   Assertiveness group in occupational therapy department
3.00pm   Write up group, discuss with co-therapists and plan next week's group
3.30pm   See one new client for initial interview
4.00pm   Write notes, complete Korner forms and carry out any other administrative duties
4.30pm   Go home.

From this sample working day, it can be seen that this senior occupational therapist's two main roles for the day are those of therapist and student supervisor.

The day-hospital setting

9.00am   Arrive at office base in the occupational therapy department in the psychiatric unit
          Check diary for day's appointments
          Check agenda items for planning meeting in the afternoon
9.30am   Go to day hospital, also based in the psychiatric unit
          Check that clients for occupational therapy have arrived

Meal planning and budgetting session with two female clients. The clients go to the local shops, while the therapist stays in the day hospital

10.00am   Meet new client; initial interview to introduce self and explain what occupational therapy is

10.30am   Begin to prepare midday meal with the two female clients when they return from shopping

11.45am   Discuss new client with day-hospital nurses while the two female clients have their lunch.

12.15pm   Return to occupational therapy department
Sandwich lunch
Discuss orders for stock and equipment with occupational therapy staff

1.00pm   Return to day hospital for clients' meeting about leisure opportunities

2.30pm   Talk to two clients who would like help to develop a leisure group

3.00pm   Attend Heads of Department meeting in District Occupational Therapist's office on the hospital site

4.15pm   Supervision session with senior occupational therapist who works on the acute psychiatric wards

5pm   Go home.

This Head Occupational Therapist has managerial duties in addition to her role as therapist in the day hospital. Management skills are covered in more detail in Chapter 26. Certain administrative tasks, such as ordering stock, can be delegated to other members of the department but require the Head's ratification. Creek and Wells (1988) describe a strategy for redefining staff roles so that time-consuming administrative duties are shared out, leaving the Head with more time for clinical work.

The community-service setting

9.00am   Arrive at team base
Attend to correspondence
Check diary for the day's appointments

Make telephone call and take two calls
Discuss afternoon relaxation group with team colleague

10.00am   Represent team at a meeting in town to discuss forthcoming 'roadshow' to promote awareness of mental health services in the local community

11.45am   Visit client at home to continue programme for decreasing her anxiety when shopping. Shop together for lunch and return to client's home to eat

2.00pm   Meet team colleague at local library to prepare room upstairs for relaxation session

2.15pm   Five clients arrive for relaxation

3.00pm   End of relaxation session; have coffee and discussion with clients and colleague

4.00pm   Return to team base
Complete Korner forms and write up notes
Telephone secretary of local occupational therapy special interest group, in capacity of chairperson, to plan the next meeting

5.00pm   Go home

Personal time management is different in a community setting and a hospital/acute-service setting. Time has to be allowed for travelling between appointments, whilst at the same time, the therapist must ensure that time as a resource is used as efficiently and effectively as possible. There is often only one member of each profession in community-based teams, therefore the therapist will often find herself in the role of team representative.

RESEARCH

A further role of some occupational therapists is that of researcher. All health service personnel are required to be more accountable for their work than they have been in previous years, hence the current emphasis on quality assurance. Accordingly, more occupational therapists are moving into the field of research, either as an addition to their clinical work or in specifically created research posts. Research serves an important function for occupational therapy, helping it 'to be a dynamic profession able to meet the ever-changing needs of society' (Mosey 1981). This is further reflected in the aspects of occupational therapy training that encourage the use of research methods in producing project work.

The subject of research is covered in more detail in Chapter 30.

The next section reviews the concept of multi-disciplinary teams, and the occupational therapist's role as team member.

THE MULTIDISCIPLINARY TEAM

Groups of different professional people who work together to provide a direct client-care service are known as multidisciplinary teams or multiprofessional teams. Occupational therapists are part of such teams, regardless of what clinical specialty they work in.

Those team members who have some contact with every client in the service are often known as 'core' team members. The composition of the core team varies from district to district but will include nurses, doctors and, usually, social workers. Clients may be referred to other professionals as appropriate. For example, community-based teams, such as community mental-health teams, might share therapists and psychologists with other teams from the same health authority. Other teams may be fortunate enough to have one or more of these professionals as core members. The occupational therapist, therefore, could find herself as a full-time member of a team, or might have a split commitment.

In addition, where there is an occupational therapy department in a hospital setting, the therapist will be a member of the occupational therapy team as well as the multidisciplinary team.

The following discusses the concept of teams, who the team members are and issues relevant to the effectiveness of a team, such as communication, leadership and responsibilities.

WHAT IS A TEAM?

The Collins dictionary defines team work as 'Cooperative work by a team acting as a unit.'

An occupational therapist could be a part of one of three types of team:

1. a large multidisciplinary team in a hospital setting
2. a smaller multidisciplinary team based in a community setting, for example, a community mental-health team
3. a team of occupational therapy staff.

Multiprofessional care teams developed as professions in addition to nursing and medicine emerged. Because a client's problems are often multi-faceted, it is appropriate that a specialist person is trained and sufficiently experienced to be able to deal specifically with the presenting problem. Each of those specialists has to prove a real commitment to the team to which he or she belongs, in order that they become a team in practice as well as in name. The creation and maintenance of an effective team also requires much hard work and self-responsibility from each of its members. The following section reviews the membership of the team.

The client

Without the client, there would be no purpose for a team, so the client can be seen as the centre of the team and must be involved in the decision-making process at every stage of the service he receives (Fig. 8.1). This focus on the client is crucial to the effectiveness of the therapy and is reflected in the College of Occupational Therapists' statement on referral (COT 1987b) 'the client shall be involved in programme/ treatment objectives.'

The carer

The carer, or client's family or close friends, are also part of the team, as they provide emotional and practical support to the client in the home setting. The 'Care in the Community' policy means that people are increasingly being treated and sup-

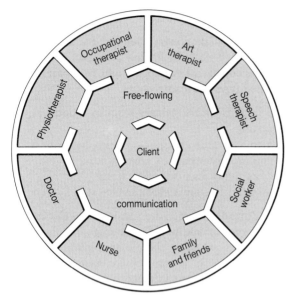

Fig. 8.1 A communication wheel, showing the client as the centre of the team, with other members as equal contributors to the total service.

ported in their own home environments, therefore the role of the carer is becoming more important. Health services are responding to the needs of carers by encouraging, initiating and/or supporting the setting up of carers' support groups, such as the Alzheimers Disease Society.

Creative therapists

This section provides only a brief overview of the team members, therefore the creative therapists are grouped together although they make up several separate professions including:

- art therapists
- drama therapists
- music therapists
- dance therapists.

There are similarities between these professions in training and in the use of the arts as treatment media.

Creative therapists are few in number and work in a variety of hospital, community, day-service and educational settings, with all client groups. Some teams have one or more of the creative

therapists working as full team members, while others share therapists between teams.

Training of the different creative-therapy professions varies. Some require a relevant degree, for example in psychology, sociology or arts. Most give preference to students who have 1 or 2 years' relevant work experience, for example, as a nursing assistant, residential social worker or occupational therapy helper. Courses may be part time of full time and lead to the award of a diploma. For example, an art therapist will have obtained a preliminary qualification of diploma or degree standard, probably had a year or more's experience working in the field of mental health and have successfully completed training to obtain a post-graduate diploma in art therapy.

All creative therapists use their particular arts medium, combined with a therapeutic approach, to enhance a person's self-expression, facilitate emotional development, promote awareness and trigger personal growth. They may work at either a pre-verbal or verbal level.

The physiotherapist

The recognition that physical exercise can make an important contribution towards good mental health is reflected in the increasing numbers of physiotherapists who are employed in a wide variety of mental-health and mental-handicap settings.

Some physiotherapists work as full-time team members, some work between teams, some work in both hospital and community-based teams.

Following a full-time 3- or 4-year training course at a physiotherapy school, qualified physiotherapists usually begin their working life in rotational posts where they spend 3 to 6 months in several different work settings. At Senior I level, specialisation is opted for, and a mental-health or mental-handicap setting is one such option.

Physiotherapists working in acute mental-health settings organise and run individual and group sessions, using physical exercise as their treatment medium. Treatment may also be given for specific physical problems, such as chest infections or mobility problems. Involvement in relaxation, sport and recreation provides an opportunity for joint working between physiotherapists and occupational therapists.

Many physiotherapists work with elderly people who have mental health problems, encouraging movement to prevent stiffening of ageing joints and muscles.

The speech therapist

There are a larger number of speech therapists working with people who have a mental handicap then there are working in mental-health settings. However, they have value in the latter, in the assessment and treatment of communication difficulties, especially disorders of language, in which the use and understanding of the spoken and written word may be impaired. In some clients admitted to a psychiatric ward, it is difficult to ascertain whether irregular language use is a symptom of their illness, or not at all related. The speech therapist can here provide an expert contribution towards the team's total assessment of the client.

Speech therapists working with people who have a mental handicap are either in a hospital or in a community setting. They offer people who are frustrated by communication difficulties the opportunity to improve their skills in order to develop more effective communicative abilities.

Training of speech therapists is over 3 or 4 years full time at polytechnics or universities.

Nurses

Nurses work in acute and long-stay wards, in day services and in community team settings. As the care and treatment of people who have mental illness or mental handicap has changed over the years, so has the role of the nurse in these settings. Nurses work in a holistic way, assessing people's strengths and needs rather than focusing only on problems. Nurses have adopted a broad span of duties and interventions, making overlap with other team members a frequent occurrence.

Qualified nurses who work in mental health have followed a 3-year course, successful completion of which makes them Registered Mental Nurses (RMNs). The qualification of a nurse working in mental handicap is the Registered Nurse for the Mentally Handicapped (RNMH). Additional training is required to work in the community.

Nurses make up the largest in number of any one profession on the team and are found on all hospital and community teams.

The clinical psychologist

Clinical psychologists in a hospital setting usually work from a psychology department. They offer treatment on an outpatient basis, bringing people into their department for sessions, as well as having input to wards and day hospitals.

Psychologists also work with people who have mental handicap, often, though not exclusively, using a behavioural approach. They are involved in advising colleagues on appropriate working methods and techniques in addition to having a direct clinical role.

The training for a clinical psychologist is long, and places are few, with the result that there are staff shortages. An honours degree in psychology is followed by a 3-year in-service course, and competition for places is fierce. The qualification in Britain is the British Psychological Society Diploma in Clinical Psychology.

The social worker

Social workers are employed by local social-services departments and are based either in hospitals or at area social-service departments. Those social workers, who work on community teams will often base themselves with the team, sharing office accommodation.

The social worker's role is broad and includes:

- liaison between the client and services available
- working towards empowering people to create change in their own lives
- statutory duties such as the protection of children and the enactment of the Mental Health Act.

Training to become a social worker can follow several routes:

- a 2-year, full-time Certificate of Qualification in Social Work (CQSW) course
- a 3-year, part-time Certificate in Social Services (CSS) course, done while working in a social-service establishment
- a relevant degree, for example Sociology, followed by a 1-year CQSW course.

This training leads to a generic qualification in social work, and social workers may opt to specialise following training.

Having a social worker as part of the multidisciplinary team provides a valuable link with social-service departments.

The doctor

In a hospital setting, the doctor of consultant status is invariably the leader of the multidisciplinary team. This is accepted because it is the consultant who has the power to admit and discharge clients and who carries ultimate responsibility for them. The consultant makes a diagnosis and assessment of the client, using medical knowledge gained through training, and using the joint assessments of the other team members.

In a community team setting, the doctor is more likely to be an equal team member. He may be involved in individual and group work, for example, anxiety management groups.

The doctor, in all settings, prescribes and monitors appropriate medication and administers treatment such as electroconvulsive therapy.

Following their 5-year training at medical school, doctors work in a hospital setting for several years as junior and senior house officers, then junior and senior registrars. Following their time as house officers they might choose to specialise in the psychiatric field or the field of mental handicap, and pursue further training in this direction.

Support workers

Support workers, or residential social workers, require no formal qualification and are employed by local social-service departments. They work in residential and day-service settings, assisting the people they work with in daily living activies and encouraging personal growth and development.

The whole of their working day (and night, in residential settings) is spent with the client. The occupational therapist and other team members will often find themselves in close liaison with the support worker, gaining information about a client, and subsequently advising on ways of working with people.

A client might come into direct or indirect contact with other professionals in the mental health and handicap settings who are not regular team members but whose services can be called on. They include:

- psychotherapist, who will be a full team member in a specialist psychotherapy unit
- dietician   these people might give
- chiropodist   direct advice or treatment
- health promotion   to a client, or may advise
  officer   other staff, such as the
                             occupational therapist
- ambulance crew, particularly in bringing elderly mentally-ill people to and from day hospitals
- ancillary staff: domestic staff, porters and clerical staff will come into direct contact with a client, especially in the hospital setting.

This brief outline of the people likely to be part of a multidisciplinary team has highlighted each member's contribution to the team process of care for the client, and also the possible overlaps in role, one of the issues discussed next.

TEAM WORK

Many of the issues that influence the working of an effective team are identified by Reed (1987). She discusses six key issues, which she claims should be addressed during the planning stage of any new health care team:

1. *Programme philosophy of the team:* this refers to the agreed role and function of the team; how they will receive referrals, how they will monitor the intervention the client receives and the discharge procedure.

2. *Client focus:* this emphasises the reason for

the team's existence, and the fact the team's working hours should be flexible in order to cater specifically for the client's needs.

3. *Role clarification:* it is important for each team member to have a clearly identifiable role within the team, in order that the service provided is both comprehensive and adheres closely to the needs of the client.

4. *Collaboration and information sharing:* 'A communication strategy must be mapped out that facilitates formal, informal and spontaneous information sharing within the team.' Team meetings are the most effective way of achieving this aim. Informal communication can be achieved through many channels, for example, during a coffee break.

5. *Policies and procedures* must be determined to give structure and identity to the team but must be reviewed and changed when appropriate.

6. *Staff support* is essential and can be gained from within the team, provided that each member commits himself to becoming a team player and does not alienate himself from the team.

The knowledge and skills that occupational therapists gain in their training can be applied to team work. They include group-work skills, role theory, the concept of leadership, and interpersonal relationships.

Team building

Team-building exercises aim to help the team to become effective and are useful for both new and established teams. The team might cancel all clinical commitments for a day and move from its base to a neutral place where staff can work through an agreed agenda of issues for discussion. The issues would cover those identified by Reed (1987), for example, review of the team's philosophy, clarification of roles and communication networks. Team-building exercises also aim to remove any barriers that might be present and that hinder effective team working.

Team leadership

Team leadership can be one such barrier, if members are dissatisfied with the way their team is led. Hospital teams usually accept the consultant as the team leader, while community teams usually prefer the use of a democratic style of working, with autonomy for each profession. In community teams, leaders sometimes emerge, or are appointed as coordinators. Their role involves the initiation, direction and coordination of team activity in order that an effective balance of client needs and team resources is achieved.

It has been mentioned that each team member must prove a commitment to the team of which he is a part. This is necessary for the team to work but, at the same time, it is also important to maintain the professional identity of each staff member.

A genuine commitment to, and understanding of, how an effective team works, is fundamental to the skills of an occupational therapist, who will always be practising as a team member. This can begin in the occupational therapy student's training, when efforts made on clinical placement to discover the role and work of other team members will provide valuable information and foundations on which team work skills can be built.

Overlapping of roles

All members of the health-care team are working towards the same overall goal, the well-being of

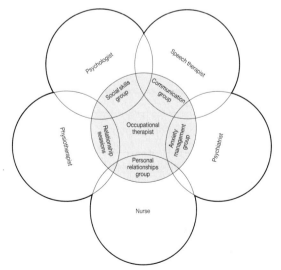

Fig. 8.2 Overlap of roles: examples of groupwork where the role of the occupational therapist overlaps with that of another team member.

the client, therefore overlapping of roles is inevitable. This can be positive for both client and staff, in that it provides opportunities to gain insight into each other's role (see Fig. 8.2) and ensures that all areas of client need are met.

However, professional rivalry and fear of overlap does occur in some health-care teams. This may be the result of poor communication between team members, as well as a lack of knowledge about each other's professions.

Stephens (1986) described the way in which staff came to acknowledge positively the overlapping of roles between nurses and therapists in a large psychiatric hospital: 'Constant discussion between nurses and occupational therapists, jointly agreeing policies, means that gradually we are breaking down the barriers that appeared to exist between nursing and occupational therapy staff .... together we are aiming to maximise our skills'.

SUMMARY

This chapter has aimed to illustrate how our working environment can affect our role as occupational therapists. In doing this, it has looked closely at the types of settings we work in, the concept of role and the roles taken by the occupational therapist, and the importance of an effective multidisciplinary team.

It is hoped that by using the information in this chapter, and indeed the rest of this book, occupational therapists will find the identification and development of their role an easier and an enjoyable experience.

REFERENCES

Craik C 1988 Stress in occupational therapy: how to cope. British Journal of Occupational Therapy 51(2): 40–43

Creek J, Wells G 1988 Points of view on working together: qualified and unqualified staff in an occupational therapy department for adults with a mental handicap. British Journal of Occupational Therapy 51(8): 204–206

Dasler P J 1987 De-institutionalising the occupational therapist. In: Cromwell F S (ed) The changing roles of occupational therapist in the 1980s. Haworth Press, New York

Mosey A C 1981 Occupational therapy: configuration of a profession. Raven Press, New York

Reed S M 1987 Occupational therapists in the interdisciplinary team setting. In: Cromwell F S (ed) The changing roles of occupational therapists in the 1980s Haworth Press New York

Stephens N 1986 Time to work together. Nursing Times 24 September 1986. 50–51

FURTHER READING

Blake R et al 1987 Spectacular teamwork, Sidgewick and Jackson

College of Occupational Therapists 1986 Management training needs of occupational therapists. COT, London

College of Occupational Therapists 1987a Policy Statement: Access to patients' notes. COT, London

College of Occupational Therapists 1987b Statement: Occupational therapy referral. COT, London

Hopkins H L, Smith 1988 H D Willard and Spackman's occupational therapy, 7th edn. Lippincott, Philadelphia

Jackson J A 1972 Role. Cambridge University Press

North East Thames Regional Health Authority 1987 Current occupational therapy practice: the core skills. NETRHA, London

9

Ethics

Ian E. Thompson

INTRODUCTION

The wit who cynically observed that 'Ethics covers a multitude of sins' was probably referring to the apparent tendency of doctors, lawyers, therapists—any professional group—to rationalise and defend their actions by appealing to the 'ethics' of their profession. But ethics is much more than a means of self-defence. In its widest sense ethics embraces the whole of man's quest for meaning and value in life (Macintyre 1967).

The purpose of this chapter is to explore the ethical basis of occupational therapy. However, this cannot be undertaken without first establishing some general points—such as what we mean by ethics and what ethical principles underpin modern health care—so the first part of the chapter looks at these two questions. We then move from the general to the specific, in exploring the ethical basis of occupational therapy and its codes. Some ethical and moral problems encountered by carers and therapists are examined in conclusion.

WHAT IS ETHICS?

A useful way to begin is to look at what we mean by 'morals', 'ethics' and 'rules'. The distinction between ethics and morals is difficult to draw precisely, because we sometimes tend to use the two words interchangeably.

MORALS

The word 'morals' derives from the Latin *mores* — meaning established social custom, convention or etiquette. In common usage, it retains the general sense of relating to the *personal* conduct of individuals or groups of people. When we describe actions as 'moral' or 'immoral', we are usually referring to personal beliefs and actions.

ETHICS

The word 'ethics' derives from the Greek word *ethos* which, in addition to meaning 'habit', 'custom', 'usage' (and thus being very similar to *mores*), also refers to the 'disposition' or 'character' of an individual or the 'spirit of a community'. The study of ethics covers:

- *the range of values* we endorse or regard as 'good' or 'bad'
- *the rules* by which we judge actions to be 'right' or wrong.

Thus any actions infringing the rules of a profession are generally described as 'unethical'.

RULES

The word 'rules' comes via Old French from the Latin verb regulare, to regulate or control. Rules are the means we use to control human behaviour and are always subject to change if they seem unjust.

Ethics incorporates both values and rules, it is the 'science of morals,' concerned with the theoretical study and practical application of our personal values and society's rules of conduct.

MAN'S SEARCH FOR MEANING AND VALUE

But why do people feel the need to have values, make rules, establish ethical principles? The explanation is linked to the natural human tendency to try to make sense of our lives, whether we are healthy or unhealthy, whole or injured, employed or unemployed, institutionalised or living in the community, to wrestle with fundamental questions of meaning and value.

The philosopher Paul Tillich wrote in 1957, 'Man is that being who is essentially concerned with his being and meaning'. The French philosopher Merleau Ponty echoed this sentiment in 1962 when he observed, 'Man is a meaning-maker' as did his contemporary Jean-Paul Sartre, writing in 1969', 'Man makes himself by his decisions'.

ETHICS AND HEALTH CARE

Man's inclination to establish personal values translates naturally to the group's desire to agree on social values. Most societies acknowledge that human beings have a fundamental right to life and to bodily integrity. Regarding health care, they accept the principles embodied in the constitution of the World Health Organization (WHO).

SOCIAL ETHICS

In its constitution, the WHO defined health as '*complete* physical, mental and social well-being, and not merely the absence of disease or infirmity' (WHO 1947). To appreciate the ethical principles underlying this definition, we must first examine the meaning of the words 'health' and 'disease'.

'Health' and 'disease' defined

How we define 'health' and 'disease' has varied over the centuries. Classical medicine saw health as the maintenance of an internal state of homeostasis (or balance) between functioning body systems. Disease was the disturbance or disruption of this balance by trauma, invasion by foreign organisms or mental disorder. No definition can be perfectly free of implied values, however this classical definition is rather one-dimensional, placing too much emphasis on maintaining the desirable state of homeostasis, to the detriment of other aspects of health. Modern attempts to define health in terms of the 'optimum function or dysfunction of an organism' (Oxford 1980) are similarly biased towards 'technical' measures of health.

Returning again to the 1947 WHO definition, its significance lies in its recognition of the dimension of *meaning and value* in health. It indicates a shift from a predominantly 'medical model' of health, biased towards homeostasis, to one in which behavioural, social and economic factors are more clearly recognised. The effects on WHO policy of this concept of health are at last being seen, for example, in the development of a new concept of public health. This means less emphasis on disease prevention and more on health promotion, less on authoritarian health education and more on promotion of lay competence, less on a clinical model and more on behavioural and sociological models, less on a purely technical and scientific approach and more on recognising moral and political factors, less on individual behaviour change and more on promoting community development and encouraging life-styles conducive to health. Further, the definition has recently been reaffirmed in the Declaration of Alma Ata (WHO 1978) when it became the focus of the campaign to achieve Health for All by the Year 2000.

INDIVIDUAL ETHICS

So far, we have been describing moral values prevailing in most societies. On a more personal level, the ethics of health care is concerned with:

- *caring* for people: recognising and respecting their *potential* and uniqueness as human beings
- *preparing* people to help themselves, whether children or vulnerable adults, is about protecting, nurturing and developing their potential, thereby *empowering* them to take greater control of their lives
- *sharing* means using our own *power* (including knowledge, skills, strength, resources and authority) to the mutual benefit of all.

THE ETHICAL BASIS OF OCCUPATIONAL THERAPY

With this background in mind, we can now move on to explaining some more direct links between ethics and occupational therapy.

On a superficial level, occupational therapy is about helping people to cope by finding something meaningful to do. Any creative activity can enable people to rediscover some sense of meaning or purpose in their lives. At a more profound level, occupational therapy is concerned with what health and disease mean to the individual. Occupational therapists are directly and practically concerned with helping people to make sense of their lives.

The role of occupational therapy, and what is in many ways the justification for its continued existence as a profession, lies in its link with man's basic need for occupation. The value of occupational therapy is therefore crucially linked to the role of activity, work and occupation in integrating the physical, psychological and social functions of human beings.

Reilly (1962), in a classic paper exploring the justification for the continued existence of occupational therapy, puts forward the hypothesis, 'Man through the use of his hands, as they are energized by mind and will, can influence the state of his own health.'

She cites the philosopher Fromm (1960), who said that the need to work is an imperative part of man's nature because man has to eat, drink, sleep and protect himself from his enemies and, in order to ensure his self-preservation, must work and produce. She points to the demoralising effect of unemployment or enforced inactivity in confinement, or the impact of forced retirement on the health and well-being of people, and argues that occupation is a basic human need. 'Man has a vital need for occupation for his central nervous system demands the rich and varied stimuli that solving life problems provides for him. This is the basic need occupational therapy ought to be servicing'.

Nuse Clark (1979) develops a more complex and sophisticated model for understanding 'occupation'. She sees occupational therapy attempting to maintain the balance between the different kinds of activities associated with self-maintenance, work and play:

- *self-maintenance* includes rest and sleep, with areas of overlap with work in physical self-care and with play in recreative activity
- *work* includes home management, education

and training, and employment, overlapping with self-maintenance in the acquisition of new skills and with play in creative self-expression
- *play* includes games, symbolic self-expression and exploration, overlapping with self-maintenance in recreative exercise and with work in artistic creation.

Both authors stand in a respectable lineage of philosophers, going back to the earliest origins of Western culture:

- the Judeo-Christian religion's celebration of man as 'homo faber': man the doer, maker, creator, whose created creativity mimics that of the Creator God
- Aristotle's metaphysical distinction between man's potential powers of being (dynamis) and effective energy (energeia) with work (ergon) as a necessary condition for potential powers to be actualised or realised
- Aquinas' writings in the 13th century 'Homo habet rationem et manum' (Man has both reason and hands)
- Marx's celebration of man the worker, defining *homo faber* in terms of his capacity for creative work, his capacity to transform the world and humanise it.

CODES OF ETHICS IN OCCUPATIONAL THERAPY

We can see that occupational therapy has a strong ethical underpinning in the 'philosophy of work'. Nevertheless, all professions, including occupational therapy, find it useful, indeed essential, to state in writing the general ethical principles that govern practice. These take the form of 'codes'. Codes attempt to do the following:

- state the duties of professionals, and emphasise their role in protecting often vulnerable clients
- set limits to professional responsibility
- protect and maintain standards (for example, education and training)

- establish ways of regulating professional conduct.

Although codes are primarily established to serve the interests of a profession, they do have another purpose, that of informing the public about what they can expect of the practitioners whose help they seek.

The code of the World Federation of Occupational Therapists (WFOT 1985) and that of the British Association of Occupational Therapists (BAOT 1985) are both modelled on the ancient Hippocratic Oath (470 BC), the oldest known code of professional ethics, which was written for physicians.

THE GENERAL PRINCIPLES OF THE HIPPOCRATIC OATH

The Hippocratic Oath (Duncan et al 1977) falls into several parts dealing with:

- responsibilities to fellow doctors
- maintenance of professional identity and standards
- responsibilities to clients
- professional integrity
- accountability before society and its gods.

After the invocation of the gods of medicine and surgery and the goddesses of cure-all and prevention, the first part of the Oath discusses professional loyalty, including mutual financial support (the first trade union!) professional monitoring of knowledge, clinical skills and standards of practice.

Responsibilities to clients include respect for life (including the proscription of abortion and euthanasia): the duty to do good and not to do ill to patients (beneficence and non-maleficence): honesty (in avoidance of quackery): non-exploitation of vulnerable patients; non-discrimination against men or women, free-men or slaves (requirements of justice) and the strict commitment of confidentiality with clients' secrets (based on respect for persons).

Finally, the doctor acknowledges his accountability to society and to the gods for the maintenance of his professional integrity and care of his patients. Thus three essential principles underlie this ancient code:

- respect for persons
- justice
- beneficence.

WFOT CODE

The code of ethics of the World Federation of Occupational Therapists (WFOT 1985) is typical of simple codes that paraphrase the Hippocratic Oath. It omits specific reference to medical treatment and emphasises the role of occupational therapists in cooperating with, accepting referrals from and consulting other professions involved in client care. It acknowledges the responsibility of the profession to maintain standards and promote its development through research and the sharing of expertise, and it notes the importance of good recordkeeping.

BAOT CODE OF PROFESSIONAL CONDUCT

The 'Code of Professional Conduct' of the British Association of Occupational Therapists (BAOT 1985) follows the format of the Royal College of Nursing's (RCN'S) Code of Professional Conduct (1976) in giving both general principles and notes on their application. However, it follows the form of the Hippocratic Oath, if not in its order, in the wording of its principal headings. In summary:

1. *Relationship with and responsibilities to clients* including statements on confidentiality, disapproval of cruelty, refraining from exploitative relationships, respect for people's rights, and not putting clients at risk by withdrawal of services.

2. *Maintaining professional integrity* by not soliciting or advertising for personal gain, acting generally within the requirements of law and morality, not discriminating against clients and avoiding the abuse of alcohol and other drugs.

3. *Relating to professional relationships and responsibilities* including loyalty to colleagues, cooperating with and respecting the expertise of other professionals and promoting professional development in occupational therapy.

4. *Maintenance of professional standards* by developing appropriate clinical competence including understanding of the professional's own limits, by accepting referrals from other professionals as well as self-referred clients and by keeping accurate and confidential records.

LIMITATIONS OF CODES

Professional codes are undoubtedly useful but they do have some common failings:

- They have traditionally been developed as a basis for justifying professional intervention in crisis situations. At such times clients are often in desperate need of help and very dependent. With this crisis or problem focus, they often ignore the more positive duties of professionals, such as positive health promotion.
- Codes can perpetuate a patronising attitude towards clients. Again, this occurs because most codes view the carer as the one in control (in the time of crisis) and the client as dependent. Overprotective care can conflict with the fundamental moral duty underlying rehabilitation, namely promotion of client autonomy.

To illustrate this point we can look at the BAOT code again. As we know, one of the primary responsibilities of the occupational therapist is to work to restore *autonomy* to those who have lost it by virtue of disease, injury or mental disorder and yet the responsibility for rehabilitation is not explicitly recognised even in the otherwise excellent BAOT Code. The code discusses clients' *negative* rights, such as the right not to be abused, but says nothing about *positive* rights. (The RCN Code of Professional Conduct [1976] does emphasise rehabilitation as the primary moral responsibility of the nurse).

CARERS' DUTIES AND CLIENTS' RIGHTS

Our brief examination of occupational therapy codes of practice has shown that the caring professions rightly emphasise the *duty* of professions to protect clients' interests and ensure that their *rights* are not infringed. But what are the principal duties of health-care workers? And what are the key *rights* of clients? We should be as specific as possible about this important subject.

CARERS' DUTIES

The principal *duties* of health-care workers include:

- giving people adequate information and resources to enable them to make responsible choices for themselves and to maintain control over their own lives
- promoting people's growth and autonomy to enable them to develop their full human potential and to enjoy good health (physical, mental and social well-being and not just the absence of disease)
- consulting people about their needs, sharing power and resources with them to ensure that they enjoy equal opportunities and do not suffer discrimination, while avoiding turning them into dependants
- recognising the need of vulnerable people to have their *rights* protected.

CLIENTS' RIGHTS

So we return again to *clients' rights*. These include:

- the right to know
- the right to privacy
- the right to care and treatment.

Each of these fundamental rights deserves closer scrutiny.

The right to know

It is a fundamental truism that 'knowledge is power'. However, we do not often recognise that the converse is also true, namely, that to be kept in a state of ignorance is to be kept in a state of impotence and dependency. The ability to control information is a powerful tool. If used responsibly, it can restore dignity and enable clients to share in decision making about their lives and futures.

Sharing of knowledge (skills, expertise) is about sharing power; it empowers others to be more independent. It is not merely about the right to adequate information to make informed choices and to give voluntary consent (to treatment, for example). It includes the rights to be informed of one's diagnosis as a client and the proposed course of treatment, indeed, the right to be informed of one's rights!

Whether clients should always be told everything about their diagnosis is, however, controversial. Doctors and other carers often feel they have a duty to withhold information for the client's own good. Others would argue that the client, having voluntarily sought help, always has the right to be told everything about his condition.

The right to privacy

Invasion of privacy strikes at the heart of a person's dignity. The right to privacy includes:

- respect for a person's physical privacy; his 'body space'
- respect for the person's intimate secrets; his sexual behaviour, psychological experience and social life
- respect for confidential information; professionals should be very cautious about, for example, sharing such information with colleagues, even 'for the client's own good'.

Professionals may demand that these personal areas of privacy be exposed to critical examination as part of the medical, psychiatric and social investigations that precede treatment. They therefore have a duty to protect the privacy and confidences of vulnerable clients.

The right to care and treatment

In the United Kingdom and in many other countries we have decided that all citizens have a moral and legal right to free medical care and treatment but putting this right into practice is not easy. Care and treatment includes everything from highly technical surgery to 'tender-loving-care' and occupational therapy. Who decides which clients have the right to occupational therapy? On what criterion is it decided how many occupational therapists there should be? Many would argue that society has not satisfactorily resolved the ethical dilemma of how to balance the right of clients to therapy with the responsible use of public resources to employ sufficient occupational therapists.

Another example shows the difficulties that can be encountered in providing adequate care and treatment. Therapists often make decisions based on their own values. Because they are unaware of this bias in their value judgements they often find it impossible to separate them from their clinical judgements. For instance, what the therapist decides is 'for the client's own good', regarding the desirable outcome of treatment or the quality of life to be aimed for on the client's behalf, may reflect the therapist's values more than the client's.

VIOLATIONS OF CLIENTS' RIGHTS

The rights of clients with mental disorder (whether mental illness, mental handicap or mental incompetence) are all too easily compromised. The Mental Health Acts (HMSO 1983 and 1984) empower health professionals to detain and treat clients compulsorily (held 'On Section'), thus abrogating the clients' rights to freedom of movement, to be kept informed and to give voluntary consent (including the otherwise absolute right to refuse treatment). Many other more subtle rights are also threatened.

Some examples of possible violations of rights are as follows.

- The 'right to know' may be denied to psychiatric clients who have been labelled 'mentally incompetent' merely because they are held under the Act, not because they are actually incapable of understanding.
- Physical privacy may be widely compromised in mixed wards.
- Confidentiality may be violated in team management where extended confidentiality is the order of the day, or by the therapists' reading correspondence and closely observing visitors and family interactions as part of treatment.
- 'Consent to treatment', even when given by

voluntary or informal clients, can be interpreted so broadly that clients may be constrained to join in group therapy, dance therapy or whatever else is on offer.

Caring staff working in psychiatric settings are very often placed in the difficult position of being required to be at once an advocate of clients' rights, and society's agent to control and restrict the client's freedom. They must try to reconcile their commitment to clients' rights with their responsibility to society; a daunting ethical dilemma for occupational therapists. Examples of other ethical problems encountered by occupational therapists follow in Boxes 9.1, 9.2 and 9.3.

BOX 9.1 THE RIGHT TO CARE AND TREATMENT

An occupational therapy department had a shortage of qualified staff. They faced the choice of insisting on giving effective and specific intervention to a small number of clients or taking the easier path of supplying a diversional service to a larger number.

Pressure was applied from all quarters:

- the managers wanted to keep the numbers up for statistical purposes
- nursing staff, also understaffed, demanded that the occupational therapy department accommodate as many people as possible to ease the burden on them
- medical staff expected all the people they referred to be offered treatment
- the clients themselves often complained if they were not included in occupational therapy
- occupational therapy helpers complained as well (rather surprisingly) because they felt their role was being undervalued if fewer clients were treated.

In the face of such opposition it was difficult for the small number of therapists to remain convinced of the value of what they were doing and to continue to offer what they saw as effective treatment.

BOX 9.2 THE RIGHT TO KNOW

In one Health Authority in England, an occupational therapy department formulated a policy statement that included the ethical principles underlying the service.

The department claimed to give clients: 'the right to know what their treatment is for and what it will involve, and the right to make an informed choice about whether or not to receive treatment'.

Shortly after this document was adopted, the Health Authority circulated a draft code of practice for the confidentiality of client information. Although the code was meant to protect clients' interests, the section on 'information to be given to patients' included the following statement:

> The medical staff responsible for the care of the patient shall have absolute discretion to decide what medical information should be disclosed to the patient . . . other professional staff will require to pass information to the patient about assessment or therapeutic procedures in which they are engaged. Such information should be related specifically to procedures within the professional competence of the staff concerned . . . Written clinical records shall not be disclosed to patients.

Any member of staff who violated this code of practice was subject to disciplinary action and yet it was not made clear what information was purely medical and what came 'within the professional competence' of the occupational therapist. (In some cases clients may have needed certain medical information to make an informed choice about whether to accept occupational therapy).

The occupational therapist working in this department could have been faced with a choice between violating the occupational therapy department's ethical principles (by withholding medical information) or facing disciplinary action (by disclosing medical information).

BOX 9.3 THE RIGHT TO PRIVACY

The professional staff in the occupational therapy department of a psychiatric day hospital became concerned that a wide range of unqualified staff had access to clients' notes. Because the hospital was situated in a small community, clients and staff often knew each other personally and maintaining confidentiality was a problem.

To help safeguard clients' privacy some qualified staff refused to write confidential material in the clients' notes but their managers pointed out that if anything went wrong they could be held legally responsible for withholding information. Staff had to choose between protecting their clients or themselves.

PROBLEMS AND DILEMMAS IN OCCUPATIONAL THERAPY

The reader will by now be aware of the difficulties of translating principles into practice. Many of the problems we have mentioned, for example those concerned with clients' rights, are shared by all health-care workers but working with psychiatric clients places very particular demands on the therapist's ethical and moral code.

The treatment of clients who are mentally disordered may be virtually indistinguishable from that of prisoners, except that their 'sentences' are indeterminate. The deviant behaviour of the mentally ill results in social sanctions and restrictions on personal liberty.

The conscientious therapist may often feel uneasy when society denies a client his freedom and may well ask whether society has the right to lock up clients and give them treatment against their will 'for their own good', in the belief that it will help restore their autonomy.

The diagnosis of mental disorder as an illness, with labels such as 'schizophrenic', 'psychopath', 'manic-depressive' or 'neurotic', is both a blessing and curse. It is a blessing because it allows the client access to care and treatment. It is a curse because the client is stigmatised, set apart and regarded as different from other people. Many observers feel it would benefit clients to find ways to take mental illness out of the medical domain, to eliminate medical labels that connote disease but such a step could be disastrous, if mentally disordered offenders were given penal treatment rather than the much more appropriate medical treatment, nursing care and rehabilitation.

SPECIFIC PROBLEMS AND DILEMMAS

The following problems and dilemmas further illustrate the tensions that can arise between our personal principles or those of our profession and the rights of clients.

Discharge of psychiatric or mentally handicapped clients from hospital

Here, the conflict is between the duty to protect the client and at the same time respect his rights. The problem is even more acute when the client is a suicide risk or has a history of violent behaviour, or when there is fear that he may be unable to cope with life in the community. Assessments of dangerousness or social competence are notoriously fallible and even arbitrary.

Carers' reluctance to allow clients to take risks or to make mistakes

Over-protectiveness may be rationalised as in the client's interest but may be a form of self-protection for the carer, who does not wish to accept responsibility if things go wrong. People only learn if they are allowed to try and fail and perhaps try again. Clients will never find out whether they can cope outside if they are kept in an artificial, safe environment and never allowed to make mistakes.

Social class attitudes and values in occupational therapy

The therapist's definition of 'coping, 'social skills' or 'self-care' may not match the client's social background. There is always a risk that therapists hold up to the client inappropriate social norms, whether in domestic matters, employment or patterns of social and sexual interaction (Freidson 1970).

COPING WITH PROBLEMS AND DILEMMAS

Most moral problems faced by therapists in everyday practice can be discussed and resolved satisfactorily if the time is taken to look at them carefully. The therapist who is least likely to resolve such problems is the one who is ignorant of their existence, hence the need for this chapter! Fortunately, it is rare for therapists to be caught in a true dilemma, in which there is a direct clash between two equally valid moral principles or duties (Thompson et al 1987).

Moral decision making is not an occult spiritual process. In simple terms, it is the exercise of one's conscience and involves the application in the moral sphere of the same problem-solving skills used in other areas. The therapist must:
- *assess* the evidence and weigh up the principles involved
- *plan* treatment based on knowledge of possible outcomes
- *implement* that plan and monitor the process, looking out for the unexpected in particular
- *evaluate* and modify practice in the light of actual consequences (Thompson et al 1987).

SUMMARY

This chapter first examined the nature of ethics, defining 'morals', 'ethics' and 'rules' and considering man's need for value.

The ethics of health care were then investigated, followed by consideration of how ethical principles apply to occupational therapists. The main ethical codes were briefly outlined and their limitations discussed.

The specific duties of the carer and the rights of the client were then considered, with examples of problematic situations.

Finally, specific ethical problems arising in occupational therapy and methods of coping with these dilemmas were looked at.

REFERENCES

Beauchamp T, Childress J 1979 Principles of bio-medical ethics. Oxford University Press, Oxford

British Association of Occupational Therapists 1985 Code of professional conduct. BAOT, London

Downie R S 1980 "Ethics, Morals and Moral Philosophy" Journal of Medical Ethics, Vol 6, No 1

Downie R S et al 1987 Healthy respect: ethics in health care. Faber & Faber, London

Duncan A S et al 1977 Dictionary of medical ethics. Darton, Longman & Todd, London

Freidson E 1970 The profession of medicine. Dodd and Mead, New York

Fromm E 1960 The Fear of Freedom. Routledge & Kegan Paul, London

Her Majesty's Stationery Office 1983 Mental health act. HMSO, London

Her Majesty's Stationery Office 1984 Mental health (Scotland) act. HMSO, London

Macintyre 1967 A short history of ethics. Routledge & Kegan Paul, London

Merleau-Ponty M 1962 The phenomenology of perception. Routledge & Kegan-Paul, London

Nuse-Clark 1979 Human development through occupation: A philosophy and conceptual model for practice. American Journal of Occupational Therapy 33 (8 and 9)

Reilly M 1962 Occupational Therapy can be one of the great ideas of Twentieth Century medicine. American Journal of Occupational Therapy 16 (1)

Royal College of Nursing 1976 Code of professional conduct. RCN, London

Sartre J P 1969 Being and nothingness. Methuen, London

Thompson I E et al 1987 Nursing ethics, 2nd edn. Churchill Livingstone, Edinburgh

Thompson I E 1987 Fundamental ethical principles in health care. British Medical Journal

Tillich P 1957 Systematic theology, vol 1. Nisbet, London

World Federation of Occupational Therapists 1985 Code of ethics for occupational therapists. WFOT, South Africa

World Health Organization 1947 Constitution of the World Health Organization. Chronicle of the WHO 1 (3.1)

World Health Organization 1978 Primary health care. Report; International conference on primary health care, Alma Ata, USSR, 6–12 September 1978. WHO, Geneva

Part 2

SECTION 5
Occupational therapy media and methods

10

Developing physical fitness to promote mental health

Hazel Bracegirdle

INTRODUCTION

In 1984 the American National Institute of Mental Health stated that physical fitness is positively associated with mental health and well-being, that exercise is associated with a reduction in anxiety and depression, and that long-term exercise is associated with fewer neurotic traits. The Institute also recommended that exercise should be used as an adjunct to physical treatments for severe depression and that physically healthy people receiving psychotropic medication could exercise safely under medical supervision. Exercise was said to result in reduction in various stress indices, including neuromuscular tension, resting heart rate and some stress hormones, and was thought to benefit people of both sexes and all ages.

To understand why these statements were made, the therapist needs to consider the evidence of a number of disciplines. The history of exercise as a treatment for mental illness is followed by an account of the philosophical debate on the mind–body relationship and its implications for psychiatry. A brief summary of motor development is followed by a look at biochemical research into the endogenous opioids and their functions. Some psychological research is briefly reviewed and the experience of exercise is described. The physical problems that people suffering from mental illness or mental handicap may have are listed and guidelines are given for organising clients' exercise sessions. Finally, a variety of activities is mentioned and an account of running a gym club for people with mental handicaps is given.

THE HISTORY OF EXERCISE AS THERAPY

Macdonald (1976) assured us that the use of physically demanding occupations, sports and exercises to lessen the effects of physical and mental illness and handicap has a long and respectable history. Hippocrates himself emphasised 'the body–mind link in all treatment' and 'recommended wrestling, riding and labour'. Later, Galen favoured digging, ploughing and building as treatments. During the Renaissance period, 'exercises . . . for toughening-up and for enjoyment were recommended by physicians and educationalists' alike. In 1705 Francis Fuller wrote a popular treatise on 'Medical Gymnastics' in 'The Cure of Several Distempers' especially the 'Hysterick or Hypochondriat Case.' His claim that a 'sedentary life' resulted in 'Effete and Languid . . . Nerves' sounds extraordinarily modern. (Hunter and Macalpine 1963).

The following 'consensus statements' were issued by The (American) National Institute of Mental Health in 1984:

- Physical fitness is positively associated with mental health and well-being.
- Exercise is associated with the reduction of stress emotions, such as anxiety.
- Anxiety and depression are common symptoms of failure to cope with mental stress, and exercise has been associated with a decreased level of mild-to-moderate depression and anxiety.
- Long-term exercise is usually associated with reductions in traits such as neuroticism and anxiety.
- Severe depression usually requires professional treatment, which may include medication, electroconvulsive therapy and/or psychotherapy, with exercise as an adjunct.
- Appropriate exercise results in reductions in various stress indices, such as neuromuscular tension, resting heart rate and some stress hormones.
- Current clinical opinion holds that exercise has beneficial emotional effects across all ages and in both sexes.
- Physically healthy people who require psychotropic medication may safely exercise when exercise and medication are titrated under close medical supervision.

THE MIND–BODY RELATIONSHIP

The idea that the body and mind (or soul) are separate, the body containing and controlling the mind, is common to many religions. Whilst the body undoubtedly dies and decays, a separate mind or soul is assured immortality by religious doctrines, from eternal bliss in the heaven of Christianity to the reincarnations of Hinduism (James 1960). The body is usually considered inferior to the soul and, in the ascetic religions, it may be subjected to practices designed to subdue its passions from fasting to the self-torture associated with saintliness. Popular superstitions reinforce this view and most ordinary people believe they have *both* a body and a mind. Philosopher Gilbert Ryle calls this the 'official doctrine' that 'with the doubtful exception of idiots and infants in arms, every human being has both a body and a mind harnessed together'. (Ryle 1949).

However, philosophers disagree on whether or not the mind is a part or aspect of the body, or a non-physical entity. Two separate philosophical theories (Hanfling 1980) prevail, that of 'dualism' (two entities) and that of 'monism' (one entity). An understanding of this distinction is central to our faith in the power of bodily action for promoting mental well-being. Let us consider a brief historical survey of the philosophers' findings, bearing in mind that these findings inform and direct our current scientific investigations by influencing the basic assumptions that scientists make about the nature of body–mind.

DUALISM

The ancient Greeks tackled the problem of a mind–body relationship in this way. Aristotle distinguished three separate entities:

1. mind was highest, because less bound by the body

2. soul was in the intermediate position
3. body was at the base.

The soul undertook the business of moving the body about, perceiving and having feelings, whereas the mind was capable of thinking, understanding abstractions and participating in a higher, immortal, collective world of reason.

Plato described death as the separation of the soul and body. Soul was the seat of reason and reality while the body was the source of sensory perception and illusion. The body was considered a hindrance to the acquisition of knowledge and an endless source of troubles and lusts, from which the soul fled, relieved, at death. The dualistic beliefs of Aristotle and Plato were partly responsible for the asceticism of later, Christian, morality.

Cartesian theory

Descartes, a formidable 17th-century thinker and scientist, asserted that mind and body are two totally different *types* of entity, made up of different kinds of substance. Although the relationship between body and mind was close, closer than that of a ship and its pilot, this early dualist insisted that the soul or mind was the essential person, the body being less important. Descartes arrived at this position by reasoning that, because he could doubt the existence of his body but not of his thoughts, he must essentially be mind, not body. He also suggested that mind and body had separate functions and that the precise anatomical point at which the mind processes were translated into bodily functions was the pineal gland. (Russel 1945).

MONISM

In the 17th century, Spinoza described mind–body as attributes of one and the same entity, which was known as god, substance or nature. Rather than being separate entities, mind–body are aspects of the same thing, related through 'parallelism'. This means that, if something happens in the spiritual or mind aspect, a corresponding event occurs in the body, and vice versa. Two other schools of thought, which may be briefly considered, also tend to support the monist position.

Materialism

Materialists claim that human beings, along with the rest of nature, are made of physical matter alone. That which has been called spirit or mind is really the result of brain processes, which are simply physical events and subject to the physical laws of a physical universe. The world is seen as a single, physical system, which will, ultimately, be described and explained by one science, a 'super physics', which will subsume all our modern, separate sciences including psychology and sociology.

This viewpoint assumes that we can eventually understand even inner, personal human experiences by breaking them down into simple, physical units. The commonsense evidence for this position is that we *do* mostly tend to locate our mind and selves in our heads and when we talk about somebody being 'brainless', 'brainy' or 'bigheaded' we are talking about mental attributes as though they were located in the brain. Finally, modern research into the function of the brain demonstrates that the complexity of our inner mental lives is mirrored in the intricacy and subtlety of the neuro-anatomy and physiology of the brain (Popkin et al 1956).

Epiphenomenalism

Epiphenomenalism is a modified form of materialism that suggests the mind is a 'by-product' of purely physical events, a sort of running commentary on our actions. Idealism states that everything, including body–mind, is actually mental rather than physical, in precisely the opposite way from materialism. Body is believed to be made up of mind substance, instead of mind being basically physical.

PSYCHIATRY AND THE MIND–BODY RELATIONSHIP

The implications of the mind–body relationship

for the practice and theory of psychiatry are well known. Currently, there is an ideological battle between those who, in the words of Anthony Clare (1976), 'insist that all genuine psychiatric disorders rest upon a physical basis' and those who are sceptical of this biological or medical model, preferring psychosocial, cultural and political explanations of mental disorder.

Fortunately, the value of physical exercise in psychiatric occupational therapy can be explained in either dualist or materialist terms. Materialists can claim that the mind–body benefits from physical work because of resulting improvements in physical function, including brain blood circulation and neurotransmitter activity. Perhaps surprisingly, humanistic psychology also provides theories that stick the mind and body firmly together, thereby raising the value of the body and feelings and reacting against Christian asceticism.

Occupational therapists working within the dualist tradition may prefer to emphasise that the spirited individual can rise above physical constraints, even those imposed by organic mental illness. The emphasis here is upon mastery and control of the body; for example, yoga is an elaborate system that promotes spiritual values and even jogging requires self-discipline. Dualists may argue that, by demonstrating power and control over the body, the mind asserts and enhances itself. Equally, by cultivating a healthy and efficient body the mind creates a vehicle that supports its own healthy functioning.

Let us now look at how the developing child gradually gains control of his body movements.

MOTOR DEVELOPMENT

Neurodevelopmental approaches to the treatment of motor control problems are based on the principle that motor development occurs sequentially (some theorists claiming that motor ontogeny recapitulates phylogeny, that is, an individual's development follows the evolution of the whole species). Generally, voluntary control of gross, mass or total movements is achieved before that of fine and discrete movements. Voluntary control of the body and limbs proceeds cephalocaudally, proximally to distally and, in the hand, ulnarly to radially. (Trombly and Scott 1977).

Although the sequence of normal motor development is roughly similar from individual to individual, there are normal exceptions. Some children, for example, never crawl but proceed from sitting through to 'bottom shuffling' to walking. All the developmental milestones described below may occur at any time within a broad range, so only the average age of each accomplishment is given (Sheridan 1973).

The movement and posture of newborn babies are dominated by primary reflexes. Head control is poor so there is marked 'head lag' when the baby is pulled into a sitting position. Gradually, the strength of the primary reflexes diminishes as the baby gains increasing control of neck and shoulder muscles by the age of 3 months. By 5 or 6 months most babies can lift head and chest when prone, supporting their weight through extended arms. They will also grasp their toes when supine and sit with support. By 9 months babies can roll over, pull themselves up to sit and sit without support. Some may have started to pull themselves up to stand (supported) and many will begin to crawl.

Babies become increasingly active and mobile as they approach their first birthday. Most by then are fast crawlers, some have even tried the stairs and most will have taken their first few steps unaided. By 18 months many toddlers can walk well independently and run safely. They will be tumbling less frequently and can usually crawl upstairs and down again, backwards, without mishap. These toddlers can elegantly pick up objects from the floor without toppling over and can sit down upon small chairs.

Two-year-olds have become graceful and competent movers. They can run well, stopping and starting safely, and some will walk upstairs unaided. By the age of 3 most children can walk downstairs (two feet onto each step) and will clamber about happily on nursery climbing apparatus and manage toy cycles. Some 3-year-olds can walk on tiptoe and jump with two feet together. The average 5-year-old appears to be far more graceful, athletic and coordinated than her parents! Five-year-olds can run up and down stairs, demonstrate various party tricks (such as handstands and forward rolls) and can hop and skip beautifully.

We need to know about normal motor development so that we can tailor exercise programmes to suit individual developmental needs. We need to know something about what happens in the brain to understand the mood changes which are associated with that exercise.

BIOMEDICAL EVIDENCE

In 1975 Hughes et al isolated the first endogenous opioids (Grossman and Sutton 1985). Endogenous opioids are chemical brain transmitters, comprising a group of opioid peptides and including endorphins, enkephalins and dysnorphins. Endogenous opioids have a chemical structure similar to that of morphine and its derivatives, which have all been used medicinally, and abused addictively, since ancient times. Endorphins are produced by the brain, pituitary gland and some other cell lines. Research into endorphin production and function in human beings usually utilises measurements of plasma levels and the demonstration of responses to opiate antagonists (notably Nalaxone) (Morgan 1985).

The action of endogenous opioids has often been described as 'morphine-like' (Morgan 1985). Although the precise physiological role of the endorphins has yet to be found and it is likely that endorphins act in conjunction with other transmitters to produce their effects, the following functions of endorphins have been proposed:

- they act as natural analgaesics
- they produce a feeling of well-being, sometimes even of euphoria
- they seem to reduce responsiveness to external stimuli
- they reduce levels of tension or anxiety
- they may also be implicated in appetite control, blood-pressure control, temperature regulation, pituitary secretions and the control of ventilation.

Because endorphins so closely resemble morphine and its derivatives, that is, drugs which both inhibit pain and produce a sense of well-being, these claims seem plausible. Endorphins may well function to reduce pain during strenuous activity. Endorphin levels in pregnant women, for example, peak during labour and delivery. There is also much anecdotal evidence of soldiers and athletes being unaware of the pain of injuries sustained during physically strenuous activity, until it has stopped. The 'runner's high', that is, the achievement of transcendental or 'peak' experiences during exercise, has been much popularised by the media. Mandell described his own altered state of consciousness in this way, 'the running literature says that if you run six miles a day for two months, you are addicted forever. I understand. A cosmic view and peace are located between six and ten miles of running.' (quoted by Morgan 1985).

However, it must be remembered that a runner's 'high' is distinguishable from that obtained by an injection of heroin, although it may lead to a form of addiction or dependence in some runners. It may be that people who exercise regularly do develop a positive addiction for their sport, which then enables them to overcome damaging addictions and maintain their well-being and calm.

The common observation that 'improved affective states accompany both acute and chronic physical activity of a vigorous nature' (Morgan 1985) may be explained by the often repeated finding that vigorous physical activity stimulates endogenous opiate production.

Farrel (1985) reviewed 12 studies, each of which clearly demonstrated a significant increase in β-endorphin levels following running. He concluded that 'exercise activates the endogenous opiate systems'. This effect can be seen both in human subjects and in animal models. Apparently, even laboratory mice can become so 'hooked' on swimming that they develop full blown morphine-like withdrawal symptoms when prevented from exercising (Christie and Chesser quoted by Morgan 1985).

Having looked at the findings of the laboratory researchers, we can now consider those of psychologists working in the clinical field.

PSYCHOLOGICAL RESEARCH FINDINGS

Recently, psychological research has demonstrated a significant, positive correlation between vigorous physical activity and improved mood, reduced anxiety and, in some instances, improved behaviour. Although studies have not proved a direct causal relationship between physical exercise and improved mental health, they do suggest that involvement in physically demanding activities is effective therapy. Moreover, improvements resulting from exercise can be shown in a variety of client groups, from behaviourally disordered children to very elderly people.

Simons (1985) reviewed seven such studies, in which people diagnosed with depression were involved in a 'multisession exercise program'. These studies all tended to support the hypothesis that depression of clinical proportions can be treated with exercise, the improvements obtained being comparable to those resulting from traditional psychotherapies. Paillard and Newak (1985) studied the effect of exercise programmes on very elderly people and Stacey (1985) looked at the effects on older adults. Both studies demonstrated a relationship between the treatment and improvement in cognitive functioning and personality, increased activity tolerance and improved affect and mood. Paillard and Newak, like Morgan (1985), emphasised that vigorous physical activity was associated with increases in self-esteem and feelings of accomplishment. Evans (1985) found improvements in selected classroom behaviours of behaviourally disordered adolescents following exercise. Schurrer's (1985) mentally handicapped subjects all showed increases in independent behaviour, work productivity and interest, as well as reductions in destructive behaviour for the duration of their physical training programme.

Controlled experiments have demonstrated associations between exercise, mood and behaviour but we need a humanistic account of the experience of physical activity to give us a richer picture.

THE EXPERIENCE OF EXERCISE

Connolly and Einzig (1986) see people as having the potential for free choice in their actions, without being unduly influenced by external factors, and having the ability to determine what they become, within certain limits. They recognise the human need for aesthetic and spiritual endeavour. They cite anthropological, historical and bio-

graphical material to support the claim that exercise provides a satisfying creative outlet and leads to the discovery of 'personal power' and giving a 'sense of freedom and autonomy'. Sport, they claim, is a force for social integration, it satisfies the need for achievement and encourages the pursuit of perfection. Participation in extremely strenuous physical activity can even, they say, give rise to transcendent spiritual experiences. Connolly and Einzig describe the following psychological benefits of exercise and sport:

- *Well-being* Recreational physical exercise, which has an element of play in it and is chosen by the subject rather than dictated by a trainer, improves the subjective experience of well-being. The routine of physical exercise seems to 'create a stable, regular framework' for fragmented modern life-styles. Setting goals and working towards them gives meaning to life.
- *Positive addiction* The release of natural endorphins as a consequence of exercise, as described above, gives rise to a 'healthy' addiction. Addiction to this 'runner's high' enables the exerciser to relinquish harmful addictions, such as drinking, smoking and eating to excess, more easily.
- *Creativity and self-expression* Nothing is more expressive of ourselves than our body movements and the language of the body can be used to communicate feelings, therefore physical activity, especially dance, is an important creative outlet. The creative experience of physical activity is based on what it feels like to move freely and beautifully.
- *Social factors* Sport, games, exercise and dance sessions all transport us to the special world of play, which is distinct from mundane ordinary life. Playing together gives rise to a sense of team spirit and comradeship, and following the rules of the game is a factor in socialisation. Participation in sport certainly gives opportunities for social interaction and spontaneous emotional expression, as anyone who has seen 'macho' footballers embrace will agree.
- *Challenge and power* Human beings seem to feel a need to overcome obstacles and confront the forces of nature, Sport and exercise provide a

channel for competitive and aggressive impulses. Self-esteem is improved by successfully meeting challenges and by realising personal potential.

• *Freedom and self-mastery* Developing personal power and physical self-mastery gives rise to a sense of freedom and autonomy. The individual no longer perceives himself as a passive object. Because our bodies change, becoming stronger, suppler and healthier by taking action, we not only express ourselves but change ourselves through physical exercise. We are no longer the victims of external circumstances but are initiating rather than reacting.

So far, exercise looks a very attractive form of therapy but many of our clients will have to overcome physical impairment before we can involve them.

PHYSICAL PROBLEMS ASSOCIATED WITH MENTAL DISORDERS

Psychiatry is a relatively young branch of medicine and so there is still much disagreement amongst practitioners about the underlying causes of mental illness. Biological, psychological and social explanations have all been given for the same associated physical phenomena. Richard Hunter, a neuropsychiatrist, carefully researched the history of psychiatry. He found that abnormal posture and movements amongst the mentally ill occurred before the introduction of neuroleptic medication (Hunter and Macalpine 1974). His observation that 'the high incidence of dystonic and dyskinetic syndromes explains why mental hospital patients the world over look and move alike, and appear to have done so since pictorial records began' tends to support his contention that all mental illness has an organic basis, yet to be established.

Conversely, Barton (1976) claimed that many motor and postural abnormalities were the direct result of a syndrome he named 'institutional neurosis.'

INSTITUTIONAL NEUROSIS

This comprises passivity, submissiveness, apathy and inactivity, together with deterioration of posture, gait and physical condition. People may become mute, losing motivation and interest in the outside world and ceasing to care for their appearance. They lose all sense of individuality as a result of living in overcrowded 'total institutions' where browbeating, petty restrictions and enforced idleness are the norm (Goffman 1961). Whatever the cause, it is well known that psychiatric inpatients and, in particular, those with a diagnosis of schizophrenia, score well below normal on 'measures related to physical activity and physical fitness' (Chamove 1985). Movements may also be affected by the side effects of commonly prescribed medicines.

THE DRUG-INDUCED DYSKINESIAS

Dopamine is a chemical messenger implicated in the integration of motor function, levels of which are affected by various drugs (Lees 1935). Amphetamine addicts develop abnormal movements, as do Parkinsonian clients receiving L-dopa, but it is the effect of neuroleptics that concerns us here. These drugs are widely used in psychiatric practice, often in heavy doses, for controlling psychotic symptoms.

In 1949 Charpentier first synthesised chlorpromazine, a neuroleptic in the phenothiazine family, which was found to induce a state of affective indifference and to reduce drive and aggressiveness without impairing memory or cognition. In 1952 Val de Grace, Delay and Deniker concluded that chlopromazine possessed antipsychotic properties. Since then it has been partly responsible for reducing the numbers of long-stay clients in institutions and has enabled general practitioners to manage acute psychotic relapses in the community.

Unfortunately, a range of distressing extrapyramidal side effects frequently occurs, some times persisting long after drug withdrawal. These include the following commonly observed disorders.

Acute movement disorders

These start within the first few days or weeks of treatment, or after an increase in dosage, and are usually reversible. They include:

• *Acute dyskinesias* These typically affect children and young adults and have an incidence of 3–10% in routine practice. Symptoms include painful dystonia, choreo-athetosis and Pisa syndrome (a postural disturbance).

• *Akathisia* This affects 10–20% of people of all ages. It consists of dysphoria and distressing motor restlessness, often seen as shuffling or foot tapping while the person is sitting down.

• *Parkinson's syndrome* Again, 10–20% of people will be affected, particularly those who are middle-aged or elderly. They show rigidity, bradykinesia and rest tremor.

• *Rabbit syndrome* Middle-aged and elderly people may be afflicted more rarely by these peri-oral 'nibbling' movements.

Late-onset movement disorder

Finally, a late onset and potentially irreversible disorder may occur up to 5 years after medication is started.

• *Tardive dyskinesia* This afflicts 10–20% of elderly people. Symptoms include bucco-lingo masticatory dyskinesia, limb choreo-athetosis and dystonia.

The occupational therapist's responsibilities

The occupational therapist is likely to have very much more face-to-face contact with the psychotic client than the psychiatrist who prescribes for him. The responsible therapist remains alert to the possibility of these disabling side effects and is quick to report their occurrence so that drug dosages may be modified or anticholinergic medication given.

Lees (1985) reports that the cosmetic impact of orofacial dyskinesias can be modified by chewing gum or sucking sweets. He also states that, be-cause the abnormal movements are often at their worst during inactivity and stress, 'physical activity and relaxation techniques should also be encouraged'.

PHYSICAL DISABILITIES ASSOCIATED WITH MENTAL HANDICAP IN ADULTHOOD

Answar (1986) states that 'mentally handicapped people have consistently been found to be inferior to non-handicapped subjects on measures of physical development, gross motor and fine motor abilities'. More-severe mental handicaps are often associated with more-severe physical disabilities, whilst moderately and mildly mentally handicapped people still have more physical difficulties to contend with than the average person.

Psychological research has established that 'there is a strong relationship between cognitive development and motor performance'. Even simple actions have to be planned in advance, the individual making predictions and inferences based on specific cues and past experience to coordinate motor behaviour.

Motor planning seems to be an intellectual function. A person uses information received from a variety of sensory receptors in order to learn new motor skills. This sensory input must be encoded and stored in a format that allows 'movement planning, execution and evaluation' to occur. Kinaesthetic and other sensory cues are compared to inner mental representations or body schemata. These representations become increasingly differentiated as the child develops and gains mastery of his bodily movements.

The complexity of this mental process perhaps explains the common observation that even moderately mentally handicapped people who have no obvious organic damage are often slow and clumsy in their movements. Furthermore, simple automatic movements such as walking and running, which are thought to present little challenge to motor planning, are well executed by this group but complex or intellectually challenging tasks cause them to become increasingly awkward and clumsy. Sporting activities can be used to engage these people's competence in gross motor performance, thus proving more successful and pleasureable than activities that demand fine motor coordination.

Many people with severe mental handicaps are limited physically not only by their cognitive deficits but also by specific areas of brain damage. For example, the physical handicaps associated with cerebral palsy in the adult ambulant population include deformities that result from the interplay of gravity, abnormal movements and lack of muscle usage over years. Mild or moderate spasticity may make one or more limbs stiff and difficult to move, with a marked 'springiness' at the extremes of joint movement. This leads to characteristic abnormal postures and gait. Individuals suffering from spasticity may have sudden, unpleasant spasms if roughly handled or exposed to unexpected noises. Pathological tonic reflexes may also persist into adulthood and can seriously impede voluntary movement.

THERAPEUTIC EXERCISE

How can we help clients to benefit from vigorous physical exercise? How do we get them up out of their chairs? Each therapist needs to develop her own dynamic, individual approach, and the following guidelines may help.

SETTING UP THERAPEUTIC EXERCISE AND SPORTS PROGRAMMES

In an ideal world, the physical activities chosen for an individual would be geared precisely to his needs and capabilities and would meet the aims and objectives of his treatment. Unfortunately, financial, organisational and social factors also affect the selection of activities. A compromise is usually made between the individual's requirements, the demands of the group, the therapist's talents and, of course, the facilities, equipment and money available. The astute therapist gains access to all the space and equipment that is available in her department, clinic or hospital. She also establishes links with local community sports and swimming facilities and liaises with appropriate charitable organisations (see 'Useful addresses', p. 158). The therapist must also keep an up-to-date file of local resources so that she can advise discharged clients about local clubs and facilities.

CONTRAINDICATIONS TO VIGOROUS EXERCISE

A study of anatomy, physiology and kinesiology equips the occupational therapist with an understanding of the body in action. However, it is also necessary to be aware of the many contraindications to physical exercise and to be ready to consult medical colleagues if a client's capacity to participate is in doubt. Such contraindications include the following:

- Vigorous physical exercise is contraindicated in heart disease, hypertension, musculo-skeletal conditions and, more rarely, bone cancers.
- Poorly controlled epilepsy may make the use of sports equipment especially dangerous.
- Some people with Down's syndrome have atlanto-axial instability and may risk neurological damage through subluxation (Collacott 1987).
- Young women suffering from anorexia nervosa, a refusal to eat combined with distorted body image, tend to abuse exercise in order to lose weight and should be excluded from sports programmes.
- People on phenothiazine medication are likely to have highly photosensitive skin and need to be protected from exposure to sunshine.

ELEMENTS OF THERAPEUTIC EXERCISE

The therapist's role

The therapist must, of course, be physically fit to lead exercise and sports groups. These activities are physically demanding and the therapist needs considerable strength and stamina.

Simple activities, such as folk dancing, soft play, keep fit or running, will be well within the capabilities of most occupational therapists. However, ideally, the therapist will have additional experience or training in chosen activities. For example, it may be necessary to rescue a floundering swimmer or to instil the discipline needed for safety on a trampoline.

The therapist should be aware of health and safety requirements and be a competent first-aider. She should be a good model, therefore her style of leadership should allow for her own participation in the activity. The effective occupational therapist is suitably dressed for action and ready to communicate her own enthusiasm for, and enjoyment of, the activity. The skilled therapist will also recruit other expert or talented staff, such as nurses and physiotherapists, to help her.

The location

Ideally, clients should carry out sports and exercise programmes in purpose-built buildings or on special playing fields, tracks or pitches, This usually involves having to leave the clinical setting and seek out appropriate community facilities (see Fig. 10.1) with all the benefits of improved social integration and reduced dependence on the in-

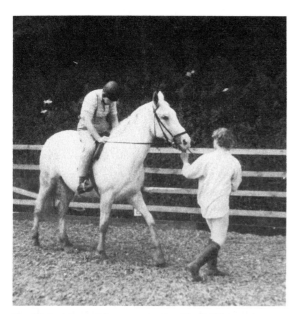

Fig. 10.1 Horse-riding uses community facilities and can boost social skills and client morale. (Source: Offerton House, Stockport)

stitution that this brings, However, playing fields, large halls and hydrotherapy pools are sometimes available within hospitals and are invaluable for those who are too fragile or ill to venture far.

Health and safety criteria must be met, whether the location is inside or outside the institution, and the environment should be well ventilated, warm and clean, The condition of the floor is particularly important; a clean, non-slip surface is imperative and special care should be taken to avoid slipping at the swimming baths.

Equipment

Many activities do not require special equipment but most sports do. Cheap and simple items, such as mats, skittles, bean bags, skipping ropes and balls should be available in every department, although the therapist may need to argue her case before larger and more expensive items, such as punch bags and table-tennis tables, are obtained. Highly specialised equipment is also highly expensive so if people want to use trampolines and ski slopes they will almost certainly have to seek them outside the hospital! All equipment should be well maintained, kept clean and stored safely. Broken, shoddy equipment is uninspiring and unattractive. A technical instructor is usually recruited to help maintain and repair such things as bicycles, and may even make simple equipment.

Kit

Everybody should be appropriately dressed for sports and exercise. Clothes should be loose-fitting, warm but absorbent and easily washed. Track suits, shorts and T-shirts are relatively inexpensive to buy and hard wearing. Most are easy to put on and take off and will fit people who are not standard shapes and sizes. People who are resident in hospitals and other institutions may need to go on a special shopping trip to obtain kit. Care should then be taken that it does not disappear in the laundry

Adequate footwear is extremely important. Advice may be obtained from the chiropodist or physiotherapist if a client has fitting problems, No one should go running without wearing proper running shoes, and pumps or lightweight sports shoes will help prevent slipping and tripping in the gym. In some activities, notably dance and yoga, the best footwear is *no* footwear. Finally, the client's kitbag should also contain soap, shampoo, towel and a comb or brush, so that he may take a shower after exercise.

Interpersonal processes

The competent therapist organises activities to give opportunities for satisfactory social interaction and to promote social skillfulness. Social aspects of exercise groups include the following.

- Managing the social factors involved in sports and exercise sessions to promote social integration and thereby enhance the individual's self-esteem.
- There is social psychological evidence to suggest that being part of a team gives rise to intragroup cooperation and identification, which produces a sense of belonging.
- Creative movement and dance groups, in particular, encourage contact and help to develop non-verbal communication skills.
- Competitive activities channel aggressive feelings productively and improve motivation to achieve and to participate.

Almost all clients who suffer from mental illness or mental handicap have some degree of impairment of social function and most have little social confidence. By focusing on the team effort and on the physical activity itself, rather than upon specific communication skills, the client's social competence is developed relatively painlessly. In the course of the sports activity he simply becomes a little closer to his team mates and is more able to express himself and to be playful with them.

RECOMMENDED ACTIVITIES

The activities described below have all been successfully incorporated into occupational-therapy programmes for the mentally ill or mentally handicapped. Each requires a minimum of specialised equipment and little expenditure, although most demand that the occupational therapist herself has a little extra training and experience. All can be adapted to meet the needs of individuals with a range of abilities and nobody needs to be particularly fit before he attempts any of them. None of the activities needs to stress competitiveness and all are suitable for groups.

Relaxation training is a valuable addition to physical exercise, therefore this is included.

Relaxation training

Vigorous physical activity undoubtedly prepares the mind and body for relaxation. Whilst reminding us that relaxation still appears to defy definition, Keable (1985) states that it is usually considered to be a mixture of reduced awareness of the environment and feelings of drowsiness and well-being. These responses are accompanied by decreases in breathing rate, skeletal blood flow, sweat output and blood pressure and are thought to be the result of parasympathetic autonomic activity.

A variety of relaxation training methods are successfully used by both therapists and clinical psychologists.

- The 'physiological' techniques, pioneered by Jacobson, emphasise learning 'to turn off tensions' as a muscular skill. This is achieved by, first, recognising the presence of minute amounts of tension. This is then 'released', proceeding muscle group by muscle group.
- Meditative techniques require a peaceful environment, the cultivation of a 'passive attitude' and, usually, some form of mantra (repetitive subvocalisation). Benson's method, for example, resulted from his observation that ancient teaching or prayer and meditation had common features (Keable 1985). His subjects were asked to subvocalise the word 'one' with every exhalation.
- Hypnotic techniques rely on the therapist's suggestion that the subject should concentrate on peaceful thoughts, experience 'warmth' and 'heaviness' in the muscles and 'witness' his own thoughts in a detached way. The actual mechanism of suggestion is unknown but many techniques include hypnotic elements, such as repetitive phrases and visualisation exercises.

Dance

Minas (1978) claims that dance has considerable therapeutic value, whether or not it is used in conjunction with traditional 'talk' therapies.

- Dancing enables the individual to become 'efficient and well coordinated' and to function 'more ably in his environment'.
- Most dance-and-movement therapy is based on the belief that free movement is a 'powerful medium for the expression of the emotions'. The body and its movements become the instrument of expression, thus allowing the release of feeling.
- Dance therapy fosters spontaneity and gives opportunities for self-exploration through creativity.
- It teaches the art of 'differential relaxation', enabling the client to master anxiety and tension in everyday life.
- Dance is a social activity that involves developing the ability to communicate non-verbally and through touch.
- It encourages participants to be aware of their use of space, including the socially important 'personal space'.
- It gives people an opportunity to have fun together without demanding of them that they communicate skillfully verbally.

Swimming

The value of hydrotherapy in the treatment of the physically disabled has long been recognised. Less formally, swimming sessions at the local baths have much to offer people with mental handicap or mental illness (see Fig. 10.2).

Swimming is a great leveller. Once in the water, people with moderate physical handicaps can participate as freely as the able-bodied. Everybody can enjoy the vigorous physical pre-swimming exercises, even if they cannot yet swim. Swimming is especially suitable for those who have arthritis, back pain or are overweight.

Most local authorities provide modern swimming pools, complete with changing rooms and snack bars, Swimming should be inexpensive; special rates may be available and swimming instruction may be available from trained attendants.

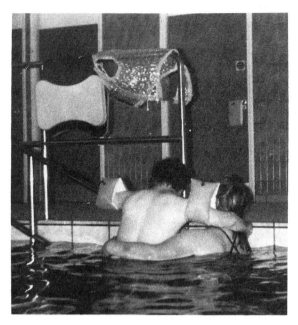

Fig. 10.2 Using local community swimming facilities. (Source: Offerton House, Stockport)

The occupational therapist in charge must, however, be a good swimmer and have passed her life-saver test. Trips to the swimming baths also encourage institutionalised people to use public transport and give the opportunity to practise self-care skills such as dressing.

Yoga

Gellharn reported that electroencephalogram changes accompany yoga trance states where 'unusual degress of mental concentration and corresponding levels of cortical excitation may be attained during complete muscular relaxation' (quoted by Keable 1985). Anderton and Winterbane (1979) stressed that yoga does not require special philosophical or religious belief and, when practised, 'increases the individual's ability for mental and physical relaxation'. Mastery of the yoga 'asanas' (postures) and breathing techniques is said to increase concentration, stimulate interest and improve body awareness.

Occupational therapists giving instruction in yoga should be adequately trained themselves but there is no shortage of yoga teachers outside the hospital and clients who develop an interest in the occupational therapy department can usually be directed to local classes.

Yoga is non-competitive, requires a peaceful atmosphere and emphasises relaxation, therefore it is of great value to the frightened and fragile mentally ill person who cannot face more boisterous activity.

Keep fit

Keep fit has been, for more than half a century, the most popular and accessible form of exercise for many people. Most clients will recognise the term and both men and women of all ages can easily be persuaded to participate. The basic occupational-therapy training equips the therapist with sufficient knowledge to run classes safely.

The keep-fit session should be well organised and disciplined but geared to the individual's needs and abilities. Recently, keep-fit teachers have introduced simple props such as balls, hoops and ribbons, and it may be appropriate to use lively music.

Again, having gained a reasonable degree of fitness and confidence in the occupational-therapy department, clients can be directed to locally available classes including 'Look after yourself' courses and 'over 60s' groups.

Walking, jogging and running

Walking is the simplest and most natural form of exercise, even for those who are very unfit. Walking trips encourage people to explore their neighbourhoods and a bus ride to the countryside offers an opportunity to enjoy nature. No special equipment is needed (unless hill walking) but a pair of stout shoes and warm socks. Ramblers Associations may meet locally and offer undemanding social contact, especially for older people.

As fitness increases, walking and jogging may be alternated provided that proper running shoes are worn and care is taken to prevent over-use injuries. Jogging and running are extremely popular, cheap and fun, and need not be solitary activities. Athletic clubs welcome runners and joggers and

may organise competitive events and 'fun runs' locally for the keen runner.

Finally, here is an account of a gym club for people with mental handicaps, that the author helped to run for $1\frac{1}{2}$ years.

A GYM CLUB FOR PEOPLE WITH MENTAL HANDICAPS

The club catered for 12 clients and enjoyed a high staff:client ratio (about 1:2.5). Apart from the trained staff (one charge nurse and one senior occupational therapist), there were up to three auxiliary nurses, additional help from students (nurses and occupational therapists) and occasional help from basic-grade physiotherapists on short placements. The club met each Friday afternoon for sessions lasting about $2\frac{1}{2}$ hours, which included walking to and from the gymnasium about half a mile from the hospital. The gym was well equipped with mats, wall bars and apparatus. Changing rooms, showers, toilets and a drinks machine were also made available to 'club' members.

THE CLIENTS

A group of 13 people, 10 residents and three day clients, was selected initially. Nine were men, four women; five people had moderate mental handicaps and the rest were diagnosed as 'severely subnormal'. The latter group included two people who had mild spasticity and associated deformities but all were ambulant. At least four participants suffered from mood disturbance and one woman had severe anxiety. Another woman had arthritis and one man suffered from frequent episodes of occulogyric crisis. Two men had Down's syndrome. Everybody else was in reasonably good health and most of the club members were in their thirties. Only one participant had to be dropped from the programme because of incontinence, which was difficult to manage in a public place.

Of the 12 remaining club members, not every person could attend every week (because of home visits, staff shortages or other treatments) but most had about three sessions each month. Just over half of the group received at least one occupational-therapy session per week and most of the others were engaged in activities run by nursing staff. Three clients were involved in no other activities at all during the week.

AIMS AND OBJECTIVES

Individual clients could be given their own, short-term objectives which could be met in the gym club context, for example, 'Bill will tolerate being with the group for the duration of the activity and will not leave the gym during the session' or 'John will put on his own trainers, independently, in response to verbal prompts.' Most people in the group also liked to have their own exercise targets and personal-best records and were applauded for their efforts to do 'just one more' sit up or, perhaps, their first proper seat drop on the trampoline. In addition to these goals, staff formulated the following broad aims of treatment.

- *Social aims*
  - to give residents a break from institutional life
  - to teach clients to find their way around the locality and use a community facility
  - to promote communication (including the use of sign language)
  - to develop a sense of belonging by increasing group cohesion.
- *Physical aims*
  - to improve coordination and spatial awareness
  - to improve general physical condition and increase cardiovascular fitness
  - to develop strength and suppleness and to improve posture and gait.
- *Personal aims*
  - to improve mood and reduce anxiety
  - to provide an outlet for aggressive impulses
  - to improve confidence and enhance self-image
  - to encourage independent personal care (especially dressing and grooming)
  - to provide opportunities for clients to face challenges and achieve success.

THE PROCEDURE

Clients were asked if they wished to attend and arrangements were made for their kit to be provided. It was determined from the beginning that only those who could be appropriately clad in the gym might attend. The party assembled at the same time and place each week and walked to the gym, following precisely the same route each time so that no-one got lost. One qualified member of staff assumed responsibility each week for the safety and well-being of club members. Once at the gym, clients and staff changed in the changing rooms, with only minimal help given.

The session began with keep-fit exercises. With everybody seated on gym mats, all joints were put through a full range of movement and muscles were warmed up and stretched. This was followed by a brief jog of five laps around the gym, then more strenuous exercises were done in a standing position. Individuals were encouraged to demonstrate or choose favourite exercises and people were asked to pair off to help each other, for example, to do sit ups. This was followed by a faster jog around the gym and, sometimes, a brisk game of tag. If there were sufficient staff to provide safe supervision, clients could then clamber up wall bars or balance on bars. The gym club members then took turns on the trampoline. Care was taken that there were enough people to 'spot' and nobody got on to the trampoline alone until he had demonstrated adequate caution when partnered by a staff member. Finally, the participants relaxed on the gym mats. Afterwards, everybody showered, dressed and had a hot drink before heading home.

LEADERSHIP

Staff used a democratic leadership style because institutionalised people are, unfortunately, often subjected to authoritarian approaches. Qualified staff took turns to explain and to demonstrate exercises and all staff joined in throughout. A playful and accepting group atmosphere was thus created and clients were encouraged to tease and cajole staff who failed to meet their own targets.

RESULTS

Eighteen months is a relatively short period for a project involving people with severe mental handicaps and yet some improvements were noted. Among the severely handicapped group, the following changes were observed.

- Two men showed a decrease in unacceptable behaviours (spitting and yelling), even outside the gym.
- Everybody in the group turned up on time each week and each exhibited a readiness to set out for the gym.
- Most people were mute and socially withdrawn but during the course of the workout they smiled and made eye-contact more often, and also made more frequent verbal utterances than usual.
- One man only began to join in consistently each week after attending for 11 months. Results were slow in coming but very worthwhile.
- Most impressive were the responses of three men who were usually to be found rocking or exhibiting other stereotypic behaviour on their own during the week, but who came alive in the gym. They frequently demonstrated greater comprehension of the spoken word and a greater willingness to interact with others during the session than at home.

Of the less-handicapped group, most of whom could, and would, express themselves verbally, nearly every person took a great deal of pride in his accomplishments. It was particularly delightful to see people who were once afraid of, for example, the trampoline developing confidence and surprising themselves by overcoming their fears. These people all said they enjoyed coming to the gym and clearly looked forward to the sessions. One woman reported feeling less anxious as a result of doing her weekly work out, and all learned to relax more.

SUMMARY

Starting with a brief look at the history of exercise in therapy, the chapter went on to outline the philosophical debate about the nature of body–mind. it then described the motor development of the normal child. Next came a look at the link between brain chemicals, mood and movement. Psychological research findings were then presented and an account was given of the experience of exercise. The chapter listed the kinds of physical impairment common amongst people suffering from mental illness or mental handicap, including the drug-induced dyskinesias. Finally, it gave guidelines for therapists to run vigorous sports and exercise programmes, illustrated by an account of the author's work with people from a mental-handicap institution.

REFERENCES

Anderton F, Winterbane A 1979 Yoga in a short stay psychiatric unit. The British Journal of Occupational Therapy 42(8)

Answar F 1986 Cognitive deficit and motor skill. In: Ellis D (ed) 1986 Sensory impairments in mentally handicapped people. Croom Helm, Kent

Ashton D, Davies B 1986 Why Exercise? Blackwell, Oxford

Barton R 1976 Institutional neurosis, 3rd edn Wright, Bristol

Chamove A S (1985) Exercise improves behaviour: a rationale for occupational therapy. British Journal of Occupational Therapy Vol 49 No. 3

Chesser E 1972 Reich and sexual freedom. Vision, London

Clare A 1976 Psychiatry in dissent. Tavistock, London

Collacott R A 1987 Atlantoaxial instability in Down's syndrome. British Medical Journal 294

Connolly C, Einzig H 1986 The fitness jungle. Century Hutchinson, London

Dale G et al 1987 Endorphin: A factor in 'fun run' collapse. British Medical Journal 294

Evans W H 1985 The effects of exercise on selected classroom behaviours of behaviourally disordered adolescents. Behavioural Disorders 11(1)

Farrel P A 1985 Exercise and endorphins: male responses. Medicine and Science in Sport and Exercise 17(1)

Goffman E 1961 Asylums. Penguin, Harmondsworth

Golding R, Goldsmith L 1986 The caring person's guide to handling the severely multiply handicapped. Macmillan, London

Grossman A, Sutton J R 1985 Endorphins: what are they? how are they measured? what is their role in exercise?

Medicine and Science in Sport and Exercise 17(1)

Grossman A 1985 Opiates for the masses. Medicine and Science in Sport and Exercise 17(1)

Hanfling O 1980 Body and mind. Open University Press, Milton Keynes

Hunter R, Macalpine I 1963 Three hundred years of psychiatry 1535–1860. Oxford University Press, Oxford

Hunter R, Macalpine I 1974 Psychiatry for the poor. Dawsons, Kent

James W (1960) The varieties of religious experience. Collins, London

Keable D 1985 Relaxation training techniques: a review, part 1. British Journal of Occupational Therapy 48(4)

Keable D 1985 Relaxation training techniques: a review, part 2. British Journal of Occupational Therapy 48(7)

Lees A J 1985 Tics and related disorders. Churchill Livingstone, Edinburgh

Lowen A 1975 Bioenergetics. Penguin, Harmondsworth

Macdonald 1976 Occupational therapy in rehabilitation, 4th edn. Balliere Tindall, London

Minas S C 1978 Dance as a therapy. British Journal of Occupational Therapy 4(3)

Morgan W P 1985 Affective benefience of vigorous physical activity. Medicine and Science in Sports and Exercise 17(1)

Paillard M, Newak K 1985 Use exercise to help older adults: clients in acute care benefit from exercise/relaxation plan. Journal of Gerontological Nursing 11(7)

Popkin R et al 1956 Philosophy made simple. W H Allen, London

Usdin E, Kvetnansky R & Koper I Catecholamines and stress; recent advances. Elsvier, North Holland, Amsterdam

Russel B 1945 A history of western philosophy. Simon and Schuster, New York

Ryle G 1949 The concept of mind. Hazell Watson & Viney, Aylesbury

Schurrer R 1985 Effects of physical training on cardiovascular fitness and behaviour patterns of mentally retarded adults. American Journal of Mental Deficiency 90(2)

Schutz W C 1967 Joy. Grove Press, Houston

Sheridan M D 1973 From birth to five years: children's developmental progress. Nelson, London

Simons A 1985 Exercise as a treatment for depression: an update. Clinical psychology Review 5(6)

Stacey C 1985 Simple cognitive and behavioural changes resulting from improved physical fitness in persons over 50 years of age. Canadian Journal on Aging 4(2)

Takagi H, Simon E J 1981 Advances in endogenous and exogenous opioids. Elsevier Biomedical, Amsterdam

Trombly C A, Scott A D 1977 Occupational therapy for physical dysfunction. Williams & Wilkins, Baltimore

FURTHER READING

Health Education Council & Sports Council, Exercise : why bother? Health Education Council, London (suitable for clients)

Gina Levette (1982) No handicap to dance Souvenir Press, London

Cotton M (1981) Out of doors with handicapped people 1981 Souvenir Press, London

Thompson N Sport and recreation provision for disabled people 1984 The Disabled Living Foundation/Sports Council The Architectural Press, London

Iyengar B K J Light on yoga 1976 Allen & Unwin, London

USEFUL ADDRESSES

The Sports Council
16 Upper Woburn Place
LONDON
WC1H OQP

Scottish Sports Council
1 St Colme Street
EDINBURGH
EH3 6AA

Central Council of Physical Recreation
Francis House

Francis Street
LONDON
SW1P 1PQ

Duke of Edinburgh's Award
5 Prince of Wales Terrace
LONDON
W8

British Sports Association for the Disabled
Hayward House
Harvey Road

Aylesbury
Buckinghamshire
HP21 8PP

Cerebral Palsy International Sports and
Recreation Association
c/o The Scottish Council for Spastics
22 Corstorphine Road
EDINBURGH
EH12 6HP

Handicapped Adventure Playground Association
Fulham Palace
Bishops Avenue
LONDON SW6

United Kingdom Sports Association for People
with Mental Handicap
c/o The Sports Council
16 Upper Woburn Place
LONDON
WC1H OQP

Society for Horticultural Therapy and Rural
Training Ltd.

Goulds Ground
Vallis Way
Frome
Somerset
BA11 1DA

SHAPE
9 Fitzroy Square
LONDON
W1P 6AE

Association of Swimming Therapy
Treetops
Swan Hill
Ellesmere
Shropshire
SY12 OLZ

National Association of Swimming Clubs for the
Handicapped
219 Preston Drive
Brighton
East Sussex
BN1 6FL

11

Sensory Integration

Shaun McCallion

INTRODUCTION

Sensory integration or sensory-integrative therapy is widely used in North America and increasingly used in the United Kingdom, Europe and Australasia in the treatment of many client groups. Ayres A J (1972a) described sensory-integration theory and therapy applied to children with learning disorders and this forms the basis from which many other therapists have derived their models of treatment. Chief amongst these is King L J (1974) who has postulated a sensory-integrative model for the treatment of adults with process or reactive schizophrenia. Many therapists have used sensory-integrative therapies based on King's work to treat schizophrenic clients (Bailey 1978, Endler and Eimon 1978, Hickerson-Christ 1979, Levine et al 1977, Rider 1978). Other therapists have adapted the work of Ayres for use in the treatment of people with mental handicap (Norton 1975, Morrison and Pothier 1972, Clark et al 1978).

Many other therapists are using sensory-integrative techniques or activities with a large sensory-integrative component in their daily treatment programmes. However, within the United Kingdom sensory integration is relatively new and is generally under-used, under-rated and only partially understood.

The aim of this chapter is to present a basic theoretical background to sensory-integration theory, to illustrate its application to different client groups and to suggest basic assessment and treatment principles that might be used in therapy. The author also hopes to promote discussion on the value of sensory-integrative therapy and on the limitations of its application. The chapter also aims to show that treatment using only a sensory-integrative model may be unsound, as it emphasises one area of deficit, and its remediation. However crucial this deficit may be in the genesis of the client's problems it is only one aspect of the multidimensional needs of the client. A more holistic view of the client's occupational needs is required. This calls for an eclectic and flexible approach to assessment and treatment based on sound models and practices of occupational therapy.

This chapter will outline what sensory integration is, how sensory integration occurs as a neurological process and the importance of the vestibular, proprioceptive and tactile systems in sensory integration. The sensory-integrative treatment model as proposed by Ayres 1972, working with children with learning disorders, will be examined to give a background to the rest of the chapter. Schizophrenia and mental handicap are then discussed, followed by suggestions on assessment and treatment. Finally, a brief section on dementia is included to show that this may involve sensory-integrative dysfunction due to the ageing process and may respond to sensory-integrative therapy.

WHAT IS SENSORY INTEGRATION?

DEFINITION OF TERMS

It is important to differentiate between sensory-integration theory and sensory-integrative therapy.

Sensory-integration theory

This describes the current knowledge of the neuroanatomical and neurophysiological functioning of the central nervous system (CNS) whose structures and mechanisms are involved in the process of sensory integration.

Sensory-integrative therapy

Sensory integrative therapy as a model is the structuring and application of sensory-integration theory to account for characteristic problems seen in client groups identified as having sensory-integrative dysfunction, using diagnostic tests designed to evaluate dysfunction in this area. Treatment is hen planned to provide direct systematic and controlled sensory-integrative therapy to remediate the underlying neural dysfuction. Enhancement of sensory-integrative function should promote more effective and adaptive occupational performance.

THE NEUROLOGICAL PROCESS

The CNS receives, filters, combines and coordinates sensory information as a continuous and dynamic process throughout the life cycle. This synthesis of sensory data from many different sensory modalities to produce meaningful packages of sensory data is known as 'sensory integration'. This enables the person to:

- monitor the environment (input)
- manipulate this information to make strategies of action (throughput)
- direct motor activity (output)
- monitor the effectiveness of his actions (feedback).

A disruption in any of these areas will disrupt function in the whole system. Dysfunction in sensory integration affects the processing of sensory input and feedback and can therefore have profound effects on effective and adaptive throughput and output.

The structure and function of the central nervous system (CNS)

Figure 11.1 gives a schematic representation of the structures and functions of the CNS; this is a simplified visual overview of the following description of the sensory-integrative process in the CNS.

The CNS can be viewed as comprising three parts:

1. the spinal cord
2. the subcortical brain structures
3. the cerebral cortex.

The spinal cord is phylogenetically the oldest

1 The cerebral cortex

Structures
- Two cerebral hemispheres
- White matter (axons)
- Basal ganglia
- Limbic system

Function
- Conscious appreciation of sensory information
- Control of volitional movement
- Cognition

2 The subcortical structures

Structures
- Thalamus
- Midbrain
- Brainstem
- Cerebellum

Function
- Subcortical integration of vestibular, proprioceptive and tactile data
- Homeostatic balance control
- Control of postural and muscle tone

3 The spinal cord

Structure
- Spinal cord
- Spinal nerve roots

Function
- Relaying of sensory data to the brain
- Mediation of the spinal reflex and inter-segmental spinal reflexes
- Relaying motor output

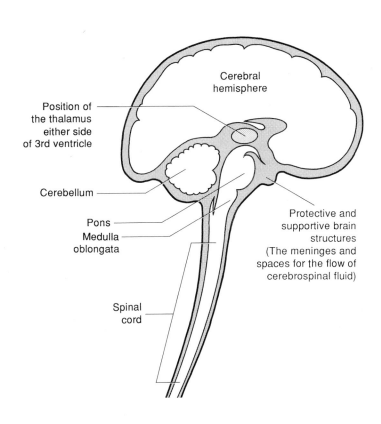

Cerebral hemisphere

Position of the thalamus either side of 3rd ventricle

Cerebellum

Pons

Medulla oblongata

Protective and supportive brain structures (The meninges and spaces for the flow of cerebrospinal fluid)

Spinal cord

Fig. 11.1   The cerebral cortex.

and simplest part, mediating the spinal reflex. The spinal reflex is the basic sensory-motor functional unit of the CNS, providing fast-acting protective responses, such as the stretch reflex (for example, the knee jerk) or the flexor-withdrawal reflex. The spinal reflex is normally under the control of higher centres of neural control, that is, the subcortical structures and the cerebral cortex.

The subcortical structures and their function

The subcortical structures are the brainstem, the midbrain and the cerebellum. The thalamus, reticular formation and limbic systems are important specific areas of sensory integration within the subcortical structures and neural mechanisms. These areas receive high input from vestibular, proprioceptive and tactile sensory neurons, and also play a major role in the control and coordination of motor output. One of the major functions of the subcortical structures appears to be the production of gross and rapid automatic motor output, which affects the body as a whole, that is, the control of posture, balance, reflex movement and the facilitation of coordinated and skilled movements against a background of automatic adjustment.

The subcortical structures of the brain are phylogenetically older than the cerebral cortex. These structures process sensory information from the vestibular, proprioceptive and tactile senses. These senses are seen as older in terms of evolution than the phylogenetically younger senses of vision and audition (hearing) associated primarily with sensory synthesis in the cerebral cortex. Maturation of the vestibular, proprioceptive and tactile sensory systems tends to be earlier than for the younger cortically controlled senses of vision and hearing. These more primitive vestibular, proprioceptive and tactile senses are integrated subcortically and are seen as crucial to the effective functioning of the more complex and discrete sensory synthesis at cortical level involving vision and hearing. This synthesis at cortical level allows for conscious perception and manipulation of sensory information to produce action strategies and volitional discrete activity. This may be motor-output activity, or cerebral activity (cognition) without motor activity.

Cortically directed purposeful and skilled movement is coordinated and mediated by the motor centres in the subcortical brain structures. The feedback on the results of these actions is primarily integrated at subcortical levels.

The structure and function of the cerebral cortex

The cerebral cortex is the largest, most complex and youngest part of the CNS. It consists of:

- the two cerebral hemispheres
- the white matter or axons connecting discrete areas within each cerebral hemisphere, connecting the hemispheres and connecting the cerebral hemispheres to the subcortical structures
- the basal ganglia (cerebral nuclei) which, in association with subcortical structures and especially the cerebellum, coordinate volitional movement against a background of automatic postural adjustment
- the limbic system or 'emotional brain' is a

cortical structure that is intimately linked with subcortical structures and is involved in sensory integration at subcortical and cortical levels.

The cerebral cortex is continuous with, and intimately linked to, the subcortical structures. The thalamus and reticular formations play a very important role in the relay of sensory information to, and adjustment of, the level of arousal in the cerebral cortex. They have a crucial role in influencing cerebral function.

The cerebral cortex is responsible for the higher-level cortical functions that are associated with 'man'. They include:

- conscious appreciation of sensory information
- skilled and purposeful movement
- perception
- cognition
  — memory
  — problem-solving abilities
  — thought
  — creativity/imagination
  — belief system
- individuality.

These higher cerebral functions are the tools that allow the person to acquire skills for interacting in an effective and adaptive manner.

Sensory integration as a neurological process can be viewed as a subcortical process primarily involving vestibular, proprioceptive and tactile modalities. A description of these systems may help clarify their importance in sensory integration and the impact that dysfunction might have on normal development and skill acquisition leading to the attainment of effective and adaptive occupational performances (skills for living).

THE VESTIBULAR SYSTEM

The vestibular system consists of two sets of receptors in the inner ear:

- receptors in the semicircular canals register head position,
- receptors in the utricle and saccule register head movements.

Both sets of receptors in both ears work together in a coordinated and balanced way. Lack of coordination and imbalance in their functioning produces vestibular dysfunction.

Neural pathways

Information on head position and movements travels along the vestibular fibres of cranial nerve VIII to the four vestibular nuclei and then on to the cerebellum. These connections help coordinate head position with the position of the body in space and postural tone in the muscles. Secondary vestibular fibres ascend to the motor nuclei of cranial nerves III, IV and VI, for the coordinated control of eye movements during changes in head position. Disturbance in one side of the vestibular input produces rhythmic oscillatory eye movements (nystagmus). Detection of abnormal nystagmus following rapid rotation of the head is indicative of vestibular dysfunction. This postrotatory nystagmus is used as a diagnostic test in sensory integration, for example, the Southern California Postrotatory Nystagmus Test (SCPNT) (Ayres A J 1972b).

The vestibular nuclei send projections to the reticular formation and limbic system. These areas are important in controlling the person's level of arousal, that is, the individual's state of alertness and ability to perceive and respond to changes in the environment.

Vestibular influences on posture and movement

The vestibular nuclei also send fibres that influence motor activity in the spinal cord. Their influence is mainly on the neck and shoulder girdle. These fibres influence primitive postural reflexes: the tonic labyrinthine reflex (TLR) and tonic neck reflex (TNR).

The TLR is evoked by a sense of falling. When the head is flexed, flexor tone is facilitated with flexion, adduction and internal rotation in the limbs; when the head is extended, extension tone is facilitated.

The TNR is elicited by turning the head to one side, producing extension in the limbs on the side to which the head is turned and flexion in the other limbs.

The TLR and TNR are normally integrated into more complex patterns of posture and movement by 9 months of age. Persistence beyond this, as demonstrated by an inability or difficulty in achieving or maintaining positions other than these, indicates vestibular dysfunction.

PROPRIOCEPTIVE SYSTEM

Proprioception is the appreciation of the relationships of body parts relative to each other. It provides a precise awareness of the position of body parts, the pattern of postural tone in the body as a whole, and the direction and quality of movement.

There are three major proprioceptive receptor groups:

1. muscle spindles (register contraction of the muscle)
2. golgi tendon organs (register stretch on tendons)
3. joint kinaesthetic receptors (register joint position).

Neural pathways

Proprioceptive information is relayed in two spinocerebellar tracts, which give a subconscious awareness of proprioception. Other tracts relay proprioceptive information to nuclei in the medulla then the thalamus. These provide discriminatory proprioception, for example, joint sensibility in the hands and precise awareness of overall limb positions. This information is relayed to the thalamus then onto the cerebral cortex for conscious perception.

Proprioceptive influences on posture and movement

Proprioception is of primary importance in providing information for the control and coordination of reciprocal innervation in the CNS. This is the basis for patterns of integrated and flexible motor output resulting in postural tone, reflex activity and skilled movements performed effectively and smoothly against a background of automatic adjustment in postural and muscle tone.

Body schema

Proprioception provides primary sensory information upon which a neurological representation or 'postural model' of the body is formed, namely body schema (Head 1926). Body schema is integrated subcortically but the conceptual awareness of body schema is a cortical process.

Body schema is the neurological basis for developing body image, which is the individual's picture of his own body and his feelings towards it (Schilder 1933, Bender and Silver 1956). Body image is important for the development of self-image. Self-image is the person's unique view of his individuality and 'being', a composite of the beliefs, attitudes and values the person holds about himself and his worth as a person to himself and to others.

TACTILE SYSTEM

Tactile receptors are distributed over all areas of the body and provide information about objects that come into contact with the body. The tactile system can be viewed as having two subsystems:

1. the protective subsystem
2. the discriminatory subsystem.

Protective subsystem (protopathic)

The protopathic receptors are found throughout the body and provide information on:

- pain
- temperature
- light moving touch.

This system protects the individual from injury. It is fast acting and influences protective reflexes, for example, a flexor withdrawal response on touching something hot or standing on a nail. These sensations are neuroanatomically intimately linked and are integrated as a functional unit in order to protect the individual.

Discriminatory subsystem (epicratic)

Epicratic receptors are located over all the body's surface and provide an appreciation of:

- localisation of touch
- two-point touch discrimination
- stereognosis (the ability to identify by feel and manual manipulation)
- graphaesthesia (the ability to recognise simple geometric shapes by feel drawn on the skin)
- pressure.

The discriminatory subsystem provides discrete information about the environment and is the sensory basis for a large part of skilled motor activity, especially manual dexterity. Functionally, the discriminatory sensory nerve fibres run together and are integrated in the thalamus and reticular formation before reaching the temporal lobes of the cortex. The information is somatopically arranged (each body part being represented); the larger the sensory area devoted to a specific body part the greater its functional significance tactually, for example, the hands and lips have the largest specific areas, whereas the trunk has only a small area.

Proprioception is also an epicratic or discriminatory sense, which is integrated with tactile information in interactions with the environment, especially joint sensibility in the hands necessary for stereognosis.

It is believed that a normal functioning tactile system represents a balance between the protective and discriminatory subsystems. The discriminatory subsystem usually supersedes the protective subsystem, enabling effective and adaptive interaction with the environment, the protective system only reestablishing dominance if an injurious contact with the environment takes place. It is suggested that, if the protective and discriminatory subsystems are disrupted by dysfunction in tactile integration, then the more primitive protective subsystem will dominate the discriminatory subsystem and respond to tactile environmental contacts as if they were adverse and injurious. When there is a normal balance or integration between the two subsystems, information on pain temperature and light moving touch augment the discriminatory subsystem.

SENSORY INTEGRATION SUMMARY

- Sensory integration is primarily a subcortical process.
- The vestibular, proprioceptive and tactile systems are viewed as the most important sensory modalities.
- The thalamus, reticular formation, limbic system and cerebellum are major areas of sensory integration.
- Subcortical sensory integration is crucial to the development of effective higher functions:
  — integration of vision and hearing
  — volitional control of movement
  — development of perception
  — cognition
  — language acquisition
  — development of individuality and personality.
- Conscious appreciation of discrete sensory information takes place in the cerebral cortex but is founded upon subcortical sensory integrative processing.
- The integration of vestibular, proprioceptive and tactile information influences the state of arousal and emotions of the individual.
- Effective sensory integration is necessary for the effective and adaptive functioning of the person and his ability to acquire skills and achieve competence in occupational performance.
- Increasingly the senses of taste and smell are being used in a multisensory approach to treatment (Farber 1982).

SENSORY-INTEGRATIVE THERAPY IN OCCUPATIONAL THERAPY

Sensory-integrative therapy as a model for treatment by occupational therapists was first presented by Ayres (1972a) in her work with children suffering from learning disorders. A brief description of Ayres' work is first given to provide a background upon which later work on sensory integration can be more easily understood. Sensory-integrative therapy as a model and treatment is then examined in relation to schizophrenia, mental handicap and very briefly in dementia.

CHILDREN WITH LEARNING DISORDERS

'Specific learning disability means a disorder in one or more of the psychological processes involved in understanding and in using language, spoken or written, which may manifest itself in an imperfect ability to listen, think, speak, read, write, spell or do mathematical calculations. The term includes such conditions as perceptual handicaps, brain injury, minimal brain dysfunction, dyslexia, developmental aphasia. The term does not include children who have learning problems which are primarily the result of visual, hearing or motor handicaps, of mental retardation, of emotional disturbance or of environmental, cultural or economic disadvantages.' (USA Department of Health, Education and Welfare 1977).

Ayres (1972) proposed, 'disordered sensory integration accounts for some aspects of learning disorders and enhancing sensory integration will make academic learning easier for those children whose problems lie in that domain. Sensory integration, or the ability to organise sensory information for use can be improved through controlling its input to active brain mechanisms'.

The sensory-integrative approach is not to teach specific skills or academic material but to enhance the brain's ability to perceive, remember and motor plan by modification of the neurological dysfunction interfering with learning and not the symptoms of the dysfunction.

Sensory integration is viewed as following the sequential development of brain structures during phylogenetic evolution, subcortical processing of vestibular, proprioceptive and tactile senses being crucial to normal sensory-integration processes and subsequent academic learning.

Ayres identified five syndromes attributed to deficits in sensory integration:

1. tactile defensiveness
2. disorders of postural and bilateral integration
3. apraxia

4. deficits in form and space perception
5. auditory/language disorders.

Tactile defensiveness

This is production of adverse responses to certain types of tactile stimuli, for example:

- light touch by others
- diminished tactile discrimination
- hypersensitivity
- poorly integrated primitive reflexes.

The behavioural correlates are hyperactivity and distractability.

This is thought to result from imbalance between the protective and discriminatory tactile subsystems, the protective subsystem disrupting the discriminatory subsystem's ability to interact effectively with the environment.

Disorders in postural and bilateral integration

- Poorly integrated postural reflexes
- immature equilibrium reactions
- poor ocular control
- difficulty in bilateral coordination
- the TLR and TNR tend to persist.

These factors combine to produce poor postural adjustment, impaired righting and equilibrium reactions and abnormal patterns of movement. This leads to abnormal posture and impaired range and flow of movement.

These problems are indicative of dysfunction in vestibular and proprioceptive integration.

Apraxia

A disorder of sensory integration that interferes with the ability to plan and execute skilled or non-habitual motor tasks; usually an inability to relate the sequences of the motions to each other. This may interfere with tasks such as walking and dressing but, especially, with fine motor skills and academic activities.

Deficits in form and space perception

A dysfunction in perceptual constancy in terms of form and spatial relationships, resulting in:

- an inability to consistently recognise forms and symbols
- difficulty in manipulating symbols
- disruption of spatial relationships resulting in poor bodily coordination, especially hand–eye coordination.

This may lead to problems in gross motor and, particularly, fine motor and academic tasks.

Auditory language disorders

The child may be slow to develop language skills, have speech problems and difficulty in learning to read and write.

ASSESSMENT OF SENSORY-INTEGRATION DYSFUNCTION IN LEARNING DISORDERS

Ayres (1972b) developed the Southern California Sensory Integration Test Battery to evaluate sensory-integration dysfunction. The test is standardised on children and widely used by therapists. The test battery evaluates the following:

- space visualisation
- figure–ground perception
- position in space
- design copying
- motor accuracy
- kinaesthesia
- manual form perception
- finger identification
- graphaesthesia
- localisation of tactile stimuli
- double tactile stimuli perception
- imitation of postures
- crossing midline of body
- bilateral motor coordination
- right–left discrimination
- standing balance, eyes open
- standing balance, eyes closed.

The Southern California Postrotatory Nystagmus Test is used in conjunction with this test battery.

TREATMENT

Treatment aims to normalise sensory integration and therefore normalise motor and perceptual responses. Activities which emphasise vestibular, tactile and proprioceptive stimulation are seen as the most effective, therefore movement is a major component in treatment. The treatments follow normal sequential development lines: non-competitive pleasurable activities are used to reduce anxiety, which interferes with sensory integration in the reticular and limbic systems by producing over-arousal.

Treatment activities

- Integration of primitive postural reflexes, especially the TLR and TNR, using:
  — scooter board
  — throwing a ball back over the head
  — pulling on ropes
  — parachute activities.
- Improvement of equilibrium and righting reactions:
  — kicking and throwing balls
  — rolling
  — crawling
  — scooter board
  — hopping
  — skipping
  — jumping.
- Improvement of bilateral integration:
  — throwing and catching balls
  — parachute activities.

These activities also improve body image, and spatial and form perception. The postural and gross motor patterns of sequential development are similar to those of Bobath and Bobath (1964). The perceptual and cognitive developmental sequence appears to follow that of Piaget (1952).

SCHIZOPHRENIA

King (1974) has developed a sensory integration frame of reference for the treatment of chronic non-paranoid schizophrenia, based on the work of Ayres.

King noted that there was a characteristic profile of postural and movement features common to chronic non-paranoid schizophrenics:

- a pronounced head–toe S-curve posture
- a shuffling gait and inability to walk in a heel–toe pattern
- an inability to raise the arms above the head, approaching the vertical
- immobility of the head and shoulder girdle
- a pattern of flexion, adduction and internal rotation in the limbs in sitting or standing
- impaired hand function, wasting of the thenar eminence, ulnar deviation of the wrist and weakness of grip.

King attributes these characteristic postural and movement patterns to sensory-integrative dysfunction in chronic non-paranoid schizophrenics. She notes that it is not the result of:

- *institutionalisation*, as other long-term clients do not exhibit this typical pattern
- *phenothiazine drugs*, as chronic paranoid clients receiving the same drugs do not exhibit the typical pattern.

King's original study involved 15 clients diagnosed as chronic non-paranoid schizophrenics, who displayed the typical postural and movement configurations she had noted, and who were treated using sensory integrative activities.

Sensory-integrative activities used by King

- standing in a circle, throwing a ball back and forth
- standing in a circle, kicking a ball around the circle
- marching to music
- stepping over ropes
- ducking under nets
- passing a ball back over the head
- jumping over ropes a few inches off the ground.

These activities were presented as non-competitive games, as the clients had no motivation to engage in work or exercise.

Results

After 2–3 weeks of treatment, the following changes were noted in the group:

- participation was more active and less sluggish
- clients turned up to the group without prompting
- increased verbalisation by clients
- improved self-care
- smiles on previously blank faces
- marked improvement in posture and mobility.

King's hypothesis

'Some individuals have defective proprioceptive feedback mechanisms, the vestibular component in particular being first under-reactive, and second, under-active in its role in the sensorimotor integration process. This deficit whether genetic, developmental, or the result of trauma constitutes an important aetiological or prodromal factor in process and reactive schizophrenia'.

From her hypothesis King interprets her findings in this study in relation to a sensory-integrative explanation of chronic non-paranoid process schizophrenia symptoms as follows:

- *Typical posture and movement patterns* produced by vestibular and proprioceptive dysfunction, causing the persistence of the TLR and TNR elicited by a fear of falling, and producing severe anxiety. Feldenkrais (1966) believes 'that all anxiety generalizes or is conditioned from a fear of falling'. Thus any anxiety will trigger the TLR-producing flexion, adduction and internal rotation in the limbs. This is uncomfortable and associated with a feeling of butterflies in the stomach and sweating. The answer is to curl up and not move further, reducing vestibular and proprioceptive feedback.
- *Lack of perceptual constancy* This is one of the characteristic signs of schizophrenia. Size and form constancy, and localisation of auditory stimuli are distorted (Chapman J 1966). This is thought to be the mechanism that may produce hallucinations.
- *Corticalisation of movement*: the need to think about moving, caused by dysfunction of the sensory-integrative process at subcortical level and the subsequent automatic adjustment, against which skilled movement takes place. This may be the cause of psychomotor retardation and of disruption and slowness in speech.
- *Blunted associational and emotional function*: the cortical processes involved in these areas may be slow, dull, with concrete thinking, inability to think in abstract terms and the presence of bizarre associations being common; emotional blunting or inappropriate emotions also being characteristic. This is thought to be due to a lack of 'tuning' in the arousal system due to poorly integrated vestibular and proprioceptive information in the reticular formation and limbic system.
- *Anxiety*, producing tension in the facial muscles, is said to reduce the ability to express emotions, producing a flattened affect, which hinders normal social interactions due to poor facial expression.

It could be hypothesised that poor sensory integration disrupts the development of body schema, the biological basis for body image and self-image. Therefore, distortions and disintegration of self-image associated with self-care may be a natural progression with the chronicity of process schizophrenia. It could also be inferred that dysfunction in tactile and proprioceptive integration disrupts the formation of a constant boundary between what constitutes the person or self and what constitutes the environment. Therefore the person's own thoughts, associations and internal commentary on his actions might be perceived by him as thought insertions, thought broadcasting or voices telling him what to do.

King's work provides an attractive and coherent model for the treatment of chronic schizophrenia that many therapists have used with some success. Their findings have been supportive of King's model although differences in study design and inherent flaws in methodology have prevented complete validations of the model.

Postural and reflex integration

Endler and Eimon (1978), assessing postural and reflex integration in schizophrenic clients, found that they showed markedly poorer integration than a control group of 'normal' people but found no difference between paranoid and non-paranoid schizophrenics. Levine et al (1977) found that evaluation of six chronic non-paranoid subjects through a battery of perceptual motor tests determined that deficits in sensory integration were present and that functioning improved following a 6-week programme of sensory-integrative therapy. Subjects' test scores improved and observable improvements in behaviour were seen:

- attendance at the group became more regular
- awareness of others increased
- evidence of enjoyment of the activities became more apparent.

Body schema

Hickerson-Christ (1979), using the Goodenough–Harris Draw-a-Person Test, found that chronic schizophrenics are significantly more immature than those of a 'normal' control group. However, following sensory-integrative treatment there was no significant improvement in the maturity of the figure drawings. The study design produced a large age discrepancy between test groups and is the likely cause of lack of support for improvement in body schema following sensory-integrative therapy. However, Levine et al (1977) reports significant improvement in figure drawing following sensory-integrative therapy.

Verbalisation

Many of the therapists using sensory-integrative therapy with chronic schizophrenics have reported improvement in the quality and frequency of verbalisation in clients, following treatment. Bailey (1978) noted significant improvement in the language content of chronic schizophrenics, following sensory-integrative therapy.

Research

Much of the work done on sensory integration in the treatment of chronic schizophrenia supports King's view that vestibular and proprioceptive dysfunction is a characteristic deficit. The work also suggests that sensory-integrative therapy improves the chronic schizophrenic's postural, motor, perceptual motor, self-care and social interaction skills. The studies have, however, been too small, contained too many methodological flaws and relied too heavily on non-standardised subjective assessments to be conclusive in validating King's model. Further research using larger study groups, standardised evaluation tools and consistent treatments and study population selection criteria are necessary before reliable and valid conclusions can be drawn.

MENTAL HANDICAP

The term 'mental handicap' will be used here instead of 'People with learning difficulties', as this term may be confused with 'People with learning disorders/disabilities', which specifically excludes mental handicap.

People with mental handicap usually have more profound problems in cognitive function, as measured by intelligence tests and academic evaluations, than people with learning disorders.

What causes mental handicap?

The majority of people labelled mentally handicapped cannot be attributed to a specific condition, for example Down's Syndrome or phenylketonuria. Non-specific cause mentally handicapped people are thought to have generalised non-specific neurological damage due to adverse conditions prevailing during CNS development in utero, for example, stress of unknown cause, or due to trauma at or around the time of birth, for example, hypoxia during a difficult labour and delivery. Caution is required in applying research from one area to another, however, in minimal brain dysfunction (MBD), soft neurological signs similar to those seen in people with mental handicap have been found. These include:

- head circumference beyond normal range
- widely spaced eyes
- epicanthal folds
- curved fifth finger
- wide gap between first and second toe.

These physical anomalies are thought to represent incomplete maturation in the CNS.

Many of the commonest characteristics seen in MBD children with learning disabilities are seen in people with mental handicap but in a more extreme form. It might be inferred that MBD is related to generalised minimal damage to the brain whereas, in mental handicap, the severity of the damage and resultant problems is more extreme.

Clements (1973) lists the 10 most common characteristics of learning-disabled children diagnosed MBD as:

- hyperactivity
- perceptual-motor impairment
- emotional lability
- general coordination deficits
- disorders of attention (short attention span, distractability, perseveration)
- impulsivity
- disorders of memory and thinking
- specific learning disabilities (reading, arithmetic, writing, spelling)
- disorders of speech and hearing
- equivocal neurological signs.

Effects of sensory integrative therapy

The application of sensory-integrative therapy to the treatment of people with mental handicap could be expected to have favourable results in improving the sensorimotor, motor perceptual, cognitive and behavioural problems of these people. However, assessment using the Southern California Sensory Integration Test (SCSIT) would only be possible with the mildly–moderately retarded person and would need the use of clinical judgement in the more profoundly handicapped person. The non-verbal and non-academic attributes of sensory-integrative treatment would lend itself to

the treatment of these more profoundly mentally handicapped people. A number of therapists have used sensory-integrative therapy with mentally handicapped people and found improvement in their clients (Norton 1975, Morrison and Pothier 1972, Clark et al 1978).

People with mental handicap may be further disadvantaged from an early age by the lack of environmental stimulus and activity opportunity offered to them. Many are institutionalised from an early age, whilst most suffer from the limitations placed on their potential by carers and professional staff who have low expectations regarding their potential for improvement.

Occupational therapists have much to offer in the assessment and remediation of the occupational needs of these clients. The provision of, and therapeutic manipulation of, environmental and activity opportunities can do much to improve the functioning and quality of life for people with mental handicap. The same statement holds true for intervention by occupational therapists in the treatment of chronic schizophrenics.

ASSESSMENT OF SCHIZOPHRENIA OR MENTAL HANDICAP

Evaluation of sensory-integrative dysfunction should not be done in isolation but as part of a comprehensive and holistic assessment of occupational performance.

Assessment should be flexible and sensitive to individual differences, for example, intelligence, age, general physical condition, degree of withdrawal from reality and social contact, and motivational level to engage in activity.

OCCUPATIONAL THERAPY ASSESSMENT

A full assessment of the person is required, not just a sensory-integrative assessment. It should include:

- an analysis of the environmental limitations

and opportunities open to the person to engage in activities and social interactions

- physical assessment
- perceptual assessment
- cognitive assessment
- ADL assessment
- assessment of social competence and interaction skills
- assessment of activity level.

Aspects of these assessments may come into sensory-integrative assessment

SENSORY-INTEGRATIVE ASSESSMENT

Standardised tests, such as the Southern California Sensory Integration Test Battery (Ayres 1972b), are available. A suggested format for assessment and treatment can be found in Ross and Burdick (1981).

The following guidelines are based on subjective experience by therapists and provide baseline information on a person's level of sensory-integrative function that can be referred to, following treatment, to evaluate that individual's response to treatment. The guidelines do not provide standardised test results and are therefore scientifically inconclusive in validating the outcome of treatment but can help in clinical management. Further development and refinement of a readily available, easily administered standardised test is required.

Tactile integration

- Observation of the person's behaviour when touched, for example, avoidance, belligerence or acceptance
- feelings about being touched
- ability to localise where he is touched
- ability to discriminate two-point touch
- ability to identify simple geometric shapes, such as a square, circle or triangle, drawn on the back of the hand (graphaesthesia)
- ability to recognise objects by feel (stereognosis), for example, a key, a coin or a teaspoon
- ability to identify an individual finger being touched, with the eyes closed.

Posture and balance

- Standing balance, eyes open
- standing balance, eyes closed
- walking a chalk line, heel–toe
- standing on one leg, right and left, for 10 seconds
- taking arms out at shoulder level, into crucifix position, with palms upwards
- can hop or jump.

Bilateral integration and coordination

- Ability to cross midline left hand to right knee, etc.
- ability to oppose thumb to forefinger in one hand without associated movement in other hand
- ability to catch and throw a large ball
- ability to draw two overlapping circles, simultaneously, with right and left hand, on a blackboard.

Body schema and fine motor skills

- Imitate postures
- identify body parts on himself
- draw-a-person
- copy-a-block design.

Auditory and visual integration

- Follow rhythms, tapping or clapping
- read newspaper headlines
- read simple paragraph
- write name
- write down a paraphrased version of a short paragraph recited to him.

Systematic clinical observation and recording of how the person performed in each subcategory should help to identify what kind of sensory-integrative problems the person is having. This will form the baseline from which treatment can be planned.

The sensory-integrative assessment has to be viewed in conjunction with the results of the other occupational therapy assessments in order to plan a suitable treatment programme.

TREATMENT OF SCHIZOPHRENIA OR MENTAL HANDICAP

It should be emphasised that sensory-integrative therapy, alone, is not the answer to the remediation of the problems experienced by people with chronic schizophrenia and mental handicap. Sensory-integrative therapy should be part of an overall treatment programme aimed at restoring competence in occupational performance.

THE ENVIRONMENT

The environment can have a major influence on the individual's performance. Many chronic schizophrenics and mentally handicapped people spend a large percentage of their lives in large hospitals. These institutions often tend to be sterile or impoverished in opportunities to experience normal sensory stimulation.

Improvement of the environmental opportunities for sensory stimulation and resultant sensory integration will enhance treatment. Pleasant surroundings of visual interest can encourage people to look and move around. Personal space with personal items can promote interest in the environment and a sense of security.

A feeling of insecurity may produce higher anxiety levels, interfering with sensory integration in the reticular and limbic systems. Houseplants provide colour and can be smelt and touched, all of which enhance experience of sensory stimulation. Pets can provide sensory-integrative stimulation, in that most regressed people would look at and follow a cat or dog's movements and would bend to stroke it (proprioceptive and tactile input). Environmental adaptation to promote a stimulating and secure surrounding can help to facilitate sensory-integrative function, as well as many other aspects of psychosocial functioning.

SUGGESTED FORMAT FOR A SENSORY-INTEGRATIVE TREATMENT SESSION

Aims

- Increase vestibular, proprioceptive and tactile stimulation
- avoid activities that demand emphasis on cortical control
- normalisation of postural reflexes, especially the TLR and TNR
- facilitation of normal motor function, especially motor planning
- emphasise body awareness to promote body schema
- use non-competitive pleasurable activities to reduce anxiety.

Treatment should be provided for 1 hour per day for 6 weeks. Sessions are presented as group activity and should have 3 phases:

1. *warm-up*: gentle exercises, with emphasis on body awareness
2. *performance phase*: emphasis on primary senses
3. *wind-down*: relaxation, positive ending.

Warm-up

This starts with people in a circle, throwing a ball and stating their name, followed by throwing a ball and naming the person to whom it is thrown. This phase is to warm up the group physically, cognitively and emotionally, and emphasises body schema and awareness of others.

Activities used include:

- tapping the fingers over head, trunk and limbs
- rubbing the trunk, arms and legs vigourously
- gentle head movements
- shrugging the shoulders
- windmill arm circling
- shaking the arms from shoulder, elbow and wrist
- clenching and unclenching the fists
- rolling and bending at waist
- shaking the legs from hip, knee and ankle
- mirror dance in pairs.

Performance phase

This depends on the mood of the group but activities are graded to promote increasing postural balance and coordination, and motor planning. Emphasis is on stimulation of the vestibular, proprioceptive and tactile systems.
Activities used include:

- rolling exercises on mats
- passing a beach ball back over the head, around the circle
- throwing, catching and kicking balls
- parachute games
  - parachute over the head
  - parachute flicked into the air
  - flicking ball around the parachute
  - running through parachute tunnels
  - being wrapped in the parachute
  - being rocked in the parachute
  - spinning, holding the parachute
- twister game
- hopping, skipping and jumping
- walking on a low-balance beam.

Wind-down

The wind-down is to relax and calm the group and to emphasise group identity.
Activities used:

- breathing in deeply with full extension of head, trunk and limbs; breathing out with flexion of head, trunk and limbs
- shake-out: limbs shaken to relax muscles
- activities to emphasise physical contact and group identity
  - pass the squeeze
  - group massage (only if group trust has been established)
- group ends with the sharing of drinks and goodbyes to group members.

PRODUCTIVE ACTIVITY

Meaningful and productive activities that have sensory-integrative stimulation inherent within them should be used in conjunction with, or on

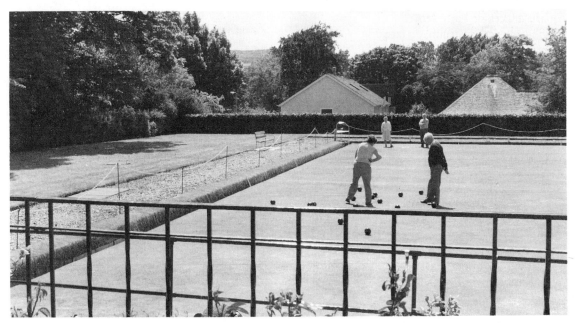

Fig. 11.2 Outdoor bowls is one leisure pursuit that promotes sensory integration. (Source: Lothian Health Board)

establishment of, basic sensory-integrative function.

Activities with inherent sensory-integrative properties

Activities of daily living

- feeding
- dressing and personal care
- cooking—especially baking
- housework.

Crafts/Arts

- woodwork
- metal scrollwork
- weaving, especially using an upright loom
- making and using puppets
- making and flying kites
- pottery
- large art work.

Leisure and games

- indoor or outdoor bowls (see Fig. 11.2)
- croquet
- square dances or barn dances
- playing musical instruments (see Fig. 11.3)
- swimming
- horse riding
- outdoor pursuits.

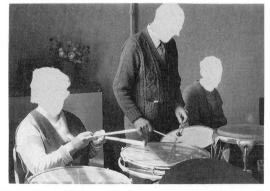

Fig. 11.3 Playing a musical instrument has inherent sensory-integrative properties. (Source: Lothian Health Board)

Horticulture and gardening

Horticultural and gardening projects (see Fig. 11.4) or hospital farms with a mixture of livestock and growing crops are excellent treatment. These activities have extremely good sensory stimulation qualities especially for vestibular, proprioceptive and tactile integration, plus the added intrinsic motivation of handling and nurturing living things.

Industrial therapy

Industrial therapy is often a major activity used with chronic schizophrenics and mentally handicapped people to provide structured and meaningful

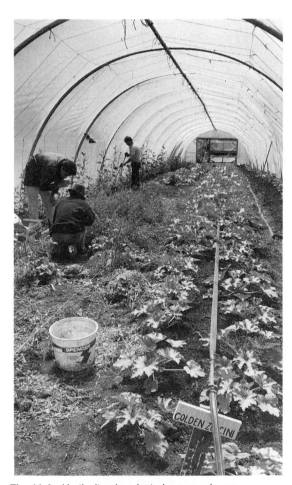

Fig. 11.4 Horticultural projects have good sensory stimulation qualities. (Source: Lothian Health Board)

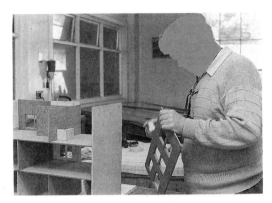

Fig. 11.5 Woodwork projects are a form of sensory-integrative industrial therapy. (Source: Lothian Health Board)

occupation. However, many of the types of activity undertaken emphasise simple, repetitive assembly tasks with emphasis on fine motor skills and are often very sedentary. Industrial therapy should probably be augmented by a daily sensory-integrative stimulation or keep-fit group if the above activities predominate.

More suitable activities would be:

- making rustic garden furniture
- making concrete paving flags, troughs etc.
- woodwork projects (see Fig. 11.5)
- metalwork projects.

DEMENTIA

The normal effects of ageing reduce the sensitivity of sensory receptors, for example, loss and impairment of the special senses and reduced efficiency of vestibular and proprioceptive senses as exhibited by increased frequency of falls in the elderly. The slowing down and reduced levels of movement and engagement in activity in the elderly also reduce the amount of sensory input they receive. This, coupled with increa ed effects of trauma and disease, for example, Parkinson's syndrome and strokes, further reduces the quality of sensory input and motor output in the elderly. Parkinson's disease, for example, is caused by degeneration of subcortical brain structures and the typical posture, noted by King (1974), can be seen. The more severe cases also display dementia.

Subjective observations have shown marked improvement in posture, balance, coordination, and functional ADL and social interactions following sensory-integrative therapy.

Dementia, in a large number of cases, is caused by Alzheimers Disease, which is organic degeneration of subcortical structures resulting in loss of contact with reality, progressive deterioration in perceptual and cognitive functions, disruption of emotional stability, deterioration in ADL and development of maladaptive behaviour: hyperactivity, distractability and the 'wanderer' problem.

It can be assumed that people with dementia previously had adequate sensory-integrative functioning but, because of progressive, accelerated or chronic degeneration of subcortical structures, there has been a consequent loss in sensory-integrative function.

Assessment and treatment

Guidelines on assessment and treatment previously mentioned hold true for the treatment of this group of clients. However, they need to be used with consideration of the effects of ageing on performance and be related to the normal occupational balance expected in elderly people.

Emphasis should be laid on using reality orientation in conjunction with sensory-integrative therapy. Previously mastered skills that have been lost should be used, for example, self-care, cooking, baking, dancing and crafts. Gustatory and olfactory stimulation should be included. Ross and Burdick (1981) provide treatment guidelines for the regressed and elderly client.

SUMMARY

Sensory-integration theory and therapy has been widely used in the treatment of many client groups. Studies suggest that it has improved the performance of many people and that it is an acceptable model of treatment. However, there needs to be considerable further study and clinical research to provide reliable and valid support for the subjective or inconclusive research results that therapists have found.

It should also be emphasised that sensory integrative therapy alone is unlikely to provide all the occupational needs of any client group. It is more logical to see sensory-integration dysfunction as one aspect (perhaps causal) of the person's problems and needs. However, occupational therapists should follow the philosophy and principles of occupational therapy and provide an holistic approach based on sound occupational-therapy models and practices to the assessment and treatment of people who have sensory-integrative problems.

REFERENCES

Ayres A J 1972a Sensory integration and learning disorders. Western Psychological Services, Los Angeles

Ayres A J 1972b Southern California Sensory Integration Test Battery. Western Psychological Services, Los Angeles

Bailey D 1978 The effects of vestibular stimulation on verbalization in chronic schizophrenics. American Journal of Occupational Therapy 32: 445–450

Bender L, Silver A 1956 Body image problems of the brain damaged child. In: Bencher L et al Psychopathology of children with organic brain disorders. Charles C Thomas, Illinois

Bobath K, Bobath B 1964 The facilitation of normal postural reactions and movements in the treatment of cerebral palsy. Physiotherapy 50: 246–262

Chapman J 1966 The early symptoms of schizophrenia. British Journal of Psychiatry 112: 225–251

Clark F et al 1978 A comparison of operant and sensory integrative methods on developmental parameters in profoundly retarded adults. American Journal of Occupational Therapy 32: 86–92

Clements S D 1973 Minimal brain dysfunction in children. In: Saipir S, Nitzburg A (eds) Children with learning problems. Brunner & Mazel, New York

Endler P, Eimon M 1978 Postural and reflex integration in schizophrenic patients. American Journal of Occupational Therapy 32(7): 456–459

Farber S 1982 Neurorehabilitation: a multisensory approach. Saunders, Philadelphia

Feldenkrais M 1966 Body and mature behaviour, anxiety, sex, gravitation and learning. New York International Universities Press, New York

Head H 1926 Aphasia and kindred disorders, 2nd edn. Cambridge University Press, Cambridge

Hickerson-Christ P 1979 Body image changes in chronic nonparanoid schizophrenics. Canadian Journal of Occupational Therapy 46(2): 61–65

King L J 1974 A sensory integrative approach to schizophrenia. American Journal of Occupational Therapy 28: 529–536

Levine I et al 1977 Sensory integration with chronic schizophrenics: a pilot study. Canadian Journal of Occupational Therapy 44(1)

Morrison D, Pothier P 1972 Two different remedial motor training programs and the development of mentally retarded preschoolers. American Journal of Mental Deficiency 77: 251–258

Norton Y 1975 Neurodevelopment and sensory integration for the profoundly retarded and multiply handicapped child. American Journal of Occupational Therapy 29: 93–100

Piaget J 1952 The origins of intelligence in children. New York International Universities Press, New York

Rider B 1978 Sensorimotor treatment of chronic schizophrenics. American Journal of Occupational Therapy 32(7): 451–455

Ross M, Burdick D 1981 Sensory Integration. Charles Slack Inc

Schilder P 1933 Image and appearance of the human body. New York International Universities Press, New York

USA Department of Health, Education and Welfare 1977, USA DHEW, Washington

12

Cognitive approaches

Jennifer Creek

INTRODUCTION

Cognition is the faculty of receiving sensory input, transforming and organising it in various ways, storing it in the memory and retrieving it for later use: 'knowing, perceiving, conceiving' (Concise Oxford Dictionary), It 'allows the individual to be oriented relative to dominant environmental features' (Mosey 1986) and to his own position in time.

Mental processes are a part of all aspects of human life, so cognition is one of the skills used in the performance of occupational roles. Most components of purposeful activity require one or more cognitive skills, and more competent cognitive performance usually contributes to greater adaptability to the environment.

The components of cognitive performance, which are thought content, cognitive structures and cognitive processes, are described in this chapter. New models of cognition are continually being suggested, as technological innovations influence the ways in which we perceive our world and ourselves. For example, 'the invention of the computer has recently given us completely new ways of thinking about the brain, displacing models based upon telephone systems' (Barley 1986). Occupational therapists have always gleaned knowledge from the field of psychology to build a model of cognition, and in this chapter we look at two of the major psychological theories of cognition. Cognitive dysfunction is defined and causes and forms are discussed. The last section describes occupational therapy intervention, giving Case examples and suggesting useful activities.

COMPONENTS OF COGNITION

The components of cognition are content, structure and processes.

- content is what the individual is thinking about
- structure includes both biological structures and cognitive schemas
- cognitive processes include attending, concentrating, retaining information, recalling, recognising, comprehending, problem solving, imagining, judging and reasoning.

CONTENT

It is postulated that the mind has both a conscious and an unconscious part, and that knowledge, beliefs, values and emotions can pass between the two. The aspect of thought content that is of interest to the therapist depends on the model of practice being used.

Knowledge

In order to survive as an independent adult, each person learns and remembers how to interact successfully with his physical and social environment. Information is received by the individual both consciously, when he pays attention, and subliminally, without him being aware of it. This includes information about himself, external objects, events and the relationships between all these. Some information is lost but some is stored in the memory in various forms (see p. 181) and is available for future use. This is called the individual's store of knowledge. It can be modified or extended in the light of further experience. People have different amounts and different fields of knowledge, depending on their genetic capacity and life experience.

The quality as well as quantity of knowledge can be increased, that is, there are different levels of knowledge (Bruce and Borg 1987):

- The most basic level is physical knowledge, for example, knowing that fire is hot.

- The next level is symbolic–representational intelligence, which is the ability to represent objects and events by symbols so that they can be analysed and communicated, for example, understanding that the figure five represents a particular number of items.
- The highest level is social cognitive development, which encompasses the rules, morals, mores and values that enable a person to interact successfully in his social environment, for example, maintaining a culturally appropriate physical distance from colleagues at work.

Beliefs and values

A belief is acceptance of the truth or existence of an object, event, fact, statement or idea. Values are the degree of worth that the individual ascribes to himself, to others, objects, activities or ideas. Everything with which the individual comes in contact is automatically given a place in his internal system of values.

Beliefs and values are developed largely from the individual's interaction with his cultural and social environment. They can be modified with changing experience but certain core beliefs are very strongly connected with the individual's sense of self and are resistant to change. Beck (1976) suggests that through experience the individual develops a personal way of anticipating the consequences of events as either likely to be positive or likely to be unpleasant and that these expectations strongly influence his mood and behaviour. Kielhofner and Burke (1980) describe people as having a sense of personal causation, which is a belief in their own degree of efficacy and which, with other factors, influences whether they take action or not.

Mosey (1986) suggests that many areas of belief, such as people's natures, their relationships to the natural world, the relationships between men and women, religion, family relationships and work, are transmitted by culture.

Emotions

Emotions are subjective feelings, as opposed to objective reasoning. Positive emotions, such as happiness, are aroused by events that satisfy the individual. Stronger emotions are usually associated with greater levels of need satisfaction. How the event is perceived affects the emotional state more than the actual degree of satisfaction or deprivation it produces (Mosey 1986). Negative emotions, such as anger or fear, are aroused by events that are perceived as not meeting the individual's needs. Beck (1976) points out that the anticipation of events can arouse emotions as effectively as the actual event.

STRUCTURE

Biological structures, such as the anatomy of the nervous system and the structure of the sense organs, are species specific. That is, the species sets limits on how far and in what way cognition can develop (Banus et al 1979). Biological structures are also individual specific, their development depending on both inheritance and environmental influences.

Cognitive schemata, or cognitive structures, underlie mental activity and coordinate cognitive functions, that is, they guide the organisation, storage and retrieval of cognitions. They develop through interaction between the individual and the environment and facilitate successful action. As the individual matures and gains experience he develops more efficient schemata and a wider range.

COGNITIVE PROCESSES

Cognitive processes are the ways in which information is changed in the mind. Some of these processes are unconscious, such as repressing unacceptable memories, while others are mainly conscious, such as remembering a shopping list. The conscious work of the mind is called thinking. The basic tools of thinking include attention, concentration, memory, concept formation, problem solving and creative thinking.

Attention and concentration

As a person grows, he learns to filter selected stimuli from the mass of information available to his senses. He learns to focus his attention on the objects or events that he chooses and to ignore the stimuli he considers irrelevant. The ability to direct the attention selectively is a prerequisite for many other cognitive functions, including developing perceptual skills, planning responses to environmental stimuli, remembering and learning through observation.

Some people can concentrate on a particular object or event for longer than others. The ability to concentrate enables the individual to learn new skills quickly and to remember information.

Since these skills are basic to many other cognitive, physical and social skills, the occupational therapist will assess and work on attention and concentration very early in treatment.

Memory

All learning is based on memory, which is usually considered to be of two types: short-term and long-term.

Short-term memory retains a small amount of information for just a few seconds. Among the multitude of stimuli bombarding us we select only a few, which are deposited in the short-term memory, either as a mental picture (visual code) or a sound (acoustic code). Since the short-term memory has only a very small capacity, any new stimuli given attention will push out the earliest information stored. Intellectual ability does not influence the capacity of the short-term memory, which is remarkably constant from person to person.

Long-term memory may retain information from a few minutes to a lifetime. Information is said to be remembered if:

- it is encoded
- it is stored in a form that will facilitate retrieval
- it can be retrieved at will.

The efficient functioning of the long-term memory depends on all three processes working and inability to remember can be due to a failure at any stage. For example, lack of attention is a common reason for memory failure as the information is never stored.

Concept formation

Concepts are processes that recognise what properties different objects, situations or events have in common. Concepts are formed through two mental processes: abstraction and generalisation.

Abstraction is observing the common properties in objects that are otherwise dissimilar. For example, all nurses care for people who cannot care for themselves, although they may or may not wear uniform and can work with many types of people in many different settings.

Generalisation is deriving a principle from varied experiences. For example, a person learns the difference between assertive and aggressive behaviour by trying out different ways of behaving in a variety of situations and observing the responses of other people.

Simple concepts may be learned by gradual acquisition through observation and experience but the formation of more-complex concepts involves an active process of hypothesis generation and testing. An occupational therapy programme designed to develop high-level skills will provide many opportunities for practice in a variety of situations.

Problem solving

People use many of the same mental processes to solve all kinds of problems. There are various problem-solving strategies, such as trial and error, which is mainly used for very simple problems. Another method is deduction, in which the solution follows logically if the premises are true. For example, Robert is older than Caitlin, and Eleanor is younger than Caitlin, therefore Robert is older than Eleanor. A third method involves insight; the individual examines the problem, then reorganises it in order to fill in the missing information. People find the experience of insight pleasurable and will seek out problems that require insight for their solution, for example, puzzles and riddles.

In insight learning, the learner is learning the relationship between a means and an end, which means that he could apply his solution in a new problem that had some of the same elements and some new elements. Occupational therapists use this process when planning a graded programme of activities to develop new skills.

Creative thinking

Creative thinking is productive work of the mind, of which two different kinds have been identified: convergent and divergent. Convergent thinking is bringing together what one knows in order to find the most appropriate solution to a problem. Divergent thinking is starting from a point and going out in as many different directions as possible. It is recognised that different individuals have different capacities and aptitudes, so some people are more able to think convergently and some divergently.

It is necessary to be able to think creatively, to some extent, in order to adapt to changing circumstances, therefore occupational therapists use creative activities in order to develop this skill.

THEORIES OF COGNITION

Two theories of cognition are widely used by occupational therapists to provide a theoretical base for understanding and treating cognitive dysfunction:

1. cognitive developmental theory, which focuses on the development of cognitive structures
2. learning theory, which focuses on the process of acquiring knowledge or skills.

COGNITIVE DEVELOPMENTAL THEORY

Cognitive development is a function of the interaction between an individual and his environment. It is dependent on and influenced by both:

- the development of other adaptive skills, such as physical and social skills
- environmental stimuli and opportunities for exploration.

Each person's pace of development is unique,

determined by these two factors, but there are patterns that are common to everyone. It is these patterns that are studied in cognitive developmental theory.

Cognition develops through a series of predictable stages that are qualitatively distinct from each other, as the nervous system matures and as the infant receives feedback on his actions from environmental stimuli. Each level of skills must be mastered before the child can move on to the next stage, and earlier skills must be integrated with new ones. Norms can be established for the age at which a child might be expected to reach each stage, depending on his cultural background. Although individual variations in the pattern might occur, no stage can be missed out if new learning is to be integrated with existing knowledge.

BOX 12.1 PIAGET'S FOUR STAGES OF COGNITIVE DEVELOPMENT

Sensorimotor stage

This normally lasts from birth to about 2 years. The infant learns about his environment by acting upon it and finding out what happens, and he begins to differentiate himself from external objects. Activity gradually changes from random, body-centred movements to goal-directed, object-centred activity. The child also learn 'object permanence', that is, that objects still exist even though he cannot see them. By the age of 2 years he can produce a mental image of objects that are not present. He begins to use trial and error to solve problems at about 12 months, and starts to think through problems by the age of 2 years.

Preoperational stage

This usually lasts from about 2 to 7 years. By the time the child enters it he will have started to use language and mental imagery. Words, images and objects are used to represent other objects, for example, a cardboard box becomes a spaceship or a house. The child's thinking is egocentric in that he interprets the world according to his own needs. This is called the preoperational stage because the child does not yet understand certain operations or rules for

Stages of cognitive development

There are many ways of looking at how cognition develops and breaking it into stages. Two alternatives are given here, one by a psychologist and one by an occupational therapist.

The Swiss psychologist, Jean Piaget, made an intensive study of children's cognitive development, from which he formulated a series of four developmental stages, as shown in Box 12.1. These stages are a useful concept for occupational therapists because they take into account both biological and psychological factors (Banus et al 1979).

transferring information from one situation to another. For example, a 2-year-old child will say that two cups of the same size contain the same amount of water but if one cupful is poured into a taller container he will then say that it contains more. The child learns to classify objects by colour, shape or size. Conservation concepts and numbers are beginning to be developed by the end of this stage.

Concrete operational stage

This normally lasts from about 7 to 11 years. The child is able to recognise relationships between objects and to use objects to help him reason syllogistically. He develops conservation concepts, first numbers, then mass and finally weight. He learns to put things in order, such as largest to smallest. The child also gains a more objective view of the environment as he becomes aware of the opinions of others. He begins to develop a concept of morality based on an understanding of right and wrong.

Abstract operational stage

This begins at about 11 years old. The child gradually develops the ability to deal with abstract concepts and to manipulate several variables in solving problems. He considers possible outcomes before acting, rather than acting first and drawing conclusions from the effect. He is able to think through a logical sequence and to tackle mathematical problems.

Mosey (1986) defines mature cognitive skill as 'the ability to perceive, represent and organise objects, events and their relationship in a manner that is considered appropriate by one's cultural group.' She breaks this mature skill down into 33 sub-skills that are developed sequentially in nine stages, as shown in Box 12.2. The various components of cognition develop in their own sequence but are dependent on the development of other components. Each strand of sub-skills becomes more mature and integrated at each successive level of development but lower-level skills are not lost and may continue to be used.

BOX 12.2 MOSEY'S STAGES OF COGNITIVE DEVELOPMENT

Use inherent behavioural patterns for environmental interaction
Babies are born with inherent behavioural patterns which provide a base for developing other sub-skills, for example, from birth to 1 month the baby is able to attend and respond to environmental stimuli, such as the nipple. Inherent behaviour patterns that lead to pleasurable consequences tend to be repeated.

Interrelating visual, manual, auditory and oral responses
Between the ages of 1 and 4 months the baby begins to look and listen actively, to make anticipatory responses to cues that suggest food, to explore objects with hands, eyes and mouth and to respond with smiling to the human face. He can imitate actions he observes if he already has the physical skill.

Attending to the environmental consequences of actions with interest
From 4 to 9 months of age the baby actively explores the environment within his reach by looking and touching. Actions which have an effect are repeated with variations.

Representing objects in an exceptual manner
The baby is able to remember stimuli in terms of the action he used to elicit them, such as the action of banging a toy on the table to produce noise, or in terms of the response he made, such as crying when he heard a loud noise.

Experiencing objects
Through handling objects the baby learns that they have some permanence of existence and of shape. Before the age of 9 months he does not recognise their existence independent of his own.

Acting on the basis of egocentric causality
The baby believes that his actions are the sole cause of events around him. This stage, which is playful and magical, lasts from 4 to 9 months.

Understanding seriate events in which the self is involved
The baby is aware of sequences of events in which he is repeatedly involved and begins to understand the concepts of before and after.

Establishing a goal and intentionally carrying out means
From the age of 9 months to 1 year the child learns to set simple goals and plan short sequences of actions that will lead to them. For example, the child will move objects out of the way to reach something he wants.

Recognising the independent existence of objects
Between 9 and 12 months the child learns that objects exist even when he is not looking at them or handling them, and will search for an object that has been covered in his presence. He also recognises that the self has a separate existence.

Interpreting signs
The child learns to anticipate what will happen next from cues given in the present. For example, he may cry when put in his cot because he knows mother will now go away.

Imitating new behaviour
The 9- to 12-month-old child learns to imitate simple behaviour that he observes and that is not already in his repertoire.

Exploring the influence of space
The child actively explores size, shape and spacial relationships but they are not fully understood before the age of 1 year.

Perceiving other objects as partially causal
The child believes that his actions initiate all events but recognises that other objects play a part in bringing about results. For example, he throws himself into his mother's arms to initiate a session of physical play.

Using trial-and-error problem solving
Between the ages of 1 year and 18 months the child tries new and unfamiliar ways of manipulating objects to bring about desired results. He will experiment until he succeeds and then lose interest in the object.

Using tools
The 1-year-old child learns to use one object to manipulate another, rather than using his hand directly. This is the difference between using finger paints and a brush for painting.

Perceiving variability in spatial positions
By the age of 18 months the child is able to try various ways of reaching his destination, other than going in a straight line.

Remembering seriate events in which the self is not involved
The child is able to remember a simple series of events that he has observed rather than participated in. This is shown by the ability to repeat a simple sequence of actions that he has seen.

Perceiving the causality of objects
After the age of 1 year the child realises that other people can initiate action and that the environment can act on him independently. For example, he recognises the effect of gravity.

Representing objects in an image manner
Between 18 months and 2 years the child is able to remember stimuli in the form of visual images. He recognises the relationship between pictures and the objects they represent.

Making-believe
From the age of 18 months the child begins to distinguish between what is real and what is pretended. He enjoys playing different roles and acting out real situations, using play objects to represent real objects, such as a cardboard box for a bed.

Inferring a cause from its effect
The 2-year-old child knows that inanimate objects do not move spontaneously and will search for the cause of movement.

Acting on the basis of combined spatial relations
By the age of 2 the child can estimate roughly whether one object will fit into another and manipulate objects, such as jigsaw pieces, to make them fit.

Attributing omnipotence to others
The 2-year-old child is beginning to realise that he is not omnipotent and to believe that others are. He expects other people to know what he is thinking and to be able to carry out his wishes.

Perceiving objects as permanent in time and place
The child recognises that objects exist consistently in time and space, independently of him.

Representing objects in endoceptual manner
Between the ages of 2 and 5 the child learns to remember experiences in terms of the feelings he had at the time.

Differentiating between thought and action
The child begins to realise that thoughts do not carry direct consequences in the way that actions do. Dreams and fantasies are recognised as make-believe and the child no longer thinks others can read his thoughts.

Recognising the need for causal sources
The child searches for a cause to explain every effect but may settle on a cause that seems illogical within his cultural group. Finding a cause that satisfies him seems more important than being right in the eyes of others.

Representing objects in a denotive manner
Between the ages of 6 and 7 the child learns to use words to represent objects and to use

language in remembering. There is an increasing use of language in reading, classifying objects and expressing similarities and differences.

Perceiving the viewpoint of others
The 7-year-old child is able to see that other people might have points of view that differ from his own and to consider alternative ways of looking at situations.

Decentring
The child is able to distinguish several characteristics of an object rather than recognising it by a single outstanding feature.

Representing objects in a connotative manner
Between the ages of 11 and 13 the child learns to classify objects by their common charac-

teristics and to use words to describe and remember object groupings. He also recognises that several different words may be used to represent the same phenomenon. This stage is characterised by flexibility of thinking.

Using formal logic
The 11- to 13-year-old child is able to work through a sequence of reasoning to support a point in a manner that is acceptable to his cultural group. Thought and action are based on an understanding of cause and effect.

Working in the realms of the hypothetical
The 13-year-old child is able to think about the future or other unknowns and imagine different possibilities. He can look at a range of possibilities and work out which is most likely, given his present information.

People under stress or suffering from an organic mental illness may regress to an earlier level of functioning, for example, schizophrenia can cause a person to believe, like a young baby, that his actions influence events in the environment in a magical way (egocentric causality). Understanding psychotic illness in developmental terms helps the occupational therapist to plan intervention that will allow the client to regain lost skills, for example, opportunities can be provided to test beliefs in a non-threatening way.

Conditions for normal development

'Human development is determined by a continuous interaction between heredity and environment' (Hilgard et al 1979). Humans have a very complex nervous system that takes many years to reach maturity, during which time the child remains dependent on his parents for the satisfaction of most of his physical needs. Children brought up in a stimulating, loving and responsive environment have been found to develop much faster than children in a deprived environment. Deprivation includes lack of attention and environmental stimulation, and a failure to meet physical needs adequately, so that the child is

preoccupied with having his survival needs met and does not have the time or energy for developmental play. Mosey (1986) suggests that play is an attitude as well as an occupation and that a playful cognitive style fosters creative thinking.

Environmental deprivation may be caused by the child having a disability that prevents him exploring without help or it may be that the human or non-human environment is empty and monotonous. While motor skills can usually catch up, given improved circumstances, early deprivation probably has lasting effects on the development of cognitive skills.

LEARNING THEORY

Learning may be defined as a change in behaviour that occurs as the result of experience.

Learning theory offers an explanation of how individuals reach a particular level of competence in cognitive performance, rather than looking at patterns common to all. The overall level of competence achieved is seen as important rather than the age at which skills are developed.

A major difference between cognitive developmental theory and learning theory is that, in the latter, skills are thought to be acquired through the individual's interaction with the environment and are not dependent on prior learning of more basic skills.

Learning theory presents a model of how skills are learned and also suggests ways in which learning can be facilitated. Learning is seen to take place through a variety of experiences, including:

- habituation
- conditioning
- transfer of learning.

Habituation

Habituation is learning not to react to stimuli that are constant or irrelevant, for example, not to listen to the background hum of traffic noise. New sights and sounds attract immediate attention but, once the judgement is made that they are irrelevant, the individual learns to ignore them.

This has implications for the design of a therapeutic environment. Small changes, such as turning off the radio, can be used to reactivate clients' attention.

Conditioning

Conditioning is the acquisition of conditioned responses, or the making of new associations between elements in the environment. There are two types of conditioning: classical conditioning and operant conditioning. Both these techniques are extensively used to change people's behaviour, that is, to teach new skills.

In classical conditioning, a behaviour normally produced in response to one stimulus is transferred to another stimulus, for example, a client with severe mental handicap feels pleasure when he drinks coffee. By always giving him a cup of coffee at the end of a treatment session the therapist teaches him to associate therapy with coffee and he learns to feel pleasure when attending a treatment session.

Operant conditioning increases or decreases the likelihood of a behaviour being repeated by applying a positive or negative stimulus immediately after the behaviour. For example, if the therapist praises a client every time he performs a task, he is more likely to repeat it. If she ignores him when he shouts inappropriately, he is less likely to

shout. Behaviour can be shaped towards a desired pattern by rewarding any operant behaviour that approximates to the desired behaviour.

Transfer of learning

Learning one skill often affects the learning of other skills, either by facilitating or by interfering with their acquisition. When earlier learning has a positive effect on later learning it is called transfer of learning, for example, learning to use a gas stove in the occupational therapy department will help a person to learn to use the gas cooker in his new flat. When the effect is negative it is called negative transfer, for example, learning how to use one make of microcomputer in occupational therapy can make it difficult to get used to a different make at home. Negative transfer effects can slow down the learning process when new skills are being learned but they do not usually persist.

Transfer occurs because of similarity of content, the way in which the skill is learned, and the principle behind solving the problems, or a combination of these.

Simulated tasks give preliminary practice when dangerous skills are being learned or when the real situation is inaccessible. However, simulation is only useful if there is positive transfer from the simulated task to the real one and no negative transfer (Munn 1966). For example, an occupational therapist designed an Activities of Daily Living (ADL) assessment unit for stroke victims, in which all figments were adjustable so that the essential features of the home environment could be simulated. It was found that even confused clients responded automatically to familiarly positioned features, demonstrating that learning was transferred from the home environment to the unit. It could therefore be assumed that further learning would transfer from the unit to the home environment, and this was found to be the case (Smith 1979).

COGNITIVE DYSFUNCTION

Cognitive dysfunction is a temporary or permanent failure to achieve a level of cognitive functioning that is within normal limits for the individual's age and cultural background. The dysfunction may be primary, as in mental handicap, or secondary to another disorder, such as anxiety neurosis. Environmental factors have a major influence on the degree of cognitive dysfunction that results from whatever cause.

Causes of cognitive dysfunction can be divided into three categories:

1. developmental delay
2. affective disorder
3. organic impairment.

DEVELOPMENTAL DELAY

Cognitive developmental delay is caused by mentally handicapping conditions, such as Down's syndrome. A person who has a mental handicap does not develop as quickly as other people and is unlikely ever to attain normal mental capacities. However, people can be helped to develop to their maximum potential if appropriate intervention is made from an early age and continued into adulthood.

The causes, effects and treatment of mental handicap are covered in Chapter 23.

AFFECTIVE DISORDER

Affective disorders are extremes of mood, such as anxiety and depression. Cognitive impairment can be severe during the acute stages but the effects are rarely permanent and cognitive functioning returns to normal as the individual recovers. For example, an acute anxiety attack limits the individual's ability to attend and concentrate, therefore his memory will be impaired. This effect disappears as his anxiety level drops.

Cognitive processes play an important part in generating and controlling emotion, for example, thinking about being in an anxiety-provoking situation will produce the symptoms of anxiety: a churning feeling in the stomach, an increase in sweating, breathlessness, a dry mouth, etc. Some theories of affective disorder regard exaggerated or pathological emotional states as being directly caused by the sufferers' own thoughts and beliefs.

One cognitive theory of depression is that it occurs as a result of committing logical errors in thinking (Beck 1976). This theory is based on Beck's observation that depressed clients tend to have a distorted perception of reality, which gives all their experiences a negative flavour. He feels that this distortion is the cause, and not the result, of a primary emotional disturbance. For example, a man buying a house finds he has been gazumped. A non-depressed person would probably be angry, disappointed and frustrated but he would either accept the experience as 'just one of those things' or firmly blame someone else in the deal for letting it happen. The depressed person, on the other hand, might decide that no-one will ever sell a house to him (arbitrary inference: a conclusion based on little or no evidence), or he might think that the deal fell through because the sellers have taken a dislike to him (selective abstraction; a conclusion that ignores the role of the many other elements and people in the situation), or he may feel that he is an absolute failure at everything (overgeneralisation: a sweeping conclusion on the basis of one event only), or he may feel as though he has made such a fool of himself that he will never be able to look his friends in the face again (magnification: a gross error in evaluating his performance).

There is a model of depression following bereavement, based on learning theory, that is relevant for occupational therapists. Depression is often associated with loss; the loss of a loved one, of health, of a job, of beauty, or of social status can all be precipitating factors. However, this theory suggests that the aspect of loss that is central to depression is the reduction in activity that follows bereavement and the resultant loss of positive reinforcement that activity would normally elicit. Part of this reduction will be caused by the absence of the lost person or role and part will be due to the bereaved person ceasing to do, or be expected to do, the activities that he was accustomed to be involved in.

Occupational therapy for people with acute disorders is covered in Chapter 18.

ORGANIC IMPAIRMENT

Organic impairment, such as that caused by dementia or head injury, causes permanent loss of cognitive function, although there may be some recovery if the disease is not progressive. Higher mental functions are usually lost first so that the sufferer shows regression to an earlier level of development in both intellect and behaviour.

The effects of organic impairment can be exacerbated by environmental factors. The treatment of dementia is discussed in Chapter 21.

Sometimes a person can be left with a serious cognitive deficit following a functional illness, without any apparent organic damage. This is seen when a person has had schizophrenia for many years, the so-called 'burnt-out schizophrenia', in which the disease process is dormant but the individual's cognitive functioning is regressed and inflexible.

OCCUPATIONAL THERAPY FOR COGNITIVE DYSFUNCTION

Occupational therapists are concerned with cognitive dysfunction when it interferes with the individual's capacity to perform tasks competently and to fulfil his normal life roles. Formal cognitive assessments are rarely used, but the therapist assesses cognitive functioning from the client's performance of tasks. In this section we look at the cognitive requirements of occupational performance, and at occupational therapy intervention for cognitive dysfunction.

COGNITIVE REQUIREMENTS FOR OCCUPATIONAL PERFORMANCE

Successful performance of occupations requires:

- a mental image of the self as a competent performer
- a plan of action, including the goal and the steps to be taken
- skills for carrying out the plan.

Cognitive functions are required for each stage of performance, including:

- knowledge about the task
- cognitive schemata to coordinate the plan
- cognitive processes such as concentration, memory and problem solving.

If the client has a primary cognitive deficit then basic skills may never have been developed. For example, a severely handicapped person who has lived all his life in an institution may never have had the opportunity to make a choice and may not have developed the skills of recognising and choosing between options. New skills should be developed in a normal sequence, starting with the most basic ones. A person with severe handicap may also have had limited life experiences and require help to build up a store of knowledge.

A client whose cognitive deficit is caused by an acute disorder that is expected to be temporary will not require direct intervention but may need help once the acute phase is over to rebuild confidence and a positive self-image. Once the self-image is damaged a person's capacity for competent performance is reduced, leading to further failures and confirmation of the poor self-image. Intervention may be necessary to reverse this process.

Cognitive deficit may be the result of skills having been lost due to illness or injury. Treatment then aims:

- to restore the lost skills, for example, practising cookery after a head injury
- to use remaining skills to compensate for the loss, for example, learning to make lists to compensate for loss of memory
- to make adjustments in life-style so the lost skills are not needed, for example, moving into a hostel where meals will be provided.

TREATMENT

Occupational therapists believe that people have the right to try to understand and solve their own problems, and to make their own mistakes. Treatment does not provide ready-made solutions but helps people to find answers that suit them. Cognitive function is developed as part of the treatment of the whole person and cognitive skills are rarely taught in isolation. They are taught as an integral part of achieving competence in occupational performance.

The first requirement for competent performance is a positive self-image and this can be developed through engagement in activities, as shown in the following example.

CASE EXAMPLE 12.1   DEVELOPING A POSITIVE SELF-IMAGE

Alan, a 37-year-old man, was referred to the occupational therapist for help in separating from his mother and building up his self-confidence. He had been off work for over a year with anxiety and was about to lose his job. At the initial interview he presented as a poorly groomed, unattractive young man with an unexpressive voice and a flat facial expression. He had never had a friend of either sex, had no hobbies and had always done a low-grade clerical job. He could not identify any personal goals, except to be happier.

Alan was offered a place in an assertiveness group, where he could improve his social skills, begin to identify his own interests and learn the skills necessary for separating emotionally from his mother if he chose to do so. He was also offered a place in an activity group, where he could explore his interests and skills in a practical way, but he declined this. He continued to see the therapist once a week, individually.

At first, the individual sessions were used for completing an occupational role history and for exploring current interests in a semi-structured interview format. The therapist gave Alan unconditional positive regard and expressed interest in everything he told her. Gradually, he began to talk more spontaneously about himself and his feelings. He felt that people found him boring and avoided his company but he could not see how to change. However, in the assertiveness-training group he quickly developed new social skills and other members began to respond more positively to him. This success gave him the confidence to ask a fellow day-patient out for a drink and this led to further social outings. He began to explore interests away from the hospital, such as a film club and a walking group. Alan's appearance improved, his face became animated and he laughed a lot.

These changes caused conflicts at home and there were times when Alan felt that he was slipping back into his old ways. The individual sessions were continued to give him support through these times. Eventually, Alan found a voluntary job and stopped attending occupational therapy regularly. He continued to contact the therapist occasionally for a chat when he needed support.

CASE EXAMPLE 12.2   PLANNING FOR ACTION

Several people were referred to occupational therapy for help with time structuring and exploration of leisure interests. They all had difficulty finding a satisfying balance of activities in daily life, although their presenting problems varied, including alcoholism, anxiety neurosis following redundancy, process schizophrenia and chronic depression.

A group of seven people was formed, with one therapist and a technical instructor. The first four sessions were spent looking at each person's present life roles, balance of activities, occupational history, interests and motivation. Everyone set personal goals to be worked for in the group, such as finding a voluntary job or making new friends. The group then decided to start exploring local resources, such as leisure centres, art galleries, parks, voluntary work, adult education and information sources.

One session was spent collecting information from libraries and information centres. The next session was used to plan a 3-month programme to try out a different activity each week. Group members chose activities to meet their particular interests and needs, and different people volunteered to plan and coordinate each outing. The programme included swimming, visiting a market, having tea at smart hotel, going to the theatre one evening, and a variety of other outings. The technical instructor was interested in fantasy games, so the group decided to have four sessions of game playing.

At the end of 3 months a meeting was held to review each person's progress and to discuss whether the group was satisfactory. One person was unhappy with the group and decided to leave, one had stopped attending, three people found voluntary work and left, one person had found a part-time paid job and left and one person decided to come back for the next group.

The second requirement for competent performance is being able to set goals and formulate a plan of action. The following example is of a group designed to develop these skills.

The third requirement for competent performance is having sufficient skills at an adequate level. The process of learning skills usually takes place in three stages:

1. playful exploration in order to learn as much as possible about the situation and to build up confidence
2. skill practice in a variety of settings for as long as necessary until a level of competence is reached
3. application of the skill to achieve personal goals.

This process can be illustrated by another example of a therapeutic group.

CASE EXAMPLE 12.3 AN
ASSERTIVENESS-TRAINING GROUP

The need for an assertiveness-training group was established for six outpatients attending a psychiatric service, all of whom had relationship problems and very poor self-confidence. The group initially met for six weekly sessions of $1\frac{1}{2}$ hours but all the members were given the option of continuing as an 'advanced' group for an indefinite period at the end of the course.

The first two sessions were used to give factual information about styles of communication and what is meant by assertive behaviour. People were asked to observe their own and other people's behaviour during the week and to remember any interesting examples. This gave members the chance to get to know each other, to gain knowledge about the subject and to start working in a very non-threatening way.

In the third session, a structured game was introduced to start people interacting in a playful way. Games were used in all the subsequent sessions, becoming progressively less structured as people became more confident. At the beginning of each session group members were asked if there was anything in particular they would like to work on and they were encouraged to use their own examples of ineffectual communication for role-playing games.

Gradually, people began to bring their own problems into the games, and to look for ways of solving them. When a more satisfactory way of behaving was found they were allowed to practice until they felt comfortable with it. They were then encouraged to try out these new ways of behaving in their everyday life, starting with less-threatening situations, and to report back to the group about how they got on.

The group continued for a further eight sessions after the initial six, then most of the members felt they did not need it any more. The two remaining members joined another advanced group at a later date but both eventually left when they felt confident enough.

Activities for developing cognitive skills

Although cognition is normally seen as a component of all activities, some activities are used more specifically for developing cognitive processes, such as:

- crafts, which are useful for developing concentration, creative thinking and planning
- quizzes and table games, for developing concentration, memory and problem-solving skills
- art and pottery, for developing creative thinking and imagination
- play-reading or discussion, to develop language skills, concentration and memory
- creative writing, to develop creative thinking, language skills and concept formation
- reality orientation, to develop memory, attention, concentration and orientation.

SUMMARY

Occupational therapists rarely make cognitive function the primary focus of their work; this is more in the domain of clinical psychologists. However, cognition is an important component of competent occupational performance and, as such, it is the concern of the occupational therapist.

This chapter defined cognition and briefly described its three components, content, structure and processes, highlighting their relevance within occupational therapy. Two theories of cognition were then described: cognitive developmental theory and learning theory, both of which are widely used by occupational therapists. The section on cognitive dysfunction discussed three categories: developmental delay, affective disorder causing temporary dysfunction and organic impairment.

The final section of the chapter looked at the three requirements for competent occupational performance; a positive self-image, a plan of action and skills; and looked at some of the cognitive functions needed to meet these requirements. The chapter finished by showing some of the ways in which occupational therapists help people to develop cognitive skills and suggested useful therapeutic activities.

REFERENCES

Banus B S et al 1979 Development of the child. In: Banus B S (ed) The developmental therapist. Slack, New Jersey

Barley N 1986 A plague of caterpillars. Viking Penguin Books, Harmondsworth

Beck A T 1976 Cognitive therapy and the emotional disorders. Meridian, New York

Bruce M A, Borg B 1987 Frames of reference in psychosocial occupational therapy. Slack, New Jersey

Hilgard E R et al 1979 Introduction to psychology, 7th edn. Harcourt Brace Jovanovich, New York

Kielhofner G, Burke J P 1980 A model of human occupation, part 1. Conceptual framework and content. American Journal of occupational therapy 34: 9

Mosey A C 1986 Psychosocial components of occupational therapy. Raven Press, New York

Munn N L 1966 Psychology: the fundamentals of human adjustment, 5th edn. Houghton Mifflin, Boston

Smith M E 1979 Familiar daily living activities as a measure of neurological deficit after stroke. Unpublished fellowship thesis for the College of Occupational Therapists, London

13

Occupational therapy and group psychotherapy

Sheena Blair

INTRODUCTION

Within psychiatry, it is generally accepted that occupational therapy offers a combination of activities which, when used in conjunction with verbal means, enrich the therapeutic experience for individuals crippled by interpersonal and emotional problems. The treatment of choice for many of these people is psychotherapy, which refers to treatment for disorders of the mind by psychological means. It is a broad term that covers a variety of methods of treatment for both individuals and groups. Various theoretical frameworks are used as a basis for psychotherapy, including psycho-analytical theory, object relations, transactional analysis and humanistic psychology. Specific methods of intervention that come under this heading include analytical psychotherapy, supportive psychotherapy and projective techniques.

Group therapy probably provides the greater part of long-term psychotherapy in the National Health Service in Britain (Brown & Pedder 1979). Frank (1961) summarises the task of a therapeutic group as that of fostering a sense of belonging in its members. This is achieved by providing a common focus that encourages people to interact. Many people find a totally verbal culture restricting and, since one of the aims of psychotherapy is to help the client experiment with new possibilities, there is a responsibility for the therapist to create a rich social matrix.

All groups should have a clearly identified task and the methods used to achieve this aim may encompass movement, listening, acting, reading or producing an object. The degree to which the activity occurring in the group is interpreted or used to achieve change is determined by:

- the prevailing culture of the unit
- the skill of the clinicians
- the quality of staff supervision.

The opening section of this chapter traces the development of group work in both supportive and explorative approaches and highlights the different levels at which psychotherapy can be practised. A central theme is that talking is not an end in itself but must produce willingness to change and enhanced self-understanding, with opportunities to rehearse new behaviour. The section on occupational therapy approaches to group psychotherapy discusses the skills required for such work and the settings where it takes place. The value of the arts in group psychotherapy is discussed, noting the special characteristics of each medium, and the benefits of this type of therapy are reviewed.

The remainder of this chapter describes the partnership of occupational therapy and group psychotherapy in work with adult psychiatric patients. Occupational therapists use both supportive and explorative approaches, sometimes within the same setting. Some of the skills used in each approach are the same, such as facilitating group interaction, while other skills are specific to the explorative approach, such as using creative media projectively. This chapter mainly describes the more specialised approach of explorative psychotherapy, through the use of examples and case histories, but attempts are made to indicate the differences between the supportive and explorative styles of psychotherapy.

The closing section of the chapter deals with methods of assessment and communication, and highlights the need to develop reliable evaluation tools.

The media and tasks described in this chapter accentuate the complementary features of occupational therapy and group therapy. Attempts are also made to dispel the early concerns of some traditional psychotherapists that group activity should be considered separately from group psychotherapy.

WHAT ARE THERAPEUTIC GROUPS?

Human life revolves around membership of various groups. At birth individuals either become part of a group or create one by changing a couple into a family. The spontaneous joining of groups occurs throughout the lifespan, from the secret societies of childhood to the special interest or self-help groups of adulthood. Social development occurs as a result of involvement in group activities associated with play, leisure and education. Groups are, therefore, intrinsic to our existence as human beings, although they may vary in type, intensity or degree of commitment. Many indications of ill health are shown in groups, both in disturbance of interpersonal relationships and in disruption of the normal balance of activity.

There is a wide variety of groups operating within the health care services and in voluntary self-help areas but most of these fall into two categories, supportive and explorative.

Supportive group psychotherapy

Encouragement and mutual support are the fundamental features of supportive group work. Those who are referred or selected for such an approach have obvious difficulties with interpersonal relationships. Aims of the group include:

- offering encouragement
- providing mutual support
- exchanging information about resources
- providing a place to air problems
- helping to relieve anxiety
- giving opportunities to consider new ways of dealing with problems.

There may be clarification of the source of the problem, but the emphasis is on finding ways of coping.

Bloch (1977), describing individual psychotherapy, explained that the main aim of supportive psychotherapy is to maintain or restore the status quo in two distinct groups of clients:

- those in crisis, for example, bereavement, divorce, or family difficulties where defences have been fragile or have collapsed

- those who are severely handicapped emotionally or interpersonally and suffer from psychotic illness or severe personality disorder.

The purpose of intervention is to strengthen defences, not to explore underlying beliefs and areas of trauma; to keep anxiety to a minimum; and to use practical advice where appropriate.

This type of group is commonly open to new members, although a core of stable membership is advised. Staff are involved as leader, co-therapist and participant observers, and it is helpful if they can be consistent in attendance.

Explorative group psychotherapy

Explorative psychotherapy is normally confined to a closed group, that is, the group meets regularly and maintains the same membership over a specified period of time, for example, an out-patient group or a group of selected inpatients. In this setting a treatment contract is negotiated and the aim is not merely to relieve symptoms but to change attitudes, promote insight, resolve conflicts, integrate the conscious with the unconscious mind and strengthen the ability to make interpersonal relationships. Ego defences are confronted and the role of transference and unconscious motivation may be explored. The therapeutic processes are intensified because several people are participating and the opportunity for multiple transference is provided. This means that each person may transfer feelings onto fellow group members, the therapist or the group itself. For example, a client may act as if fellow clients are siblings in competition for the leader/parent's attention, or may project unacceptable parts of himself onto others. These behaviours can be used to generate discussion within explorative group therapy and, as understanding develops about why the individual needs to react in this way, it becomes possible to find ways of changing. Thus, the network of interaction provides possibilities for ego-defence mechanisms to be explored and the complexities of human motivation to be studied. In this form of group psychotherapy, change is encouraged through greater self-understanding.

The following principles apply when using an explorative approach:

- If the frame of reference or model of treatment is geared towards sealing over unconscious material and strengthening ego-defence mechanisms, then this approach is contraindicated.
- The momentum and pace of therapy is largely dictated by the client.
- Validation of information that has been raised and discussed during sessions is required.
- Explorative activities are demanding and tiring, and need to be interspersed with ego-supportive activities such as sports and leisure pursuits.
- A contract of confidentiality must be adhered to about material discussed or produced by the group. For example, permission must be sought to use paintings or clay work for teaching purposes.

Controversies surrounding an explorative approach

Concern over the specialisation of occupational therapy in this field centres on three main areas of criticism, reflecting different professional biases:

- Some occupational therapists are concerned that the explorative approach represents a departure from the main ethos of occupational therapy into pseudopsychotherapy.
- Traditional psychotherapists fear that the effectiveness of psychotherapy is diluted by using groups and employing activities.
- Creative therapy specialists feel that using creative media, such as paint and clay, in a structured manner blocks the expression of innate creativity.

THE HISTORY OF THE GROUP MOVEMENT

EARLY HISTORY

All large psychiatric hospitals will have early records stating that groups of clients worked together on common projects involving agriculture, craft or leisure. This subscribed to the moral philosophy of treatment of the mid-18th to mid-19th century and incorporated the view that involvement in occupation contributed towards mental health.

Sigmund Freud 1856–1939 did not work in groups himself but he did write about the relationship of groups with their leaders, particularly in the church and army (Freud 1921).

The first use of therapeutic groups in a clinical setting is attributed to Pratt (1907), a physician who believed in treating the person rather than the disease and who held weekly meetings for tuberculosis patients. Positive results from this approach included reduced social isolation and a consequent increase in morale.

From the 1920s to 1930s a number of psychiatrists experimented with group approaches, however it was Moreno (1948), best known for his development of psychodrama, who first used the term 'group therapy.'

1940 TO THE PRESENT

In Britain the potency of groups was most effectively demonstrated during the Second World War through the work of Bion (1961) and Foulkes (1964) at the Northfield Military Hospital in Birmingham. Those Northfield experiments provided the impetus for social therapy and the growth of the therapeutic community movement.

As the effects of the work in groups became known, different therapeutic and training groups, such as encounter, gestalt, psychodrama, transactional analysis, behavioural psychotherapy and analytical psychotherapy developed.

Significant changes in attitude and design of treatment emerged from the therapeutic community movement whose pioneers were Main (1946), Jones (1968) and Clark (1977). Most noticeable was the formation of a multildisciplinary clinical team that:

- reduced isolation of professions by better coordination of clinical care
- intensified and improved treatment by pooling resources
- facilitated better communication, resulting in a mutual education of professions.

HOW OCCUPATIONAL THERAPISTS BEGAN TO USE GROUPS

Activity groups have been used in occupational therapy throughout its history. The 'task-orientated group' is the original and perhaps most basic kind of occupational therapy group. The 'task' ranges widely in nature, from preparing food in a lunch group, to four people combining their efforts to produce a children's toy or a number of people organised round a table to do simple contract work. These examples require parallel participation in completion of a task but may not acknowledge group processes or dynamics. McFeely (1985) traces the use of groups in occupational therapy from cooperation to produce an end product, through treating the individual in a group setting for econonomic reasons, to a period in the 1960s when active use of group dynamics began to be employed by occupational therapists.

An analytical approach was energetically advocated in the work of the Azimas (1959) in the USA, who outlined a theory of occupational therapy based upon psychodynamic principles. The concept of projective group therapy was described for the first time, and the technique was defined as 'a group therapeutic situation in which some parts of the relating of ego system and need system are sought in and through representation in an available external medium, for example, plasticine, crayon and paper etc.' Projection means putting a fantasy distance between ego and need.

In Scotland Batchelor (1970) echoed the earlier reasoning of the Azimas' work and stated that occupational therapy could be differentiated from other forms of psychotherapy by the presence of objects, ready made, offered or created.

Throughout the 1960s and 1970s a number of occupational therapists described work in groups using action techniques such as music, art, poetry and pottery in an explorative manner. The aim was to contribute towards psychotherapy by offering improved communication and different routes towards better understanding of self. Personal change was seen to occur in a situation that combined activity with talking and this facilitated what Robinson (1984) described as the 'working through process' in emotional conflict. In the last

10 years there has been an ambivalence about terminology and fears about excessive specialisation. Stockwell (1984) stresses that although the origins of creative therapy came from psychoanalysis, psychodrama and analytical psychology 'it has yet to identify its own discrete theoretical framework'.

This ambivalence has provided the momentum for modern theorists in occupational therapy to explore a paradigm that unites the many facets of the profession within a common philosophy. Professional confidence is growing, helped by changes in the education system. The occupational therapist working in psychiatry today has to be flexible in both thinking and approach. Group work encompasses many approaches and techniques; the crucial task for the occupational therapist is to select the task that encourages adaptive behaviour.

THE OCCUPATIONAL THERAPY APPROACH WITHIN GROUP PSYCHOTHERAPY

Groups used by occupational therapists range from supportive methods to those involving an increasing depth of exploration. De Mare and Kreegar (1974) suggested that groups can operate at three different levels:

- psychotherapeutic
- communicational
- recreational.

Occupational therapists may find themselves in a situation where they use all three levels of intervention within the same admission ward. A selected and closed group may meet for psychotherapeutic group work, another group has the express purpose of encouraging communication and finding ways to learn more about the individual members, while the recreation group unites the total unit and contributes to the living and learning milieu of the ward.

Occupational therapy focuses upon the integration of feeling, thought and action. It studies those factors that prevent individuals from adapt-

ing and realising their potential, and contributes to the adaptive spiral (Yalom 1970), in which the patient's interpersonal distortions become reduced as self-esteem and coping ability increase.

Although the reduced length of hospital admissions that has followed the development of modern drugs means people have less time in hospital to effect sustained change in attitude (Walton 1971) many inpatient psychotherapy units do attempt to create a therapeutic milieu, that is, there is a deliberate attempt by the staff of a unit to manipulate the whole environment to provide a 'living and learning' experience that facilitates change.

Mutual therapeutic properties shared by psychotherapy and occupational therapy include:

- belief in people's potential to effect change in themselves and others
- catering for different levels of intensity of treatment according to the needs of the client
- opportunities for intrapersonal and interpersonal learning
- acknowledgement that change in feeling leads to change in behaviour and adaptation to life
- promoting individual responsibility while concurrently providing emotional support.

USING A SUPPORTIVE APPROACH

Supportive group psychotherapy is used when explorative psychotherapy is not available or is contraindicated. Its function is to strengthen ego-defence mechanisms and help people to cope with long-term problems such as chronic anxiety, depressive psychosis or process schizophrenia. Supportive psychotherapy groups are held in various settings, including:

- inpatient units where psychotherapy is not the main form of treatment
- day hospitals and day centres
- outpatient groups.

Groups are often open, that is some members leave and new people come in during the life of the group. This way, groups can run for a long time and there will be no list of clients waiting for a new group to begin.

Many supportive groups use only verbal methods of psychotherapy but occupational therapists use a variety of media. Robinson (1984) makes a distinction between the use of arts media as projective techniques for working in depth within a psychotherapeutic setting, and using the same media in a creative manner without exploring in order to encourage communication. Meyerowitz (1979) examines art activities under the heading of expressive media and indicates their use for promoting self-expression, exploring and developing creative potential, and enhancing the awareness of self and others. She believes that the task-orientated group is employed to foster a 'facilitative and growth-promoting therapeutic atmosphere.' Brown & Pedder (1979) also described the value of alternative means of expression for those unused to talking about themselves and their feelings and explained that self-discovery has to be parallel with integration, change and adaptive behaviour.

USING AN EXPLORATIVE APPROACH

Explorative groups are used in various settings, including:

- specialised units that use group psychotherapy as the main frame of reference
- therapeutic communities
- psychiatric admission wards where screening is carried out by the team or therapists to select those who would benefit from this approach
- family groups
- outpatient groups.

In all of these settings, supervision by an experienced practitioner is essential to examine the intervention by staff, the application of media and consequent results.

The occupational therapist who works in a group psychotherapy unit is a member of the clinical team and affects the therapeutic milieu of the unit. She therefore has a responsibility to contribute to the ward culture by designing a complementary and balanced treatment programme.

It requires skill and discerning judgement to:

- understand the philosophy of the group setting, whether it is supportive or explorative, orientated towards a behavioural approach or an analytical frame of reference
- analyse the expectations of staff and patients and consider whether they are compatible with occupational therapy philosophy
- understand the selection procedures for all therapeutic groups, and the objectives of each session
- analyse activities in terms of psychotherapeutic potential and design treatment plans accordingly.

In order to carry out these functions effectively, occupational therapists need to have a working knowledge of:

- Freud's theory of personality, unconscious motivation and ego-defence mechanisms
- the normal sequence of personality development
- the psychology of groups (Tuckman 1965)
- dynamic theory of occupational therapy (Fidler and Fidler 1963)
- activity analysis and treatment planning (see Ch. 6).

All channels of commincation need to be used both to learn from other staff about changes in clients and to contribute specific information to the team from occupational therapy groups.

The work of an explorative group psychotherapy unit concentrates on ever-changing group dynamics and identity. Various stages in the life of the group have been defined by Tuckman (1965) as:

- forming—the initiation of a group
- storming—testing out of boundaries
- norming—group cohesion develops with emerging norms and the growth of mutual support
- performing—realisation of a working group where possibilities for solving difficulties emerge.

Feeling states alter, for example, a sense of

autonomy emerges to replace dependency, defensive patterns of behaviour become manifest and the joint responsibility of staff and clients is to reflect and work on emerging issues. Each group is therefore reviewed by the staff, usually with the objective appraisal of a member of staff who has not been in the session. During the review, predominant themes are elicited, for example, difficulty in expressing anger, fear of rejection or parental conflict. These may be used as the central focus for the next session in occupational therapy.

Case example 13.1 indicates the process of staff discussion that is used in explorative group psychotherapy to reach an understanding of the group dynamics and to formulate the theme around which the occupational therapist will plan her next session. Although the group is analysed to select a common theme it must be remembered that each individual within the group has specific treatment aims that will have been discussed with him individually.

CASE EXAMPLE 13.1

A group was unable to work after receiving the information that two staff members were to leave the ward in a few weeks. Members of the formal psychotherapy group in the morning displayed angry non-verbal behaviour and two young women discussed fear of rejection and disenchantment with parental example. Another member had volunteered that it was 'safer' to be self-reliant than to become 'dependent' upon another person or group. Sparse interaction occurred and a retreat into self was apparent.

In reviewing this session, the team decided that ambivalence about trusting and dependency were features of the group and that the central theme was 'parents'. The task for the occupational therapist was identified as being to take 'parents' as the theme for exploration and, using the three-dimensional aspects of clay, to invite the group to model each person's family group in its present state.

Organising an explorative group

The organisation of a session involves careful preparation of the environment and materials. Seating, tools and equipment are arranged beforehand to ensure that the session begins without time-wasting preliminaries.

When all group members and staff are present, the therapist will introduce the theme and explain the amount of time that will be used for the practical activity and when discussion will commence.

Sessions last for up to 2 hours, depending upon the size of the group. The pattern of events is as follows.

- The introduction, which allows for questions and is used to set the climate of the group.
- Participation time, where the main activity is carried out.
- Individuals' explanations of their work.
- Group interaction following, and arising out of, individual participation. This draws similarities between people's work and gives an opportunity for mutual support. The discussion constantly refers to the work done and its significance for the individual or group.
- The summary is usually made by the therapist, who reiterates the theme and reasons for its choice. Main points are drawn together, with acknowledgements of the work done in the group. Some therapists prefer to ask a group member to sum up, which can be equally useful.

THE ARTS IN EXPLORATIVE GROUP PSYCHOTHERAPY

The arts range of activities, including music, art, clay work, poetry and drama, lends itself well to explorative measures, providing ways of bringing people together and exploring the self. The method of applying these activities is commonly referred to as 'projective techniques'. Remocker and Storch (1982) define these as 'methods used to discover an individual's attitudes, motivations, defensive manoeuvres and characteristic ways of responding, through analysis of their responses to unstructured ambiguous stimuli'. Blair (1974) describes such techniques as a system that uses the arts range of activity to allow the person further

Daily Programme For Psychotherapy Unit			
9.00 – 9.30	Ward report	2.00 – 3.30	Occupational therapy: Monday – Pottery Tuesday – Art Wednesday – Relaxation/ recreation Thursday – Psychodrama Friday – Outing (until 5pm)
9.30 – 10.30	Group psychotherapy meeting (all patients and team) taken in rotation by consultants, medical staff or nursing staff as therapist, with other staff as co-therapists	3.30 – 4.00	Informal feedback of occupational therapy session
10.30 – 11.30	Group review by staff to monitor therapists' perceptions of the content of the group, together with evaluation of client and staff interaction and staff intervention	4.00 – 5.00	Group psychotherapy meeting (all patients); meeting led by nursing staff as therapist with other staff acting as co-therapists
11.00 – 12.00	Consultants' ward rounds, or admission and discharge meeting, or discussion of psychoanalytical theory	5.00 – 5.15	Group review as above
1.30 – 2.00	Nurses' meetings or clients' administration meeting; or students' meeting, or staff meeting	8.00 – 8.30	Supper group: informal psychotherapy session

Fig. 13.1 A daily programme for a psychotherapy unit.

exploration of feeling and understanding of self. As a group treatment they make use of the spontaneous creative work of each client. For example, group members make and analyse drawings, which often express their underlying emotional conflicts.

Activities that can be used in an explorative manner fall into three types:

- those using verbal means but including additional media, for example, poetry and music

- those using a practical and doing element, for example, art and sculpture
- those including an element of movement, such as some forms of remedial drama.

Thus, a number of behaviours, such as reading, listening, painting, sculpting, touching or enacting, are involved, enriching the group experience. Group work has been compared to working in a hall of mirrors, meaning that people are involved in multiple transferences. A profile of each person can be constructed by learning from the individual's participation in a number of explorative sessions, in addition to other more educative or recreational activities. A typical weekly ward programme, which aims at a balanced milieu, is shown in Figure 13.1.

Two important features permeate the use of the arts in an explorative manner by occupational therapists:

- activities are analysed for their meaning and therapeutic potential (Fidler & Fidler 1963) and applied within a group psychotherapy setting
- the balance of activities is considered not only within the arts range but complemented by other more ego-supportive activities such as yoga or baking.

While it is understood that the arts can be used in many different ways, this section considers the use of painting, clay modelling, poetry and music from an interpretive perspective. Drama is covered in Chapter 14.

Painting

The use of painting as therapy with different client groups is widely documented. Within occupational therapy the early work of Azima and Azima (1959) and Azima, Cramer and Wittkower (1957) was instrumental in forming our understanding of group art therapy. Their work was based on psychoanalytical principles and they emphasised the therapeutic benefit of free association around the paintings that were produced. The aim was to 'penetrate ego defences, to uncover underlying conflict and to serve as indicators of change in personality structure'.

Painting has the potential to serve a number of purposes (Malcolm 1975):

- to aid diagnosis
- to provide a forum for learning about emotional conflict
- to lead to understanding of ego defences
- to be a vehicle for self-expression.

Additional advantages of using painting as an explorative medium are that:

- it provides a wealth of material that

contributes to the overall profile of the client and helps towards understanding of his difficulties
- used in conjunction with group psychotherapy it intensifies the group experience
- there are numerous techniques in art that offer different ways of communicating
- previous experience with art is neither a help nor a hindrance to the group participant
- pictorial interpretation by the individual with the help of the group and the therapist allows access to distress, low self-esteem and strength of feeling that the patient may have difficulty expressing verbally
- the simplest paintings are often the most meaningful, for example, a tiny featureless man drawn in stick-figure style in the middle of a vast sheet of white paper allows projection of many feelings by group members
- if paintings are kept, changes can be seen over the course of time. For example, a person may progress from very concrete or defensive forms to freer use of materials. Frequently a resurrection of defences can be seen as people are about to be discharged, in the form of idyllic scenes, rosy futures or a phoenix rising
- the organisation of the session allows for maximum participation.

Organising a painting session

Prior to a painting group, consultation with the treatment team takes place to identify the predominant themes that the group needs to work on and to decide what theme the group's attention could most usefully be directed towards. Paper and paint are supplied and the room is arranged to accommodate the correct number of people. Valuable group time can be wasted by ignoring basic organisation.

When the group assembles, the occupational therapist explains the choice of theme, sets the time limit for the painting part of the session and answers any questions. During painting, informal conversation continues and those who want help may seek out the therapist. Each group lasts 1½ hours, with the time being divided fairly equally between painting and discussion. Upon completion of the practical part of the activity the paintings are put up on a pin board for all to see while they talk about them.

Some therapists prefer to ask each patient individually about his work and its significance, while others reiterate the theme and wait for spontaneous participation. It is at this stage that group phenomena become evident through the paintings, in similar interpretations of the theme, use of colour, a tendency to use particular symbols, or splitting the paper into halves or quarters with different aspects portrayed in each section. It is useful to draw attention to these features for mutual reflection, and the visual language often has an enabling effect on the group.

At the end of the group, a summary is given by the therapist about the use of the theme and significant features that occurred in the group. The therapist also requests to be allowed to keep the paintings so they can be reviewed by the team prior to the next group.

Useful work can also be done with the client at some stage of treatment by showing him the series of paintings he has produced during his membership of the group and reviewing any progress and change of behaviour and attitude he has made.

Poetry

Leedy (1960) is probably the best known exponent of poetry as therapy and his books are comprehensive texts on the various client groups who can be helped using poetry. In group psychotherapy the aim is to achieve the maximum therapeutic effect by using selected poems as a focus for the group. Clarification of feelings, recognition of mutual difficulties or stimulation of alternative viewpoints or

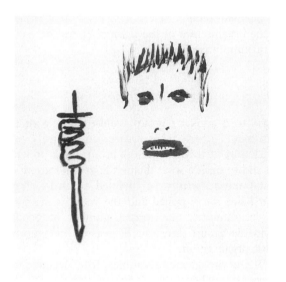

Fig. 13.2 A painting that allowed projection by all members and raised the questions of whether the painting conveyed rage or anger, was suicidal or homicidal. Contrast was made between the quiet unassuming stance of the man who painted this and the pictorial evidence before the group.

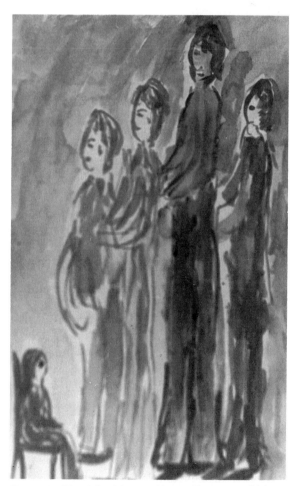

Fig. 13.3 Pictorial evidence of low self-esteem, which illustrates how this girl felt in relation to high-achieving siblings.

insight can occur. Affleck (1977) described the use of poetry, in a unit for the treatment of alcoholism, as a catalyst to assist self-understanding.

Literature contains a vast number of poems that describe every nuance of emotion and relationship. Poems are selected by the therapist, in discussion with other staff, for a specific purpose to coincide with the group's development, pace and learning potential. Selection depends upon the skill of the therapist in accurately interpreting the group dynamics.

The special characteristics of poetry as therapy are that:

- poetry allows an exploration of individual feeling and group dynamics
- the session offers the participants something concrete, which puts them at ease in the group
- the poem gives words to describe concepts, situations or events with which people can identify
- skilful choice of material can accelerate the pace of a group and leads to an awareness of the potential for change.

Organising a poetry session

A poetry session may be run in different ways but, most commonly, two poems are presented. They may highlight different relationship needs, indicate conflicting feelings or show a progression from one feeling state to another. Members read both poems silently and make a choice, and a consensus decision is taken on which poem to use. At this point the therapist asks someone to read the poem aloud and thereafter conducts the group with the assistance of the co-therapist and other staff.

Music

Music is often considered to be the most universal of all the arts. Its influence on the mind and body has been recorded from the earliest time. Music affects mood, and is therefore particularly suited to a context in which feelings are explored and communication with others encouraged.

Alvin (1966) states, 'the group offers an opportunity to observe individual and group reactions and interpersonal relationships within a collective musical experience.' She describes psychological responses to music, including stimulation of communication, identification with the feeling state, and imagery. Tears, discomfort and fidgeting, or panic may be evoked in response to music, depending upon its association with memories or moods.

CASE EXAMPLE 13.2

This small group consisted of seven clients specifically selected from an acute admission ward to explore common issues.

The aim of the session was to introduce poems that might get in touch with feelings underlying the group's insecurity, in particular, loneliness and ambivalence.

The poems chosen by the therapist were:

- 'Loneliness' by Sarah Churchill
- 'Questions', which had been written by a client some weeks previously.

The poem 'Questions' was chosen by the majority, although the decision was taken to discuss the other poem if time permitted.

Nina read the poem and stated that she was unsure of what she had to do in order to change. This statement precipitated the emergence of one of the main group themes: change. Is it necessary, do we want to change and is it worth it? Main participants were Jean, Jessie, Dorothy and John.

On the staff's comments that the group was finding communication difficult, there seemed to be a determined effort to make the group work, with many people volunteering information about themselves through the poem. Many used the poet's description of his feelings to describe their own situation, particularly in relation to marital difficulties.

Caroline was invited to speak by Jean and said that she was confused by the line 'How can I curb a wandering mind?' She began to cry and rushed to the door. She was prevented from leaving by two group members, but was trembling and tearful.

Others shared feelings of being lost and vulnerable, and the sense of panic arising from being aware of bad feelings but doing one's utmost to avoid them.

The group concluded on a sharing warm note of empathy.

In the Uffculme clinic in Birmingham in the 1970s music was used to augment group psychotherapy in the treatment of specific groups of neurotic clients. The main objective was to provoke fantasies, release emotion and enable the client to verbalise strong feelings.

Music can recall to mind sensations such as smell, touch or even colour. 'Desert Island Discs', the popular radio programme, brought out the associative power of music in both guest and audience.

Imagery and fantasy responses are also frequent, and are described as visual images, for example:

- Mr X described the music as evoking images of waves engulfing him, until the end of the piece when he managed to break free and then felt himself to be running through a thick wood and battling to get out
- Mrs Y described a lonely hillside with a far horizon upon which her family were lined up, far away and unattainable but able to watch her.

The cathartic effect of music allows emotional release. Sometimes it reawakens a feeling for beauty, an unexpected ability to respond or nostalgia. Music often provokes verbalisation in a group, so that each member shares a common experience although the personal interpretation of the music is purely subjective.

Organising a music session

An analysis of the group is necessary before choosing a piece of music. Identifying the prevailing mood, feeling and stage of the group requires skill and close cooperation with the treatment team. A piece of music may be chosen to match the current group mood and encourage work on a specific topic or it may be required to change the mood in order to get the group past a block.

The room used should be quiet, warm and comfortable, with no distractions or interruptions. Members are invited to sit quietly and are given time to relax before the music is played. A good-quality cassette player is an advantage. The music is played for approximately 5 minutes, during which time a variety of behaviours may be seen. Rhythm may be followed by finger-or toe-tapping,

and direct emotional response or discomfort may be witnessed.

Following the music, there are a variety of ways of conducting the session depending upon the therapist's skill and style or on the culture of the unit. Each person may describe his response in turn, followed by general group discussion, or free-floating discussion may begin on completion of the music.

CASE EXAMPLE 13.3

Five patients met with the therapist, co-therapist and two students to use music in an attempt to understand why the group was having problems with communication.

The music chosen was 'Meditation' from 'Thais' by Massanet.

Each individual in the group responded to the music in his own way.

- *Kate* was in tears as soon as the music started and remained so throughout the music. Her mother had come back from holiday once and given her a musical doll which played the same tune, which now raised painful memories for her.
- *John* found the music very moving and as he spoke tears rolled down his face. He described seeing his wife sitting at the bottom of their garden, seeming so real it was hard to believe she was dead. He described how his wife had always been there at home for him to go back to—a peaceful person. He found it difficult to describe how he felt about her or to put it into words. He talked about the facade he built up after her death and how he hid his grief, only being able to cry alone. He continually fought back tears as he spoke.
- *Gordon*, also in tears, said he really felt for John. This great big man in tears was too much for him. The music made him see his wife walking away from the hospital as she had done the previous evening, walking out of his life.
- *Mhorag* tried to sympathise with John but she said that she could not appreciate how he felt. She subsequently withdrew from the group, saying the music conjured up no images for her, and she pointedly pretended to fall asleep.
- *Sadie* was silent for the majority of the session, after describing a forest scene where the sun shone only rarely through the branches.

This piece of music allowed a group to unblock their emotions. Information shared was important, personal and permitted a closeness that fuelled future groups towards useful change.

Clay modelling

Pottery has always been viewed as a very important activity in occupational therapy. Used in an explorative manner it yields a wealth of information about the inner life of a person.

Clay modelling features prominently in evaluative procedures developed by Shoemyen (1982) as part of the Shoemyen battery, which also includes finger painting, mosaic-tile work and sculpture. It is also part of the Goodman battery (Hemphill l982), which evaluates ego assets and deficits. This test includes copying a mosaic design, spontaneous drawing, figure drawing and, finally, the clay task.

Clay has considerable potential in enabling expression of inner feelings, the ease with which form can be changed or reversed being its most valuable feature. One interesting feature of clay work is the possibility of moving pieces of finished work around in relation to each other and looking at their relationships. A review of family relationships can be tackled in this way. Another interesting aspect of clay is the way that people suffering from eating disorders frequently model themselves as either grossly fat or small, formless and asexual.

Meares (1960) describes the therapeutic value of clay and some of the ways in which it can be used to achieve greater understanding of different client groups.

The significant features of clay modelling as a therapeutic medium are:

- it is three dimensional
- it is malleable
- it is passive and indestructible
- no technique or skill is required
- the tactile nature provides additional sensory and emotional benefits.

Organising a clay modelling session

A theme for the session is selected by the therapist, in consultation with the team, and described to the group. Time is allowed for knocking the clay into a suitable texture for working, then the practical manipulation of the clay begins.

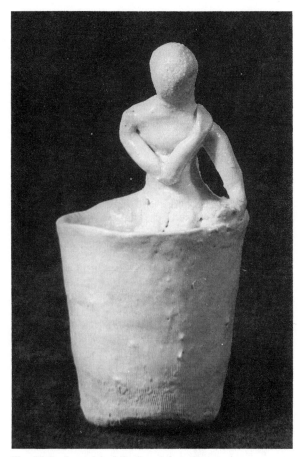

Fig. 13.4 A model of 'feeling defenseless and vulnerable'. The face has no features. The person who modelled this described it as 'a featureless character' who was like her.

After approximately 20 minutes items are placed in a central position in full view of all members, to be discussed.

This example shows how members of the group can use clay to make a variety of representations. Symbols are commonly used, for example a fearless lion, but lifelike figures are very often made. The 'angry mass' type of model, although not easy to interpret by the group, often contains the most potential for exploration and understanding of the individual.

WHO BENEFITS?

It is often felt by psychiatrists and other professionals that the only people who can benefit

CASE EXAMPLE 13.4

Five clients from an acute admission unit, diagnosed reactive depression, chronic anxiety, phobic states and personality disorder, were selected for explorative work in a small group.

The group was asked to model feelings that had been predominantly on their minds during the last week. Members seemed restless and excitable but, after initial reluctance, began to work.

- *Ann* modelled two figures, one smaller than the other, representing her husband and son. They looked stooped, dishevelled and dejected. She felt they missed her, and she, in turn, was missing them.
- *Teresa* modelled an abstract mass that she could not leave alone but angrily kept sticking her fingers or modelling tools into. She stated that this was 'festering anger'.
- *Bob* modelled a scene in which his own figure was strong and well proportioned. His wife was distorted, with two faces: one blank and one with an enigmatic expression. The figures were separated by a wall and a dead tree, which he interpreted as meaning that 'life is not a bed of roses'. He described feeling guilty because his wife was always full of sad resignation.
- *Fiona* modelled a lone figure that was youthful and vulnerable in appearance (Fiona was 53 years old).
- *Paul* modelled a lion, which, although outwardly fearless, was as cowardly as the lion from 'The Wizard of Oz.'

from psychotherapy are the young, intelligent and articulate but this assumption requires careful examination.

First, the work of psychotherapy is more emotional than intellectual and at no time in the life cycle do emotions cease to be important.

Second, many young people have difficulty in expressing feelings verbally but can often demonstrate, illustrate or talk through a variety of media.

The settings in which the combination of group psychotherapy and occupational therapy occur has already been described, including the types of problem found in those settings. However, as Luborsky et al (1975) conclude in their large-scale study of psychotherapy, it is difficult to prove scientifically which groups of people benefit most from a psychotherapeutic approach. It does seem that people suffering from neurotic conditions or personality disorders are most likely to improve with this approach. However, the elderly should not be excluded on the grounds of personality rigidity, sensory loss or inability to learn. The stereotypes of both psychotherapy and the elderly can prevent a lot of useful work being done.

Personal change is not the monopoly of one stratum of society. Case example 13.5 outlines the effect of a combination of group psychotherapy and occupational therapy on a shy, insecure girl, who had great difficulty expressing feelings.

What is evident from the example of Beatrice is that change is not a distinct event. Rather, the individual needs to reflect continually upon alterations in feeling and behaviour. Practice is needed to bring faulty responses under control until they become part of a more healthy adjustment.

EVALUATIVE MEASURES

METHODS OF ASSESSMENT

The most comprehensive account of methods of evaluating the explorative use of activities is to be found in Hemphill (1982) in the section on projective instruments. The Azima battery, introduced in 1960, attempted to explain the individual's inner world by encouraging the free creation of objects using three media: drawing, clay and finger painting. The scale was divided into:

1. organisation of mood
2. organisation of drives
3. organisation of ego
4. organisation of object relations.

This assessment is based on a psychodynamic frame of reference. The results can be used to help in treatment planning, differential diagnosis and prognosis.

The Shoemyen battery is an extensive and labour-intensive test involving four activities taking a maximum of 45 minutes each. It is well

CASE EXAMPLE 13.5

Beatrice was 22 years old. She worked in a sweet factory and lived with her parents, three brothers and two sisters. Her father was a butcher, described as pleasant, and her mother was a housewife who 'kept herself to herself', Beatrice was described as bossy at home, often dominating her parents.

A history of isolation at work, feelings of desperation and difficulties in her reaction to men were intensified by the sexual innuendo that featured in normal conversations at work. Over 3 years her problems had become worse. She had two hospital admissions within the last year, and stated her problems as:

- abuse of tablets
- loss of weight, vomitting, amenorrhoea and over-exercising
- poor social relationships
- an immature, dependent relationship with parents.

Beatrice was initially nervous and tense in the group, afraid and suspicious of staff and clients. In art sessions she would leave the paper blank. She stated that she had no response to music and that poetry was for schoolchildren. However, she enjoyed recreation, outings and yoga. At the end of her second week in the unit changes were noticeable. She began to write on the paper in art sessions and risked a few comments in the discussion part of the pottery group. As she gradually integrated into the group and her relationship with her individual therapist strengthened, defences began to weaken and, in the course of discussion, new features of the family came to light. In pottery she modelled her parents with numerous presents beside them, which she had given to buy their love.

At this stage she dressed in tomboyish clothes, although she made a considerable effort to look feminine for one ward social. When this was noticed and compliments came from fellow patients and one male staff member she rushed off to change and reappeared dressed in baggy trousers.

Information steadily accumulated about Beatrice, making her present coping mechanisms understandable. She began to trust, to take risks in approaching others and, with the group's support, to try out new forms of behaviour.

A development could be traced, particularly in her art work, from initial resistance, through tentative participation in treatment, to recognition of how she contributed to her own problems.

Beatrice became an important member of the group, and felt the experience allowed her to grow up. New confidence emerged, revealing a girl who had been under-achieving. Subsequently she began to apply for auxiliary nursing posts and decided to take further education.

The basic goals achieved by Beatrice were that she was able, with support from the group, to explore areas of confusion and ambivalence in her family relationships. Paint, clay and psychodrama were particularly useful in helping her to look at painful feelings. The outcome of therapy was an emotional re-education that enabled Beatrice to overcome her problems.

---

documented with detailed case histories (Hemphill 1982).

The Goodman battery (Hemphill 1982) also uses four media and in each the patient's ability to understand and organise the task is recorded.

A group evaluation was developed by Ehronberg (1982) in which the completion of each task required different degrees of group interaction. In essence it was an aid to treatment, planning and assessment and the group offered an increased number of behaviours that could be used to test functional ability.

Standardisation remains the biggest difficulty for rating scales, and for this a knowledge of research methodology is required. Increasingly, oc-cupational therapists are taking up training opportunities in research and it is now a part of most basic training courses in occupational therapy.

METHODS OF REPORTING AND RECORDING

Recording groups is very difficult because it is necessary to recall what was said and any important interactions, while at the same time interpreting the sequence of events. There are problems in deciding what was important enough to be recorded, noting therapists' reactions and detecting the feeling state of both individuals and the total group.

Different types of reporting and recording are needed for different aspects of the group. These can be divided into verbal and written accounts.

Verbal methods

Verbal methods of reporting depend on cultivation of a good memory for the sequence of events. It is often difficult to recall a group accurately, due to personal bias. Different staff members will often have different perceptions of the same event. Consequently, it is most useful to give a verbatim account of the group as far as possible, including what, where and how staff interjected or participated. This may seem tedious but it is necessary for the supervisor and other members of the team who were not present to receive as impartial an account as possible.

Staff review sessions

Following each organised session, feedback to significant team members takes place. Frequently the co-therapist or another staff member takes this responsibility, leaving the conductor the opportunity to receive feedback about the group from other staff who were there. A verbal report would include:

- a brief description of the task the group was given
- the group's reaction to the therapist's introduction
- how each group member responded to the medium used
- the level of individual participation
- the main interactions and dynamics within the group
- how the group was concluded.

Wherever possible, visual material in art, pottery or creative writing is shown at the review. A staff discussion ensues to allow understanding of the group, whether the aims were achieved and what the current stage of the group is.

This review session has an educational function for all staff by giving an opportunity for them to reflect upon their own participation or learn about the techniques of other disciplines.

Ward rounds

During a ward round the therapist needs to be able to summarise the involvement and progress of clients from the material gathered over a series of sessions. She may also be asked to give an opinion about a specific aspect of the client. Ideally, she will know beforehand who is to be discussed and go prepared, having read through all her notes.

Written methods

Different methods can be employed for permanent records of individual clients and of each group.

Kardex

Brief reports of each individual's participation, feeling state and relevant change will be entered into this personal record of the patient.

A profile is constructed to allow the objective reader an understanding of the response to treatment.

Group therapy interaction chronogram

This was devised by Cox (1973) who reviewed different techniques of recording group-therapy sessions. It is a visual aid that allows, at a glance, an awareness of who stays silent, whether the group was leader dominated or where the focus of activity stayed. For students, it is particularly useful in recognising patterns that occur in groups, and the significance of interactions.

Detailed group reports

In these reports, all observable phenomena are recorded. Group interactions, defensive form of behaviour and reactions to interpretations are written in sequence. This written account is of particular value for supervision sessions.

Following an explorative session, the following points are recorded:

- aims of the session

- media and the theme chosen
- what occurred during the activity period
- detailed accounts of the use of media plus discussion and interaction
- conclusions, including the sum-up at the end by the therapist.

Group reports are kept together in a folder or book and read by staff to familiarise themselves with the stage of the group (Tuckman 1965) or to find clues to understanding current group phenomena.

THE CHALLENGE OF RESEARCH

There is a paucity of reliable research findings in the combination of group psychotherapy and occupational therapy.

Luborsky et al (1975) extensively recorded comparisons of the psychotherapies against one another and against other treatments, and indicated the difficulties in conclusively proving success for any one treatment approach.

In 1980, Crown discussed the future of psychotherapy and, while acknowledging formidable methodological problems, felt that the ideal setting for continued research was in teaching hospitals or in the psychiatric wards of general hospitals. He also stressed the need for a multidisciplinary research group.

Thousands of people are treated as outpatients using group psychotherapy, another area where activity and pursuit of self-awareness could be combined. Areas for research include considering which clients might benefit from this approach and for how long, and what the selection process might be.

Traditionally, the middle aged and the elderly were considered unsuitable for a psychotherapeutic approach. The value of combining reminiscence with activity for the elderly intensifies the experience and suggests another potential research area.

SUMMARY

This chapter has sought to clarify the different levels at which psychotherapy, and in particular group psychotherapy, can be used, from a supportive approach to an explorative one. All these levels of approach are used by occupational therapists, and the chapter has attempted to explain the relationship between group psychotherapy and some techniques used in occupational therapy. Important points include:

- the history and nature of group psychotherapy
- the complementary nature of occupational therapy and group psychotherapy
- the contribution of occupational therapy to the ethos in an explorative psychotherapy unit
- the individual characteristics of a variety of creative media used as projective techniques
- the necessity for supervision from an experienced practitioner when using techniques in an explorative manner
- the importance of effective communication between team members working in group psychotherapy
- the need for accurate records of group events and progress.

Personal change requires that a balance be maintained between the wish to adapt and the need for time to adjust to change. Occupational therapy in the context of explorative group psychotherapy is offered as an opportunity to rehearse emotional changes, to integrate the conscious with the unconscious mind and to strengthen the personality.

REFERENCES

Affleck I 1977 Poetry as medium in a unit for the treatment of alcoholism. British Journal of Occupational Therapy 40: 11

Alvin J 1966 Music Therapy. W & J Mackay, Kent

Azima H, Cramer F, Wittkower E D 1957 Analytic group art therapy. International Journal of Group Psychotherapy 7: 243–260

Azima G, Azima J 1959 Outline of a dynamic theory of occupational therapy. American Journal of Occupational Therapy 13: 5

Batchelor L J 1970 The occupational therapist as therapeutic medium. Scottish Journal of Occupational Therapy. 83: 16–28

Bion W. R 1961 Experience in groups. Tavistock Publications, London

Blair S. E. E. 1974 Projective techniques:—their application within a group psychotherapy situation. Transcript of the proceedings of the World Federation of Occupational Therapists' Congress, Canada

Bloch S 1977 Supportive psychotherapy. British Journal of Hospital Medicine 16: 637

Brown D, Pedder J 1979 Introduction to psychotherapy. Tavistock, London

Clark D H 1977 The therapeutic community. British Journal of Psychiatry 131: 553–564

Cox M 1973 The group therapy interaction chronogram. British Journal of Social Work 3: 2

Crown S 1980 The future of the psychotherapies. In: M Lader (ed) Priorities in psychiatric research. John Wiley

De Mare P B, Kreegar L C 1974 Introduction to group treatments in psychiatry. Butterworth, London

Ehronberg F 1982 Comprehensive assessment process: a group evaluation. In: Hemphill (ed) The evaluation process in psychiatric occupational therapy. Slack, New Jersey

Fidler G, Fidler J 1963 Occupational therapy: a communication process in psychiatry. MacMillan, New York

Foulkes S H 1964 Therapeutic group analysis. Allen & Unwin, London

Frank J O 1961 Persuasion and healing. Johns Hopkins, Baltimore

Freud S 1921 Group psychology and the analysis of the ego. In: Civilization, society and religion. Penguin, Harmondsworth

Hemphill B J 1982 The evaluation process in psychiatric occupational therapy. Slack, New Jersey

Jones M 1968 Social psychiatry in practice: the idea of the therapeutic community. Penguin, Harmondsworth

Leedy J J 1960 Poetry therapy. Lippincott, Philadelphia

Luborsky L, Singer B, Luborsky 1975 Comparative studies of psychotherapy. Archives of General Psychiatry 32, August 1975

McFeely G 1985 The primary activity group: projective techniques in the psychoanalytic setting. Unpublished project held at Department of Occupational Therapy, Queen Margaret College, Edinburgh

Main T F 1946 The hospital as a therapeutic institution. Bulletin of Menninger Clinic 10: 66–70

Malcolm M 1975 Art as a projective technique. British Journal of Occupational Therapy 38: 7

Meares A 1960 Shapes of sanity. Charles C Thomas, Illinois

Meyerowitz K 1979 Group therapy: philosophical and practical considerations. South African Journal of Occupational Therapy May 1979

Moreno J L 1948 Psychodrama. Beacon, New York

Pratt J H 1907 The class method of treating consumption in the homes of the poor. Journal of the American Medical Association 49: 755–59

Remocker A J, Storch E T 1982 Action speaks louder. Churchill Livingstone, Edinburgh

Robinson E 1984 The role of the occupational therapist in a psychotherapeutic setting. British Journal of Occupational Therapy 47(4)

Shoemyen C 1982 The Shoemyen battery in the evaluative process. In: Hemphill B the evaluative process in psychiatric occupational therapy. Slack, New Jersey

Stockwell R 1984 Creative therapies. In: Moya Willson (ed) Occupational therapy in short-term psychiatry. Churchill Livingstone, Edinburgh

Tuckman 1965 Development sequence in small groups. Psychological Bulletin 63: 384

Walton H (ed) 1971. Small group psychotherapy. Penguin, Harmondsworth

Yalom I D 1970 Theory and practice of group psychotherapy. Basic Books, New York

Drama and occupational therapy

Teresa Brown

INTRODUCTION

Drama has been defined as 'A composition in prose or verse, adapted to be acted on the stage in which a story is related by means of dialogue and action, and is represented with accompanying gesture, costume and scenery as in real life.' (OED)

Using drama as a medium allows the therapist to treat a wide range of disorders because it does not depend on the intellectual or emotional development of the client group.

Drama techniques can be used to treat young or old, mentally or physically disabled. They can be employed in teaching and training with the professions.

Drama provides the possibility to identify not only the presenting difficulties but also the means to work through the feelings and emotions involved and it is a vehicle for change. The individual has the opportunity to conduct a 'rehearsal for life' within the dramatic setting. He can create his own world and experience it afresh with a view to exploring new methods of coping and being.

DRAMA IN OCCUPATIONAL THERAPY

Drama is about people: communication and creativity. It was created by the Ancient Greeks and used in the teaching of religion throughout the centuries.

'By its very nature, drama presupposes communication—and this is the primary social process' (Courtney 1974).

A HISTORICAL PERSPECTIVE

Drama was used to soothe the sick as early as the 5th century AD, but the modern use of drama as treatment can be credited to Moreno. With the development of psychiatry and the emergence of psychoanalytical techniques in the early part of the 20th century Moreno began to define psychodrama formally. He claims to have enacted the first psychodrama on 1 April 1921 between 7 and 10 p.m. before an audience of 1000 people from varying cultures and backgrounds in a theatre in postwar Vienna. His inspiration for the use of drama as therapy came from watching children in a Viennese park. He observed the ease with which they acted out the roles of society within their microcosm.

Many techniques used in group psychotherapy, Gestalt therapy, play therapy and drama therapy have their roots in the psychodrama developed by Moreno.

The development of drama as therapy

The 1960s and the 1970s saw a great vogue for drama as a therapeutic medium. Occupational therapists were already using the arts as a therapeutic tool and by the nature of their work, particularly in psychiatry, they were beginning to incorporate drama into the treatment programme.

During this time occupational therapists were encouraged in the use of projective techniques in their training and in their work with clients. In Freudian theory projection is an ego defence mechanism where the subject invests another person with desired qualities or externalises on to the non-self those things that are unacceptable in the self.

Therein lies the rationale for the use of the arts to establish a therapeutic relationship with the client through involvement in activities such as art, poetry, music, pottery, dance and drama. Clients were encouraged within a group setting to project their feelings into an art theme, a poem, a piece of clay or action in drama and by doing so would gain insight and understanding into their personalities, behaviour and communication processes. The use of drama by occupational therapists was part of an established tradition of teaching recognising that the activity mirrored the persona.

THERAPEUTIC RATIONALE

Therapy is any treatment aimed at curing or reducing the effects of a physical or mental disorder. The occupational therapist is trained in a holistic approach to the client and tailors the available techniques to the individual's needs.

The ability for self-expression is often reduced or absent in the client encountered by the occupational therapist. By using drama the therapist can set the scene for the client to enact and express the emotion that might otherwise remain suppressed. Drama is one of the few media that allow the individual a freedom of expression irrespective of communication skills or sensory disabilities.

Rogers (1984) emphasised the need for a client-centred approach and believed in the full potential of each individual.

The creation of a supportive and caring environment allows the individual to recognise his needs and difficulties and to begin the process of healing. This facilitates an awareness of responsibility and a degree of self-reliance for the client, which fosters a sense of independence.

Nevertheless, within the foregoing structure important underlying dynamic issues, such as ego defence mechanisms and unresolved parental issues require understanding. Given the opportunity to effect change, the individual is often forced to confront unresolved conflicts and emotional issues that are so far unarticulated.

Psychodrama

A psychoanalytical approach works with the unconscious and suggests that the client 'tell me' about the problem; a psychodramatic approach allows him to 'show me'. In 'showing', by enacting his difficulties, the client experiences a number of differing aspects of himself and his relationship with others.

A psychodynamic and a psychodramatic approach to the individual can be combined, as the individual's enactment is the most realistic way of expressing the problem to himself and others. It generates a great sense of self-awareness that is often not achieved in other forms of therapy.

The therapist must, however, possess detailed knowledge of psychoanalytical principles. Without any theory or guidance to identify the source and disorder of the individual's personality development, the therapist will be working in a vacuum. There is little point in directing the drama if the action fails to reach a critical audience.

Drama as a creative therapy

'Creative therapy' is a relatively modern term that encompasses a vast array of artistic media, such as poetry, art, pottery, dance, music and drama. These creative therapies differ from the projective techniques in that they may not rely solely·on psychoanalytical principles. Indeed, many therapists may find themselves using creative therapies within a medical model of psychiatry that pays little or no heed to Freudian psychodynamics.

The therapist must adopt an eclectic approach and may decide to work within a developmental or occupational behaviour type of model. Most occupational therapists cannot afford the luxury of a rigid psychiatric school of thought; instead adopting a broad-based approach to the client in treatment can help to offset some of the more dogmatic views arising elsewhere in the treatment programme.

USING DRAMA IN OCCUPATIONAL THERAPY

The clients

Clients are selected according to their needs; this does not preclude psychotically ill clients but the recovering schizophrenic is more likely to benefit from drama in therapy than the overtly manic or floridly schizophrenic individual who is admitted in a psychotic state.

Referral patterns may vary and admission into the occupational therapist's treatment programme can be anything from blanket referral to specific individual referrals.

Broadly speaking the decision to engage the client in drama therapy will depend on the occupational therapist and her relationship with the multidisciplinary team. She may choose to run the drama therapy with a member of the team as it is preferable not to work in isolation. The therapist must communicate with the other members of the treatment team the client interacts with in order to treat the individual completely.

There is hardly an area of occupational therapy that a therapist cannot adapt and use in or for drama in therapy. Drama can be used with people who have physical or emotional illness or mental handicap, and with the elderly, children and adolescents. It is a therapeutic tool that can be used and applied within the occupational therapist's treatment programme in a variety of ways. It is not possible to identify all of these in one chapter but a wealth of literature is available (Langley 1983, Jennings 1987, Blatner 1980, Remocker and Storch 1987, Jennings 1983).

COMMUNICATING WITH OTHER PROFESSIONALS

The groups described in the following sections all take place once a week in a ward-based programme. They are an integrated part of ward life and each one is written up either in a group book or the individual's involvement, response and progress is written up in the nursing Kardex. Groups are always reported back to each multidisciplinary team meeting every week and to the nurses on shift at the end of each group. Much of the work of groups, particularly drama-oriented groups, happens in the spaces between the groups; in the quiet of the evening or the loneliness of a weekend on the ward. In this time, the nurses have one-to-one involvement with the client and need feedback from the occupational therapy sessions to integrate the work together. It is, therefore, almost impossible, and certainly not advisable, to work in isolation.

Despite the difficulties of professional envy and role blurring it should be possible to find ways of communicating in the staff team, otherwise client care will suffer and little progress will be made. The therapist using drama in therapy is working towards enabling the individual to reach his full potential, to be independent within himself, to make his own decisions and to be responsible for himself as far as possible. This is not always easy in a medical-model ward where, by the very nature of the treatments on offer, the individual sometimes is encouraged to be dependent rather than independent. It is therefore even more important that clients have a place in the ward to call their own, to find their voices and to be enabled to take part in their own recovery.

Treatment programmes

The four sections that follow look at two types of treatment programme.

1. A ward-based treatment programme in an acute admission setting, with sections on three types of group:
   - a contact group
   - an art group
   - a group for the elderly.
   These groups have been selected to show how drama can be used with a wide range of age groups and client types.
2. A day-care programme in an analytical psychotherapy unit, describing a psychodrama group.

A CONTACT GROUP

The group is suitable for an acute admission ward, with its rapid turnover and wide variety of clients. It gives the therapist a useful setting in which to observe clients' interpersonal skills, as well as giving clients an opportunity to explore their own problems.

Aims

This group is designed to:

- provide a structured and supportive environment, in which the individual can be encouraged to identify his needs
- create opportunities for the client to learn about how he relates to others and how they relate to him
- explore new methods of coping
- improve social interaction skills.

CLIENT SELECTION

The clients for this type of group can be drawn from most of the neurotic illnesses, some phases of psychotic illness and other problems found in an acute admissions ward, such as eating disorders and drug and alcohol dependence.

A useful precursor is an open access group consisting of Keep Fit and Relaxation. These techniques involve physical activity and provide a valuable monitor for the motivation of the individual, as well as allowing the therapist to assess the mood, behaviour and communication of each person and the dynamics of the group as a whole.

COMMUNICATION OF AIMS

Having selected suitable clients, the therapist must then explain the aims of the group at the outset, for example, by saying, 'This is the contact group. It is designed to bring you into contact with each other in the ward. It is your group and your time to talk with each other and learn about what brought you into hospital and what part you can play in your recovery'.

This information may need to be repeated at every meeting because the therapist will carry the burden of engendering trust within the group, which, by its nature, will change in character and population as clients are admitted and discharged from the unit.

GROUP COMPOSITION

The group must accommodate an age spectrum from adolescence to elderly, and the therapist must select her dramatic material accordingly. The ideal number of people in a group is 8–12 but there may often be as many as 15 in a contact group, depending on need.

ORGANISING THE GROUP

The group should meet twice a week, for 1–1½ hours, depending on the needs of the clients, as an integrated part of the treatment programme.

In the contact group, it is important to keep the time, place and person leading the group consistent. It may be useful to have a contact group at the beginning and at the end of a week. Most wards operate on a principle of weekend passes and individuals need space, time and opportunity to talk about how the connection between hospital and home has been made.

It is very helpful to have a day-care programme integrated into the ward programme where clients can be discharged from inpatient care to day patient care for a graded period of time, for example, 2 weeks, then 3 days for 3 weeks, then 2 days, etc. until the transition is completed in as helpful a way to the client as possible.

An individual's time in hospital can range from 6 weeks to 2 months or more, during which time he may experience weekend passes and slowly build up his confidence to return to his world of family, job, commitment, unemployment or fear and loneliness. He needs time, discussion and constructive help in working towards the independence necessary for the transition between hospital and home. In the contact group he may now have established himself as a person in his own right, made positive relationships with others, yet still be lacking in self-esteem. The therapist may adopt the following approach.

RUNNING THE GROUP

Open groups, that is, groups with a changing membership, go through various phases in their life cycle:

● *forming:* when new members become engaged in the group, communication processes are set up and trust is established

● *working:* the established group is able to focus on individuals' problems and work through them
● *separating:* in an established group at any time there may be clients in the process of leaving.

Whatever stage the group is at, each session is in three parts:

1. *warm-ups:* these can be verbal and/or physical
2. *working:* this usually takes the form of exercises and games that follow the warm-ups
3. *winding down:* group members must be given the opportunity to recover from any strong feelings before leaving the group.

Warm-ups

The purpose of a warm-up is to get the group members used to being together, concentrating, listening and sharing. Warm-ups can take as long as needed to get the individual engaged in action, usually a minimum of 15 minutes. If there is a particular emotion present in the group, for example, sadness, the warm-up can be used to promote awareness of this and other related feelings in a constructive and supportive manner.

Warm-ups are selected by the therapist and tailored to suit the needs of the individuals in the group. There may be an overall group theme, particularly connected to the life of the ward, for example, change of staff. Perhaps a well-respected and important member of the treatment team has moved to another job; the therapist's task would be to get in touch with the group members' feelings of loss, anger and disappointment, to choose a warm-up to elicit these feelings and to create an atmosphere in which they can be safely shared and discussed. She may choose to connect the feelings of concrete loss on the ward with feelings of loss in each individual's life. This theme may be pursued in subsequent groups.

Many warm-ups, can be used to involve people in action; talking is a form of action but doing and enacting the person's individual drama is going a step further. The individual learns through experiencing, and may gain insight into his behaviour and methods of communicating. He also needs to feel accepted by others, to feel he is being listened to, and he must get feedback from other people about how he behaves and interacts, in order to make changes if he chooses to.

The therapist may use a verbal warm-up to open the group. Verbal warm-ups are designed to focus clients' attention on the here-and-now reality of being in the group. Examples of such warm-ups include:

- 'Introduce yourself by name and say how you feel today.'
- 'Introduce the neighbour on your left and say how you think he might be feeling today.'
- 'Make one statement about the ward/hospital/day room.'

Once the therapist has established a therapeutic relationship within the new group she may use any of the examples above to start the group before moving on to engage clients in more spontaneous, playful exercises.

Working

When the therapist feels that the group is sufficiently warmed up, that is, the members feel comfortable enough to focus on more personal issues, she will use exercises designed to engage the imagination and the creative child within each individual. Examples of such exercises might be:

- The therapist instructs the group to 'Imagine you have a magic box. It can be any shape or form and it can contain anything you want at this present time: a feeling, a desire or an object'.

The therapist may choose to demonstrate by identifying her own box, outlining its shape and form and declaring its contents to the group. If group members are struggling with the use of imagination the therapist can ask them to help each other, for example, an individual may be suffering from poverty of thought or difficulty in concentrating. It is by trying to help a neighbour that each individual finds himself behaving spontaneously.

- The therapist instructs the group to 'Think of a flower/fish/tree/bird. Look around the group to see which person most resembles this flower/fish/tree/bird and give one reason why'.

Individuals may offer this information spontaneously, depending on the mood of the group, or a round robin can be used.

The therapist uses these exercises to promote self-awareness, awareness of others and interaction within the group. She may choose to take them a step further into action and invite the members to enact a verbal exercise physically, for example:

- 'Show us your magic box. Stand up and let us see the size and shape. Does it have a lid? Is it locked? Where is the key?'

The therapist can invite other group members to ask about the box and its contents. She may ask the individual to choose another group member to show his box to when he is finished.

If the individual is experiencing difficulty in expressing himself then the therapist must make it safe for him to express himself without fear of judgement, ridicule or laughter. She may do this by entering into his world, with his permission, and working with him using her own inner child and spontaneity.

In an established contact group some clients may be in the process of leaving. This can be dealt with in the safe environment of the group by using a combination of verbal and physical exercises as follows:

- 'Make a statement about home, saying how it is different from hospital.'
- 'What is difficult about home for you, at present?'

Physical warm-up

The therapist may decide to divide people into pairs to discuss these themes in more detail. She may select the pairs herself, according to the abilities and needs of the individuals in the group, or she may invite the group members to select a partner. She gives them between 10 and 15 minutes to discuss the themes, and may need to keep herself objective and 'float' between the pairs, checking out their progress, or she may need to take on the least able or most disturbed or vulnerable person in the group. If she is fortunate enough to have a co-worker or visiting student

CASE EXAMPLE 14.1

After a verbal and a physical warm-up, as described above, the paired clients are invited to come back into sitting in a circle in the group and each half of a pair is invited to share their partner's fears and hopes.

Bill and Betty were paired off together. Bill introduced Betty and shared that she had told him she had been in hospital before on several occasions, as she had an illness marked by severe mood swings. On this occasion she had been depressed, followed by a period of elation. She was particularly worried about the debt she had incurred during her 'high', the embarrassment she had caused her friends, family and herself and the overriding fear that she would 'break down' again. When hearing her own thoughts spoken aloud she became more aware of them and despite her anxiety was able to share with the group her further fears concerning the wellbeing of the family: 'How was she going to cope when she went home?'

The group were invited to share their thoughts and feelings with Betty. Some remained silent, some identified openly with her and talked of their own experiences of hospitalisation and the joy mixed with the trauma of returning home to the responsibility of taking control of one's own life.

Betty then shared Bill's fears and hopes. He was a policeman who dreaded going back to work. He recognised that he had become almost mute prior to being admitted and had worked hard at the beginning not to talk about himself and his feelings. He was particularly worried about going back to work and facing his colleagues.

At this point, if there is sufficient time, the therapist can offer Bill the opportunity of experiencing his work scene if he wants to, as a rehearsal for living. If she and the group work together with the client's active permission and interaction they can create a space for learning through action.

For example, the therapist may say, 'Bill we hear you talk about your fear of going back to work. Can you show us?' She then asks Bill to set up his work scene and to show the group the room, using one area of the therapy room as a stage, (This may sound like psychodrama to the reader; it is a *part* of psychodrama tailored to suit the needs of this particular group. We will look at psychodrama in detail later on.)

The main aim of setting the scene and engaging the client in doing so is to desensitise him to an anxiety-provoking situation, that is, going back to work. The therapist can engage Bill and the other group members in the act of playing together in safety, experiencing the difficulties together. In this instance the therapist is focussing on the behaviour and communication of the clients involved. She is not necessarily looking for catharsis, as in psychodrama. However she needs to be aware of the underlying emotions and dynamics of the scene. Therapeutic drama is not about creating a crisis; it is designed to create a spontaneous space for people to be aware of their feelings, others' feelings and to acknowledge their strengths and weaknesses. The therapist must be aware of how to defuse a potentially inflammatory situation with skill, humour and professionalism.

In the scene with Bill he has been warmed up already by the action of pairing with Betty to discuss his difficulties about going home.

When he has set up his office, using the available furniture in the room, the main aim is to allow him to meet his fear in his own way. It is essential to check on how he feels throughout the drama. The therapist may ask Bill if he needs to meet someone in the office, and if so, 'Who is it?' 'Can we meet him?'

The therapist then invites Bill to be this person in role for a few minutes. If she senses he is reluctant she must look for the reason for his apprehension. It may be that the person he has chosen to role play is a powerful and difficult figure for him, perhaps a father figure. The therapist must use her clinical skill to ascertain whether it is useful to pursue this role or whether to encourage Bill to choose one person he feels supported by in his workplace. It is better to go with the client from a position of strength. If the therapist can encourage Bill to take on the role of someone for whom he has positive regard it can also put him in touch with that role within himself, that is the part of himself that he can still feel positive about. By allowing Bill to be this person in role she is enabling him to experience and experiment with the healing part of his psyche.

How does the therapist do this? She asks Bill to be the person and then interviews him in role by inviting other group members to ask questions. She may start by asking, 'Who are you?' 'What's your name?' 'How old are you?' and 'Where are you just now?' until Bill is in

(Continued on p. 218.)

(Case example 14.1 continued)

role as his friend. Another alternative is to say, 'Tell me about yourself', 'How would you describe yourself?'

It is important to engage the other group members in this process so that they are also involved in the communication and spontaneity of the action.

Once in role as his friend Joe, Bill became 'alive' and talked about his work in the police force, his family and his life. He was then asked about Bill and, for a brief moment in time, through action and by enacting his situation dramatically, he was freed to express that part of himself that was also like Joe. The therapist then reversed roles and the group talked to Bill about himself, acknowledging with him that he himself did possess these positive thoughts and feelings.

they can share the task. (Visiting students from differing disciplines need to know, prior to the group starting, that they may be involved in the pairing off.)

Individuals are asked to share with each other their fears and hopes about going home and are asked to remember their discussion as it will be shared in the group.

There are many ways to go on the journey with the client. The therapist can only work with him in relation to how far she has come herself, for example, it is very difficult to meet death in drama if we have not experienced it ourselves. We learn from the client, our relationship with him and the journey we take together.

With Bill, in Case example 14.1, it was enough, at that time to experience the positive aspects of his relationship, himself, with Joe. It also fuelled the sharing process in the group with others and enabled them, by the drama they were involved in, to get in touch with some of the positive aspects of themselves.

It is important to acknowledge the limitations of the individual members, the group process and the therapist's own limitations and expectations of herself, and her expectations of the client group.

Winding down

The last few minutes of the session are spent in helping clients to calm down and prepare to leave the room. If the group has been particularly emotional, the winding down period will need to be longer, although in a supportive inpatient setting the winding down may actually be continued after the session ends.

Winding down exercises are often verbal, such as formally giving each person a chance to say how he feels. The therapist may summarise the events of the session, helping members to understand and integrate what has been happening, or she may invite a group member to give a summary.

Many drama exercises are designed to incorporate their own winding down period. For example, the discussion at the end of a role-play gives group members a chance to get out of role and return to the here and now.

Sometimes a non-verbal exercise is used to express a particular dynamic that has been important in the session, for example, a group hug could symbolise the warmth and sharing that has been evident between members. Laughter is also a very useful way to diffuse tense or difficult feelings that have not been adequately dealt with, and a non-verbal warm-up, such as a group tangle, can leave the group helpless with laughter.

An experienced therapist has a repertoire of winding down exercises so that she can use her skill and judgement to select an appropriate one or two with which to end the session.

Within the group described in Case example 14.1 there were eight people, suffering in different degrees from disturbances in thought, volition, mood, behaviour and communication. Careful selection ensured that no clients in this group were overtly psychotic, and yet these people also require treatment. The following section shows how this can be given.

AN ART GROUP

An activity that has been found most useful to the overtly psychotic client is the art group. Acting out is done mainly on paper rather than with the whole body, since this would be very threatening for this particular client group. In fact, clients may attend this group until they are well enough to join the contact group described above. The warm-ups and exercises used are carefully graded to meet individual client needs in the same way that any activities are graded.

With the actively psychotic client, the therapist must be aware of the following factors:

- the group must be structured, and yet free enough to allow spontaneity to develop
- warm-ups and exercises should be concrete and simple to follow, and reality orientated
- verbal and non-verbal support must be given by the therapist; because of the nature of psychosis, the individual's thought processes, methods of communicating and behaviour may affect his active participation in the activity
- the activity must be low key; people with psychosis are easily overstimulated by too much activity, interaction and emotion.

Bearing these factors in mind the therapist can create a group specifically tailored to suit the needs of this particular client type.

ORGANISING THE GROUP

This is a flexible group that can last from 45 minutes to $1\frac{1}{2}$ hours. When a client is newly admitted the therapist meets with him, however briefly, and introduces herself and the treatment programme. From that moment, each time she engages with him is important as it is the route to engaging him in the therapeutic relationship.

At the beginning of new group the therapist may leave the door open, encourage the selected group members to work together in setting up the room, inviting them to push the tables together to make one big table and to set up the paints, pencils, crayons and paper. It is within her discretion to set up prior to the group starting, depending on the needs of the clients.

She needs to recognise that some individuals may only stay for 5 minutes, some longer. It is essential to provide an atmosphere of calm, acceptance and trust in order to enable the person to feel safe with the reality of the room and the activity therein.

RUNNING THE GROUP

The therapist may introduce a new art group in the following manner, 'This is the art group. It meets once a week, every Wednesday afternoon. It is your group where you can talk with each other, paint, listen to music or learn about yourselves and your relationships with others'.

A useful exercise with a new group is to invite each member to write or paint his own name in any way he chooses. This acts as a warm-up and orientates the group to the activity. She may then invite them to create a group collage on a theme, for example, 'likes and dislikes', making it concrete by giving a concrete example of her own, such as 'I like spring but I don't like winter'.

The group may use magazines and clients may search through them, cutting out suitable pictures of their own likes and dislikes. The activity becomes a means for communicating in the here and now, for example, simple requests, such as, 'Can I borrow the scissors?', 'Can I have some glue?' or 'Where's the paper?' are all orientated towards keeping the psychotically ill person aware of the present and communicating appropriately within the group.

The group decides how to create the collage. The therapist gently facilitates interaction among members by asking questions, such as, 'How can we do this?' 'Where will we put the paper—on the table or on the wall?', until the members are able to engage in working together for themselves.

Once the therapeutic relationship has been established the therapist may start a session by introducing a theme for clients to express on paper in their own way. She will rarely have a completely new set of clients and can encourage the more longstanding members to help the new ones.

A theme should be selected in the planning session prior to the group. A simple approach is to list the names of the proposed members of the group and beside each name make a clear statement about his present needs and how best to meet them, bearing in mind his diagnosis and stage of treatment and whether or not he is on medication. From this list, it becomes clearer what theme to suggest, for example, 'Myself at home', or 'Myself in hospital'.

CASE EXAMPLE 14.2 AN ESTABLISHED GROUP

Once an art group had been established and was continuing to work, in the fourth week, the therapist decided to introduce a theme for writing.

Each person was given a piece of paper (about the size of a sheet of writing paper) and invited to write about one of the following:

- the season of the year (they are presently in)
- a person I know
- a favourite pastime, possession, television programme or piece of music.

The theme was selected according to where the clients were in their treatment and progress.

One young man, Michael, admitted over a period of years for assessment and treatment of his psychotic behaviour and self-mutilation, wrote the following poem on the theme of 'A person I know'.

Two and two make three

Two and two made three
that's what bothered me.
In my life I searched to see
who was hiding the hidden key.

Maybe mum, maybe dad
whoever it was was very bad
that's what bothered me.
I often thought, 'Don't live anymore'

unless I could make my sum into four;
But no matter how I tried
no matter how I cried
My two and two made three;
that's what bothered me.

Life has got much better now
I don't really know the score,
Today when counting two and two
My two made four.

I've only just discovered,
After all this search of mine
The one who had it all along was me
I've had it all the time.

After writing this Michael was encouraged to share his thoughts and feelings about it within the group. Others were able to identify with him and talk through their own fears and feelings.

Michael was a very difficult client to treat. He repeatedly hurt himself and his family and yet it was obvious from the poem that he had insight and, however painful his life was, still possessed remarkable creativity. The drama is in the writing; the therapy is in the enactment of his feelings on paper and in the discussion that followed within the group. When last heard of, Michael was.well and working in a kibbutz in Israel.

A GROUP FOR THE ELDERLY

In an admission ward the therapist will be required to treat clients who have organic impairment in addition to the psychiatric problem they were admitted for. She may encounter people suffering from strokes, sensory impairment, burnt-out schizophrenia and dementia, as well as depression, paranoia, anxiety or other affective disorders.

This group is suitable for all clients aged 55 or over who have a combination of the above problems. It is designed to meet as many needs as possible in the client group. The group is usually in two stages, as described below.

ORGANISING THE GROUP

The session should consist of two parts:

- music and movement for 30–40 minutes
- a break for 10 minutes, for tea
- a discussion for 20–30 minutes.

The session lasts approximately 1½ hours in total.

Setting up the room

The therapist is advised to set up the room 15 minutes before the group starts because of the practicalities of motivating and encouraging the client to move from his bed/sitting room/chair to the group room, and to allow the less able time to walk there or be helped there.

The therapist should set out the correct number of chairs in a circle; her choice of music, using a tape recorder or record player; and tea, coffee, biscuits, cups, saucers, kettle, etc.

It is useful to have a room with a lock, to keep

other clients out, not the current group in. The therapist should always let the group members know there is a lock and ask their permission to use it, stating why, for example, 'We need to be free from interruption in this session. This is the lock. This is how it works. Does anyone mind if we use it for this treatment session?' If there are objections, the lock should not be used.

It is also useful to have curtains or blinds to shut out the light. Again, do not assume this is all right with the client group. Explain why you are closing the curtains, for example, 'We are closing the curtains during relaxation to shut out the light and encourage people to relax in a calmer, darkened room by shutting out the external stimuli.' Always speak to the client in language that will be acceptable to him and understood by him.

RUNNING THE GROUP

It is essential, when working with this very disabled group of clients, to choose a non-threatening activity, such as movement to music, that is familiar to everyone. There is a range of activities that can be selected from the general category of music and movement, keep-fit and relaxation. The therapist should note the following points when making her selection.

- Choose simple exercises that can be carried out while sitting in a chair. The therapist will use herself as a model and encourage each individual to mirror her.
- Choose music of an era that the clients will identify with, for example, the Glen Miller Orchestra, which has a good beat and is familiar to the clients.
- Warm the group up by engaging each person individually while doing the exercises.
- Make the exercises repetitive but simple, and concentrate on each area of the body in turn. This, in itself, orientates each individual to the activity and allows them to enter reality safely.
- Not everyone will be able to do everything so pitch it at the level of the least able initially and grade it accordingly to the needs of the individuals.

Part 1: Movement and music

The therapist may begin a session by stating the following:

'This is the group for the older members of the ward/young at heart.' or 'This is a special group for the people in it.'

'Our first task is to loosen up the stiffness in the joints from sitting in chairs and lying in bed, to feel our bodies working again, and then to talk with each other about how it feels to be in hospital, away from home.' In this way, the therapist uses music and movement as a warm-up to the discussion.

A useful warm-up, after the basic exercises, might be for the therapist to say, 'Can we have a movement from everyone? It doesn't matter what kind of movement, from the little finger to the big toe. Any movement that the group can follow.'

If someone finds it difficult to begin, the therapist may start herself and then say to the person on her left or right, 'Let's see your movement'. This engenders involvement, participation and stimulation. The more able can help the least able in as unobtrusive a way as possible. The group dynamics mean that clients are rarely allowed to opt out.

This exercise can be adapted in many ways, for example, if there are approximately 10 people in the group there are a lot of exercises to remember, but it can become a memory game, for example, 'Can the group remember who started today? What was their movement? Who finished last?'

It is helpful to use a similar piece of music each week as it stimulates the individual to remember. Music can be a very useful tool. It can be used in reminiscence work, to stimulate discussion and to engage spontaneity.

The tea break

It is often enough in the way of stimulation and concentration to have all members together for the first 30 minutes and then break for tea. During the tea break the more overtly disturbed and less-orientated clients may enjoy the social aspect of tea and spontaneous communication before leaving to allow the others time and freedom to talk without having to accommodate repetitive behaviour and communication difficulties.

Much can be picked up and assessed as to the mood of the group during the tea-break. Individuals should be encouraged to organise it themselves: make the tea, set the tables and put out the biscuits. It is in these little rituals that people gain self-awareness, self-esteem and security in a strange environment. It is also interesting to note who takes on what task and role within the group process.

Part 2: The discussion

The therapist may choose to pick up the threads of what is discussed over tea and use it in her selection of a medium and theme for the second part of the session, the discussion. She may choose a poem for the group members to discuss, or a piece of music selected by a member of the group. An ongoing theme is also useful, for example, following the seasons of the year, using music, poetry and drama to enact them.

CASE EXAMPLE 14.3   USING ROLE PLAY

During a discussion amongst a group of five elderly individuals in the ward it came to light that William felt his grandson just did not understand him. This was a source of great sorrow and anger to William and the moment of spontaneity arrived in which the space was available for movement and action.

The therapist invited William to be his grandson for a moment:

'Be John. Let us meet John'

and, in the method explained earlier in the chapter, the group met their own grandchildren and family through William's meeting John.

When the therapist reversed roles and John became William again there was a greater understanding of the ever-present adolescent within William (as in everyone) and an insight into the communication breakdown between the two people concerned.

There was an active discussion after this role play, in which the group members reminisced about their own youths and exploits, and experienced the joy, pleasure and anguish of being young and now growing old, to face dependence, ill-health, loss and death.

By being enabled to get in touch with their own inner strength, they were able to face the future with a little more optimism in view of what they had achieved in the past.

PSYCHODRAMA IN AN ANALYTICAL PSYCHOTHERAPY DAY UNIT

'Psychodrama is the method by which a person can be helped to explore the psychological dimensions of his problems through the *enactment of* his conflict situations, rather than by talking about them.' (Blatner 1980).

The development of psychodrama was essentially the work of one man, Dr Jacob Levy Moreno (1892–1969).

Psychodrama started off in Vienna and was introduced in the USA in 1925. Since then a number of clinical methods have been developed which owe their origins and beginnings to the work of Moreno: the therapeutic psychodrama, the sociodrama, gestalt therapy, dramatherapy, role playing and various modifications of these.

Psychodrama has a theoretical base which integrates psychodynamic theory with the dimensions of experiential and participatory involvement. Like occupational therapy, it is an eclectic form of therapy, based on the recognition that each client has a unique set of challenges, abilities and needs requiring a variety of methods of intervention.

THE CLIENTS

In the psychotherapy day unit clients are carefully selected and assessed according to their needs, difficulties and ego strengths. Clients are usually referred by their general practitioner, consultant psychiatrists or members of the treatment team. Clients usually present with forms of neurosis, such as anxiety, depression or agoraphobia, and understand that their main difficulties lie in their relationships with others.

The group described in this section is using psychodrama in conjunction with analytical psychotherapy; clients range from 24–36 years of age, number approximately 6–10 people of mixed sex, and stay from 6 months to 2 years, attending for 3 days per week. Leaving is a group and a personal decision, which is the hardest part of being in the group.

In a psychotherapy day unit the clients are in an open group, in the sense that, although people do leave, a group is usually together for 6 months before new people arrive. The clients become reasonably sophisticated in the use of psychodrama and analytical group work and this approach seems to work well in giving the individual the opportunity for a rehearsal for living.

THE PSYCHODRAMA

The chief participants in a therapeutic psychodrama are the protagonist or subject, the director or chief therapist, the auxiliary egos, and the group or audience.

The protagonist may emerge from the warm-up at the start of the psychodrama session and he may be in touch with an issue pertinent to his personal life or to the group life. The work of the director and auxiliary egos and audience is to help the protagonist bring his personal conflict to life by enacting the event and it is through the experience of enacting that the protagonist gains insight and understanding of his conflict.

Psychodrama has 3 stages:

1. the warm-up
2. the action
3. the sharing.
   Each session lasts $2\frac{1}{2}$–3 hours.

The warm-up

The main aim of the warm-up is to create a supportive environment in which creativity and spontaneity are freed, by engaging the participant in a physical or verbal exercise tuned in to the aim of the particular group and the need of individuals within it.

In an analytical psychodrama, the director does not impose an organised warm-up on the group; she allows the group to sit (preferably on soft cushions surrounding the stage area) and the unconscious material is allowed to surface in its own time, a group form of free association. From this a protagonist emerges and, with the group's permission, is enabled to work. This can take from 10 to 35 minutes.

The therapist or director's main role during this time is to identify the group themes, contain the unexpressed feelings and enable the group to verbalise the repressed material in as safe a way as possible. She is using her skills to get in touch with the collective group theme as well as the individual's emotions. The director can use transference and counter-transference but it is more useful to bring it into the reality of the group as well as linking it into earlier parental relationships.

The therapist is often seen as 'mother' in the group and this must be recognised and articulated, for example, 'I recognise that you see me as mother here but in order to be director in your psychodrama it is important to separate the two. Here are two empty chairs. Make a clear statement to myself as your mother and myself as your director.' This enables the protagonist to separate the two, to shift some of the resistance around and to make it safer. The director appeals to the healthy person within the protagonist and each group member to work in action.

The action

Moreno (1985) expressed the importance of having a stage set on three levels to create the power of the enactment.

Most therapists create a stage area in the treatment room and use the furniture at their disposal. It is very useful to have both large and small cushions, mattresses, a stage and theatrical lighting but not everyone is so fortunate. Occupational therapists are adaptable.

In the action the therapist or director has worked with the group to create a supportive and enabling environment for the protagonist to work in. It is important to identify strengths, as well as weaknesses, and the essence of where the psychodrama will go in interviewing the protagonist.

The director may ask the protagonist. 'Where do we need to start? I notice you were warmed up earlier in the session when we were discussing absent fathers. Is that still with you?' She may choose to begin by engaging the protagonist with one person. It is important that she encourages the protagonist to set the scene and helps him to warm up to it, for example, by saying, 'Where are the windows and doors?, 'What time of the year is it?', 'Is it in the present or are we in the past?' The therapist encourages the protagonist to set the scene and meet with his past/present/future conflict. When identifying roles in his life, she encourages the protagonist to be the known role, for example, if Jim is meeting his mother in his own kitchen, he must be his mother first as it is his perception the therapist is working with. This also warms up the group or audience to be ready to take on the role.

So the scene is set, action has begun. When the protagonist asks his mother a question, or pauses, or spontaneity is lacking, roles are reversed until the protagonist is engaged. The director or the audience can act as double, which effectively means standing behind the protagonist and echoing his thoughts and feelings or getting in touch with the *unsaid* statement; helping the protagonist to release repressed material, words, information and, most of all, feelings. If the protagonist does not feel what the double is saying on his behalf then he must be encouraged to say so.

Moreno (1985) defines the phenomenon of catharsis as being central to the development of psychodrama and the purpose of building the scene, reversing roles, doubling and mirroring is to create the spontaneity and space for the release of emotion. This begins in the protagonist as he enacts his own drama, scene after scene, and can be the expression of sadness, anger, distress. It does not have to be explosive and dramatic, it can be in a fleeting moment or a gentle exchange; whatever is enough for the protagonist at the time of enactment.

The sharing

The third and final part of psychodrama is the sharing and closure. This is when the protagonist has the opportunity to recover and reintegrate some of the feelings he has repressed. It is also the time to de-role the auxiliary egos. This is done by encouraging everyone in the group to share what touched them in the psychodrama in relation to their own life experience and feelings, and to let go of the role, they were invited to play by the protagonist. Moreno believed in 'tele', in which it is no coincidence that there is always a connection, however tenous, between the role the person is asked to play and the person himself.

The above was a very brief description of the basics of psychodrama. The Further Reading list at the end of the chapter suggests sources of further information.

Occupational therapists are particularly suited to working with psychodrama, which is about the psyche in action. Further training is necessary and it would be difficult to work in this area without it, especially if there is no psychodramatist from whom to learn.

HANDLING CLIENT PROBLEMS

Whatever the group the therapist will inevitably meet the following:

- the distressed and tearful client
- the angry client
- the unpredictable client
- the uncommunicative client.

Before considering methods of dealing with the above clients, the therapist must look to herself and her own understanding of these feelings within herself. Is she aware of her own anger and sadness? Is she sometimes unpredictable and uncommunicative? She needs to have an awareness and understanding of her own inner world, and to have a degree of insight into what belongs to her own psyche and what belongs to the client.

The therapist is trained to use her skills in observation, listening, empathy and understanding, and in applying her theoretical knowledge. A client does not often exhibit the above feelings without prompting either by the effect of the group process, the warm-up or the action itself, so there are usually clues to follow, cues to pick up on and others to consider and work with.

THE DISTRESSED AND TEARFUL CLIENT

The therapist may choose to allow the client time and space to cry in, to enable others in the group to recognise the distress and to support him if he can tolerate it. Any expression of emotion needs space, time and permission to happen.

The temptation to rush in and confront the distressed client is enormous but the therapist must be aware of the source of the distress, the immediate needs of the client and the needs of the group. Each person has their own boundaries, physical and emotional, and they need to be respected.

The tears may indicate the presence of much pain, sadness and distress but they may also be an expression of anger, frustration and rage. The client expressing these emotions may also be unconsciously expressing the underlying feelings of the group members. It is therefore essential to share the sadness and accompanying feelings in the group with the group until a level of understanding has been reached.

THE ANGRY CLIENT

Anger can be a powerful and frightening emotion both to express and to receive. In a drama group, as in other forms of therapy, physical violence and damage to property is not allowed. Depending on the client group, it is often useful to remind group members of this rule. It provides a structure and limits, which any group needs. When a person expresses emotion, particularly anger, there is often a sense of losing control of the self. This can be very frightening and unnerving for the individual and the group.

The therapist needs to communicate a sense of authoritative, rather than authoritarian, leadership and be aware of her own feelings in relation to anger. Anger may occur spontaneously, as a result of personal interaction, in response to a warm-up

or in role within someone's drama work. It merits the same response as other expressed emotions: it needs to be recognised, explored and understood by the individual concerned and the group involved.

THE UNPREDICTABLE CLIENT

The schizophrenic, organically impaired, or psychotically depressed person may present as unpredictable in behaviour, communication and response to external stimuli.

The client may not be in touch with reality as the therapist and other group members know it and may react to his own world rather than to the world of the group. He may exhibit this in many ways, such as total absorption in self. To the outsider he may appear withdrawn, isolated and 'on another planet'. He may be heard talking to himself and suddenly appear to act in an odd manner, totally inappropriate to the group he is in. He may identify a person or an object in the room as something other than it is, for example, 'I'm not sitting in that chair. The devil's sitting there'.

The therapist may be tempted to dissuade him from this belief, or to collude with it; she needs to hear what he is saying and find a way of being in both the world of the group and the client's world simultaneously. She may identify his distress and involve the other group members in gently bringing him into the reality of the work in progress. She may say, 'I can see you're really disturbed. Can anyone in the group identify with Jim's feelings at the moment?' Someone else may say that they can't see the devil in the chair but they do understand the fear of that.

Sometimes, if there is sufficient trust and acceptance in the group, other members may share similar experiences, for example, one young man said he used to see the devil but that it had now changed to the Mafia and he moved on to describe in detail his delusional experience of being smuggled on an aeroplane, inside a washing machine to a secret destination. The group members listened and were aware of his fear and intense anxiety. At the end of his description one member said, 'That must have been a very frightening experience. Was it real to you or do you think it was your

tion?' Jim replied, 'Now that I'm saying it aloud I realise that sometimes I really believe it's happening to me and sometimes I know it's a dream. I think it's connected to feeling sick and well.' The group moved on, with the careful guidance of the therapist, to discuss how each person felt about being sick and being well.

Some therapists would not choose to work in this manner, believing that allowing the person permission to acknowledge his delusional system may reinforce his belief in it, but I have found the opposite to be true. Everyone has psychotic and neurotic parts, as well as healthy parts, and therefore when labelling someone as neurotic there is already an assumption that he will behave and communicate in a certain way. The same applies to psychotic behaviour. It is important to recognise and accept the client as a person with needs, feelings and psychotic and neurotic parts. Only then can you be free as a therapist to enable the person to grow and mature in a healthy and useful manner.

THE UNCOMMUNICATIVE CLIENT

'Uncommunicative' here means with no expression, verbal or non-verbal. Sometimes the client's only method of expressing himself and the intensity of his need is to become completely mute and apparently inaccessible. The adolescent client may often present in this way.

A useful exercise provided in the context of a supportive and caring environment is 'mirroring'. The therapist sits opposite the client and mirrors his exact posture. She may choose to ask the group (if he has reached the stage of being in a group) to mirror the client's posture and also make a statement about the feelings they guess are underneath. This can also be very threatening so the therapist must be selective and aware of the individual's needs and the group dynamics.

Sometimes it is helpful for the client to remain in his adopted stance and hear how others see him. Drama is a therapeutic tool and, as with any tool, the user needs to know how it works and how to use it constructively and sensitively. Everyone has their own defence system and it is there for a

reason. The therapist needs to be aware of how to engage the client without disarming him of all his defences at once. He needs to feel safe enough to show his defences and to keep them in place if he needs to.

Another useful exercise is the blind partnership game. The therapist invites the group members to stand up, push their chairs back and choose a partner.

1. One partner is to be 'blind' first. The pair are invited to make a decision together about who goes first. The 'blind' person must close his eyes.

2. The sighted person has the job of leading the 'blind' person around the room and introducing him to objects to see if he can guess what they are. 'Use your imagination and encourage your partner to experience the touch, the feel of textures, temperatures, for example, the coldness of the window or the warmth of the heater, or the sensation of cold or warm water being poured onto the hand. Be aware of how you lead your partner around the room.'

3. If it is appropriate to the group, introduce your partner to other people by first of all guiding him to shake hands with this new person. The introduction can be to a 'sighted' or 'blind' person. If you can get the person's permission you can touch his face and hair, then try to guess who it is. Try to do this without talking so that the voices don't give it away.

4. Move onto another person. How many people do you really know in this group?

5. Now change partners, reverse the roles and follow the same procedure. The newly sighted must introduce their partners to objects first and, when instructed, to people in the room.

This exercise must obviously be adapted to suit the needs of the individuals but it provides a variety of experiences. It stimulates individuals to become aware of the world outside themselves, to become aware of the sensation of touch, the use of the eyes and the value of speech, and crystallises these experiences into one exercise.

The group discussion after the exercise can be facilitated to move in a variety of ways according to the aims of treatment and the time available.

For example, with the more psychotically disturbed it would be useful to keep the group in touch with the reality of objects in the room and the other people. The more explorative work may identify the role of leader and follower: Where were people most comfortable/uncomfortable? How does this link up with your life outside of hospital, in your relationships with others?

The aims change as the group changes in population, insight, awareness and personal growth.

SUMMARY

Drama in therapy offers much, not only to clients in inpatient and outpatient settings, but to teachers, educationalists and managers. It is a tool that can be utilised in many different and rewarding ways but it must be used with care, consideration and skill, and with a real understanding as to why it is being used and how best to use it.

Most of all it can be fun. Therapy can be enjoyable in the sense of the real joy experienced when the client engages with his true self and is safe to express himself openly and spontaneously, even for a moment, in the process of the group. It is hoped that after experiencing this in the security of the therapy session he can experience it in his own life and learn to feel able to take control of his life to whatever degree he is able within the limitations of his illness and the expectations of himself.

REFERENCES

Blatner H A 1980 Acting in. Springer, New York
Courtney R 1974 Play, drama and thought: the intellectual background to drama in education. Cassell, London
Jennings S (ed) 1983 Creative therapy. Kemble Press, Oxford
Jennings S (ed) 1987 Dramatherapy: theory and practice for teachers and clinicians. Croom Helm, London
Langley D M 1983 Dramatherapy and psychiatry. Croom Helm, London

Moreno J L 1985 Psychodrama. Beacon House, New York, vol 1
Remocker A J, Storch E T 1987 Action speaks louder, 4th edn. Churchill Livingstone, Edinburgh
Rogers C 1984 Client-centred therapy: its current practice, implications and theory. Houghton Mifflin, Boston

FURTHER READING

Anzieu D 1984 The group and the unconscious. Routledge, London
Bion W R 1961 Experience in the groups. Tavistock, London
Bruce M A, Borg B 1987 Frames of reference in psychosocial occupational therapy. Slack, New Jersey
Casement P 1985 On learning from the patient. Tavistock, New York
Foulkes S H, Anthony E J 1965 Group psychotherapy: the psychoanalytic approach. Penguin, Harmondsworth
Goldman A, Morrison B 1984 Psychodrama: experience and process. Kendall-Hunt, Dubuque
Green H 1967 I never promised you a rose garden. Pan, London
Howe M C, Schwartzberg S L 1986 A functional approach to group work in occupational therapy. J B Lippincott, Philadelphia

Mosey A C 1986 Psychosocial components of occupational therapy. Raven Press, New York.
Mullen H, Rosenbaum M 1978 Group psychotherapy: theory and practice, 2nd edn. Free Press, New York
Starr A 1977 Psychodrama: rehearsal for living. Nelson Hall, Chicago
Symington N 1986 The analytic experience. Free Association Books, London
Walton H 1974 Small group psychotherapy. Penguin, Harmondsworth
Whittaker D S 1985 Using groups to help people. Routledge & Kegan, London
Worden J W 1982 Grief counselling and grief therapy. Tavistock, London
Yalom I D 1975 The theory and practice of group psychotherapy. Basic Books, New York
Yalom I D 1983 In-patient group psychotherapy. Basic Books, New York

15

Social skills training

Linda Franklin

INTRODUCTION

What are social skills? For most of us, the majority of our waking hours are spent talking to, looking at, listening to and touching other people. This has been labelled social behaviour, face-to-face interaction, interpersonal behaviour and, recently, social skill. It includes such everyday actions as greeting, asking questions, explaining, encouraging, discouraging, persuading and resisting. At a more detailed level it includes the words we use, the nods of our heads and the winks of our eyes.

An obvious, but significant, distinction has been made between verbal and non-verbal behaviour as components of interpersonal communication. We communicate our intentions and opinions not just through the words we use but also through facial expressions, gestures, bodily movements and posture. Some non-verbal behaviour, for example smiles, nods and gestures, may be as consciously controlled as words. Other behaviour may 'leak' our feelings unconsciously, for example, drumming fingers and crossing legs. Verbal and non-verbal, conscious and unconscious behaviour; these are the ingredients of social skills and the material for social skills training.

This chapter will look at the elements of social skills in some detail and discuss social skills deficits, that is, lack of competence in culturally appropriate social skills to support life roles. The causes of social skills deficits are discussed and two approaches to social skills training are outlined.

SOCIAL INADEQUACY

What are the characteristics of social inadequacy? A person can be regarded as socially inadequate if he is unable to affect the behaviour and feelings of others in the way that he intends and that society accepts. Such a person may appear annoying, unforthcoming, uninteresting, cold, isolated, inept, bad-tempered or destructive and others will generally find him unrewarding to be with. These impressions are conveyed to others by the ways in which he uses elements of verbal and non-verbal behaviour. The socially inadequate person has difficulty in using these skills and understanding other people's use of them. Many people who are not psychiatric clients may also have poor social skills but what distinguishes them from clients is usually the degree of deficit and the extent to which their inadequacy disrupts social life.

Many clients are immediately recognisable as such through abnormalities of social behaviour. These may be:

- failure to communicate with others
- difficulties in the field of interaction and interpersonal relationships
- peculiarities of appearance, posture, gesture, facial expression, tone of voice, etc.
- incoherent speech
- lack of affect, that is, failure to express emotions appropriately
- poor perception of others' needs and responses
- low empathic ability, that is, difficulty in entering into others' feelings.

Many of these characteristics have been found in people with schizophrenia and some kinds of personality disorders. People with chronic schizophrenia show the most extreme forms of social inadequacy. Others displaying forms of social inadequacy are not easily classified into diagnostic categories.

Later in this chapter we shall look more closely at different aspects of failure to develop social competence and the elements of behaviour involved.

SOCIAL SKILLS TRAINING

The aim of social skills training is to help people to enter into and be more effective in, social situations. It is based on the idea that skills are learned and can be taught to those who lack them, enabling them to influence their environment sufficiently to attain basic personal goals. The most comprehensive approach to social skills training for clients with neurotic personality disorders is that of Michael Argyle and his colleagues (as presented in Trower et al 1978). Clients with chronic schizophrenia, with gross deficiency of skills, require a different form of approach, however, as the key factor affecting training programmes is their general lack of motivation to engage in social situations. Both training approaches will be described.

Goldsmith and McFall (1975) wrote 'in contrast to the therapies aimed primarily at the elimination of "maladaptive" behaviours, skills training emphasises the positive, educational aspects of treatment . . . Whatever the origins of deficit (e.g. lack of experience, faulty learning, biological dysfunction) it often may be overcome or partially compensated for through appropriate training in more skilful response alternatives'.

SKILLS NECESSARY FOR SOCIAL COMPETENCE

Successful social interaction depends on having a level of competence in social skills that allows the individual to influence other people in a socially acceptable way. The greater the repertoire of skills a person has, the greater will be his sense of competence in a variety of social situations. Such skills continue to be learned throughout life.

In this section, we will look at the range of skills that make up competent social behaviour: non-verbal communication skills, verbal communication skills and the rules governing social interaction.

NON-VERBAL COMMUNICATION

Non-verbal communication involves any means other than language. It includes communication through body movement and body posture, gaze, voice qualities, manipulation of space, arrangement of environmental props and personal appearance, including the use of clothing and cosmetics. During social behaviour every part of our body is active. However, certain parts of the body convey more information than others and do so in distinctive ways (Trower et al 1978).

Face

The face is the most important and most complex body area for non-verbal signalling. Its two main functions are expression of emotion and attitude, and speech accompaniments.

- *Expression of emotion and attitude* There are six primary emotions: surprise, anger, disgust, fear, happiness and sadness. Expression of these is said to be innate and universal but is modified by cultural learning in four ways: intensified, weakened, masked or mixed.
- *Speech accompaniment* A rapid sequence of facial movements accompanies, and is subordinate to, speech and is used by speakers to emphasise, frame and in other ways elaborate the spoken word, for example, a smile given with a word of praise shows that the speaker is pleased about the success he is praising. Listeners use facial movements to encourage or discourage the speaker and to comment upon his utterances. Information about personality and identity is also conveyed, for example, by typical and idiosyncratic expressions.

Gestures

There is a close link between hand movements and speech. The hands communicate by illustrating the object of discussion, by pointing and by sign language. Hands also indicate the level of physiological and emotional arousal and display truncated acts of touching, such as fist shaking, which is a gesture symbolic of hitting. 'Autistic' gestures of self-touching, thought to show attitudes towards the self, are used. Some may simply satisfy bodily needs, for example, scratching, but others 'leak' information about feelings that are concealed by face and voice, for example, picking at the skin can show nervousness and lack of self-confidence.

Other parts of the body function in different ways. Nodding the head, for example, indicates agreement or willingness for the other to continue speaking and acts as reinforcement. Bodily posture mainly shows how tense or relaxed someone is and signifies attitudes and emotions. The feet do not convey much information, although they can indicate the level of arousal.

Gaze

Gaze is unique in being both a channel (receiver) and signal (sender). The main function of gaze is to receive non-verbal signals from others. In addition, the amount and type of gaze communicate interpersonal attitudes. Gaze is closely coordinated with speech and serves to add emphasis, provide feedback, indicate attention and manage speaking turns. These different functions are combined and a glance used to collect information also sends information to the other person.

Spatial behaviour

Two factors are involved in spatial behaviour:

- proximity, or the distance between people
- orientation, or the angle at which people's bodies are in relation to each other.

The distance between two people can show how intimate or formal they are. People can communicate their liking for another by sitting or standing nearer. Orientation shows the degree of intimacy or formality in much the same way as proximity. For example, a face-to-face orientation signifies a more intimate relationship than a side-by-side orientation. People can also control the behaviour of others by changing spatial arrangements, for example, by the position of a desk.

Non-verbal aspects of speech

The same words can be delivered in quite different ways by varying pitch, stress and timing. Linguists distinguish between two types of sounds:

- prosodic sounds, which affect the meaning of utterances, for example pauses, stress and timing

- paralinguistic sounds, which convey emotions by tone of voice and suggest personality characteristics by voice quality, for example, volume, pitch and clarity.

Bodily contact

This is the earliest form of communication used by infants and is a powerful signal in later life, indicating sexual, affiliative or aggressive attitudes. Bodily contact is controlled by elaborate social rules. For example, in some countries physical contact is only permitted in the family, at greetings and in situations where crowds make people anonymous.

Appearance

This is used primarily to send messages about the self. Styles of dress and hair, cosmetics and jewellery convey information about social status, occupation and personality and constitute one of the main forms of self-presentation. Appearance also signals social attitudes, such as sexual availability, affiliation to a particular social group, such as punks, or emotional state. The meaning of these signals changes rapidly with time and fashion.

VERBAL COMMUNICATION

Verbal utterances affect the behaviour of others as well as having meaning in themselves. They consist of two elements:

- content of speech, which is the words spoken and their purpose
- form of speech, which is the way language is used to meet the speaker's aims.

Content of speech

There are several different kinds of utterance which function in different ways, as outlined by Trower et al (1978).

- Instructions and directions are intended to influence the behaviour of others directly. These can be specific instructions, varying from mild suggestions to commands, or 'structuring' utterances, as when a teacher indicates the nature of the next teaching episode.
- Questions are intended to influence verbal behaviour, that is, to elicit appropriate replies. Questions are also used to initiate encounters: a reply indicates willingness to engage in an encounter. Questions can also indicate interest in or concern for the other person.
- Comments, suggestions and factual information are given in response to questions, as independent comments on other utterances and on special social occasions, such as meetings and lectures.
- A great deal of social behaviour consists of idle chat, gossip and jokes, where little information is exchanged and behaviour is unaffected. The purpose of these utterances is to establish, sustain and enjoy social relationships.
- Performative utterances are those that have an immediate social consequence, for example, apologising.
- Social routines, such as greetings, farewells or thanks, involve standardised verbal components that have no meaning in isolation.
- Emotional states can be expressed in words ('I feel angry') but are more effectively expressed non-verbally, by facial expression and tone of voice. Similarly, attitudes to others who are present can be expressed in words but non-verbal signals have more impact. Attitudes to people who are not present, however, are more commonly put into words.
- The same information or questions can be expressed in a large variety of ways. This gives the potential for sending a further, implied message, called a 'latent message', by choosing a particular method of expression. For example, if a customer complains to the manager about poor service the manager must reprimand the shop assistant involved. However, he can do it in a way that implies the customer was really at fault. Latent messages may be intentional or unintentional.

Forms of verbal communication

Words are put together into increasingly complex

sequences that make up the building blocks of conversation. The elements of conversation include speech, listening, and interaction sequences (Trower et al 1978).

- *Length* The amount of speech contributes very significantly to an overall impression of social skill. The longer the speech, the more skilled the speaker appears, and vice versa.
- *Generality* Speech may vary in generality from vague, brief and uninformative, at one extreme, to overinclusive, detailed and uninteresting, at the other.
- *Formality* The intimate–formal dimension has various sub-components:
  — disclosures of factual information about self or others, from personal to impersonal in nature
  — verbal expression of emotion and opinion, from weak to strong
  — informal talk of a chatty kind to formal talk using third-person pronouns.
- *Variety* This does not necessarily imply change of topic but rather variety of type of social discourse, including humour, storytelling, factual information and expression of opinion.
- *Non-verbal 'grammar'* Non-verbal elements punctuate, clarify and colour speech. (See 'Non-verbal communication' on p 230.)
- *Feedback* Different kinds of listener feedback have an effect on the speaker's output:
  — Attention feedback is the listener signalling attention, which means 'I'm listening, understand and approve'. This is given by nodding, verbal affirmatives, eye contact and posture.
  — Reflective feedback is seen as empathic and rewarding. It may include expressions of surprise, amusement and so on, by verbal or non-verbal means.
- *Meshing* Speakers synchronise their periods of talk by negotiation but, when this fails, two kinds of breakdown can occur: simultaneous talking (interruptions) and latencies (periods of non-response).
- *Turn taking* Speakers negotiate their speaking turns by a multichannel system of signals, such as verbal content, intonation and gesture.

Problems may arise in taking up or handing over the conversation, either of which may be insufficient or excessive.
- *Direct questions* and indirect questions are essential for getting conversation going, eliciting information, showing an interest in others and affecting the behaviour of others.
- *Supportive routines* There are a number of social conventions that are made up of a sequence of verbal and non-verbal acts, which may be called routines. Some of the important ones are: greetings, partings, giving thanks, giving praise, paying compliments, apologising and offering sympathy.
- *Initiative and assertion routines* Some assertion routines are essential to avoid being offended or insulted, or to alter an undesirable social situation. Examples of these routines include making complaints, requests or demands, disagreeing and refusing.
- *Behaviour in public* Social conventions govern behaviour in public situations where little or no interaction takes place, for example, standing in a queue. Conventions of this kind include avoiding contact and respecting personal space.

RULES GOVERNING SOCIAL INTERACTION

The verbal and non-verbal elements of communication described above combine to form social behaviour. However, social behaviour takes place in specific social situations and for each situation there are a restricted number of social acts, or moves, that are relevant and acceptable. In every culture there are rules governing behaviour for most common situations, since rules provide a satisfactory way of handling interaction in particular situations. These rules govern:

- who may be present
- the appropriate setting or equipment
- the task and how it should be done
- approved topics and style of conversation
- interpersonal relationships and emotional tone
- sometimes, the clothes to be worn.

The distinction between rules and conventions is an important one, as rules seem to be obligatory in each situation whereas conventions are not. For example, a guest at a meal will be forgiven for using the wrong knife and fork (convention) but not for refusing to eat or being rude to the other guests (rules) (Argyle 1975).

Rules governing the sequence of individual utterances in different social situations are less obvious but four different sequences have been distinguished (Jones and Gerard 1967).

1. *Reactive contingency* Each person responds to the last move by the other. This rule applies in most impromptu social conversation.

2. Asymmetrical contingency—A reacts to B but B is following a plan of his own and does not react to A. This rule applies in some kinds of teaching or speech making. Socially inadequate people often appear to treat situations as if they are all of this type, that is, they always react to others and fail to pursue plans of their own.

3. *Mutual contingency* Each person reacts to the other but also has a plan. This rule applies in joint discussion or therapy.

4. *Pseudo-contingency* Each person is not really responding to the other, except to coordinate timing, but is acting out a learned sequence. This rule applies in highly structured interactions such as exchanging greetings or performing a ritual.

Each sequence of utterances is bounded by a theme, such as a topic of conversation. The rules governing behaviour within it are strictly observed and the sequence is highly predictable. Participants cooperate to perform the sequence as a joint social act.

The particular situation is important in determining behaviour and individuals will respond differently in different situations. Behaviour is a function of people, of situations and of person–situation interaction. Problems can arise if people fail to change their behaviour to suit the different situation. This was discovered in a sample of psychiatric clients, who were first found to be more consistent in their behaviour than is normal, but who became more flexible as they recovered (Moos 1969).

SOCIAL SKILLS DEFICITS

A repertoire of social skills is normally built up throughout life as circumstances, roles and society's expectations change. In order to understand how an individual can fail to develop a sufficient range of skills, it is necessary to have a model of how skills are acquired through normal development.

In this section, two such models are described; the behavioural model, which is based on learning theory, and the skills model, which takes into account personal goals and motivations. Consideration is then given to the social skills problems of psychiatric clients in general and clients with chronic schizophrenia in particular.

HOW SKILLS ARE ACQUIRED

When studying a complex subject such as social skills development it is helpful to use a model to structure the information available. The model chosen will include a definition of skills, an idea of the way in which skills are acquired and a view of competence. If the model is to be used for social skills training then it will include a way of identifying deficit, that is, lack of skill or inadequate competence in skills performance, and the purpose and techniques of intervention.

BEHAVIOURAL MODEL

A behaviourist view of learning suggests that evidence should be confined to those features of the learner and his environment that can easily be observed. Two major approaches to changing behaviour have emerged within this tradition, 'classical conditioning' and 'operant conditioning' (see Ch. 13, p. 187). Both approaches try to understand learning in terms of observable behaviour and environmental conditions.

Classical conditioning is concerned with the ways in which behaviour elicited by one stimulus may, in time, be elicited by another stimulus, which becomes associated with the original one. Pavlov's famous experiment (1927) showed that a dog that salivates in response to being given meat may be 'conditioned' to salivate at the sound of a bell that is regularly rung just before the meat is presented.

Operant conditioning uses the way in which the stimulus that follows an action may affect the probability of a particular behaviour recurring. Skinner (1983) used rats pressing a bar to demonstrate that the behaviour is more likely to be repeated if food appears immediately after the bar is pressed. Attempts to promote learning through procedures based on these two areas of work are described as 'behaviour modification'.

SKILLS MODEL

The skills model has been particularly influential in the development of training programmes for the acquisition of motor skills (Fitts & Posner, 1967; Welford 1968). It was first applied to account for the acquisition of social skills by Argyle & Kendon (1967). This model sees people as pursuing social and other goals, acting according to rules and monitoring their performance in the light of continuous feedback from the environment. The

model is a sequence of five parts, as illustrated in Figure 15.1.

Motivation

People have social goals, such as to make friends, to gain knowledge or to give information. These goals are desired because they satisfy basic needs; affiliation, achievement, etc. Social goals are hierarchically organised into sub-goals, leading to an overall goal, each of which is achieved by a sequence of behaviour. Short sequences of goal-directed behaviour are habitual and mainly unconscious. Longer sequences are controlled by plans that are conscious and may be put into words. For example, the social goal may be to join an evening class. A plan is made to go to college, with the necessary fee, on the correct evening and to enrol. This goal and plan can be expressed in words. Sub-goals are to dress appropriately for going out on a cool evening, walk to the bus stop, catch the right bus, walk to the college, find the enrolment counter, wait in a queue, enrol and go home again. Most of these sub-goals require behaviour that is habitual, so that very little thought is required to put them into action.

Perception

In any social situation a person selects, from the mass of stimuli bombarding him, what he attends to, on the basis of:

- his plans and motives
- how well he knows the other people involved
- how familiar the situation is
- his social stereotypes
- his beliefs about the motives and plans of others.

This selective attention has a major influence on how he perceives the situation.

Translation

Perceptions are 'translated' into performances. The translation stage is a cognitive process that involves solving problems and making decisions. The individual draws upon his available store of

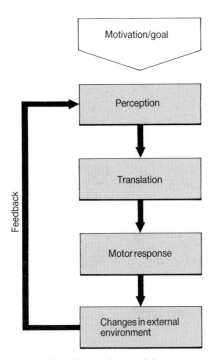

Fig. 15.1 A social skills training model.

knowledge about possible causes of action, considers alternatives and selects what he thinks is the best option in the light of previous experience.

Motor responses

A repertoire of skilled behavioural responses is required, so that translation-stage decisions can be implemented. These social responses are hierarchically organised, with large units being composed of smaller units. For example, interviewing a job applicant is a large unit of behaviour that is made up of smaller units such as appropriate eye-contact and body language, asking questions and listening.

Changes in the external environment

Any action by the individual will have an effect on the human and non-human environment, either temporary or permanent. For example, moving a chess piece will change its position and will also cue one's opponent to consider his next move. Some effects are not immediately visible and the result is either seen later or not at all, for example, the chess opponent may take a long time to make his move. The more skills a person has, the greater will be his ability to produce the environmental changes that he desires.

Feedback

Feedback is received on the effect of actions and is continuously monitored so that allowances can be made for variations in the situation or errors in the initial plan of action.

Primary failure to develop social competence

The social skills model assumes that skills are acquired through various forms of learning, such as imitation, reinforcement and instruction. For learning to take place, it is necessary to have exposure to a wide variety of environmental opportunities and to skilled models such as parents, siblings and peers. Failure to acquire skills may be due to a lack of either skilled models or social opportunities, although it is not possible to separate

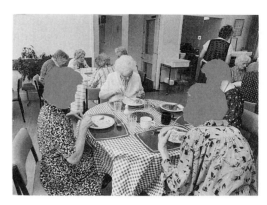

Fig. 15.2 Communal mealtimes provide an opportunity to practise communication and social skills. (Source: Lothian Health Board)

these two influences in reality. There has been little specific research in this area and only partial substantiation of links between parent–child relationships and environmental experiences, and the development of social skills. However, it seems probable that socially unskilled parents have less accurate perceptions of what appropriate behaviour is and are therefore less likely to teach and reinforce skilled responses to their children.

The social skills model proposes that cognitive abilities are used for processing information, making inferences about the consequences of courses of action, taking the role of the other person, etc. Parents who lack empathic or problem-solving skills will not be able to promote the development of these skills in their children.

It seems likely that the rudiments of social skills develop, or fail to develop, in early childhood. However, Clarke & Clarke (1972) have warned against assuming that early experience necessarily predetermines the course of later development. It is now generally acknowledged that a change from an adverse environment into a better one tends to be followed by desirable changes in behaviour. It is nevertheless possible that social skills for influencing the behaviour of others, acquired in the early years, may increase both the range of later experiences and the quality of learning that occurs in them.

Studies suggest that both innate and environmental factors play their part in the acquisition of social behaviour.

SOCIAL INADEQUACY AND PSYCHIATRY

Social inadequacy is defined by social norms and is therefore subjective and hard to define precisely but some forms of mental disorder may be caused or exacerbated by lack of social competence. There are two possible sequences of events.

1. Failure of social competence is primary, as described above, leading to rejection by society and isolation, which in turn produces a disturbed mental state.

2. Mental illness affects all areas of behaviour, including social performance. The secondary social inadequacy that this brings about results in rejection by society and isolation, thus adding to the original sources of stress and leading to deterioration of mental condition.

Social skills problems in psychiatric clients

Some of the most extensive research into the characteristics of social inadequacy among psychiatric outpatients found that socially inadequate clients tend to show a particular style of behaviour (Trower et al 1978). 'They will probably appear rather cold, unassertive and unrewarding to others, will show little expressive variation in face, voice and posture, will look rather infrequently at the other person, will make little effort to produce a spontaneous and interesting flow of speech, and will take little part in the management of conversations'.

Socially inadequate clients are likely to have a history of poor mixing with others, lack of boyfriends or girlfriends and considerable difficulty in a wide range of social situations, in particular those involving actively seeking contact with relative strangers, especially those of the opposite sex.

While social withdrawal is commonly found in schizophrenic clients, there is little evidence to associate lack of social skill with other specific diagnoses.

However, there may be an interrelationship between anxiety,·depression and social difficulties.

Depressed clients show verbal behaviour of a flat, passive and expressionless kind, they lack initiative in conversation, adopt a helpless attitude to the environment and may lose interest in friends and social life. However, when their symptoms lessen the clients usually return to normal. Depression in men, particularly those who are single, may be an indicator of social inadequacy.

Anxious clients may have rapid and breathy speech, which is interrupted by speech disturbances, and in tense posture and jerky, poorly controlled gestures.

They are often oversensitive to the reactions of others, fear they are doing the wrong thing and dread being the centre of attention. Some may develop phobias to specific social situations.

Other characteristics of socially inadequate clients include:

- 'egocentricity', that is, lack of the empathic ability to perceive themselves and the world from another's viewpoint
- disturbed goals in their encounters with other people, for example, aggressive or destructive
- distorted perceptions of their environment, for example, paranoid interpretations of events.

Social skills deficits and schizophrenia

People with chronic schizophrenia show the most extreme forms of social inadequacy. Often, they display social withdrawal, engaging in behaviours that avoid contact with other people. It is important that we examine theories relating to this social isolation in people with schizophrenia in order to understand how the problem is different from that of other socially inadequate clients.

There is evidence to suggest that people with chronic schizophrenia exhibit elevated states of cortical arousal, which are strongly associated with a reduced capacity to select the appropriate stimuli from the environment when processing information. Spratt and Gale (1979) demonstrated that there are clear links between the degree of arousal, the extent of observable pathology, and the person's capacity to process simple visual information.

Inability to selectively screen out background stimuli may be the cause of non-specific central nervous system arousal. This view of cortical hyper-arousal fits in with the ideas initially proposed by Venables (1964). That is, in order to reduce hyper-arousal, the most effective behavioural strategy is to cut oneself off from all stimuli perceived as arousing. Withdrawal by people with chronic schizophrenia is selective and is away from stimuli that are classified as 'social', and that have greater arousal potential than other classes of stimuli. The person with chronic schizophrenia may be attempting to avoid sensory input, particularly social sensory input, merely to remain comfortable.

This has important implications for any social skills training programme, as the client will lack the motivation to participate in social situations. His ability to concentrate and attend to information will be seriously affected and his learning ability will be impaired.

SOCIAL SKILLS TRAINING

There are many approaches to training social skills, based on the various models that have been developed. Some approaches are more suited to certain problems than others. This section covers the general principles of skills training, outlines an approach for use with socially inadequate clients and provides a model for use with people with chronic schizophrenia.

PRINCIPLES OF SKILLS TRAINING

The principles of skills teaching, or 'training,' are demonstration, guidance, practice and feedback.

- Demonstration has three main functions:
  1. it can draw attention to, and magnify, important components in a task
  2. the demonstration of a task serves to set a standard for future attempts
  3. it serves as a basis for imitation or a 'model'.
- Guidance refers to information given about the task to help the subjects perform correctly in

the initial stages of learning. Guidance can be given verbally, visually or by physical positioning. A major issue is the degree to which subjects should be allowed to experience errors in order to learn more effectively. If learners become too dependent on receiving additional information, then their progress will be impaired in the long run.

- Practice is necessary for skills acquisition but the amount needed will depend on the complexity of the skill to be learned. Very complex tasks may have to be learned in parts; the learner first acquires the necessary skills for successful performance and then combines them into a 'whole.' Simple skills may not need to be learned in this way.
- Feedback is information about the consequences of actions that can be used to develop and improve skilled behaviour. Practice alone is not enough. Information on performance may come from carrying out the task itself and is then called 'intrinsic feedback'. Alternatively, information may be supplied by factors external to the task and then it is called 'extrinsic feedback'. Extrinsic feedback is most useful when received at the end of a task and presented in such a way as to highlight the intrinsic feedback in the task. Extrinsic feedback presented during task performance may produce initial improvements but may also obscure feedback in the task itself, resulting in poor skills acquisition in the long term.

TRAINING SOCIALLY INADEQUATE CLIENTS

The most comprehensive approach to social skills training for socially inadequate clients is that of Michael Argyle and his colleagues (Trower et al 1978). The following provides a summary of the assessment and training procedures involved and gives an outline of a training programme. If more detailed information is required, further reading is recommended.

ASSESSMENT

Information is needed both to identify clients who

lack social skills and to plan training programmes. This information falls into three main areas.

1. *Past and current relationships* This area concerns difficulties of an enduring nature that are experienced with various kinds of people in various settings.

2. *Social situations* This information is about difficulties in specific social situations.

3. *Behaviour* This refers to inadequate social performance in social situations.

Information on the first and second areas is obtained mainly from interviewing the client. Information on the third area is from direct observation, either in real situations or in role plays.

INDIVIDUAL VERSUS GROUP TRAINING

A social skills training programme can be tailored to individual needs and organised around a particular client's social problems. Alternatively, the programme can be based on a standard 'package' for which clients are selected. People with observable social skill deficits (socially inadequate) and those who have adequate skills but whose performance is disrupted by anxiety (socially phobic) can be usefully mixed in a group training programme. Some clients, if very regressed, need to receive individual training first then can eventually be placed in a group.

The standard group training programme is a predesigned course that deals systematically with most of the important basic social skills, one or more of which form the theme of each session. Training in groups has several advantages.

- The group is a ready-made social situation, in which participants undergoing training can practise on each other. The chances of new social behaviour generalising to other social situations is greater when the skills are learned in a group than if they are taught one-to-one.
- Clients tend to feel less inhibited in a group of people in a similar situation to themselves
- Group training is a cost-effective use of the therapist's time.

Disadvantages of training in groups include the following.

- Members may be poor models for each other, although this can be partly overcome by having a high ratio of therapists to clients.
- Individuals' particular problems may not receive specific attention.

Ideally, social skills training groups consist of six clients and two therapists so that they can divide into two 'work triads', each with a therapist. Sessions should last no more than 1 hour once a week, or 1 hour twice a week.

SPECIFIC SKILLS COVERED

The elements of social skills that are included in a training programme have been listed by Trower et al (1978) and include both verbal and non-verbal skills.

Verbal:

- asking and answering questions
- giving and seeking information
- giving instructions
- offering and seeking opinions or suggestions
- greeting, bidding farewell
- apologising, explaining
- telling jokes
- agreeing, disagreeing
- thanking.

Non-verbal:

- gaze, mutual gaze, glance
- facial expression
- proximity and orientation
- voice quality: pitch, loudness, speed, accent
- gestures accompanying speech and expressing emotions
- posture: relaxed–tense, dominant–submissive
- appearance: image conveyed by grooming, hair, clothes.

These elements are combined into skills that Trower et al (1978) present in eight sets, with suggestions for training exercises given for each. The eight sets of skills are:

1. Observation skills:
   - getting information about a situation
   - getting information about the other's attitudes and feelings
   - clarifying the causes of others' behaviour
   - observing own behaviour
   - recognising emotions
   - recognising attitudes.
2. Listening skills:
   - reflecting feelings and mood matching
   - attention feedback (includes nodding, etc.)
   - listener commentary (includes verbal and non-verbal response)
   - questioning.
3. Speaking skills:
   - disclosing factual information
   - disclosing feelings
   - fluency of speech and non-verbal characteristics and accompaniments of speech.
4. Meshing skills:
   - content and change of content
   - timing.
5. Expression of attitudes:
   - matching the other's style and choosing a different style in order to influence him.
6. Social routines:
   - giving greetings
   - making farewells
   - making requests
   - gaining access to strangers
   - offering compliments, praise, encouragement, congratulations, sympathy
   - giving explanations
   - making apologies
   - saving face
   - asserting oneself.
7. Tactics and strategies:
   - bringing together previously learned skills and considering alternative ways of behaving.
8. Situation training:
   - putting skills into practice in particular situations.

THE TRAINING PROGRAMME

The social skills training programme runs for a set number of sessions that have been designed to deal with the most common problems. It is a group programme but is flexible enough to meet the needs of individual participants through the use of personal goals and homework assignments.

Goals

Training is only successful if the therapist specifies desired goals that the client has consistently failed to achieve because of inadequate skills. The therapist must secure the client's agreement on the relevance of goals to his everyday social interaction. These goals can be grouped under general titles, such as 'Sustaining a conversation' or 'Requesting a service'. The situations are then rated for their importance as desired goals, for the level of anxiety they produce and for the anticipated level of competence to be achieved.

Contracts

Obtaining a contract or a 'promise' from the client encourages him to regulate his own behaviour towards mutually agreed objectives. The contract is used mainly for homework assignments.

Revision

Each session, except the first, begins with a revision of the main points of the previous training session and a report from the client on his successes and failures during the week. The client's successes are praised and information on the precise nature of the failures is obtained in order to provide corrective training.

Learning points

Each session has a theme, which the therapist analyses into a sequence of behavioural elements. These serve as learning points and are written down and memorised by the client. The therapist explains how the skills sequence functions in everyday interaction, the effect it has and how it will help the client.

Demonstration

Demonstration, or modelling, of skills should be clear and follow the learning points closely. The model should give performance that copes with, rather than masters, the situation, showing that he has difficulties but still manages to be effective. The demonstration should be repeated several times, preferably by other models. Demonstrations can be prepared using videotape but live models are usually more personal and realistic.

Imitation

The client is invited to perform the skill that has been modelled; to 'role-play' the model. His first attempt should be as exact an imitation as possible, using the same or similar dialogue or situation.

Feedback

The therapist praises the good aspects of the performance, focussing on the task rather than on the person. Feedback should be detailed and specific, referring to actual performance and directed at those aspects relevant to the learning points given in that particular session. Other aspects that are not closely related to the theme of the session can be dealt with later. Feedback should be given as promptly as possible after the observed behaviour and there should be proportionately more praise and positive expectation than criticism. Feedback can also be given by the use of audio and video equipment. This gives the client an opportunity to comment on his own performance as well as hearing comments from his role partner and other group members.

Practice

From the feedback comments, a few correction points can be identified. The client practises these aspects in detail and with continuous encouragement and guidance from the therapist. He is also invited to improvise more and more, making the responses 'his' as he progressively shapes the action into his own style. The application of these skills in real settings is preceded by role-play simulations of actual or possible real-life encounters. The client describes a situation and allocates roles to himself and other group members.

Homework assignments

These are an integral part of social skills training, in that the client can put into practice the skills learned during therapy sessions, thus generalising the skills to real situations. The client suggests times, places and situations where he can put into practice the skill, and states his intention to do so. In groups, these commitments are made out loud and members made answerable to each other to keep them. In addition, clients might also keep a daily diary, recording all social events they observed or participated in, and what they felt about them. These diaries can provide an important source of material for training exercises.

When the advantages and disadvantages of this group programme for teaching social skills are weighed up, it is found to be a useful method of helping the large numbers of people with social skills problems that occupational therapists encounter in their work.

A TRAINING MODEL FOR CHRONIC SCHIZOPHRENICS

People with chronic schizophrenia lack the motivation to participate in social situations, with associated social withdrawal and serious deterioration in verbal and non-verbal skill levels. These people also experience difficulties in concentrating and in processing information, so a social skills training programme needs to be directed at simple targets or goals. Rather than trying to teach people specific skills, such as how to have eye contact, appropriate posture or clarity of voice, it will concentrate on getting clients to generate approach behaviours, such as initiating a conversation, and talking and listening behaviours in order to achieve simple goals. Aspects of quality in social responses are not ignored but they receive less emphasis than the production of behaviours likely to achieve social goals.

THE PROBLEM-SOLVING APPROACH

This model of social skills training has been developed over a 10-year period by Dr Graham Spratt, clinical psychologist, and myself. It uses a problem-solving approach to motivate clients to participate, to identify the behaviour required and to teach new skills.

What is problem solving?

Problem solving is a part of everyday life. In order to satisfy basic needs we all have to face questions such as 'How do I make myself understood in order to communicate my needs?', 'How do I make friends in order to get support?'. A major problem for people with chronic mental illness is that the perceived obstacles between the statement of a problem and its solution loom so large that clients tend to resort to inaction rather than choosing between different actions. This is seen in such behaviours as avoidance of others, withdrawal when given instructions, lack of communication and sleeping during the day. Problem solving gives them a chance to learn, within their capacities and limitations, a range of strategies by which action rather than inaction will succeed.

A major assumption of this approach is that achieving solutions through action, without external help, is a way of judging one's competence to interact successfully with the world. Words like competence, success, confidence and assuredness are clearly the labels of self-reward and are stimulated by reliance on one's own behaviours in solving problems.

Since we are dealing with major defects in behavioural capacity, it seems unrealistic to expect people to demonstrate qualitatively normal social behaviours. It is more reasonable to aim for getting people to initiate and sustain communication as a beginning, however incompetently, before time is spent in tutoring the 'fine tuning' of such behaviours.

Problem-solving activity as a training technique

In the past, strict behavioural regimes such as 'token economy' have been used as the main forms of treatment for chronic schizophrenic inpatients. This involves setting a scale of behaviours that can earn varying numbers of tokens, for example, making one's own bed earns one token. At the end of the week the tokens can be used to buy privileges such as cigarettes or outings. Behavioural targets are usually self-care and social interaction. These regimes are effective in improving behaviours within the token economy unit but major problems or relapses often occur upon discharge.

At the simplest level, this failure may be because reinforcement schedules increase and maintain the occurrence of particular behaviours in the training environment but when the reinforcement ends on discharge, the improved behaviour undergoes gradual extinction. This problem led to the formulation of an alternative training strategy to promote behaviours that may be more likely to be retained after discharge.

In a new environment, the individual meets a number of choices but the reward offered (extrinsic reinforcement) has gone. However, if the client is involved in behaviours which lead to self-reward (intrinsic reinforcement), he might develop more confidence in his own ability and rely less upon extrinsic rewards.

Taking this a stage further, a capacity to sustain behaviour through self-reward, in the absence of external reward, must improve the capacity to cope with the choices of the new environment.

Training is designed to reinforce self-generated behaviours that produce engagement with others on a social level, for example, approach, use of speech, gesture and attention to appearance. First, desirable behaviours are identified for reinforcement. Then a range of problem-solving activities is used to stimulate their development and enable the clients to practise freely without fearing negative consequences if he makes a mistake.

Practical features

Social skills training for the person with chronic schizophrenia is based on group, rather than individual, treatment with the following design features.

• Problem-solving activities and behaviour modification techniques are used.

• Treatment sessions take place on a daily basis, for the duration of 1 hour. The degree of deficit coupled with the impaired learning ability of this client group makes frequent practice essential.

• The group is 'open' so that people can join and leave at any point. This is necessary as clients will change slowly and the rehabilitation period required by an individual will vary from 3 months to 2 years.

• The group consists of between 6 and 9 clients and 2 or 3 therapists.

For the purposes of this programme, a definition of problem solving includes the following features.

• Problems require action rather than inaction.

• Target behaviours are identified by the way the problem is described. Starting from a baseline of the existing behaviours, it is necessary to identify a target, discern ways to reach it and select the most appropriate solution.

• The solution is unambiguous and easily discerned.

• The solution may be achieved by a number of different strategies.

Sequence of activities

The activity programme, which is based on the problem-solving process outlined above, is organised into a structured sequence.

• *Behaviour required* Select the type of behaviour you want the person to engage in and practise it for most of the session. This will be a specific social-interaction skill involving communication, such as asking someone to pass something at the table.

• *Size and constitution of group* Estimate the size of group likely to participate and the amount of practice required by each individual.

• *Level of skills deficit* Review the overall level of problems displayed by the group and decide the level of difficulty of the problem design. This should be a level that can be solved by most of the group.

• *Problem* Construct a problem that will elicit the target behaviour and present it in the form of a verbal instruction. This should contain all the information the person is likely to need to reach a solution. For example, 'You require the jam and Fred is the only person who can reach it. He is not looking at you so you will have to attract his attention and let him know what you want.' Decide the degree to which problems can increase in difficulty to allow for improved performance as a result of practice on earlier problems.

• *Number of problems* Estimate the number of problems that can be solved in the time available and design sufficient to cover this time period.

There are certain important features in the design of this activity.

• The instructions are simple.

• Target behaviours are relevant for overcoming the behavioural deficits characteristic of people with chronic schizophrenia.

• The problems can be repeated on numerous occasions using different practical situations.

• The activity encourages maximum engagement of all clients in the task for the time period set.

• The ratio of action to instruction is maintained at a high level.

• The complexity of the problem can be varied to cater for any level of defect likely to be encountered. The range of problems that can be set is limited only by the therapist's ingenuity in designing them. A helpful tip is to incorporate the use of simple props as a focus for the problem-solving activity, for example, packs of cards, Monopoly money, Scrabble letters or other props made by the therapist.

A SAMPLE ACTIVITY

The following is a sample activity showing the stages of its design.

• *Behaviour required* Individuals to approach one another and engage in social information exchange in an effective way.

• *Size and constitution of group* There are nine clients for this half-hour session, each requiring to be involved in as much of the required activity as is reasonable.

- *Level of skills deficit* All members have the physical and cognitive competence to engage in this activity but display varying degrees of social avoidance, social anxiety, ineffective social exchange and poor memory.
- *Problem* The problems set could vary in difficulty between the two extremes indicated by the following instructions:
  — 'Find out how many people in the group had breakfast this morning.'
  — 'Find out how everyone in this group spent their time over the weekend.'
- *Number of problems* Starting with a simple problem, the activity is repeated for the time period specified, progressing to more-complex concepts if the group is successful in solving each one.

TRAINING TECHNIQUES

The problem-solving technique described above is the vehicle by which change is promoted. The success of this technique depends, first, on motivating the clients to attempt the problem-solving exercise, and then on eliciting appropriate behaviours. To build behaviours from the deficits exhibited by people with chronic illness, the therapist needs an appropriate combination of extinction and selective reinforcement.

Extinction is reducing the occurrence of a behaviour by giving no reinforcement. This is theoretically straightforward but rather more difficult to apply in practice, as it means making no response to disruptive behaviours that the client exhibits, such as constant requests for cigarettes.

Selective reinforcement means that an attempt is made to extinguish inappropriate behaviours whilst at the same time reinforcing appropriate behaviours.

The process of changing behaviour is in three stages:

1. eliciting behaviour by a system of instructions, cues and prompts
2. modelling strategies solving the problem that has been set

3. shaping elicited and modelled behaviours through social reinforcement, which is contingent on the required behaviour being exhibited.

Instructions, cues and prompts

Certain important principles of instruction must be observed in setting up the statement of the problem. The clients involved will have difficulties with attention, concentration and recall, therefore instructions have to be clear, unambiguous and with a low information content. The emphasis is upon clients understanding the demands of the problem before the exercise proceeds to the next stage.

The activity is specifically chosen to elicit target behaviours with which the client has difficulty or is unacquainted, therefore poor performance is to be expected. Defects in performance may be manifest either as inaction or inappropriate action, at which point cues are required to stimulate appropriate behaviours. Indirect prompting is used to give some information as to the expectations of behaviour, without indicating precisely what is required, for example, 'What should you be doing now?' Direct prompting, for example, 'Go and ask him a question', should be avoided as it reduces the clients' reliance upon their own behavioural skills.

It is important to be consistent in maintaining the mode of cueing, since inadvertent slips into directional prompting act as partial reinforcement for the most pronounced behaviour of this client group, that of inaction.

Modelling

Frequently, a person's behaviour fails to meet the demands of the problem-solving situation and this might be due to an absence of effective behaviours from his repertoire. Modelling is used to present new behaviours in a form that can be copied and practised by the client. The behaviour might be modelled in its complete form or, more usually, broken down into its component parts, which are demonstrated, in turn, as a chain of behaviours that lead to the solution of the problem.

Shaping

The aim is not to reinforce the appearance of a particular level of performance, but to reinforce a particular level of 'effort', which is inferred from observed behaviours. Social reward is given for the following types of behaviour.

- Any spontaneously generated behaviour that is related to the demands of the problems-solving situation, for example, any interpersonal engagement.
- A level of performance that indicates effortful concentration, such as remembering past events or repeating actions to elicit a response from others.
- Any overt signs of effortful concentration, such as arriving at a solution to the problem.

OBSERVED RESULTS OF THE PROBLEM-SOLVING TECHNIQUE

- Improvements were closely linked to the complexity of problems that the clients could cope with.
- Improvement was closely related to an increase in spontaneous self-generated behaviours, especially in the area of social communication.
- Once the group had become established, the 'warm-up' period of each activity session would be run by the clients themselves, with little input from the therapists.
- During activity periods there was a markedly low incidence of inappropriate behaviours.
- Clients began to demonstrate valuable supportive behaviours by becoming models and reinforcers for other group members.
- Clients displayed tolerance for either high or low competence in a very discriminating way. Those of a high capacity were given far less tolerance for inappropriate behaviours than those of a low capacity.
- Clients began to show evidence of taking responsibility for organising the pace of their own programme.
- Most clients displayed improvements in communication, appearance and self-care without a corresponding improvement in clinical state.

EVALUATION OF SOCIAL SKILL TRAINING

Unfortunately, there have been too few studies done on the effectiveness of social skills training with psychiatric clients. Studies, to date, show that as many questions have been raised as answered and point to the need for better designs and measures in a field that is proving to be very difficult and yet extremely promising.

Studies of inpatients provide encouraging evidence that, at least in the short-term, social skills training can produce improvements in behaviour and subjective feelings of comfort in social situations, sometimes within a very short period of time and in clients with widely differing diagnoses.

In a 3-month controlled study with chronic clients the problem-solving model was compared with a more traditional activity programme. 'It showed that patients in the problem-solving group demonstrated more spontaneous speech and the amount of speech between group participants was also greater' (Spratt, 1984).

Studies of outpatients show that social skills training can produce improvements in general social functioning for persons described as 'socially inadequate'. 'These improvements seemed to be lasting ones, at least over the follow-up period. The training also appeared to be of clinical benefit and to make a real contribution towards expanding the social life of the patients and reducing their need for further treatment.' (Trower et al 1978).

It is only in recent years that training methods for treating social problems have developed to any degree. As in any new development, it is difficult to find clear evidence for the effectiveness of skills training until a substantial body of research has been carried out. Future research should be directed towards:

- establishing methods of maintaining new behaviour and generalising it to real life
- investigating the various components of training, such as modelling and role-playing
- investigating the various training approaches being used, in particular those used with chronic clients.

SUMMARY

This chapter looked in detail at what we mean by social behaviour and at the skills necessary for successful social interaction. It then discussed two models of how social skills are acquired and looked at failure to develop competence in social behaviour, leading to social inadequacy. The principles of social skills training were discussed and two training programmes described: training people with social inadequacy, using a technique developed by Argyle and colleagues; and training people with chronic schizophrenia, using a problem-solving approach. The chapter concluded with an evaluation of social skills training as a therapeutic technique.

REFERENCES

Argyle M 1975 Bodily communication. London, Methuen

Argyle M, Kendon A 1967 The experimental analysis of social performance. Advances in Experimental Social Psychology, vol 3. Academic Press. New York

Clarke A D B, Clarke A M 1972 Consistency and variability in the growth of human characteristics. Advances in Educational Psychology London, University Press, London

Fitts P, Posner M 1967 Human performance. Brooks-Cole, Monterey

Goldsmith J B, McFall R M 1975 Development and evaluation of an interpersonal skill training programme for psychiatric in patients. Journal of Abnormal Psychology, 84: 51–8

Jones E E, Gerard H B 1967 Foundations of social psychology. Wiley, New York

Moos R H 1969 Sources of variance in responses to questionnaires and in behaviour. Journal of Abnormal Psychology 7: 405–412

Pavlov I P 1927 Conditioned reflexes. Oxford University Press, New York

Skinner B F 1938 The behaviour of organisms. Appleton Century Crofts, New York

Spratt G 1984 Personal communication

Spratt G, Gale A 1979 An EEG study of visual attention in schizophrenic patients. Biological Psychology 9: 249–269

Trower P et al 1978 Social skills and mental health. Methuen, London

Welford A 1968 Fundamentals of skill. Methuen, London

Venables P H 1964 Input dysfunction in schizophrenia. Progress in experimental personality research, vol 1. Academic Press, New York

16

Play therapy

Lily I H Jeffrey

INTRODUCTION

What is play therapy? Why is it used? Who uses play therapy? Who needs this form of therapy? When is it used? Where can it be obtained? How is it used? This chapter attempts to answer these questions and in addition seeks to describe how beneficial this type of therapy can be when it is prescribed correctly.

In this present century, child analysts and later child psychiatrists have focussed their skills on devising treatment strategies to help disturbed children. Occupational therapists working with children have continued this tradition. The occupational therapy profession with its threefold approach of:

1. therapeutic relationship
2. therapeutic techniques
3. therapeutic activity

has developed its own philosophy on the use of the therapeutic medium of play, to help children with emotional and behavioural disorders.

Young children are unable to express their emotional needs and conflicts with the verbal ability of adults, who use intricate thought concepts and sophisticated language. Childhood has a language of its own, that is, play. This chapter considers play, which assists the normal development of the child in relation to its healing value in everyday situations. It then considers the therapeutic value of play when it is used as a treatment intervention. The use of play therapy in the context of the multidisciplinary team approach is discussed in relation to children who are under stress for a variety of reasons. The theoretical rationales of the different types of play therapy are outlined in relation to correct prescription. Practical guidelines for therapists are given and the wealth of recent play-therapy research is described.

PLAY

For therapists wanting to understand and help emotionally and behaviourally disturbed children, it is essential to learn their 'play language', in all its developmental aspects, so that the child can communicate freely with the adult. The child is constantly communicating through his play. The therapist needs to be skilled at tuning into and interpreting this complex language of childhood.

From the persistent attempts to reach and grasp his first rattle to the current sophisticated computer games of infinite variety and complexity, the years of childhood, for the normal healthy child, are filled with a rich variety of experiences as he engages in play activity of one kind or another throughout most of his waking hours. The study of play illustrates the complex nature of this activity (Bruner et al 1976, Miller 1973) and focusing on the purpose of play in childhood has produced numerous theories (Ellis 1973).

THE THERAPEUTIC VALUE OF NORMAL PLAY

Play assists and enhances all aspects of development: physical, emotional, social, cognitive, perceptual, sensory integration and language. It is a medium for forming and sharing relationships, either the mother–child, or parent–child relationships, extending to siblings and peers. Play time provides the child with his own 'space' to work out his own problems, often at an unconscious level, for example, repeating certain play themes over and over again and so mastering his anxiety. As he symbollically expresses his fears and fantasies, he becomes the ruler of his play world and so works through his inner turmoil. Through

play he is able to express (and so become aware of) his own feelings, especially towards safe inanimate objects that do not retaliate. He becomes aware of his potentials and limitations in regard to different play materials. He has his own likes and dislikes, he forms his own self-awareness and identity. He receives praise and recognition from the various skills he acquires. This builds up his confidence in his own abilities and establishes a positive self-image.

Research into the various facets of play has escalated in recent years. The significance of this research for the play therapist is in how play can enhance the various aspects of development of the child, for example, the relationship between infant play with inanimate objects and social interest in mother (Harman et al 1982), play of mothers with babies, some relationships between maternal personality and early attachment and developmental processes (Weininger 1983), parent–child play interaction and interactive competence (MacDonald et al 1984), and the relations of play and sensorimotor behaviour to language in the second year (Ungerer et al 1984).

PLAY AS A MEDIUM FOR THERAPY

Occupational therapy has been defined as 'the treatment of physical and psychiatric conditions through specific selected activities in order to help people reach their maximum level of function and independence in all aspects of daily life' (COT 1981). Occupational therapists working with disturbed children use therapeutic play and therapeutic techniques 'in order to help them reach either their full potential or to help them to adjust to and function at the highest level possible with whatever residual incapacity remains' (Jeffrey 1982a).

Play has many purposes in the therapy session. It is used to establish a therapeutic relationship with a child by providing a neutral shared experience. The inanimate play object provides a link between therapist and child without, at this stage, feelings being revealed. The play assists the assessment processes, that is, diagnostic, behavioural, developmental and continuous assessment. The child, through different play activities, can regress and use play symbolically to release tension and aggression. His unconscious and conscious needs and conflicts can be enacted with the play materials, as well as expressing fears, fantasies, etc. By interpreting all these activities the therapist helps the child to gain insight and he can alter his attitudes, improve his way of relating to adults and peers, and practise these new skills in the social setting of play-group therapy. The child develops new skills, and uses his creativity, which can sublimate basic needs in a socially acceptable way and he receives praise and recognition so that his confidence and self-image are improved.

PLAY THERAPY: AN INTRODUCTION

The use of play as a therapeutic medium to help emotionally and behaviourally disturbed children is a complex area of work. The field ranges from play therapy as a method of communicating effectively with a child, to the use of play within the context of a transference relationship, which promotes emotional growth. Many children with a multitude of disorders benefit from these types of intervention. Different types of play therapy are practised by many professions. It is one of the many therapeutic strategies used in the field of child psychiatry and needs to be complementary to other forms of treatment. This chapter seeks to clarify some of the issues involved in the correct referral, choice of different types of play therapy for effective outcomes and the need to evaluate the application of these techniques.

CHILDREN WHO NEED PLAY THERAPY

Every child experiences stress of some kind in his life. This is normally worked through by the child himself, with help from his parents and extended family, his peers, teachers at school, or other significant adults that he meets in the community. These children usually have access to rich play en-

vironments and supportive relationships. The child needs to play out upsetting experiences, with the support of a trusted adult, just as an adult would need to talk about such events with colleagues, friends or relatives.

Some children, for a variety of reasons, develop distressing psychological symptomatology and need to be referred to the multidisciplinary team in a child psychiatry unit. Play therapy is one form of treatment available in this setting.

THE PSYCHOLOGICAL DISORDERS OF CHILDHOOD AND ADOLESCENCE

1. *Neurotic disorders*, such as anxiety states, phobias, obsessions, compulsions, hysterical disorders, depression, hypochondriasis, school refusal.
2. *Developmental disorders*, including learning disorders, speech and language delay, perceptual problems, abnormal clumsiness.
3. *Hyperkinetic syndrome/attention deficit disorder.*
4. *Epilepsy.*
5. *Eneurisis and encopresis.*
6. *Psychoses*, including infantile autism, schizophrenia, disintegrative psychoses, folie à deux, affective psychoses.
7. *Psychosomatic disorders* such as asthma, eczema, ulcerative colitis.
8. *Anorexia nervosa, bulimia, obesity.*
9. *Conduct disorders.*
10. *Non-accidentally injured children.*
11. *Sexually abused children.*
12. *Elective mutism.*
13. *Stammering.*
14. *Tics.*
15. *Gilles de la Tourette syndrome.*

PLAY THERAPY FOR CHILDREN UNDER STRESS

Play therapy can help any child who is under stress, such as the child who is admitted to hospital, perhaps as an emergency, or with an illness that requires prolonged or painful treatment. Play therapy in its various forms can help by allowing the child to express his fears. Through play, staff can explain the complicated procedures necessary in treatment.

Play therapy helps the chronic sick child and the child with a permanent physical handicap to make the necessary emotional adjustments to cope with life with a handicap, by allowing expression of frustrations and exploring methods of deriving satisfaction from alternative activities. Child therapists have also described their work with dying children.

Children coping with difficult family situations, including separated or divorced parents, and children taken into care need to communicate their anxieties and frustrations at these situations. Within the context of a therapeutic relationship with a trusting adult, play therapy provides a means of communication so that these children can express their feelings of despair that the parental situation cannot be altered. It also provides a situation where the child can be helped to adapt to these circumstances, for example, the child can be prepared for the necessary adjustments needed for successful fostering or adoption and also provides support in the months after this event to ensure that a smooth transition is made. The neutral adult (child therapist) provides the support and opportunity for expression of frustrated feelings, which the child is unable to express in the new parental situation. Children who are physically or sexually abused need this type of help to work through all the feelings associated with this traumatic experience, which, if left unheeded, would scar them emotionally for the rest of their lives. The child in a bereaved family needs help with his adjustment to the tragic event and often his needs are overlooked by the grieving adults around him.

THE MULTIDISCIPLINARY TEAM

Who practices play therapy? The roots of play therapy are firmly grounded in child analysis. Play therapy in its various forms is practised by many people. In relation to child psychiatric disorders, this involves the whole clinical team, child psychiatrists, clinical and educational psychologists, social workers, occupational therapists, speech therapists and nursing staff.

The multifactorial aetiology of the psychological disorders of childhood needs to be investigated by a team of professionals. Traditionally, diagnosis and formulation of problems was carried out by a tripartite group, composed of child psychiatrist, child psychologist and psychiatric social worker and, in some settings, a child psychotherapist joined the team. With the development of the day and residential units for treatment, teachers, nurses and occupational therapists were incorporated and as the complexities of the illnesses emerged, speech therapists, EEG technicians, etc., were all asked to contribute their knowledge and skills.

The role of the play therapist in this distinguished team is to be the voice of the child. The omission of this key person in the team means that no-one investigates the presenting problems solely from the child's point of view. Without their thorough investigation by communicating effectively with the child in the play setting, the diagnostic symptomatology, behaviour, developmental play level and other vital play communication is not conveyed to the team on behalf of the child.

PLAY THERAPY AND OTHER FORMS OF TREATMENT

How are children with emotional and behavioural problems helped? As the causes of these disturbances are so numerous and variable, the types of treatment available are many.

Beginning with the child himself, he may have individual or group psychotherapy (often in the form of play therapy) or it may be necessary to seek a new accepting environment in a residential unit, so that relief is given to both child and parents and the destructive emotional climate is not perpetuated in the home. The child may need specific remedial and educational help and attendance at the unit school either as an inpatient or on a daily basis in a day unit may be essential. Some units focus on behavioural problems and use a variety of behavioural techniques to reduce or eliminate these problems. The use of chemotherapy in child psychiatry is minimal.

Parents, too, need help. This could be in the form of supportive psychotherapy on an individual or group basis, or perhaps specific marital help is required. More frequently, the approach is to treat the whole family in family therapy using a variety of models.

Play therapy is an essential adjunct to all these different types of approaches, as it is the main method of communicating the child's view of the difficulties and is also the basic way of providing individual treatment for the child to solve his own psychosocial and developmental problems.

REFERRAL FOR PLAY THERAPY

Many children are referred for play therapy. What are the expectations of the medical staff when a referral is made? What can the play therapist offer under this blanket term? What are the child's current specific needs? Can play therapy really help the child with these difficulties?

Those who practise play therapy must:

- know the types of play therapy that are available
- become proficient in the knowledge and practice of some of the techniques
- convey what can be offered to the referring agencies and other staff and give detailed explanations of the goals of treatment.

Indiscriminate prescription of play therapy in the past has led to its being undervalued today as its effectiveness has not been proved. Its importance can therefore be overlooked when selecting different types of therapy for the child. This sets up a vicious circle, that is, the undervaluing of play therapy means that as a form of treatment it is not always prescribed. Those making referrals do not always appreciate the goals of treatment and realistically understand what can be achieved.

Training in play therapy in its various forms is sparse in this country and research into the effectiveness of different therapeutic techniques with children with different disorders is very limited. Still less research has been carried out into the essential components that combine to provide the play-therapy experience and the actual process of therapy.

THEORETICAL FRAMEWORKS FOR DIFFERENT TYPES OF PLAY THERAPY

In the 1930s child psychiatrists and psychologists, recognising the natural therapeutic qualities in the play of 'normal' children, began to exploit these play devices to provide therapy for children with emotional and behavioural problems. Today the list of different play techniques used for therapeutic purposes is endless. The following sections of this chapter outline a few of the main types of play therapy but the practitioner must explore the vast literature that has accumulated, to add relevant techniques to his or her own therapeutic repertoire. As the aetiology of childhood disorders is so complex, no one method of play therapy can be used effectively with all disorders and an eclectic therapeutic approach is useful to provide the correct help for the child.

TYPES OF PLAY THERAPY

The major types of play therapy are:

- psychoanalytically orientated
- non-directive
- relationship
- developmental
- directed
- group
- family.

PSYCHOANALYTICALLY ORIENTATED

In this type of play therapy, the therapist is dealing with the child's unconscious anxieties and defences. These are clearly demonstrated in the transference relationship that develops between the child and the therapist. In this relationship the child experiences unconscious needs that were unmet and unconscious conflicts that were unresolved with significant figures (parents) in his early life. The transference relationship reflects the emotional level that the child has reached and is fixated at. The aim of the therapy is to resolve these past conflicts and unmet needs and to help the child to progress from the fixated level, through the normal phases of emotional development until he attains the correct emotional level for his chronological age.

Through the accepting transference relationship, the child displays and experiences his needs as he is no longer required to repress them in his daily life. This experience brings awareness and, with interpretation, insight is gained and, within the relationship, he is helped to mature. Klein (1932) indicated that in the analysis of children the free play of the child is a direct substitute for the verbal free association of the adult in psychoanalysis. The child produces unconscious material in his symbolic play and reveals his inner world. The acceptance of this material by the therapist and her interpretation helps the child to gain insight into his fears, frustrations, conflicts, needs, anxieties, and fantasies and helps him work through and integrate his feelings.

Often, the child participates in role reversal with the therapist, in a symbolic way. The child becomes a significant adult figure in his life and the therapist is directed to take on the role of the child. The child then masters his fears and conflicts in the real relationship by acting out the adult's role as he sees it or as he would like to see it. Freud (1920) described how, in play, the child no longer accepts the inevitable control of his life by adults but takes control of his own play world and reconstructs disturbing situations with the play material, where he directs the course of action and so masters his anxieties.

The repetition of a particular play theme illustrates the child's unconscious anxiety about a particular situation and the therapist interpreting the anxieties helps them to diminish. The repetition helps the child to integrate his feelings and anxieties into his general experience, just as an adult would think over or talk over a particularly upsetting experience, probably elaborating and describing how he would have liked to have handled the situation.

The theoretical approaches of Sigmund Freud, Melanie Klein, Anna Freud, Margaret Lowenfeld, Donald Winnicott, etc. should be studied by all who interpret children's play. However, it is important that this is supplemented with training and case supervision from experienced practitioners or membership of a self-help peer group to support the therapist who is starting to use these techniques. (See the Further Reading list at the end of the Chapter.)

NON-DIRECTIVE

This is probably the most common form of play therapy used in this country and in North America. It was devised for children by Virginia Axline (Axline 1947) from the therapeutic work of Carl Rogers with adults, that is, client-centred therapy (Rogers 1967).

Axline's work is based on her theory that the child's innate drive to achieve maturity must be given the optimum facilitating environment to achieve that goal. She suggests that this can be achieved in the following ways.

- By providing an 'ideal' play environment so that the child can play out all his bewildering feelings and by doing this, become aware of them, acknowledge them, and eventually direct and control them.
- By providing an adult who accepts and understands all these feelings completely, reflecting back the feelings so that they are clarified for the child.

The therapist does not direct the child's play in any way, limit setting is minimal, and the therapist presents a concerned, consistent approach, aware of all that the child is communicating in his play and ensuring that the child realises that he is accepted, whatever feelings he displays. She allows the child to be himself. This increases his confidence and self-esteem. The child is completely free to realise his potentialities and so he matures. By learning to understand and accept himself, he learns to understand and accept others.

RELATIONSHIP

Relationship therapy emphasises the therapeutic relationship between child and therapist. The focus of sessions is on the 'here and now' relationship. The therapy begins at the presenting level of emotional development of the child and the feelings expressed in the therapy sessions towards the therapist form the basis of the maturational experience. This type of therapy is suitable for any age range but for younger children a play experience is added for communication purposes.

The nature of the therapeutic relationship

Practitioners new to the field often query the differences between relationship therapy and non-directive therapy. The difference lies in the nature of the therapeutic relationship. In non-directive therapy, the therapist has a quiescent approach, using reflection of feelings as the main form of communication, whereas relationship therapy uses the 'here and now' feelings of the child for the therapist to explore the child's level of emotional functioning. In relationship therapy the accepting therapist allows the child to express these feelings and actively explains (interprets) their significance in the relationship and so helps the child to mature.

DEVELOPMENTAL

Developmental play therapy is a model which is based on developmental theories, that is, Hellersberg's Psychophysical Theory of Development and Freud and Peller's Psychosexual Theories of Development (Hellersberg 1955, Peller 1952, Hall 1954). See Table 16.1. These theories explain the complex play patterns which the child presents in play therapy sessions. Jeffrey (1984) has outlined how a knowledge of these three theories, in relation to the child's play in therapy, provides the therapist with a sound theoretical rationale for providing an initial assessment that gives a baseline of the child's emotional state and subsequently, as therapy proceeds, provides a method of measuring progress. For this to be achieved, the play takes place in the context of relationship therapy using non-directive play.

The aim of this therapy is to allow the child, within the context of the therapeutic relationship and with the use of appropriate play activities, to achieve his appropriate level of emotional development for his chronological age. This method of therapy is based on developmental theories that suggest that, for healthy personality development to occur, the child needs to progress through each stage of emotional development successfully, before tackling a further phase. If the child's needs at one stage are not satisfied, he is fixated at that particular level, he does not mature and does not become a well-integrated adult who can cope with the ordinary stresses and strains of life.

It is essential, therefore, that the therapeutic experience provides a good therapeutic relationship that permits the child to relate to the therapist and play out the particular level of emotional development he has reached. The child is free to choose whatever activities he wishes to participate in. He is not expected to achieve, as he would be in the school situation, nor is he expected to conform to a particular standard of behaviour. In this atmosphere of therapeutic freedom, he is enabled to demonstrate his particular problems. The therapist empathetically accepts, explores and clarifies his feelings and interprets the type of relationship he forms with her and also the behaviour he

Table 16.1 Developmental play therapy (Adapted from Jeffrey 1984. Reproduced with permission from the British Journal of Occupational Therapy.)

Phases of therapy	Psychophysical (Hellersberg)	Psychoanalytical (Freud)	Psychosexual (Peller)
Phase 1	Sensory/Tactile	Oral	Narcissistic
Phase 2	Motor	Anal	Pre-Oedipal
Phase 3	Representational	Phallic	Oedipal
Phase 4	Constructive	Latency	Post-Oedipal

produces. However, more important, in this type of therapy it is by allowing the child to use the play material as he wishes, reflecting his stage of emotional development, that this phase is worked through. This is because the child's needs are satisfied both by the type of relationship he is experiencing and the type of therapeutic play he can indulge in. The child, by this bio-psychosocial approach reexperiences his early development, makes up the deficiences and hence achieves emotional maturity.

DIRECTED

Directed play therapy is used when the therapist decides to use the play medium for a specific therapeutic aim and directs the use of the play materials by the child, so that, if possible, the objective is achieved. Often this involves contriving, through play, the reenactment of past, present or future disturbing events in the child's life, for example, using therapy dolls to help express her guilt and fear of being sexually abused by her father, or helping the child express feelings about separation from a loved parent, when parents have just divorced, or rehearsing feelings about particular painful procedures if the child is about to be admitted to hospital, explaining the need for the procedures and exactly what is to be done.

Directed play techniques have been used for over 50 years with a multitude of aims and objectives. An early paper on the subject (Levy 1939) described how, in imaginative play, the normal child copes with anxiety. Levy harnessed this in 'release therapy'. With older children he encouraged them to reenact a situation that had particularly troubled them and was a precipitating factor in their particular symptomatology. For younger children he did not explore actual events but allowed them to indulge in play of a primitive nature, for example, messy sand, water and clay, which the child used in a variety of ways. This expression of basic aggressive feelings and accompanying regressive play released the child from the controls of a too-strict upbringing, when too high expectations and demands were made of him.

The main keys to the use of directed play therapy are practice, experience and evaluation.

There is an extensive literature of different techniques, and the therapist, having determined a child's specific need, will consider that one of these techniques would help, then try that specific technique and carefully evaluate its effectiveness on the child's therapy.

There are a wealth of directed techniques for different types of psychological disorders in childhood,

● Theraplay (Jernberg 1979) for children who for a variety of reasons have either missed or not responded to normal sensory motor play in the first 2 years of life.

● Gardner (1971) has used his 'Mutual Storytelling Technique' to help children with all types of psychological problems. He uses both audio-tapes and video-tapes of the child and recommends the use of these items of equipment rather than toy props, as the child enjoys participating in the adult world of communication, and is not distracted by fantasy material, and so produces his own imaginative creations in verbal form.

● Gardner has also devised the 'Talking, Feeling and Doing' game, specifically for children who find it difficult, even with his story technique to express their needs and conflicts (Gardner 1975).

● O'Connor (1982) has also suggested that the older child needs to verbalise, rather than just play out, feelings and has devised the 'Colour Your Life Technique', so that feelings are expressed verbally through the use of significant colours.

GROUP

Group therapy for emotionally disturbed children in the form of Activity Group Therapy was first introduced by Slavson (Slavson and Schiffer, 1975). His colleague Schiffer (1971) introduced this form of therapy for the younger age group, naming it 'Therapeutic Play Groups'.

Group therapy can never be a substitute for individual therapy. Group therapy has different aims and objectives and, although it is a very useful adjunct to individual therapy, it cannot replace the one-to-one therapeutic relationship, if that is what the disturbed child requires for his particular disorder. It is also essential that children placed in groups must have a potential for social development and social play, whatever their chronological age and that they are not fixated at an earlier level of development.

The group with the adult therapist or therapists and the peer group of children, reflects the family situation with parents and siblings or reflects the school situation with teachers and classmates. From an assessment point of view, the child interacts in this new 'family' or new 'school' set-up as he has done in the previous settings. The child plays one adult against another, as he does at home. His sibling rivalry difficulties are reflected in the new 'family' setting. Within the warm, empathetic, atmosphere of the group, his difficulties are displayed and accepted. In the group, adults do not repeat emotionally charged parental interaction and peers are encouraged to understand the child's difficulties, just as their own difficulties are being accepted and tolerated. So, in this therapeutic situation, the child can try out new ways of behaving and relating. As the child feels more accepted, a positive self-image develops, he accepts more responsibility for his behaviour, becomes more independent and matures.

Certain children do not benefit from group therapy, for example, severely deprived children, autistic children, severely neurotic children, and some psychotic and brain damaged children. The child with a mental handicap should not be placed in a therapeutic group of this nature as he is scapegoated.

FAMILY

When considering the different models for family therapy, it is important to remember the young child in this setting. Some family therapists make provision for the child by having play materials available. However, it is also important to understand how the young child is affected by the family dynamics within the group, hence, the importance of having a play therapist present who can organise play materials that allow the child to communicate at his correct maturational age and emotional developmental level. The child does not have the verbal abilities of the adults present but he will communicate through his play. The play

therapist's role in this setting is to draw the attention of the family and family therapist to the communication of the young child. She must also help the child by clarifying the adults' communication at a level he can understand.

Therapists have derived different approaches to including children in this setting, for example, conjoint play therapy for the young child and his parent (Safer 1965); the specific participation of the child in family therapy (Villeneuve 1979), etc.

PRACTICAL GUIDELINES

The child, having been assessed by the multidisciplinary team, is referred for play therapy. To ensure a successful outcome of treatment many practical considerations need to be examined at this stage. This includes the roles of the participants, the child himself, the parents, the therapist and the play environment. As already described, choosing the therapeutic technique is of paramount importance. All the therapies need careful introduction, handling throughout the course of treatment and successful termination.

THE ROLE OF THE PARENTS

It is vital initially that the parents understand the child's need for therapy. It is also important to gain their cooperation and commitment to bringing the child for regular sessions.

Parental commitment

Children who are inpatients or day patients in a unit with a play therapist can easily attend for sessions. This is not so with outpatients. Often parents or other caretakers find the weekly or more-frequent commitment of bringing the child to the unit a considerable drain on their time. It helps if it can be arranged that the parent sees medical and social-work staff at the same time as the child is having therapy and so are having their own needs attended to.

Some units have devised imaginative programmes with occupational therapists providing individual or group sessions for the children and having activity groups, for example, for depressed young mothers who are isolated from close and extended family. Supportive coffee and chat groups with another member of staff when practical handling problems, etc. can be discussed are an alternative.

Introducing play therapy to parents

It is useful to give a handout to the parents, explaining the general principles of play therapy. The doctor referring the child, or the social worker involved, can discuss this sheet with the parent and clarify any difficulties and will involve the play therapist, if necessary.

The sheet should explain how playing out problems for the child is a substitute for the talking out of problems by the adult and that the child needs a therapeutic relationship with the play therapist, a neutral figure, away from his ordinary daily living activities. The length of treatment (difficult to predict but often long) must be indicated and it must be stressed that the parents' commitment is vital, especially in relation to bringing the child regularly.

Parents are naturally very curious about what takes place in the play room. Clear guidelines must be given to avoid rivalry developing between the parents and therapist. It is important to let the parents see the playroom and meet the play therapist on their introductory visit. However, it is essential to convey that the play sessions are confidential and indicate that questions such as, has the child had a good time and what has he been playing with, will often be ignored by the child.

The parent will want to know how the child is progressing in play therapy. This should be discussed with the social worker, rather than approaching the play therapist at the end of the session when the child is present.

From a practical point of view, it is important to emphasise to parents that all types of activities are used, including messy paint and clay, and that they can help by allowing the child to come to the unit in clothing suitable for these activities.

THE ROLE OF THE OCCUPATIONAL THERAPIST

Therapists planning treatment for children will be influenced by their training, knowledge, skills and experience. It is essential for therapists to focus on the difficulties that the individual child is presenting in his home, at school, etc. Therapists must provide a play environment that enables the child to communicate his views of the problem.

Assessment

The initial phase of the intervention has several purposes.

● It is therapeutic, as the child builds up a relationship with the therapist in a permissive, trusting atmosphere.

● In this accepting situation, the child reveals his problems as he sees them. Again, self-revelation accompanied by ventilation of feelings is therapeutic.

● The child's maturational level is assessed.

● His behaviour in the setting is noted.

● The emotional stage that the child has reached is determined by the type of play he uses in a non-directive setting and the type of relationship he forms with the therapist.

This essential information must then be conveyed to the multidisciplinary team by the therapist, so that future management can be planned.

Treatment

Once the therapist is aware of the child's emotional developmental level and has the knowledge of the child's specific problems, play therapy sessions can now take place in the context of a suitably chosen therapeutic technique.

Supervision

The way each therapist approaches treatment for a particular child will differ. This is inevitable, for, even if the therapists were trained in a particular theory of development and applied the same therapeutic technique, they each approach the child from their own perspective. Their own childhood experiences and their relationships with key figures in their own lives influence their reactions to the child. Sometimes these experiences have been so prominent in their own personality development that they unconsciously identify with the child.

To enable therapists to cope with feelings roused after many years and which, if left unresolved would affect the therapy, it is helpful if the therapist can discuss the child in treatment with a senior colleague. Therapists who have practised therapy for many years still value the opportunity to discuss a child's treatment progress with an experienced senior therapist. Many children who have had fearful, painful, upsetting, depriving experiences will unload these feelings onto the therapist who needs support to cope with this onslaught and help to contain the child's overwhelming fears, anxieties, fantasies, etc.

Case supervision

Case supervision enables the therapist to discuss the child's progress. The supervisor emphasises the different developmental theories and the theoretical rationale of different techniques. He compares his own experience of handling children with similar problems. Regular weekly individual or group supervision should be available for all practising this type of therapy. For supervisors this is a very time-consuming task, yet, if they are committed to this type of approach, they will realise its importance and so devote the time to it.

Personal supervision

Personal supervision is offered by some psychiatrists and psychotherapists, enabling the child therapists to explore their own unresolved difficulties, stemming back to their own childhood experiences, and so enable the therapists to continue with therapy unimpeded by past experiences.

Recording sessions

A useful method is to record as much of the play

session as possible, either at the time or, if this is too inhibiting for the child, as soon as possible after the session. Accurate observations of the child's play are invaluable, that is, what he plays with, how he plays with the toys, his significant interactions with the therapist, what type of reaction this arouses in the therapist, etc. This material is then used in supervision to explore the play sessions in full. Often, seemingly trivial themes in the child's play in the first few sessions only become recognised as important communications after many sessions, when the child plays out this particular theme again and again.

THE ROLE OF THE CHILD

Often a child's introduction to a Child Psychiatry Unit is surrounded by anger and guilt, both for the parents and the child. The child's behaviour has become intolerable and help is needed. The parents feel they have failed in their upbringing of the child. The child may have been threatened with all sorts of dire consequences if his behaviour does not improve, so it is very important when meeting him to begin immediately to clarify the role of the unit and the play therapy itself.

Introducing the child to therapy

At the introductory visit it is important for both child and parent to meet the play therapist and see the play therapy room. It must be stressed immediately that the play therapist knows that the child has been having some difficulties and his life has not been happy (there is no need to discuss the problems in detail) and that the play therapist is there to help him. The procedure for attending sessions should be explained, for example, the parent will be seeing the social worker, while the child comes for his 45-minute session with the play therapist.

The play therapist will collect him from the waiting room and they will return there at the end of the session.

The initial phase

The first session may be clouded with separation

difficulties for both parent and child, and this must be worked through. Sometimes this can take several sessions and occasionally the child finds the situation so threatening that the parent needs to remain in the room. It is best, at this point, just to use the time to introduce the child to all the play materials available and allow him to enjoy himself and be at ease, rather than focus on the therapy when the parent is present.

For the child who can separate, the play therapist indicates that she knows the child has been having problems, again there is no need to elaborate. The child will communicate his view of the problems in his own time. The therapist must explain that coming for regular sessions to play in this room with her will help. The child is then introduced to the play materials and given permission to play with anything he likes. Children vary in the time they take to settle into the play situation, usually depending on their previous separation experiences and degree of anxiety, but the therapist conveying her interest and approval in what they are doing gives the secure framework necessary.

It is important, in the initial sessions, to clarify any fantasies the child may have about the unit, for example, one distressed child enquired when the therapist was going to give him the 'needle'. Another fearful child wanted to know where the 'operations room' was. This child had undergone surgery several times in his young life. The therapist and child spent the first session exploring every room in the building to reassure him that he was not there for any physical reasons.

Often in the first few sessions the child (usually depending on his age) will become anxious after a time, this is partly normal separation anxiety but sometimes children have been threatened that they will be sent away and feel that they will not be taken back to their parents at the end of the session. If a child becomes very anxious, it is best to terminate the session at this point and take him back to his parents.

Setting limits

Even in non-directive play therapy some limits are essential. First, the therapist must be in control of the play situation. If she is not, the child finds this a very threatening experience. Next, many disturbed children have not had consistent experiences in their lives. The variations of the same adult's reactions to single factors of their behaviour has left them confused, with no idea of which behaviour is approved and which is not. The limits within the therapy situation provide this consistent approach by the therapist and so order can be given to the child's life, during the play session. Later this generalises to the rest of his life.

Limits also demonstrate the concern that the therapist has for the child. They are there for the child's wellbeing, for example, he must not harm the fabric of the room, the therapist, the other children or himself, and he must not destroy the toys. If the child does break these limits, he is out of control, the situation is frightening for him and later he experiences considerable guilt. The limit is set at the appropriate time when this deviant behaviour is displayed.

Sometimes the child wishes to take the play materials home with him. This expresses a need to take the play-situation home. This must be interpreted to the child in terms of a simple explanation, that the work of therapy takes place in the session and is not repeated in other situations. Some therapists suggest that the very young child needs a toy to take home as a 'transitional object' to remind the small child that the play experience is there and will return.

Some therapists do not display paintings and other projective work and do not allow it to be removed from the playroom. Again, remember that this is not ordinary play, but therapy, and children need to know that the feelings expressed in the play room are confidential and are contained there by the therapist, that is, the therapist takes care of the child's picture, etc., which is stored in his own drawer.

Testing out the therapist

The child also tests out the therapist by using certain types of behaviour, for example, running out of the room, deliberately flooding the sand tray, putting the lights on and off, painting the floor, walls or furniture, throwing toys at the therapist, deliberately hurting another child, etc.

Careful management techniques need to be worked out to handle this acting out. As well as interpreting the child's need to use this behaviour, realistic explanations should be given as to why he cannot carry it out and limits firmly set.

One of the most difficult situations to handle is when the child tries to play off the therapist against the parent. This needs careful handling at the time by the play therapist and often the parents need support from their social worker to help them handle this type of behaviour from the child. If unresolved, rivalry could develop between the parents and the play therapist.

Terminating therapy

The child, having worked through his problems, must be given ample warning that therapy will end. He needs time to work through leaving what has been an intense relationship with the therapist. The child is helped in this process by reviewing his original reason for referral and indicating how he has progressed and helping him with plans for the future. The child may produce symptoms again in an attempt to retain the therapy situation but, by careful preparation, he will be ready for the discharge date. Sometimes children in a residential unit continue to attend the unit for outpatient play therapy while they settle into their new surroundings or return to their original home and school. Again, termination must be judged with care, when the child no longer needs the support offered.

THE PLAY ENVIRONMENT

The entire aim of creating the child-centred play environment is to allow the child to communicate. Through the play medium, with toys and other play activities, he obtains the therapeutic experience he requires to restore his emotional wellbeing.

A CHILD-CENTRED ENVIRONMENT

A room should preferably be specifically designed for play therapy and reserved solely for this purpose. The child needs to feel free to be himself in that room and does not want the atmosphere clouded with previous memories and associations, for example, a classroom, a medical room in the school, or a room previously used when parents have been interviewed.

The room must be completely child centred, with child-sized furniture of various heights. The therapist's office should preferably be elsewhere as a desk, telephone, filing cabinets and notes do not enhance the play atmosphere.

A useful arrangement is a partly carpeted area so that both child and therapist can sit on the floor, with the rest of the room having a vinyl covering for sand, water, paint, clay and other messy activities. An easy chair is an asset, as therapists who use 'reading therapy' will find that the story atmosphere created by this setting is a very useful way of ending sessions. The room must convey a sense of privacy, for example, windows should be of frosted glass to a certain height if there is the likelihood of the sessions being observed from outside. It is important that the child feels he can trust the play environment. If the therapist wishes to use one-way screens, sound recording or videotape equipment, this must always be fully explained to the child.

Display and storage of toys

Display of toys, other play materials, books, etc. must always be considered carefully. Open shelving is required for the display of toys, all readily accessible to the child. In some instances, there is a need to restrict certain play materials and there should be lockable storage cupboards, so that the therapist can control the play environment.

Some therapists like to exhibit the children's pictures and other products of play sessions on pinboards or in display cabinets. This really should be the child's decision; remember that he is revealing his inner emotions through these media and may not want them to be displayed for all to see. In contrast, other children need recognition for their efforts.

Safety

Tools must be kept in a lockable cupboard with shadowboards for easy identification and checking at the end of the session. Paint, glue, turps, etc. should be stored in a lockable metal cupboard.

The therapist must be able to control the water and electricity supply to the room. Enclosed strip lighting should be installed for safety purposes.

Sand and water play

When planning the 'messy' play area, careful thought is needed in relation to the sitting of the sand tray, or trays, in relation to the sink. It is important that they should not be constantly flooded as this impedes the play of other children attending that day. Ideally, three types of sand in separated trays should be available:

1. dry sand for pouring
2. damp ordinary sand for modelling
3. very messy wet sand.

A useful arrangement, if it is not possible to have three sand trays or if space is scarce, is to have one sand tray stand, with one tray in place, and underneath two stackable trays with the other types of sand available and exchanged when necessary. Two lids are also useful to cover the sand tray and the top container, to control the use of this material. Some therapists prefer a sandpit at floor level. A play sink (child height) so that the child can indulge in water play, without being constricted to a small handbasin, is an essential feature. It is useful if this sink is at a height for comfortable sitting for child and therapist, that is, knee room must be available.

The correct play environment is essential and this can be illustrated by describing the settings for two types of therapy.

1. A non-directive play room would have all play materials displayed with easy access for the child.
2. In contrast, an autistic child or a hyperactive child would need a stimulus-free environment. In this instance, furniture, curtains, wall and floor coverings would be in soft shades and tones, so that there is no distraction from the selected task in hand. Toys and other play materials would be stored away.

Space is very important and a cluttered atmosphere confuses the child. A playroom with restricted materials is often far more effective than one where the child is overwhelmed by too much to choose from. Remember the room is designed to facilitate communication and if a good therapeutic relationship is established the child will convey his 'inner world' with the limited materials available. An overstocked playroom is more for the therapist's security than to cater for the child's needs.

TOYS AND PLAY MATERIALS

The toys and play materials used are all available to allow the child to communicate and express his feelings. They are also needed to assess the child's emotional development level and to allow him to fixate, regress and eventually mature emotionally through the relationship experience and participation in the play activity.

Different types of play therapy require different play materials, but the following selection based on the developmental play therapy model should cater for most children's needs. (See the section on Developmental play therapy p. 253 Hellersberg 1955, Hall 1954, Peller 1952).

General equipment

- overalls, or plastic aprons
- sponges for quick mopping up
- dustpan, brush
- squeezy mop
- paper towels, wastepaper bins.

Phase 1: Sensory/Tactile/Oral/Narcissistic

- Materials for bubble blowing: a suitable container for a mixture of washing-up liquid and water. Bubble masters, as these give instant success.
- Food activity of some sort (see Fig. 16.1), for example, simple sweet-making with instant icing,

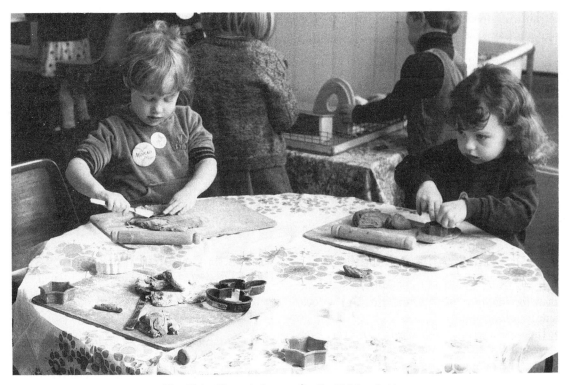

Fig. 16.1   Phase 1: Sensory/tactile. Children baking.

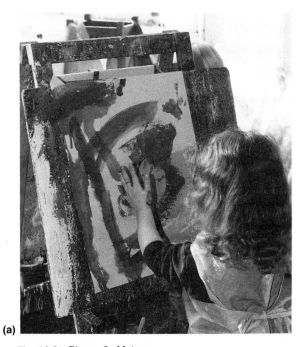

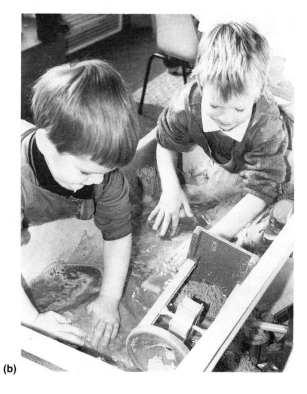

(a)

Fig. 16.2   Phase 2: Motor.
(a) Finger printing.   (b) Wet, soggy sand.   (b)

or introducing food into the session, for example, orange juice and biscuits.

- Tea-party toys for dolls and small children: cups, saucers, spoons, teapot, milk jug, etc.
- For the older child, still fixated at this stage, food preparation at a more sophisticated level and using the department's kitchen, if this is appropriate.
- Musical instruments and singing activities. It is useful to have a suitable selection of tapes.
- Dry sand for pouring, sand tray and toys for sand play.
- A variety of toys for object-related play, for example, a post box, inset trays, etc.

Phase 2: Motor/Anal/Pre-Oedipal

- If available, an outside adventure playground is ideal for this type of play, or visits to the local adventure playground.
- Indoors, a gym is also ideal. However, even in a restricted space, movement games can be devised, for example, a play tunnel.
- Hammer toys and simple woodwork activity also provides suitable movement activities.
- Water play in the sink is important at this stage, with suitable water-play toys for pouring, etc.
- Clay should be available for smearing at this stage. Finger painting, with water paste and liquid paint is ideal (Fig. 16.2(a)).
- Play dough (home made) is excellent, with boards, rolling pins and cutters.
- Dolls, with cot, clothes, feeding bottles (real size), bath, potty, etc.
- A sand tray and toys for wet, messy sand play (Fig. 16.2(b)).

Phase 3: Representational/Phallic/Oedipal

- A selection of fairy stories, with the text on one page and illustration on the opposite page.
- A dolls house, dolls and furniture.
- A farm and layout (Fig. 16.3). Domestic animal families.
- Wild model animals. Fantasy animals, for example, dragons.

- A play mat with a garage and transport toys, police cars, ambulance, aeroplanes, motor bikes, cars, helicopters, a fire brigade, a train set, etc.
- Miniature figures: policemen, firemen, ambulance driver, etc.
- Domestic play equipment and play dough.
- A Wendy house, cot, doll bed, chairs, table, cooker, doll family.
- Dressing up clothes and other props for imaginative play. A toy telephone.
- Puppets and a puppet theatre.
- A miniature hospital. Play toys.
- Drawing materials: paper, pencils, crayons, felt-tip pens, brushes, liquid paint and palettes.

Phase 4: Constructive/Latency/Post-Oedipal.

A selection of constructive and creative activities for use in a group, as follows.

- Construction toys: Duplo, Lego, Helter-Skelter (Fig. 16.4(a)).
- Table games: picture lotto, picture dominoes (Fig. 16.4(b)).
- Clay or plasticine for modelling.
- Materials for collage: glue, paint, etc.

To equip a new play therapy room, a selection of toys should be made from each of these phases.

PLAY-THERAPY RESEARCH

Early research in play therapy was reviewed by Ginott (1961). In the 25 years following that summary, the literature on play-therapy research has escalated.

The whole field of normal play and play-therapy research invades every aspect of the child's mental health, from assisting normal development, health maintenance and prevention, to early intervention and treatment strategies required to eliminate severe pathology.

As has been noted previously, for correct prescription of play therapy, rather than a blanket referral, it is vital to:

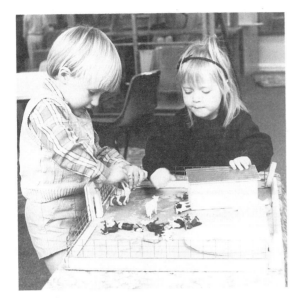

Fig. 16.3 Phase 3: Representational. A farm layout.

Fig. 16.4 Phase 4: Constructive.
(a) Lego.   **(b)** Picture dominoes.

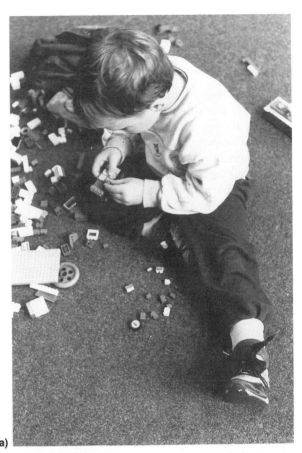

(a)

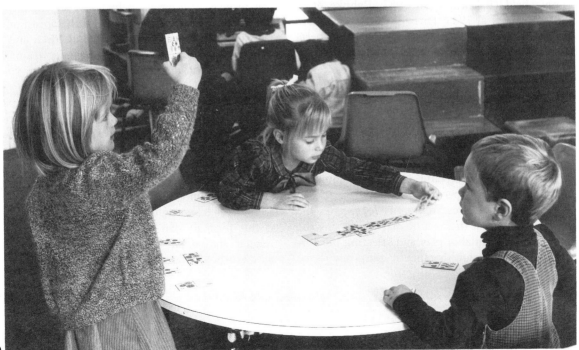

(b)

- establish the need for therapy, that is, the child's specific problem, which can be solved by play therapy
- apply the correct play-therapy technique.

Only then can comparison and evaluation of therapeutic procedures be made and consideration given to all the variables that will effect the outcome, for example, the therapist's own personality and experience, her specific expertise, knowledge, training and skills, the play materials available, the number and frequency of sessions and the age of the child.

The number of treatment techniques, especially in relation to directed therapy, increases yearly. The problems to which they are applied vary widely. The clinicians instigating these new methods are committed to, and enthusiastic about, their particular mode of treatment. It is difficult to refine research methodology to evaluate the outcome and effectiveness of the techniques used, yet it is vital, with such a scarce resource of child therapists, to establish successful treatment strategies so that they can be applied effectively to the numerous child problems created by the pressures of today's society.

An examination of the play studies in recent years indicates the range of research possibilities in this field (Baldwin et al 1982, Behnke et al 1984, Casby et al 1985, Earls et al 1983, Letts et al 1983, Lowery 1985, Purcell et al 1983, Roberts et al 1984, Terrell et al 1984, Thompson et al 1985).

An investigation of the need for research by occupational therapists working in the field of child psychiatry was undertaken in 1980 (Jeffrey 1982b). The need to establish research into the effectiveness of therapeutic techniques and therapeutic play for various disorders was evident, so that optimum therapeutic experiences could be provided in these departments.

This preliminary research study focuses on the psychodynamics of therapeutic play. Analysing the therapeutic potential of play and selecting the correct type of play for therapeutic purposes is the core of the occupational therapist's role in this field. The vast literature on the use of play in 'normal' childhood for educational and therapeutic purposes, as well as the use of play as a therapeutic tool for the treatment of disease and disability, will provide fertile terrain for the new generation of graduate therapists, to research into the developmental origins of occupations, which forms the basis of treatment for the profession.

SUMMARY

The many pressures of modern life are manifesting in various ways in today's society. Children may be either directly or indirectly affected by unemployment, divorce, reconstituted families, drug or alcohol abuse, etc.

Children who are suffering from a chronic or terminal illness, those who are taken into care, fostered or adopted, children suffering from non-accidental injury or sexual abuse, etc. suffer from excessive stress and unhappiness.

More and more adults under stress, seek help in the form of counselling, therapy or self-help groups. It is essential that children under stress can receive appropriate help too. Play therapy is one form of help necessary. Play therapists must contribute their knowledge of the children and of their problems to the multidisciplinary team. In that setting the play therapist is indeed the voice of the child.

This chapter has outlined different types of play therapy available and has given details of the practical approach to this work from the point of view of the children who need this help, their parents, the therapist and the play environment. The need for postgraduate training opportunities, necessary supervision, and careful evaluation of the different techniques has been discussed. These are essential if this form of therapy is to be established as a regular component of treatment programmes for all disturbed children.

REFERENCES

Axline V M 1947 Play therapy. Ballantine Books, New York

Baldwin C P et al 1982 Family free play interaction: the role of the patient in the family interaction. Monograph of Social Research into Child Development 47(5): 45–59

Behnke C T et al 1984 Examining the reliability and validity of the play history. American Journal of Occupational Therapy 38(2): 94–100

Bruner J S et al 1976 Play: its role in development and evolution. Penguin, Harmondsworth

Casby M W et al 1985 Symbolic play and early communication development in hearing-impaired children. Journal of Communication Disorders 18(1): 67–68

College of Occupational Therapists 1981 Diploma Course: Training in occupational therapy. College of Occupational Therapists, London

Earls F et al 1983 Play observations of three-year old children and their relationship to parental reports of behaviour problems and temperamental characteristics. Child Psychiatry and Human Development 13(4): 225–232

Ellis M J 1973 Why people play. Prentice Hall, New Jersey

Freud S 1920 Beyond the pleasure principle. In: On metapsychology, vol 2 1984. The Pelican Freud Library. Penguin, Harmondsworth

Gardner R A 1971 Therapeutic communication with children: the mutual story telling technique. Jason Aronson, New York

Gardner R A 1975 Psychotherapeutic approaches to the resistant child: the talking, feeling and doing game. Jason Aronson, New York

Ginott H G 1961 Group psychotherapy with children. McGraw-Hill, New York

Hall C S 1954 A Primer of Freudian Psychology. World Publishing Company, New York.

Harman R J et al 1982 The relationship between infant play with inanimate objects and social interest in mother. Journal of the American Academy of Child Psychiatry 21(6): 549–554

Hellersberg E F 1955 Child growth in play therapy. American Journal of Psychotherapy 9: 484–502

Jeffrey L I 1982a Occupational therapy in child and adolescent psychiatry: the future. British Journal of Occupational Therapy 45(10): 330–334

Jeffrey L I H 1982b Exploration of the use of therapeutic play in the rehabilitation of psychologically disturbed children. Fellowship thesis: Available from the British Library

Jeffrey L I H 1984 Developmental play therapy: an assessment and therapeutic technique in child psychiatry. British Journal of Occupational Therapy 47(3): 70–74

Jernberg A 1979 Theraplay. Jossey-Bass, San Francisco

Klein M 1932 The psychoanalysis of children. Hogarth Press, London

Letts M et al 1983 Puppetry and doll play as an adjunct to paediatric orthopaedics. Journal of Paediatric Orthopaedics 3(5): 605–609

Levy D 1939 Release therapy. American Journal of Orthopsychiatry 9: 713–736

Lowery E F 1985 Autistic aloofnesss reconsidered: case reports of two children in play therapy. Bulletin of the Menninger Clinic 49(2): 135–150

MacDonald K et al 1984 Bridging the gap: parent child play interaction and peer interactive competence. Child Development 55(4): 1265–1277

Miller S 1973 The psychology of play. Penguin, Harmondsworth

O'Connor K J 1982 The color your life technique. In: Schaefer C, O'Connor (eds) Handbook of play therapy. Wiley, New York

Peller L E 1952 Models of children's play. Mental Hygiene 36: 66–83

Purcell P D et al 1983 Effects of play therapy on preschool children during initial dental visits. Journal of Child Dentistry 50(6): 433–436

Roberts M A et al 1984 A playroom observational procedure for assessing hyperactive boys. Journal of Paediatric Psychology 9(2): 177–191

Rogers C R 1967 On becoming a person. Constable, London

Safer A 1965 Conjoint play therapy for the young child and his parent. Archives of General Psychiatry 13: 320–326

Schiffer M 1971 The therapeutic play group. Allen and Unwin, London

Slavson S R, Schiffer M 1975 Group psychotherapies for children. International Universities Press, New York

Smith P K 1977 Social and fantasy play in young children in: Tizard B, Harvey D (eds) Spastics International Medical Publications, London. Heinemann Medical Books

Terrell B Y et al 1984 Symbolic play in normal and language-impaired children. Journal of Speech and Hearing Research 27(3): 424–429

Thompson T J et al 1985 Stereotyped behaviour of severely disabled children in classroom and free play settings. American Journal of Mental Deficiency 89(6): 580–586

Ungerer J A et al 1984 The relation of play and sensorimotor behaviour to language in the second year. Child Development 55(4): 1448–1455

Villeneuve C 1979 The specific participation of the child in family therapy. American Academy of Child Psychiatry 44–53

Weininger O 1983 Play of mothers with babies: some relationships between maternal personality and early attachment and developmental process. Psychological Research 53(1): 27–42

FURTHER READING

OVERVIEWS OF THE FIELD

Haworth M R 1964 Child psychotherapy practise and theory. Basic Books, New York

Jeffrey L I H 1982a Occupational therapy in child and adolescent psychiatry: the future. British Journal of Occupational Therapy 45(10): 330–334

Jeffrey L I H 1982b Exploration of the use of therapeutic play in the rehabilitation of psychologically disturbed children. Fellowship thesis: available from the British Library and the College of Occupational Therapists, London

Schaefer C, O'Connor K (eds) 1962 Handbook of play therapy. Wiley, New York

Schaefer C 1976 Therapeutic use of child's play. Aronson, New York

Oaklander V 1978 Windows to our children. Real People Press, Utah

PSYCHOANALYTICALLY ORIENTATED

Boston M, Szur R 1983 Psychotherapy with severely deprived children. Routledge & Kegan Paul, London

Bettelheim B 1978 The uses of enchantment. Penguin, Harmondsworth

Copley B, Forryan C 1987 Therapeutic work with children and young people. Robert Royce, London

Daws D, Boston M 1977 The child psychotherapist and problems of young people. Wildwood House, London

Freud A 1966 Normality and pathology in childhood. Hogarth Press, London

Freud S 1909 Analysis of a phobia in a five year old boy. In: Case Histories, vol 10. 1977. The Pelican Freud Library. Penguin, Harmondsworth

Freud S 1920 Beyond the pleasure principle. In: On metapsychology, vol 11. 1984 The Pelican Freud Library. Penguin, Harmondsworth

Klein M Reprinted 1975 The psychoanalysis of children. Hogarth Press, London

Lowenfield M 1968 Play in childhood. Cedric Chivers, London

Winnicot D W 1971 Therapeutic consultations in child psychiatry. Hogarth, London

Winnicot D W 1980 The Piggle. Penguin, Harmondsworth

NON-DIRECTIVE

Axline V M 1969 Play therapy. Ballantine Books, New York

Axline V M 1971 Dibs: in search of self. Penguin Books, Harmondsworth

RELATIONSHIP

Allen F H 1942 Psychotherapy with children. Norton, New York

Menaker E 1982 Otto Rank: a rediscovered legacy. Colombia University Press, New York

Moustakas C E 1973 Children in play therapy. Aronson, New York

Moustakas C E 1979 Psychotherapy with children. Harper and Row, New York

Rank O Reprinted 1978 Truth and reality. Norton, New York

Rank O Reprinted 1978 Will therapy. Norton, New York

Taft J 1933 The dynamics of therapy in a controlled relationship. MacMillan, New York

DEVELOPMENTAL

Hall C S 1954 A primer of Freudian psychology. World Publishing, New York

Hellersberg E F 1955 Child growth in play therapy. American Journal of Psychotherapy 9: 484–502

Jeffrey L I H 1984 Developmental play therapy: an assessment and therapeutic technique in child psychiatry. British Journal of Occupational Therapy 47(3): 70–74

Peller L E 1952 Models of children's play. Mental Hygiene 36: 66–83

Peller L E 1954 Libidinal phases, ego development and play. The Psychoanalytical Study of the Child 9: 178–198

DIRECTED

Gardner R A 1971 Therapeutic communication with children: The mutual story telling technique. Aronson, New York

Jernberg A 1979 Theraplay. Josey-Bass, San Francisco

Levy D 1939 Release therapy. Journal of Orthopsychiatry 9: 713–736

Nickerson E, O'Laoughlin K (eds) 1982 Action orientated therapies. Human Resource Development Press, Amherst

O'Connor K J 1982 The color your life technique. In: Schaefer C, O'Connor K J (eds) Handbook of play Therapy. Wiley, New York

Redgrave K 1987 Child's play: direct work with the deprived child. Boys and Girls Welfare Society, Creadle

Schaefer C, Reid S (eds) 1986 Game play: therapeutic use of childhood games. Wiley, New York

GROUP

Forward G E 1965 Group therapy for the emotionally disturbed child. Occupational Therapy 28(9, 10, 11)

Ginott H G 1961 Group psychotherapy with children. McGraw-Hill, New York

Schiffer M 1971 The therapeutic play group. Allen and Unwin, London

Slavson S R 1945 An introduction to group therapy. International Universities Press, New York

Slavson S R, Schiffer M 1975 Group psychotherapies for children. International Universities Press, New York

FAMILIES

Safer A 1965 Conjoint play therapy for the young child and his parent. Archives of General Psychiatry 13: 320–326

Villeneuve C 1979 The specific participation of the child in family therapy. American Academy of Child Psychiatry 44–53

17

Computers and occupational therapy

Judith Reid

INTRODUCTION

In recent years a number of occupational therapists have begun to use microcomputers in clinical work. This chapter primarily aims to allay some of the therapist's anxieties about working with microcomputers in the treatment setting and offers a theoretical framework for their application in the field of psychiatric occupational therapy.

Clinical work is emphasised, as the place of micro-technology in administration is now well established. Database systems have been designed to collate Korner statistics (see Ch. 28), store functional and management budgeting information, and analyse research. In many departments typewriters have been replaced by word processors. Plans are being made to computerise medical records, although such developments must meet the criteria laid down in the Data Protection Act (see p. 284).

A brief guide to computers is followed by a section on selecting a computer system, covering general factors affecting such a decision, as well as the selection of each item of equipment.

We then look at how computers are used in occupational therapy, and describe Allen's (1985) six levels of cognitive function. The subsequent sections on individual work and group work use these cognitive levels as the basis for selecting appropriate software and equipment.

Work assessment, habilitation and rehabilitation are then covered, with a final section on the implications of the Data Protection Act (1984) for the occupational therapist working with computers.

SELECTING A COMPUTER SYSTEM

Technological advances are an integral function of computer systems but these will not be discussed here since there are many books and magazines on the subject. Neither will this section recommend one particular system for therapeutic use. Rather, it is intended to help the occupational therapist working in psychiatry to select the system that is most appropriate for the needs of a particular group of clients.

In deciding to purchase a microcomputer, occupational therapists should resist falling into the trap of believing that a computer bought for therapy can carry out the dual purpose of being a piece of general office equipment available to staff. It is important to separate the two concepts from the outset to prevent conflict of interests.

A BASIC GUIDE TO COMPUTERS

Computing is simply mathematical calculating. A computer is 'an automatic electronic apparatus for making calculations or controlling operations that are expressible in numerical or logical terms' (Concise English Dictionary). Computers can therefore only work on information stored within them. They cannot produce answers to questions on material not stored.

Microcomputers have a number of facilities that are capable of many different types of work, although not all have the same facilities or capacity. Some computers are dedicated word processors whereas on others, such as the BBC Master, word processing and spread sheets can also be done.

Information is entered into the microcomputer by way of a language it understands, for example, BASIC or PASCAL. For a computer to act as a word processor it will already have been given a series of instructions, stored on a microchip, which will make it respond to text and written commands. Information put into a computer is processed, stored in its memory and may be reproduced in words, figures or sound. The format in which the computer is to reproduce material must have been included in the information provided through the program.

Information is stored in the computer on ROM and RAM chips. The amount of memory or number of ROMS and RAMS needed to run a program will depend on the number and type of calculations required. Complex programs require more complex calculations than simple programs so will need a computer with a larger memory capacity.

ROM chips store information needed to operate the computer. RAM chips store the material produced while the machine is switched on. To keep long-term records of programs and data (other than those internal to the computer) material is transferred onto discs or cassette tapes, which are then stored until required.

Numerous textbooks on computing are available. When purchasing a computer it is often useful to buy a book, in addition to the computer manual, to obtain further information as to how a particular system can be used.

Appropriate training reduces some of the frustrations of learning by trial and error. Occupational therapists who are to use computers in treatment should be given the opportunity to learn to produce simple programs and word processing. Teaching sessions should include theoretical and practical work.

FACTORS AFFECTING SELECTION
Therapeutic setting

The most commonly met systems for therapeutic use are those in the personal-computer range that include a word-processing facility. These systems vary in their computing capacity and in the range and quality of software that accompanies them. The occupational therapist must decide in which therapeutic setting the system will be most used and choose a computer that will meet those needs. For example, a computer for use in work assessment or training should have a word-processing facility and business software packages that easily simulate office work.

If the system is to be used primarily for group activities or to encourage specific cognitive skills in individual clients, then the therapist should purchase a computer that will run programs applicable to these areas. Many such programs are now commercially available for the more established computer systems and others are being written especially for occupational therapists. Where the intention is to do collaborative research with other therapists, the same type of system should be purchased by each therapist taking part.

Cost

One of the main constraints that occupational therapists will face is cost and this will, to a large extent, determine the type of system. Computers at the cheaper end of the range may be as effective as more expensive models. Although the cheaper systems have a shorter life span and no maintenance agreement is offered after the first year, it may still be cheaper to replace these models when they fail than to buy a maintenance agreement for a more expensive machine. Another advantage of replacement, rather than repair, is that new models are more technologically advanced and so it is cheaper to keep up to date. However, it is important to ensure that a cheaper model will fulfill all the functions for which it will be required. Professional advice should be sought from people who teach in computing, in schools or higher education; from other users, such as occupational therapists; from groups, such as the British Computer Society Disabled Specialist Group; and from suppliers.

System components

The standard computer system usually consists of a keyboard, which houses and gives instructions to the computer, a visual display unit (VDU) or monitor, a disc drive or cassette deck, and a printer (Fig. 17.1).

Microcomputers can either be purchased as complete systems or separate components. If the decision is taken to build up a system gradually, it is important that each of the individual components is compatible with the others. This can normally be done by checking and planning consultation with the supplier but, if there is any doubt, it is wise to consult a computer teacher, an experienced user or the manufacturer. Computer magazines are also a useful source of information. It is worthwhile considering each component

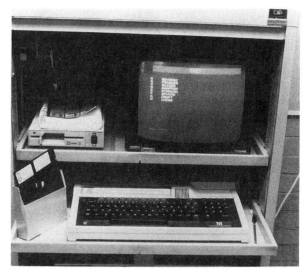

Fig. 17.1 Computer equipment, showing a VDU with coloured screen, a keyboard, a disc drive, a floppy disc holder and an operations manual.

(peripheral) in turn, that is, the computation capacity, the keyboard, the VDU, the disc drive and the printer, in order to select the most suitable equipment for specific purposes.

Computation capacity

Some computers are more powerful than others and it is important to check that the one to be purchased will be able to do the work required. The more powerful the computer, the more capacity it will have to handle different sorts of data. If, for example, clients are to write programs, the computer should have a memory capacity of at least 32 K. A computer with a smaller memory limits the software that can be used and thereby the range of therapeutic activities.

Staff training

In addition to the initial expense involved in buying the equipment there will be the cost of staff training (Fig. 17.2). Where staff turnover is high, training will become an annual expenditure and should be budgeted for, although some forms of

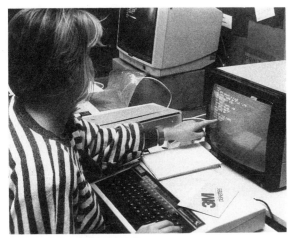

Fig. 17.2 The cost of staff training must be allowed for in the initial budget.

Table 17.1 Input devices

Input device	Advantages	Disadvantages
Keyboard	Familiar layout Wide range of compatible software	Basic literacy essential
Joystick	Easy to use for some games Drawing Literacy not essential	Limited range of compatible software
Concept keyboard	Literacy not essential	Limited range of compatible software
Mouse	Literacy not essential	Difficult to manipulate Limited range of compatible software

knowledge such as the Data Protection Act (see p. 284) can be acquired locally.

One important aspect to remember is that if a computer system is built up from separate items it is likely that each component will have its own detailed operational manual. The importance of the therapist gaining some understanding of the manuals to overcome problems that arise when working with the system cannot be overemphasised.

SELECTING THE EQUIPMENT

Input devices

The keyboard is the conventional way of communicating with the computer but it can be replaced by other types of equipment, which can form the link between the operator and the machine (see Table 17.1).

Keyboard

The keyboard is an important feature to consider. Although microcomputer keyboards have the same layout as a typewriter, the keys are sometimes quite close together. Clients who are taking psychotropic medication often have slower, less coordinated fine movements. They may also have an accommodation defect that affects near vision.

Consequently, it is necessary to ensure that the keyboard is both clearly marked and well spaced, otherwise the clients may become frustrated and lose confidence in their abilities, simply because they frequently hit the wrong keys.

Joystick

In psychiatry this most commonly replaces the keyboard in games programs, where rapid responses are needed to move up, down or across the VDU screen. It can also be used with some drawing programs to reproduce pictures on the screen.

Concept keyboard

This is an important piece of equipment for clients unable to use the convential keyboard. In psychiatry it is considered to be effective in treating very low-functioning clients and those with learning difficulties, when it is used with specially designed software. The keyboard is flat, with no apparent keys, but each part of the surface can be programmed to reproduce an image when touched. To know which part of the surface to press, a piece of squared paper is placed over it. Written or drawn in the squares are words or symbols. When a square is touched its content is reproduced on the screen or a sound is made.

Mouse

This may be used instead of a joystick as it can move an image around the screen in any direction but some clients find it difficult to manipulate because of its round shape.

The visual display unit (VDU)

Visual display units (VDUs) must also be chosen carefully. A VDU that is attached to the keyboard makes the personal computer look more sturdy and is also easy for individual clients to use because it is in a fixed position directly above the keyboard. It may, however, have a standard black-and-white monitor, not a colour display. Colour is useful for clients with visual difficulties, as is a high-resolution screen, which produces a clearer image. A monitor with a green screen also makes lettering easier to see. See Table 17.2.

A VDU that is not attached to the keyboard is better for group work since the monitor can then be placed in the most appropriate position for

everyone. It also allows the therapist more flexibility in choosing the one that is required for the particular type of treatment setting.

A further advantage of separate equipment is that if one piece breaks down it is often possible to find a replacement while it is being repaired. For example, a VDU can be temporarily replaced by another monitor or even a portable television set.

The disc drive

The purpose of a disc drive is to load the program onto the computer. Most of this section will concentrate on floppy or soft discs, which are the most common drives found in therapeutic settings. There are several aspects to be considered. If the occupational therapist intends to use discs from other centres it is advisable to purchase a 40/80 switchable disc drive. This means that you will be able to run all of the programs designed for your type of computer. An 80-track disc has the advantage of storing more data than a 40-track disc but both are in common use. Dual disc drives are more versatile than single disc drives. They are particularly useful when data is stored on two discs as the user can easily switch from one to another. They also simplify the process of making duplicate copies of existing software although it is important that the therapist is aware of any copyright agreements.

Hard disc drives are used more for business purposes and are found in offices where a large amount of information needs to be stored. They are much more expensive than soft disc drives but are useful in psychiatric settings for several reasons. One is that floppy discs are easily damaged, and there is an increased risk of damage to soft discs where multiple users are involved. Clients on medication are not always aware of the way in which they are holding a floppy disc and sometimes use them roughly. Hard discs are enclosed in a casing and cannot be touched.

Another handicap is that floppy discs have a limited amount of storage space and data may have to be stored on several discs. A hard disc drive has much more space available to store information and is therefore more useful for simulating office

Table 17.2 VDUs and monitors

Screen	Advantages	Disadvantages
Green	Easy to read text	No colour to differentiate items
		More expensive
Black and white	Cheaper	More difficult to read text over long periods of time
		No colour to differentiate items
Colour	Items can be highlighted by colour	More expensive
		More difficult to read text over long periods of time
	Good for games	

Table 17.3 Disc drives and cassette decks

Device	Advantages	Disadvantages
Floppy soft disc drive	Cheaper than hard disc Back-up copies made on same equipment	Easily damaged Less storage capacity than hard disc
Hard disc drive	Less easily damaged More storage capacity	Expensive Back-up copies must be made on floppy disc; necessary to have both systems
Cassette deck	Cheapest Easily available	Slow to access/process data Limited storage capacity

Table 17.4 Printers

Printer	Advantages	Disadvantages
Dot matrix	Cheap	No colour print facility Quality of reproduction varies on different models
Daisy wheel	Good-quality reproduction	Expensive No colour print facility
Laser	Good-quality reproduction Prints in colour	Very expensive

work, where a lot of data is frequently accessed. Back-up copies of data stored on a hard disc are made on a floppy disc in case some malfunction occurs and the data is lost. A brief summary of the advantages and disadvantages of hard and soft disc drives appears in Table 17.3.

The cassette deck

This has the same function as, and can be used in place of, a disc drive. Unfortunately, it is slow to access and save data, and in treatment settings there is an increased tendency for clients to disengage from the activity during the delays in processing the material. It is suggested that the therapist only uses a cassette deck when there are mechanical problems with the disc drive or a fault in the disc itself and the back-up copy has been stored on tape.

The printer

The questions to be answered before buying a printer concern the quality of print (will it be used to type reports or letters?) and the amount of money available (is the budget limited?). Printers

can reproduce images from the screen on paper in three different ways:

- dot matrix—a series of small dots printed closely together to produce the image
- daisy wheel
- laser.

Daisy-wheel printers are less expensive than laser printers, although the latter can print in colour. The cheapest and most common are dot-matrix printers. Most of these will now automatically print to letter standard but some have to be set specially to do this. Table 17.4 compares the advantages and disadvantages of the three types of printer.

Altering the way in which the printer displays information is normally done by computer commands. This is a fairly simple process; the problem usually lies in the therapist not knowing which command or series of commands to use. If the occupational therapist is not confident in handling computer systems it is advisable to make sure the printer is easily adjusted.

USING COMPUTERS IN OCCUPATIONAL THERAPY

Computers began to appear in occupational therapy departments in Britain between 1983 and 1986 when the DHSS and the Department of

Trade and Industry (DTI) funded a project to stimulate interest in micro-technology in hospitals. This led to a number of occupational therapy departments being offered BBC microcomputers to use with clients in treatment. The opportunity to explore this new technology was seized by a number of occupational therapists working in different fields. Elizabeth Grove, the then occupational therapy representative at the DHSS, promoted and coordinated the scheme. Training was provided to the occupational therapists who were to use the equipment.

An occupational therapy Special Interest Group in Microcomputers was established in 1984.

To enable all occupational therapists to identify mentally ill people who may benefit from using a computer in therapy, Allen's (1985) mode of cognitive function is later analysed. Her model has been chosen for this chapter because the skills required to use a microcomputer are essentially cognitive and Allen's formulation of cognitive function is one occupational therapists can use easily in treatment. Other models, perhaps more familiar to occupational therapists, such as those described by Mosey (1970), Reed and Sanderson (1980) and Kielhofner (1985), lack the detail required for this purpose.

For therapy to be successful it is important that the client is given computing tasks within his range of cognitive ability. This is not simply a matter of intellectual capacity; the therapist must also consider perceptual performance, memory and, in some instances, the degree of cognitive control necessary in motor function. Within Allen's (1985) hierarchy computing could be selected as an appropriate individual activity for clients functioning at levels 4, 5 or 6 if it is to be used as a group activity.

Throughout the sections on treatment suggestions are made for software suitable for each level. Recognising that individual clients are motivated by different computer processes is essential as this allows the therapist to work in a variety of ways with clients functioning at the same level. For example, one client functioning at level 4 could use the computer in individual sessions to improve his general cognitive performance, while another at this level could be involved in a work habilitation programme.

THE LATTO AND BARNITT SURVEY (1986)

As computers from the DHSS/DTI project started to arrive in occupational therapy departments additional funding was made available to study how they were being used. Latto and Barnitt collated data from nine of the 12 centres for mentally ill people that participated. The survey, although descriptive, reflected the ways in which microcomputers were being employed and the types of clients involved. All centres had used the computer with clients from three diagnostic categories: schizophrenià, personality and behaviour disorder. The majority had also applied it in the treatment of depressed clients, manic-depressive clients and those with alcohol dependency syndrome. In only a minority of centres were neurotic clients and the elderly included with other diagnostic groupings. These findings may reflect client categories treated by occupational therapists rather than the versatility of the computer.

The results also showed that occupational therapists using microcomputers had differing aims of treatment. Six centres used the microcomputer to improve concentration, motivation and intellectual ability. Five wanted to provide intellectual stimulation, increase the clients' self-confidence and self-assertion, facilitate social reintegration and to provide work experience and training. Four centres reported that they had used their computer to reinforce or reward appropriate patterns of behaviour within a behaviour-modification programme.

The Latto and Barnitt survey is of particular interest to British occupational therapists who want to carry out additional research in order to identify the clinical areas in which microcomputers are most effective. A study that considers the application of microcomputers within a well-defined model of occupational therapy and uses precisely the International Classification of Diseases (1978) should produce such results. The systematic examination of single case studies is another way of increasing knowledge.

LEVELS OF COGNITIVE FUNCTION

Allen (1985) described a system whereby levels of

behaviour are indicative of cognitive function. This assists the therapist in selecting activities. To simplify this process of task analysis and task selection Allen's (1985) formulation of cognitive function is applied in the following sections. It will also help the occupational therapist recognise when computing can become an active part of therapy. As more occupational therapists use microcomputers with clients these broad guidelines should become more defined.

Allen's hierarchy has six levels, as described below.

Level 1 Automatic actions

Clients are able to perform very basic tasks of daily living, for example, walking, eating and dressing, but neglect personal hygiene. Their general level of activity is low, almost catatonic. They are preoccupied and do not respond to events taking place around them.

Level 2 Postural actions

Clients are beginning to take an interest in their environment and are particularly attracted to gross motor movements. At this point the client will be able to imitate the therapist, who can therefore engage his interest by demonstrating a simple activity accompanied by short, precise verbal instructions. Attention span remains extremely limited and clients are easily distracted.

Level 3 Manual actions

Clients respond to objects that catch their attention. They are not yet able to work towards a specific goal but are able to repeat actions independently. The therapist can direct these actions constructively in an activity. Concentration span remains poor but can be sustained as long as the client is motivated by the activity.

Level 4 Goal-directed actions

These clients have a basic understanding of the components of a task. They are able to recognise mistakes but may be unable to correct these independently or solve problems in an abstract way.

Level 5 Exploratory actions

Clients are able to learn through experience and to show initiative. They may, however, be unable to anticipate some difficulties that may arise within an activity but once they have gone through the process of solving a specific problem they will recognise it again in the future and be able to deal with it independently.

Level 6 Planned actions

These clients respond in a multi-dimensional way to themselves and their environment. They are able to use information to develop ideas and can anticipate problems within a task and take remedial action. They can independently plan their own goals and identify how these can be achieved.

Using Allen's hierarchy, a microcomputer can always be used in the treatment of clients from levels 3 to 6. Below level 3 each individual will need to be assessed to ensure that the degree of cognitive awareness is sufficient to perform independently on computer tasks that require a preconceived goal. If the therapist believes this to be so then it is suggested that the information provided for level-3 clients is modified as described under level 3 in the following section.

WORKING WITH INDIVIDUAL CLIENTS

Working with a microcomputer is an exciting and absorbing experience. The challenge it offers is ideally suited to occupational therapy. As with all therapeutic activities, the skill of the occupational therapist lies in the ability to exploit the medium in which she works and, through this, to engage the client. Each particular task has a variety of components that demand separate skills.

LEVEL-3 CLIENTS

Computers can be extremely effective in gaining and holding the attention of distractable patients. For the therapist treating level-3 clients, and below, an important part of treatment will be to develop concentration.

Useful hardware features

• Special input devices, such as the concept keyboard, should be used instead of the conventional keyboard as these easily reinforce stimulus–response connections.

• A high-resolution colour VDU. The image on the screen should be precise and a high-resolution monitor will provide this. Colour is an important feature in gaining and holding attention.

• A single floppy disc drive. A double disc drive may confuse the client, a hard disc drive is too complicated and a cassette deck too slow.

Selecting software

There are several programs that have been specially designed for the concept keyboard. The therapist will find that they are easy to adapt to the needs of different clients, however, the following points are important when choosing software.

• Any instructions delivered in the program should be unambiguous.

• The program should be clearly designed so that is presents information simply.

• Colours are useful in enabling the client to distinguish one part of the program from another but should be used consistently and sparingly since a plethora of colours can be confusing and distracting.

• Symbols should be easy to understand.

• When a client makes a mistake, the program should contain a visible or audible cue so that he can correct it without having to use abstract problem-solving processes.

• Concept keyboard programs, from which the client can form words, patterns, pictures or symbols on the screen, may all be used as a therapeutic activity at this level.

Using the equipment

A therapist using a microcomputer with level-3 clients and below will have to load the disc and access the software, so that the client only operates the program. Initially, the therapist should demonstrate the task and give verbal cues. She should then encourage the client to imitate, giving short, simple verbal instructions to reinforce the procedure. The client will need to be supervised by the therapist throughout the session but she should only prompt selectively so that the client's attention is focused on responding to the image on the screen.

LEVEL-4 CLIENTS

Clients functioning at level 4 will be able to use the microcomputer to achieve short-term goals but will need the therapist's help to solve the abstract problems they meet. Concentration will be improving but frustration tolerance will be low so that the therapist should control the number of times the client is exposed to difficult instructions by selecting appropriate hardware and software.

Useful hardware features

• The conventional keyboard should be used most frequently as this gives access to a wide range of programs.

• The joystick should replace the conventional keyboard when poor hand–eye coordination is thought to increase frustration, which then hinders concentration.

• A high resolution colour monitor, as for level 3.

• A single disc drive, as for level 3.

Selecting software

The therapist should follow the guidelines outlined in the section on level-3 clients, omitting only that related to the concept keyboard. In general, the therapist should evaluate the content of a program in terms of the amount of visual stimuli, the speed of delivery and the demands made on the user's memory by checking the following points.

• Programs that contain long lists of information should be rejected as these clients have difficulty in memorising complex instructions.

- The text should be simple. It is useful to have a few programs in large lettering for clients whose vision is impaired.
- The text should be delivered slowly. The therapist should buy a selection of programs that contain a facility to adjust the speed.
- Programs should reward success and not failure. A selection of simple games will provide this.

Purposely designed programs are extremely useful for some clients, particularly where the therapist wishes to increase, gradually, the duration of the task and the length of time the client spends engaged in the activity. A computer department in a local school or college may be interested in doing this.

Software suitable for level-4 clients includes simple games, basic budgeting, drawing, basic literacy and numeracy and memory programs.

Using the equipment

As with level-3 clients, a therapist using a computer in the treatment of level-4 clients should focus on the individual operating the program, rather than the hardware. Again, instructions should be clear, both in the demonstration and verbally.

The text in the software will be self-explanatory so that the therapist should give verbal instructions only where necessary.

LEVEL-5 CLIENTS

Clients at this stage will be able to use the computer independently. They will be self-motivated, show initiative and be able to learn through experience. However, they may have difficulties in foreseeing problems and so the therapist should be aware that this will limit the clients' potential in using the computer to its capacity.

Selecting software

The guidelines outlined for level-3 clients should continue to be followed. In general, software for level-5 clients should encourage them to explore the microcomputer facilities but should guide them through the process. Appropriate activities will include working through the manufacturer's introduction program, simple adventure games, social-skills packages, advanced budgeting, advanced drawing and simple programming.

Using the equipment

The therapist should teach the clients to load discs and access programs. More complex concepts, such as various computer functions, can be explained verbally. Close support and supervision is no longer necessary but the therapist should be available to give help when required.

Suitable tasks could include: computer adventure games, programming, and learning to use other computer functions such as spread sheets, word-processing and database systems.

LEVEL-6 CLIENTS

Microcomputers can offer these clients opportunities for personal development and creativity. They have the potential to develop a variety of computing skills and so can decide for themselves the activities they undertake.

Selecting software

A range of software should be available, from which the client can select appropriate material. At level 6 the client should be able to judge for himself the extent to which he wants to develop his skills.

Using the equipment

At level 6 the therapist should expect the client to be able to operate the microcomputer system with only a minimal amount of support and so clients should be independent in using both the hardware and software. Observations should continue to be made on the client's performance and any supervision should be unintrusive. As the client develops a basic understanding of the relationship between different aspects of computing, the therapist should encourage him to retain his knowledge and to solve new problems unaided.

GROUP WORK

SELECTING CLIENTS

Sharing an activity such as microcomputing depends on the individual's ability to develop a skill and work cooperatively. Unwanted behaviour is discouraged. In Allen's hierarchy only clients functioning between levels 4 and 6 may be suitable for microcomputer groups. In general, these clients can benefit from group work because of the way in which they respond both to the activity and to other people.

Single versus mixed-level groups

In using computing as a therapeutic activity it is important for clients functioning at the same level to be grouped together. This allows the therapist to channel her energies into matching the abilities of the group with the activity and enables individual group members to participate fully. Those who progress quickly can continue to work with the remaining clients to their maximum level of functioning.

Mixed-level groups rarely permit individuals functioning at the highest and lowest levels to participate actively and, consequently, the therapist running these must direct individual actions and interactions to maintain group cohesion; the task itself will not. In single-level groups the task facilitates group cohesion and the therapist can concentrate on ensuring that individual needs are met.

Open versus closed groups

Individuals take differing lengths of time to improve their functioning ability and also achieve varying ranges of skill. These issues should be considered when establishing a microcomputer group.

In the majority of occupational therapy departments open groups, which allow clients to join and leave as fits their individual therapy programme, will be more appropriate than closed groups. It is usually very difficult to run closed microcomputer groups, where the clients start and finish together,

as 'drop-out' due to discharge, or to a recurrent episode of illness and subsequent deterioration in mental state can severely reduce numbers and therefore the viability of the group.

In running open computer groups the therapist must be alert to the needs of newcomers while explaining operating techniques in ways that continue to stimulate established members. No matter how much care is taken, some clients will have a particularly low tolerance to any revision. In such instances the group can be divided into small working units, separating any intolerant clients from new members.

LEVEL-4 GROUPS

At this stage the therapist can channel the clients' actions towards a specific goal. A group of level-4 clients should all work together on the same task, which contains a single goal.

Selecting equipment

Clients at level 4 may still have difficulties in coordinating fine motor movements, therefore it is often practical to replace the conventional keyboard with a joystick. This also has the advantage of being passed easily to each member of the group and so stimulates interaction and active participation.

Selecting software

Although the clients can be taught to load and access software, the main purpose of the group is to operate the programs selected by the therapist. These will include simple quiz games to stimulate cognitive function and social interaction; basic problem-solving programs to promote abstract thought: and computer-assisted learning packages concerned with the skills of daily living.

Encouraging interaction

Social behaviour will still be returning or developing in these clients so that the therapist should focus her attention on improving only a limited repertoire of skills. Simple verbal statements between members and constructive comments on others' performance should be positively re-inforced; negative criticism should be confronted or corrected according to the clients' mental state.

LEVEL-5 GROUPS

Level 5 is the stage at which clients are ready to explore and to learn through experience. When a task has been learnt the therapist can expect the group to use it independently in the future.

Selecting equipment

In selecting the range of equipment to be used the therapist should consider the functional abilities of each member. If some individuals are suffering from the side effects of medication, in particular those caused by major tranquillisers, they may have difficulty in coordinating fine motor move-ments. Performance may be improved by using input switches other than the keyboard, such as joysticks, light pens or even touch-sensitive screens.

Initially the therapist may prefer to limit the group to using basic equipment, such as the com-puter, the disc drive, the VDU and the input switches. When the group has become proficient in using these to carry out simple activities, the printer can be included to complete the system. The printer is an extremely useful item for group work. It provides each member with a record of his activity and this can stimulate interest outside the formal sessions.

Selecting software

Software should be carefully selected by the therapist for level-5 clients to ensure that the needs of individuals are met. In general, the programs should be clearly designed. When symbols are used they should be simple and consistent. Any text should be concise and not open to varying interpretations.

The range of software used should include the following.

● Programs that teach operating procedures and test the groups' knowledge of simple com-puter techniques

● Competitive games and adventure games to encourage group interaction and to stimulate social reponses

● Problem-solving programs based on the ac-tivities of daily living and social skills training will help clients examine practical issues and their own behaviour in a group setting.

Using the equipment

It is important that the group become familiar with the techniques of loading and accessing software and this can be achieved simply by using several discs in each session. When first preparing for a level-5 group the therapist should grade the programs selected according to complexity. A range within each grading should then be stored on different discs. The therapist can then choose programs from different discs so that the clients automatically handle the equipment.

Encouraging interaction

Level-5 clients may still have some difficulty in initiating conventional social behaviours, such as starting a conversation, and programs have been designed to facilitate social interaction. However, in mental illness interaction is affected both by mental state and cognitive function, so it is im-portant that the therapist promotes interaction in a way that will not raise individual levels of frustration. Members' abilities to solve problems will vary and this is a factor to consider when preparing a session on computer games. If some clients generally respond more quickly than others, they are likely to dominate the group. In such circumstances it may be preferable that group members compete as individuals, rather than in teams, and each person is given an equal oppor-tunity to participate.

Allen (1985) suggests that level-5 clients still have difficulties in anticipating problems and find-ing solutions without assistance. In a shared ac-tivity this may not only refer to the task in hand but also to relating to the other group members. When a group member is having difficulty in un-derstanding the behaviour of others, it may be necessary for the therapist to intervene and explain. A useful technique for developing group cohesion is to encourage members to give feedback on the activity at the end of each session and to set realistic goals for the next. The therapist can then use their ideas when planning and preparing the following session.

LEVEL-6 GROUPS

Level-6 clients can set goals based on their own, as well as others' abilities. Here the therapist can expect the group to select a long-term goal and make realistic plans to achieve it. The aim should be for the group to function as independently as possible.

Introducing new members

Once the group has become established it is preferable that new members are formally interviewed by the therapist before joining. Here the therapist can inform the client of the aims of the group, of any current activities and what he can expect to gain in becoming a member. This also gives the client an opportunity to discuss his motivation for joining and any previous experience of computing. Once a client has been accepted by the therapist a starting date should be agreed.

After introducing the new member to the others in the first session each person should briefly describe his interest in computing and his task in the current activity. The new member begins by being given a task that matches his technical skill and potential. If he has little or no previous knowledge of microcomputing then one of the established members can be asked to demonstrate the basic techniques of operating the equipment.

When a level-6 group is first established, or when a number of members leave and new ones join, the therapist should avoid assuming the role of leader. In this way the group can remain as independent as the environment permits, with the therapist being used as a resource for advice or materials. This arrangement allows the group to attempt more complex tasks that may otherwise be inhibited by the therapist's own limitations. By learning together and sharing problems the group will form bonds that the therapist can use to guide the members towards an agreed goal.

Selecting software

The most suitable software for a level-6 group demands a range of relatively complex skills. Games in which accuracy and speed are important can draw on the user's abilities in hand–eye coordination and fine motor movements. Adventure games not only require logic and skill in solving problems but also a high degree of persistence and concentration. Producing a news-sheet, using one of the commercial software packages now available for some computers, offers opportunities in creative and cooperative work and programming demands a combination of logic, problem-solving skills, creativity and cooperation.

Using the equipment

Members should be familiar with all the hardware that is available for therapy. This includes the computer, VDU, cassette deck, disc drive both for floppy discs and hard discs, where available, keyboard and any additional input devices and printer. Once the group is established, members should be given the responsibility of passing on this information to newcomers. The therapist will then only assist the group in using the equipment when the chosen activity involves more complex computing techniques.

WORK ASSESSMENT, HABILITATION AND REHABILITATION

There is an obvious place for microcomputers in work programmes for mentally ill people. However, there is much confusion over the concept of work in treatment and it is important to clarify the terminology used here before discussing the place of microcomputers.

For the purposes of this section two definitions of 'work' are used:

- '*Work* is to do something involving effort (of body or mind)' and,
- '*Work* is to exert oneself for a definite purpose, particularly to produce something,

effect some useful result, or to gain one's livelihood'. (Shorter Oxford English Dictionary)

- *Habilitation*: 'To endow with ability and to render capable' (Shorter Oxford English Dictionary)
- *Rehabilitation*: 'Restoring to effectiveness or normal life' (Concise Oxford Dictionary)
- *Assessment*: 'an estimation of quality' (Concise Oxford Dictionary).

Work, as defined here, has long been associated with mental and physical well-being because it requires an ability to expend purposeful effort. Various types of work demand differing abilities in terms of cognitive functioning, manual dexterity and social skill, consequently most people gain some sense of achievement through work. One of the most valuable aspects of work is that it is a means of gaining one's livelihood and thereby maintaining or improving the quality of life.

The use of work in treatment is considered to be an important part of a normalisation programme. In Allen's (1985) hierarchy, clients with behavioural functioning at levels 4 (goal-directed), 5 (exploratory) and 6 (planned functions) may benefit from situations found in conventional work settings and it is here that microcomputers are establishing themselves as invaluable.

WORK ASSESSMENT

When considering the use of microcomputers in work assessment the therapist should first determine the purpose of the evaluation as the microcomputer techniques that estimate general work skills differ from those used to assess specific computing skills.

Estimating general work skills

Because the information that the microcomputer provides is objective, it is of considerable value to the therapist in evaluating general work skills. This complements traditional subjective approaches and helps to minimise the risk of inaccurate assessments. Where only subjective methods are used, clients with good verbal and social skills can influence the therapist to overestimate their ability on task performance. Conversely, psychotic patients, whose interpersonal skills remain limited, may be inaccurately rated in a subjective assessment and cognitive abilities may be overlooked due to poor communication skills. Microcomputers can also help the therapist monitor improvement in work skills.

A client who initially performs poorly but is then seen to improve rapidly as the equipment becomes more familiar may have suffered from a transient cognitive impairment, whereas the individual who makes little progress and repeatedly has difficulty solving the same types of problem may be suffering some organic deterioration or residual cognitive impairment.

Selecting software

Software suitable for general work-assessment purposes should consist of programs that test a wide range of cognitive performance.
These will include:

- programs that can test the client's memory, comprehension, perception and reaction time
- programs that can be used to estimate performance in literacy, numeracy, problem-solving skills and social skills.

Where the occupational therapist wishes to make a specific assessment of the individual's ability to use a microcomputer in open employment, the factors to be taken into consideration are the type of microcomputer available and the complexity of skill that can be achieved in a therapeutic setting.

Level-4 clients

Clients whose highest functioning ability remains at level 4 are unlikely to achieve open employment so the therapist will probably assess them for sheltered work or day centres. Although at this level the client's behaviour is goal directed, it would be unusual for him to be competent in more than basic computing skills. Furthermore, it should be recognised that he may have difficulty transferring any skills he has from one computer to another.

Level-5 clients

Level-5 clients may find employment using more complex computing skills, such as word processing and inputting or retrieving information from database systems. Again, the therapist may find that it is often difficult to estimate the individual's capacity to transfer skills from one computer to another. Familiarity with one computer, on which the client has learnt to recognise and solve problems, may bias the assessment and not be a real test of his ability to function independently. It is likely that the client will need further training if he is to use a different machine at work.

Level-6 clients

Where the therapist is required to estimate the capacity of a level-6 client to work with microcomputers the range of skills that need to be assessed will vary according to the type of work the client hopes to do. If he aims to find employment performing a routine skill, such as word processing or operating a database system, then the therapist should consider the factors already mentioned. Where the client is expected to return to or find employment in the field of advanced technology it is important that the therapist recognises the limitation of the systems normally found in a therapeutic environment. This can help prevent overestimating the individual's ability.

Microcomputer technology is an extremely competitive commercial field and the individual will be pressured to produce results. Such stress can lead to relapse of psychiatric illness (Brown and Birley 1968). Where the therapist is confident of the client's skill but concerned at the fragility of his mental state, strenuous efforts should be made to guide the client towards a tolerant and sympathetic employer.

WORK HABILITATION

The process of developing specific computing skills can be an integral part of a treatment programme. To formulate such a programme the therapist must first decide whether the client requires work habilitation or work rehabilitation.

Although, it is not necessary for the client to have any former knowledge of computing in the initial stages of either programme, the concept of habilitation allows for the acquisition of new skills, whereas rehabilitation suggests that the aim is to restore skills.

In habilitation the therapist's goal is to develop skills that have been in abeyance for a variety of reasons. The first task is to improve motivation and confidence in order to increase the individual's capacity in general work skills. When this has been achieved and the client is familiar with basic techniques then the therapist can prepare a treatment programme based on each individual's level of function, for example, a level-4 client may need to begin a programme with literacy and numeracy skills, a level-5 client with keyboard skills and a level-6 client with problem-solving skills.

Level-4 clients

Clients who remain at level 4 are likely to require sheltered-employment day centres or industrial therapy. In the past the type of work most often found in these units has been limited to simple manual and clerical tasks. Microcomputers have been seen to increase the range of commercial work available to these clients (Schrank 1986). Where clerical and secretarial tasks are broken down with the aid of a word processor or database system a number of individuals can work on the same item. It is then brought together again and checked before being printed and mistakes rectified simply, without the client experiencing loss of confidence or feelings of frustration. The quality and style of the end product should therefore be attractive to the commercial market.

Level-5 and -6 clients

The place of microcomputers in the work habilitation programmes for clients functioning at levels 5 and 6 will vary according to the therapeutic setting. In hospitals the individual can be introduced to a variety of basic computing skills such as word processing, computer programming and operating simple database systems (Fig. 17.3). These skills

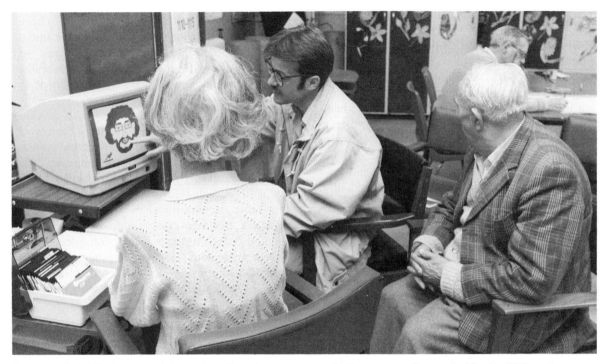

Fig. 17.3 Rehabilitation can include teaching clients how to operate simple programs. (Source: Lothian Health Board)

can be directed to specific purposes, which can themselves contribute to the management of the institution, for example, the clients' wages, or creating a simple newsletter to keep people informed of developments inside and outside the hospital. Some clients may then choose to continue microcomputing as a leisure pursuit or go on to vocational training.

WORK REHABILITATION

When using microcomputers for this purpose the aim of the therapist is to reestablish the individual's former skills and agree on a treatment programme that may contribute to their restoration. The extent to which this can be carried out will vary according to the type of skill to be restored, the equipment available and the extent to which the client is debilitated by illness. Programs should be chosen and upgraded according to changing levels of functioning ability. The therapist should select software applicable to the specific deficits from which the individual suffers.

Level-4 clients

Clients who are rehabilitated to level 4 should then follow a work habilitation programme.

Level-5 and -6 clients

Specific activities will encourage these clients to reestablish the patterns of behaviour they will be required to use outside hospital. For example, by using a combination of an ordinary typewriter and a word-processing package, it may be possible to rehabilitate someone who is usually employed as a typist or word processor (Fig. 17.4).

Using community facilities

Several areas now have specially equipped computer centres and clients can transfer to these and continue their rehabilitation programme outside hospital. Some may be specifically for disabled people and other facilities can be found in adult-education centres, polytechnics and state-funded skills centres. These services can be extremely

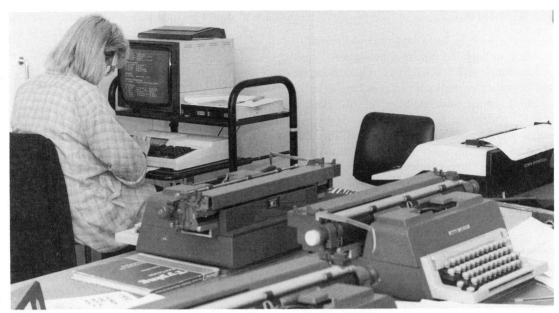

Fig. 17.4 Rehabilitation can lead to successful reemployment as a typist or word-processor operator. (Source: Lothian Health Board)

helpful as they can both offer a range of courses in computer technology and give realistic advice on career opportunities. One or two clients may choose to join a privately organised course, although these can be quite expensive.

It may be possible to arrange for clients who already have employment to which they intend to return to carry out the final stages of their rehabilitation programme in their normal working environment. In large companies this can often be done with the assistance of the personnel department, whereas in smaller firms discussion will need to take place directly with the employer.

LITERACY AND NUMERACY

Education is not considered to be a primary function of occupational therapy, however, the therapist may feel that the acquisition of knowledge is therapeutically beneficial.

Clients whose ability to function is impaired by difficulties in literacy and numeracy can be given the opportunity, during treatment, to try the computer-assisted learning software packages that are now available for adults. Improvements in literacy raise the individual's level of understanding, enabling him to execute routine tasks independently. A client who has literacy difficulties may report anxieties about travelling to and from work because he is unable to read travel information. He may have further problems at work because he cannot read hazard notices or general information concerning conditions of service and may even be ridiculed by his colleagues. By including adult-literacy software packages in a general work rehabilitation or rehabilitation programme the therapist may help the client achieve a greater level of independence and happiness.

Residential homes

Clients living in group homes can gain a knowledge of local resources and emergency services from computer-assisted learning packages. A basic software program can be produced that not only tests the clients' general knowledge on daily living subjects but also includes items specific to the home in which he is to reside.

General interest

Some people wish to learn basic microcomputing skills whilst in hospital; they may also want to continue learning after discharge. The therapist should be aware of the local facilities available for this, and have an understanding of the client's ability to undertake such a project. Some individuals will be able to carry out a self-directed learning programme, such as found in the Open University or in correspondence courses, whereas others will make better progress in a more formal setting such as an adult-education centre or polytechnic.

THE DATA PROTECTION ACT (1984)

The purpose of this section is to increase the occupational therapist's level of awareness of how the Act controls the use of computers. It is not all-embracing and should not be regarded as a substitute for the Act itself.

The Data Protection Act (1984) is 'concerned with information about individuals (Personal Data) which is processed automatically (that is, in computer systems) with those who undertake the processing (data users or computer bureaux), and with the individuals to whom the data relates (data subjects)'. The Act goes on to define, in legal terms, the type of data it covers and what it does not.

Definitions of the terminology used in the Act are given below.

TERMINOLOGY

Data

This is information that is presented in a form through which it can be processed by an automatic system.

An automatic system

The Act does not define this specifically but it is taken to include mainframe and microcomputers, word processors and punch-card processors. If you are in doubt as to whether your particular system fulfills the criteria you should seek advice from the office of the Data Protection Registrar.

Personal data

Any information about a living person. It includes expressions of opinion about people and any personal details. There are several classes of personal data, including identification, family and social circumstances, employment, finance, health, etc.

The Act also states that the sources of such information should be made clear on registration as well as to whom it is intended to be disclosed.

Data users

Any organisation or individual who controls the collection of personal data to be processed or the contents of any data that has been processed.

Computer bureaux

Any organisation or individual who processes personal data for data users or allows data users to process personal data on his equipment.

Both data users and computer bureaux are obliged under the Act to state clearly what personal data they hold and to honour a code of practice in relation to that data. Control operates through registration and occupational therapists should specify what sort of data they hold or intend to hold when applying for registration under the Act.

The NHS Data Protection Guidelines (1984) assume that the data user will usually be the Health Authority and should register as both a data user and as a computer bureau. In Local Authorities it is likewise assumed that the employee is merely acting as an agent of the employer. Under these circumstances it is unlikely that the occupational therapist would need to register separately.

Therapists who work in the private sector or for voluntary or charitable organisations should ensure that they are covered by registering individually.

The therapist could otherwise be held liable under the Act and civil action be taken against her, and a professional insurance scheme may not cover such legal proceedings.

A data subject

An individual to whom personal data relates is called a 'data subject'. It is important to remember that in occupational therapy this will include clients, members of staff and research subjects.

A data subject has legal rights under the Act. He may seek compensation through the courts for damage and any associated distress caused by the loss, destruction or unauthorised disclosure of data, or by inaccurate data. He may also apply to the courts for rectification or erasure of inaccurate data and from November 1987 the 'Subject Access' provisions entitled him to have some access to the data held about himself.

CODE OF PRACTICE

The Act outlines eight principles that constitute a Code of Practice. Their purpose is to help data users and computer bureaux operate legally.

The first principle is, 'the information to be contained in personal data shall be obtained, and personal data shall be processed, fairly and lawfully'. Data users should specify how the data will be collected, how the source of the information will be informed of its purpose and to whom it will be disclosed.

The second principle covers the purpose of holding the personal data. It states, 'personal data shall be held only for one or more specified and lawful purposes'. These specified purposes are described in the registration form. It is important to make a full declaration of the reasons for holding such data to the Registrar.

The third principle considers the use and disclosure of personal data. 'Personal data held for any purpose or purposes shall not be used or disclosed in any manner incompatible with that purpose or those purposes'. The therapist should register both the way in which the data is processed and the circumstances and manner in which it will be disclosed. Disclosure may be a screen display, computer printout, handwritten, or oral, and adequate security measures should be taken.

The fourth principle states, 'personal data held for any purpose or purposes shall be adequate, relevant and not excessive in relation to that purpose or those purposes'. Occupational therapists will, therefore, need to review the data they hold regularly to ensure that it is still required.

The fifth principle is 'personal data shall be accurate and, where necessary, kept up to date'.

The sixth principle states, 'personal data held for any purpose or purposes shall not be kept longer than is necessary for that purpose or those purposes'. There are, however, some dispensations for research data.

The seventh principle refers to disclosure and subject access. 'An individual shall be entitled at reasonable intervals and without undue delay or expense to be informed by any data user whether he holds personal data of which that individual is the subject, and to assess any such data corrected or erased'. The Secretary of State fixes the maximum fee that may be charged to subject access to ensure no 'undue expense', but 'reasonable intervals' are as yet undefined.

The eighth principle covers security measures. It states, 'appropriate security measures shall be taken against unauthorised access to, or alternatively disclosure or destruction of, personal data and against accidental loss or destruction of personal data'. Occupational therapists should make every effort to preserve the physical security of the system and, where necessary, build control codes into programs to limit access. Furthermore, they must also ensure that whoever has access to the data is reliable and respects confidentiality.

THE DATA PROTECTION COORDINATOR AND DATA CUSTODIANS

Occupational therapists will find that all large organisations have a data protection coordinator. This person is responsible for informing those who use automatic systems of the Act, establishing local policies and completing and submitting the registration. The Data Protection Coordinator will also be the person to whom data subjects apply for subject access. These applications are then referred to a data custodian whose authorisation must be obtained before data can be disclosed.

A data custodian commands the data. In large organisations several people are likely to be designated data custodians. In the Health Service this is likely to be senior officers, that is, consultants, divisional nursing officers, personnel officers or a district occupational therapist, but it will vary according to local circumstances.

It is anticipated that data protection coordinators and data custodians will work closely together, particularly in training employees and raising the general level of awareness of the Act.

BREACH OF CONFIDENCE

Therapists may find that some organisations add special clauses into the contract of any member of staff who may have access to personal data. Breaches of confidence may lead to dismissal and a civil action for damages. Many professionals involved in the collection of personal data recommend that guidelines in accordance with the code of practice are drawn up for each discrete system. Wherever automatic systems are used by occupational therapists, clear guidelines should be given on the security measures necessary to prevent loss or disclosure of personal data and operational policies should clearly define who has access to the data. In departments where the equipment is used by both staff and clients it is important that these measures are rigorously adhered to.

REGISTRATION

It is a criminal offence to hold personal data without being registered under the Act. As previously stated, large organisations will probably have a data-protection coordinator who will apply for registration on behalf of all their users. In smaller concerns it is the responsibility of the data user. Registrations can be amended as, and when, appropriate. Where two or more organisations are involved in working with the same personal data there should be written agreements concerning the control of that data. In some circumstances only one organisation need apply for registration but in others it may be more appropriate for each to register separately. Advice is available from the Office of the Data Protection Registrar.

Occupational therapists collaborating on research projects involving personal data in the provision of health care should be aware that some topics are considered sensitive and are subject to more rigorous scrutiny. These include mental illness, addiction and sexually transmitted diseases. A more extensive list can be found in the NHS Data Protection Guidelines (1984).

Exemptions

Registration can rarely be avoided. Home computers, where the personal data held only concerns the family and household affairs, are exempt. If the same system is also used for business purposes, it may come under the terms of the Act, as will work done at home for an employer. The code of practice and rules for registration will then need to be rigorously adhered to. The physical security arrangements for the equipment and the system security arrangements or codes programmed into the system to prevent general access should be strict.

Word processors used only as typewriters, to prepare letters and documents, are also exempt but if they are used to sort or analyse personal data, in any way, they fall within the scope of the Act. Mailing lists are exempt if they contain only the names and addresses, or other necessary details, purely for the purposes of distribution. If more personal data is needed to identify particular groups or individuals, then it is likely that registration will be required. Research workers may, in some cases, claim exemption from subject access, particularly if the data is not in a form by which individual subjects can be identified. For a full list of exemptions, consult the Act or seek advice from the Office of the Data Protection Registrar. The NHS Computer Policy Committee issued Data Protection Guidelines in 1984 to all Health

Authorities to help them comply with the provisions of the Act. This document describes the experiences of some Health Authorities who were used in the registration pilot.

SUMMARY

- Computers are simply calculators that store information and were introduced into occupational therapy departments in Britain between 1983 and 1986.
- To simplify the process of analysing and selecting appropriate computing tasks for clients in treatment Allen's (1985) formulation of cognitive function is applied throughout the chapter. This also enables the occupational therapist to recognise when computing can become an active part of therapy.
- It is recommended that occupational therapists designing research projects on the effectiveness of computers in treatment use the Latto and Barnitt Survey (1986), the International Classification of Diseases (1978) and a model of occupational therapy.
- To select a computer for occupational therapy the user groups should first be identified, then a system chosen to meet their needs. The advantages and disadvantages of different types of equipment have been discussed to make this task easier.
- Computers can be used in the individual treatment of clients performing at levels 3 to 6 in Allen's (1985) hierarchy of cognitive function. Appropriate hardware and software has been described for each.
- Computers can be used in group work with clients functioning between levels 4 and 6 of Allen's hierarchy of cognitive function. The advantages of establishing separate groups for each level have been emphasised.
- The equipment, software and the way these may be used to encourage interaction have been discussed.
- Computers can be used in work assessment, habilitation and rehabilitation of clients functioning between levels 4 and 6. Clients who remain at level 4 are likely to be able to use computers in a sheltered work setting or day centre. Those who function at levels 5 and 6 may wish to develop their computing skills further by attending facilities in the community, such as colleges or state skills centres.
- Literacy, numeracy and daily-living-skills programmes can be delivered through computer-assisted learning packages.
- Occupational therapists must conform to the Data Protection Act (1984) if they wish to store personal data on computer. It is a criminal offence to hold personal data without being registered.

REFERENCES

Allen C K 1985 Occupational therapy for psychiatric diseases: measurement and management of cognitive disabilities, Little, Brown & Co. Boston

Brown G W, Birley J L T 1968 Crisis and life changes and the onset of schizophrenia. Journal of Health and Social Behaviour 9: 203–214

Data Protection Act 1984 HMSO, London

Kielhofner G (ed) 1985 A model of human occupation. Williams & Wilkins, Baltimore

Latto S, Barnitt R 1986 The use of microcomputers in occupational therapy. Liverpool Institute of Higher Education, Liverpool

Mosey A C 1970 Three frames of reference in mental health. Slack, New Jersey

NHS Computer Policy Committee 1984 Data protection guidelines, Centre of Information Technology, Birmingham

Reed K, Sanderson S R 1980 Concepts of occupational therapy. Williams and Wilkins, Baltimore

Schrank W 1986 Job rehabilitation of the psychiatric disabled and their work in data processing. Proceedings of the 2nd Annual Conference, British Computer Society Disabled Specialist Group. British Computer Society, London

World Health Organization 1978 International classification of diseases, 9th revision. Mental disorders. WHO, Geneva

FURTHER READING

Foster L (1988) Writers' Workshops: The Word Processor and the Psychiatric Patient. British Journal of Occupational Therapy 51(6): 191–192

Saunders P (1984) Micros for handicapped users. Helena Press, Whitley

USEFUL ADDRESSES

Software

Software Director
Lochee Publications Ltd
Oak Villa
New Alyth
Perthshire PH11 8NN
Tel: 082 83 2154

Software Ltd
Special Needs
74 Victoria Crescent Road
Glasgow
G12 9JN
Tel: 041 357 1659

Open Software Library
164 Windsor Road
Ashton in Makerfield
Wigan WN4 9ES
Tel: 0942 712385

CASE
Department of Psychology
Keele
University of Keele
Staffordshire
ST5 5BG.

Office of the Data Protection Registrar
Springfield House
Water Lane
Wilmslow
Cheshire
SK9 5AX
Tel: 0625 535777

Equipment

Microcomputers
Suppliers in most towns.
Also available through mail order.
Look for details in computer magazines.

Concept keyboard
Star Microterminals
Unit 6
Moorside Road
Winnall
Winchester SO23 7RX
Tel: 0962 843322

Advice
Occupational Therapists Special Interest
Group in Microcomputers
c/o Mrs C V McCaul
66 Strangers Lane
Canterbury
Kent
CC1 3XG

British Computer Society
Disabled Specialist Group
13 Mansfield Street
London W1M OBP

SECTION 6
Client groups

18

Acute admission

Lesley McCallion

INTRODUCTION

Occupational therapists have, in the past, felt that acute psychiatry was a small area of concern for them, particularly where they were made to feel that their only role was as a distractor or a symptom-reliever. It is hoped that this chapter will summarise the relevant occupational therapy philosophy and practice, illustrating the unique contribution occupational therapy has to make in this field and highlighting particular areas of concern for the therapist to work upon.

The occupational therapist may be the only person in the multidisciplinary team highly skilled in assessing and treating problems underlying symptoms. If these remain undisclosed and unresolved, then symptoms are likely to recur.

The occupational therapist is fortunate in having non-medical models for practice and in not being bound by parameters of disease and sickness. Occupational therapy concerns activity of every type and is thus a shared frame of reference with clients, an instantly normalising experience.

This chapter first defines acute psychiatry and looks at the contribution to be made by the occupational therapist in this area. There is an extensive section on the range of problems and conditions the therapist is likely to meet, looking at appropriate treatment for each condition.

The comparatively newer form of therapy found in crisis intervention is then examined, using case examples to illustrate the therapist's role in this type of treatment. The chapter finally applies the occupational therapy process specifically to acute intervention, detailing the tasks involved in problem solving, data collection, assessment, setting goals, intervention, evaluation and discharge.

DEFINITION OF TERMS

The Shorter Oxford English Dictionary defines 'acute' as: 'Turning point esp. of disease; time of danger or suspense . . . from GK. krisis: decision.' Through this definition we can focus on two significant points: suddenness and crisis. Individuals may manage at home, although with some degree of difficulty, until an apparently negligible event precipitates crisis, leading to an admission.

EFFECTS OF ADMISSION

The sudden new event of admission can be quite devastating for both client and family, and shock, puzzlement and disorientation may compound existing feelings. Despite this, the individual is often expected to assimilate the alien culture of the ward and learn to live by its rules, rotas, philosophy and hierarchy. It is remarkable how quickly people do this, despite experiencing trauma. For the family there are sudden separations, they are on the periphery of a new culture, and may also feel guilt at the relief and respite the admission has brought them.

Sometimes admission to an acute unit is not a new experience, and yet another stay in hospital may bring a sense of failure, bitterness and fear. For others it may mean company, companionship and better conditions than outside in the community. Trends in psychiatry continue to move away from large institutions and long-term care but the institutionalism already engendered does not always disappear at the same rate as the institution.

OCCUPATIONAL THERAPY AND ACUTE PSYCHIATRY

TEMPORAL PERSPECTIVE

Occupational therapists perceive the individual as

CASE EXAMPLE 18.1

Barbara S, a 60-year-old lady, was admitted to an acute ward. She had lost weight, taken to her bed and ceased to eat or drink. She had worked as a secretary in the past and had sustained a number of other roles including home-maker, hobbyist, home-maintainer, family member and community figure. She had begun to suffer from agoraphobia a few years earlier and had gradually withdrawn from all roles. She now felt that parts of her body no longer existed and that she was dead. Her diagnosis was depression with nihilistic delusions.

The occupational therapist felt that she had withdrawn from the desire to interact with and explore any aspect of her environment. Occupational-therapy philosophy includes the concept that man has an innate desire to explore and interact with the environment. Barbara appeared to have almost lost this motivation and the therapist's task was somehow to engage her inborn drive to interact.

The first meeting between therapist and client took place in the lounge of the acute ward, following Barbara's refusal of a meal. She was greatly distressed, feeling that only her eyes and ears existed. She made sucking sounds and pronounced sucking gestures with her mouth. She could barely speak and to do so caused her profound distress. She felt she was not real, and any suggestions of 'proof' through her impact on the environment were equally upsetting.

The occupational therapist considered developmental theories of human psychology, particularly that of Erik Erikson, in determining the course of therapy, paired with an occupational behaviour model as a basis for treatment. It was conjectured that Barbara had ceased to feel the environment to be within her control and that she had regressed to a primitive stage of development. How or why this had occurred could not be determined at this early stage of treatment.

The therapist decided to reflect Barbara's actions, mirroring them in a subtle way. During brief treatment sessions the impact she was able to have on the therapist as part of her environment was demonstrated to her. The impact was within her control since it affected the therapist's posture and gesture. Gradually she became able to interact in other ways and established other means of exploring and controlling her environment for herself.

a person with a past, a present and future; someone whose development is taking place over a continuum of time. This temporal perspective enables occupational therapists, with their clients, to view the 'opportunity' in crisis. It also facilitates the salvaging and restitution of submerged skills, roles and goals. The temporal view has some bearing on the trust and optimism enshrined in the relationship between therapist and client. In working with clients in crisis, however distressed or regressed they are, the therapist can call upon their total experience, making it possible to reach some shared point of interaction, however basic.

THE ENVIRONMENT

Reed and Sanderson (1980) state that one of the unique aspects of occupational therapy is the possession of knowledge of 'methods of adapting people's behaviour response to the human and non-human environments, or adapting the environment to people's behaviour.' Environment includes both physical surroundings and personal situation. Occupational therapists can assist clients to 'manage' environments, for example, by taking over a proportion of responsibility for management while the individual concerned is in an acutely stressed state, unable to cope with prevailing environmental conditions. Through the occupational therapy process, the therapist uses graded planning to bring about the appropriate environment.

Long-term problems

When the individual is in an acute phase of illness or crisis the occupational therapist is not primarily concerned with symptom relief, although she may use this with the client to help him regain some sense of control over his environment, for example, learning to control and overcome feelings of anxiety. Once symptoms are more within the individual's sphere of control the primary concern is to uncover and work with the client upon the often long-term problems or dysfunctions that have brought about the symptom or crisis. Unless acute clients come back as outpatients, the task may be to relieve symptoms and begin discovering underlying longer-term problems that will be dealt with elsewhere.

TRENDS IN PSYCHIATRY

Trends in psychiatry are towards much shorter admissions, admission only as a last resort and helping acutely ill clients in the setting of a day hospital.

There are implications for occupational therapists working with the acutely ill:

- Due to shorter hospital admissions the therapist needs to develop excellence in assessing and planning quickly and accurately with the client while he is an inpatient.
- Therapists at higher and management grades need to ensure the appropriate level of staffing provision in acute psychiatry to allow this to happen.
- The therapist must use her flexibility and skills to work with one client in a variety of settings and conditions, also helping the client to adapt.
- The therapist must maintain excellent communication throughout a potential network of agencies and workers, once the client has left the ward.

THE FUTURE OF OCCUPATIONAL THERAPY IN ACUTE ADMISSION

At the time of writing there are fears that occupational therapy may be seen as a luxurious adjunct to drug therapy and hospitalisation. However, as one of the most respected writers of the profession wrote, 'Occupational therapy can be one of the great ideas of 20th century medicine' (Reilly 1962). Many other professions focus on dealing with symptoms as a primary concern but occupational therapists are concerned with the underlying difficulties and it is only when these difficulties are rectified that symptoms usually stop recurring.

Financial constraints and concerns are likely to highlight areas of work for therapists in crisis intervention and preventitive psychiatric work. An occupational therapist can help an individual perceive an unhealthy balance of activity and work with him to change that before a crisis occurs, preventing hospitalisation. Increasing choice in location and type of health care means that people are looking at alternative solutions to pills and prescriptive treatment. There is increasing awareness of, and desire for, holistic consideration from clients in difficulty. Occupational therapists in acute psychiatry already offer this. It would be very exciting to see community clinics of occupational therapists practising outside the acute unit and working in physical, emotional, learning and environmental areas with clients in their community. The fulfilment of this ideal may be some distance in the future but is slowly being realised as therapists are finding themselves more involved in crisis intervention and preventitive work.

ACUTE PROBLEMS AND CONDITIONS

Occupational therapists are not primarily concerned with the use of medical terms for mental illness, nor is diagnosis seen as an end in itself. Rather, they are concerned with function and dysfunction, the parameters being the individual within his environment. However, the ways in which people express emotional distress fall into identifiable groups. People experiencing one type of problem may respond favourably to certain therapeutic approaches and may experience the phenomena in loosely similar ways. Occupational therapy can never be 'prescribed' in terms of the activity to 'cure' a particular 'illness' but occupational therapists work with other professionals using a medical model and it is important to have an understanding of the terminology and features of specific diagnoses.

ATTEMPTED SUICIDE

Attempted suicide is the action of an individual who wishes to end his life. There may be many reasons for this decision, for example, depression,

psychosis or physical illness. The individual may be aware of severe psychic damage and may have concluded that the pain of continuing in an empty life is too great.

Treatment

The occupational therapist will be involved in helping the individual back to a state of function, from which to reconsider that decision, and may also need to help the individual understand and come to terms with pain caused to others, and personal guilt resulting from attempting what is sometimes considered a moral crime. If the individual is badly damaged or injured, the therapist may see him for some time after the event, following a period of time being physically monitored, for example. The client may have had no-one to talk to about feelings during this time and may be alienated and more deeply depressed following the attempt.

Sometimes the attempt may be an act of very great anger, which the individual could not ex-

CASE EXAMPLE 18.2

Joanne was admitted to hospital, having taken an overdose of sleeping tablets. Following a brief period on a medical observation ward, she was transferred to an acute psychiatric ward. Initially she was glad to talk to an occupational therapist in one-to-one sessions, twice weekly. The emphasis of treatment at this stage was on support, rather than exploration.

Joanne had become convinced she had AIDS as a result of her husband having an affair. She was primarily very anxious and had lately been depressed. Following two weeks' counselling and a negative AIDS blood test, the occupational therapist began to talk to Joanne about her anxiety and its possible causes. Treatment at this stage continued to involve support and now included education and insight about anxiety.

After 6 weeks of treatment, Joanne left hospital with a greater understanding of her anxiety. The couple sought marriage guidance. Joanne was not a classically depressed client but had become frantic and desperate about her situation and had not been able to request help.

press in any other way. He will need the therapist's help in recognising and understanding this and finding other ways to release the emotion.

In the short term, treatment will involve counselling or supportive psychotherapy. This helps the individual to come to terms with the traumatic events surrounding the suicide attempt and the period in hospital. The occupational therapist uses these sessions to help establish the underlying reasons for the attempt, and then works with the client to resolve the difficulties.

PARASUICIDE

Parasuicide is what often used to be called 'a cry for help'. The individual seems unable to ask for help or, when he does, is treated unsympathetically. The parasuicide is often a symbolic gesture of despair and helplessness but is not really intended to end life. For example, the person who takes sleeping tablets half an hour before he knows his partner is due home from work may be making a parasuicide attempt. People who do this may find all their behaviour becomes labelled as 'attention-seeking'.

Treatment

It is important for the occupational therapist involved to explore the individual's feelings and needs, perhaps looking closely with them at where they feel their locus of control lies.

SELF-MUTILATION

People mutilate themselves under all sorts of circumstances and for all sorts of reasons. This phenomenon crosses almost the entire spectrum of mental illness and mental handicap.

Others may harm themselves as a result of a reactive depressive psychosis, or agitated depression. This is described as 'A depressive psychosis, . . . apparently provoked by stress such as bereavement or a severe disappointment or frustration . . . The delusions are more often understandable in the context of the life experiences' (Brooke et al 1980). The individual often experi-

---

> **CASE EXAMPLE 18.3**
>
> Vivian, aged 42, was a talented professional painter and enucleated both eyes because she felt God had communicated to her that He wanted her to make this sacrifice. Vivian periodically experienced psychotic episodes where she lost touch with reality and felt God communicating with her in various ways.
>
> Once the terrible physical damage had been repaired and the psychosis had retreated following drug therapy, she was terribly depressed for a long period of time, only very gradually feeling she wanted to explore the environment and consider how she could reform lost roles.
>
> The occupational therapist's role was in giving supportive psychotherapy and in helping to enrich Vivian's environment. For example, involving her in sessions using clay, making her tapes of music she enjoyed and introducing interesting and pleasant smells, textures and contours into the day-to-day life of the ward.
>
> Vivian eventually began to visit her home and learned to live in it as a blind person. The treatment ended when Vivian took up a place on a course to train the unsighted for daily living.

ences extremely disturbed behaviour and the multilation may also be a suicide attempt.

In the initial phase of treatment the occupational therapist adopts a gentle approach, interacting with the individual for fairly brief periods. Treatment may at first involve distraction, as the individual is often very preoccupied with what they see as their own 'foulness', for example, with Eleanor (Case example 18.4), to sit with her reinforced the idea that her presence was tolerable.

Another group of people who may mutilate themselves are sometimes referred to as 'cutters'. Researchers seem unsure how to classify this phenomenon. Some feel it is a behavioural reaction, others that it is psychotic in origin and others that it is a form of emotional release similar to orgasm in experience but not in sensation. Individuals who harm themselves in this way tend to be females in their twenties, often inflicting damage to arms and legs, usually requiring stitches.

Such clients often make the staff nursing them

CASE EXAMPLE 18.4

Eleanor was a 58-year-old lady who had been widowed 3 years previously. Her son had bought her a bungalow near his family and she had moved there quite soon after her husband's death. She had become seriously depressed, convinced she was a dreadful person, and that she smelled so unbearably that no-one could tolerate her presence. She had covered herself with petrol and set light to herself, severely burning her hand and arm.

She was transferred to the acute psychiatric unit as soon as the wound was stabilised but was still very agitated, desperately distressed at having to exist. Her thoughts were further fuelled by the suppuration of the burns, which had an unpleasant smell. She was treated with electroconvulsive therapy.

Eleanor was not able to attend the occupational therapy department at first but gradually stayed for part of a ward group, for example, listening to some relaxing music. Once her worst symptoms had abated, she discharged herself and did not wish to continue her occupational therapy programme. She had several subsequent admissions to various psychiatric hospitals in the region.

feel demoralised, responsible, and split into factions with different reactions to the client and the events.

The occupational therapist may have a role in supporting fellow team members who are feeling stressed by such clients, as well as supporting the client.

Individuals who cut themselves in this way often have a desire to demonstrate to themselves where reality begins and ends, a phenomenon associated with the boundaries of self and not-self and, as such, relating to quite a primitive stage of development.

Treatment

The occupational therapy model of a person as an open system has clearly defined boundaries but examines the reciprocal relationship between individual and environment. This, used in conjunction with psychodynamic theories, may help the therapist work towards therapeutic intervention with such clients.

ANXIETY NEUROSIS

An anxiety state has been defined as 'A state of continual irrational anxiety and apprehension, sometimes flaring up into acute fear amounting to panic, accompanied by symptoms of autonomic and endocrine disturbance; with secondary effects on such other mental functions as concentration, attention, memory, and judgement' (Stafford-Clark and Smith 1974).

Anxiety is part of the normal range of human feelings. It stems from a saving reaction, designed to alert the individual to dangers, helping him take evasive action for self-preservation.

In someone who is suffering from anxiety neurosis the reaction occurs either constantly, too frequently, or in a way that interferes with the individual's skills, habits and, ultimately, with his desire to act and feeling of efficacy in action.

Treatment

In acute psychiatry the occupational therapist will meet individuals who feel at the mercy of anxiety 'attacks' and have retreated from any activity that could possibly bring one on. There are a number of useful areas of work for the therapist, who may initially help the individual to bring symptoms under his own control by teaching relaxation. This will help the individual feel more in control and may enable him to control the anxiety once it is occurring but does not directly do anything to rectify underlying difficulties.

There is usually a disruption of, and lack of, activity in those suffering from anxiety, as well as problems of general lack of confidence and low self-esteem. Planned structuring of time may be used in conjunction with examining the balance of activity, and the underlying causes of anxiety. In later stages of treatment the therapist may use other adaptive methods to help the individual deal with severe anxiety in the future, for example, examining motivation, recognition of stressors prior to experiencing bouts of anxiety, life-style change and enhancement.

CASE EXAMPLE 18.5

Alison G, a 31-year-old lady, was referred to the occupational therapist for help with anxiety. She had given birth to her second daughter by Caesarian section 6 weeks prior to the referral. She was suffering panic attacks, felt she could not leave the house or see friends and family, was not sleeping well and was lying awake or in a state of panic for long periods during the night.

After taking a brief history the therapist began the intervention by helping Alison to sleep. Together with the therapist, Alison and her husband coordinated the baby's feeding rota so that Alison was free to sleep after 11 p.m. The therapist taught Alison some relaxation techniques specifically to encourage sleep and encouraged her to use and establish a 'winding down' routine 2 hours before sleeping. She encouraged Alison and her husband to use massage and relaxing aromatherapy oils and provided them with commonly available information about foods and drinks containing stimulants and additives. Alison responded very well to this approach and her sleeping pattern rapidly improved, giving her a greater feeling of resilience during the day.

Following this stage, the therapist continued to assess the client and also helped her to structure her time, achieving a balance of activity and reducing anxiety through planning. In the latter part of treatment, the therapist encouraged the client to examine how she viewed the environment and how she felt others viewed her. This involved work in the area of self-awareness, confidence building, and assertiveness. It also involved allowing her to express anger about certain life events that Alison had in the past felt she must 'forgive' others for, rather than seeking resolution.

PHOBIA

Phobia refers to anxiety that is focused on particular objects, events or situations. It is a specific form of anxiety. There are many examples of phobias including agoraphobia, (a fear of going out or away from home) fear of flying, fear of fish, cats, snakes, birds, dogs; phobias seldom exist in isolation but tend to act as the trigger for activating an underlying state of anxiety caused by many factors.

CASE EXAMPLE 18.6

Gavin was a 48-year-old businessman who had to make regular trips to Europe. He was admitted to hospital with panic attacks. It appeared he had begun to experience anxiety about flying some 6 months previously but had tried to control this by trying to ignore the feeling and making use of the in-flight drinks trolley. He had been due to fly to Stockholm the day of his admission but had been admitted to hospital following a severe panic attack that Gavin and his wife had feared was cardiac failure.

Following physical tests, Gavin was reassured that his heart was normal. On interview, he admitted he had become terrified of flying. Images of planes on television could now increase his heart rate and cause his mouth to become dry. It also emerged that Gavin was under pressure at work, was increasing his hours of work and that the marriage was suffering as a consequence.

Gavin needed to return to work quickly but was able to arrange to work from the office for 6 months. He was swiftly discharged from hospital and saw the therapist as an outpatient. He had individual appointments and also attended a group to learn about anxiety and how to overcome it.

In individual sessions the therapist explored with Gavin the way he used his time and took a full occupational role history. Some of his constant worry about 'keeping up' at work seemed linked to a period at the age of 7 where he had been off school for 8 months following a fracture and had felt behind his peer group in academic terms and as though he had lost friendship.

Gavin became able to relate former patterns of behaviour to his recent desire to 'stay ahead' and be popular with others within the firm. Using time structuring, he realised that most of his activity had begun to fall within the category of 'work'.

At the same time, the therapist began a programme to desensitise Gavin's fear of flying. A graded programme over the 6 months involved chatting about flying, looking at images of aeroplanes, visiting the airport, and eventually taking a shuttle flight to London and back.

The occupational therapist had taught Gavin relaxation techniques to use during stressful situations and meanwhile he had made a number of life-style changes, for example, having a much healthier balance of activity.

After 6 months he was able to return fully to his job. He continued to feel mildly anxious about flying but the panic attacks did not recur.

Treatment

The occupational therapy approach would be multifaceted, including time structuring, teaching methods of anxiety control, modelling behaviour and supportive psychotherapy, all used within the framework of an appropriate occupational therapy model.

ACUTE PSYCHOSIS

Psychosis is defined by the Oxford English Dictionary as 'severe mental derangement involving the whole personality'.

Difficulties arising from severe mental illness manifest themselves in functional psychoses. There is a complex interplay in these conditions between the workings of the individual's body and mind, his environment, and stress interacting with his 'open system'. There are three areas of psychosis:

- schizophrenic psychosis
- severe depression
- mania.

Schizophrenic psychosis

This involves the progressive deterioration of the personality and its relationship with the environment. It is a term usually confined to long lasting and recurring mental states. Using an occupational therapy model, schizophrenia could be regarded as a difficulty with perception, initially, and with volition, latterly, as the individual experiences increasing disparity with others and becomes increasingly isolated from his environment.

In the acute setting, individuals with schizophrenia may have found that stress triggers experiences of unreality, merged with reality. The essential features of schizophrenia include disorders of thinking, which include delusions, for example, the individual knows himself to be special, royalty, or in receipt of information beamed down from space. There may be feelings of passivity, for example, MI5 or spacemen are able to read the individual's mind, and contact with reality may be lost in the form of experiencing visual and/or auditory hallucinations. The individual's emotions may appear disordered as may movement, thought and behaviour.

Treatment

The therapist will also consider treatment to organise and 'normalise' perception and consolidate and strengthen existing skills, habits and roles. She may also help the individual reduce stresses likely to precipitate further acute attacks through planning and education.

Psychosis of this sort is usually treated by the use of major tranquillisers, which suppress hallucinations and delusions. The individual will require supportive psychotherapy to help him gain rapport with the therapist.

Severe depression

Severe depression sometimes becomes psychotic. It may occur as a reaction to troubling life events, that is, a reactive depression. Alternatively the depression may be of an endogenous nature, perhaps as part of a syndrome involving mania as well. A hereditary cause is suspected in this type of disorder, which does not always seem to be precipitated by stressful life events. The experience of depression is characterised by:

- feelings of guilt, anguish and despair
- loss of temporal orientation in relation to one's past and future self
- anger that is turned against oneself
- somatic experiences including
  — insomnia
  — anxiety
  — poor appetite
  — total exhaustion
  — constipation
  — bodily discomfort, which is often described by sufferers as being similar to symptoms of influenza.

The depression either appears spontaneously, that is, it is endogenous, or represents a reaction to life events that goes on for longer or is more intensely felt than is normal for that individual. It is quite normal to feel depressed following a death, or the ending of a significant relationship. This classification of depression is rather simplistic and occupational therapists will always be concerned with underlying causes and the individual's environmental history as well as current events.

Therapists sometimes find they are seeing clients who have had repeated admissions for depression. The medication prescribed, in some cases 20 or 30 years previously, has helped to dull distressing symptoms but has left the clients unable to resolve maturational crises.

Treatment

The therapist can help the client come to terms with distant life events as well as current ones. Medical treatment for symptoms can be important since, during the acute phase, the client cannot easily focus thoughts and actions other than upon the internal distress and trauma.

CASE EXAMPLE 18.7

Mary, aged 32, had become severely depressed, with a decline in appetite and sleep, increasing distress and self-hatred. She had a history of depressive episodes.

On one visit she was convinced that the occupational therapist had a tape-recorder in her bag and was conspiring to have the client's child put into care. The therapist emptied out her handbag for the client, as practical, concrete, ways of sharing reality are important in acute stages of illness; continued seeing the client to give her support; and arranged an immediate review of medication.

The client was given additional drug therapy, which controlled the worst symptoms and enabled her to continue changing underlying patterns of doing and thinking.

Other types of psychosis include agitated depression, which was described in Case example 18.1. It is characterised by extreme agitation and profound severance from reality with sufferers at great risk of harming themselves.

Mania

In some individuals, periods of depression alternate with periods of elation or mania. This phenomenon is called manic-depressive psychosis. The depressive phase is characterised by loss of judgement, severance from reality and sometimes by delusions or hallucinations. The phase of elation may involve aggression, ceaseless activity, hilarity, restlessness and sleeplessness. The individual is apparently divorced from his usual self and may do things that are entirely out of character.

CASE EXAMPLE 18.8

Frances, a 29-year-old woman, was a very respected research graduate involved in teaching at a university. She formed an interest in a particular popular singer and began to write to him, offering to sing with him when he came to her town and, in reality, creating embarrassing scenes when he did visit. She felt she should become a pop star and experienced feelings of being able to do her research work much more quickly.

She could read entire books in a night and began to stay up all night to do so, though she could retain very little of the information contained within the books. She felt she had a superior intellect and qualities to her peers which made her feel quite contemptuous of most people around her.

Individuals experiencing this dysfunction often have great difficulty in completing planned activities and may find it very hard to do only one thing at once. They may have tremendously ambitious plans to alter world politics or extend their house, for example, yet in reality often have difficulty in completing simple daily routines.

Treatment

As well as helping with cognitive elements, the therapist may need to give the client supportive psychotherapy and latterly possibly support in repairing damaged relationships and in coming to terms with events prior to admission.

EATING DISORDERS

Compulsive eating and dieting, bulimia and anorexia nervosa have been described as epidemic among women (Chernin 1985). Comparatively few men experience eating disorders.

In eating disorders, the body is used as a means to express past and present conflict in a three-dimensional way. The occupational therapist working with clients experiencing such phenomena will be interested in using three-dimensional media to help them resolve such conflicts. For example, clay, drama, movement, sculpting and modelling may all be useful and significant media for such clients.

Eating disorders appear to relate to early unresolved conflicts focussing on the child's autonomy and separateness. Anorexia nervosa could be said to involve some form of perceptual disorder in the individual's convictions about her body boundaries. Chernin (1985) associates eating with the struggle for a submerged identity aggravated by present social pressures to extend and challenge the boundaries of female roles beyond traditional expectations. Identity, rage and sexuality may all be bound within a complex relationship women have with food. Chernin (1985) suggests that food obsession contains all the elements of a rite of passage that normally precipitates the individual into the next life cycle or maturational crisis but that this has sometimes never reached resolution with neither sufferer nor healer having a clear understanding of what the complex relationship with food really means.

Bulimia

Bulimia is characterised by bouts of over-eating, followed by purging in the form of vomiting, which is self-induced, and sometimes also the abuse of laxatives. Bulimic individuals tend to be of an average body weight and size.

Anorexia nervosa

Anorexia nervosa involves extremely rigid rules about food and dieting, with the individual ex-periencing terror that food taken in will make her fat. In some cases people experiencing anorexia will also become bulimic. Anorexic individuals are more likely to be admitted to acute psychiatric units because of the danger to life involved in the very low body weight sometimes reached by such clients.

Treatment of eating disorders

Difficulties with eating are very often treated in a behavioural way in acute units, with the difficulty being interpreted as a learnt behaviour that can be changed by a routine and a structured programme involving rewards and increasingly greater freedom.

However, there are a number of areas with which the occupational therapist may also be concerned, for example in bulimia the individual may need support and help in planning and resolving financial difficulties since the individual frequently incurs large debts to finance the eating binges. The individual may also be experiencing severe depression since there is usually an awareness and acknowledgement by the client that the problem exists, with the sufferer being suffused by self-doubt and loathing of their inability to control themselves. By contrast, anorexic individuals frequently deny that a problem exists, feeling that they are still fat despite appearing to others to be emaciated.

GRIEF REACTION

Grief is a process rather than an illness. It is a natural way in which people cope with bereavement and loss, particularly where a bond of love is severed. Symptoms may be physical, including exhaustion, numbness and sickness. Losses are often referred to as a 'blow' or a 'wound'. The individual will also usually experience a reactive depression with its characteristic symptoms. There may be experiences of anxiety and fear because of the separation from the loved one. Bereavement and loss can include losing a partner, a child, an animal, a limb, a special place and may also en-compass experiences such as abortion. The in-dividual characteristically goes through stages of shock and disbelief followed by yearning for the loved one, depression and feelings of futility ultimately followed by resolution.

There is no set time during which individuals should resolve each stage although complications may arise where individuals are not able to complete each stage of grief. Grieving clients may have a great need to talk; this may be denied them either because they are alone or because their family discourages it.

Treatment

The occupational therapist may have an important preventative role in helping the individual and his family through the grieving process at home and giving extra support to grieving individuals who also experience regular episodes of depression, mania or schizophrenia.

CONFUSIONAL STATES

A state of confusion is a feature of very many emotional phenomena including grief reaction and psychotic depression. However, there are a recognisable group of transient organic psychotic conditions which are described thus:

'States characterised by clouded consciousness, confusion, disorientation, illusions and often vivid hallucinations. They are usually due to some intra- or extra-cerebral toxic, infectious, metabolic or other systemic disturbance and are generally reversible. Depressive and paranoid symptoms may also be present but are not the main feature.' (Brooke et al 1980).

Confusional states may also be observed in those suffering senile dementia and subcortical dementia. Both concern the pathological atrophy of brain tissue. Individuals may also experience transient acute confusional states lasting hours or days.

These may take many forms and may be associated with physical states such as endocrine disorders, epilepsy and reaction to medication.

Treatment

An important role for the occupational therapist would be in assessment, defining the confused thought and behaviour so that unnecessary medication and diagnoses are avoided.

CASE EXAMPLE 18.9

Ethel, a 58-year-old lady was admitted to an acute ward. She had taken to her bed, and had not got up for 6 weeks. On assessment she complained of 'attacks', in which she fell, and described sorrow at having to give up her role as shopper and housekeeper in her family. A possible diagnosis of illness behaviour was made but additional tests were done.

The occupational therapist conducted a neurological assessment as well as testing motivation and taking a full occupational history. She felt there were some signs of neurological damage and this, paired with a motivation the client had to continue her role and her profound fear of the falls and attacks, led the therapist to question the proposed diagnosis. Following a computed tomography (CT) scan the client was found to be suffering from subcortical dementia.

SEXUAL PROBLEMS

Clients admitted to acute units seldom have sexual difficulty as a primary cause of their admission. Rather, it is the profound depression and anxiety brought about by the underlying difficulty that leads to their admission. Sexual dysfunction may be a feature of anxiety and depression where the individual's drive is likely to decline. Recovery from anxiety and depression and resolution of underlying difficulties may help.

Treatment

Because it is a sensitive area of discussion, the occupational therapist will approach mentioning emotional and physical relationships with care. Having discovered a sexual difficulty beneath an initial problem of anxiety the therapist may go on to discover further problems in the client's history, for example, the client is unable to enjoy a sexual relationship with his current partner and there is a history of the client being sexually abused as a child. These difficulties require supportive counselling in a trusting environment. The individual suffering such abuse may frequently be left holding the 'terrible secret' long after the abuser has died. There are a number of specialist groups and organisations to help survivors of incest or abuse and the therapist should make herself aware of these, in case the client would prefer their help.

Sexual orientation becomes a difficulty only when the individual or their significant figures are unable to accept this and no longer give the individual unconditional love and support and the individual is not self-sufficient.

For example, a female patient in her twenties had begun to abuse alcohol. She had always felt unhappy, apart from a brief period when she openly lived with another woman as her partner. Her family pressurised her to conform and she did so, marrying a former boyfriend of whom her mother approved. She became increasingly low and began drinking. There were sexual difficulties in the marriage.

The occupational therapist should be aware of practical physical difficulties and be prepared to help people with these, for example, individuals may experience tension in relationships and depression because of intercourse that is painful or unsatisfactory. Provision of information about foreplay, vaginal dryness, etc. may help resolve emotional difficulties. The therapist should provide information as long as she feels comfortable with the topic and should refer the client on to other agencies where appropriate, for example, if she feels embarrassed about discussing sexuality.

Sexuality is commonly oriented only around specific acts of physical union and the drive for sexual gratification. It is, however, only one aspect of intimacy with emotional and intellectual intimacy having as significant a meaning in the individual's development as physical intimacy. Sexual needs should not be repressed. However, those who chose celibacy do not necessarily have sexual problems.

PERSONALITY DISORDERS

This group of difficulties involves individuals who have very deeply ingrained patterns of maladaptive behaviour. The behaviour is usually recognised by adolescence and often fades in middle age and later life.

The personality of the individual is abnormal in one or more ways, which may include personality components, quality or expression or all of these.

Certain personality disorders are described as sociopathic or asocial, manifesting themselves in a complete lack of regard for the usual social rules and obligations, lack of feeling for others and impetuous violence or total unconcern for others' distress. The individual's behaviour is grossly disparate from accepted social norms and does not change through experience, which may include punishment as a criminal.

Other personality disorders may be characterised by behaviour indicative of an excess of normal personality traits. For example, a paranoid personality disorder is suffered by the individual who is immensely sensitive to setbacks or apparent humiliations. There is a tendency to misconstrue friendly gestures as suspicious or hostile. The individual may be aggressive, while feeling humiliated and put upon.

Other trait personality disorders include affective, schizoid, explosive, and hysterical personalities. Less intractable than sociopathic disorders, they may respond to help in analysing what is occurring in the environment, and how those phenomena are processed within the open system. Such individuals may change and respond to appropriate environmental conditions.

ACUTE STATES OF ALCOHOLISM AND DRUG ABUSE

Individuals who abuse alcohol or substances are often admitted to specialised acute units or to small areas of general acute units because their difficulty appears different from other aspects of psychological dysfunction. Initially, the individual may be withdrawing from a dependency on alcohol and drugs requiring a withdrawal programme with the substitution of Heminevrin for alcohol, for example.

Dependency on alcohol or drugs can be physical or psychological. Some people can use alcohol in quite large quantities without actually becoming dependent, although they undoubtedly risk their health by doing so.

Dependence on alcohol involves behavioural and other responses that always include the compulsion to take alcohol to experience its psychic effect or avoid its absence. Drug dependence works in a similar way and may involve prescribed or illicit drugs.

Clients may abuse alcohol or drugs for a number of reasons. These include social inadequacy and anxiety, and difficulties in planning and structuring time. For example, one client's interests focussed only around his job of playing in a band in a club. He was constantly exposed to alcohol and eventually became dependent upon it. To change involved totally restructuring his interests and leisure activities. For others, drugs and alcohol may drive away problems in reality, which are all the more painful once the effects of the drug or alcohol have worn off.

Treatment

The occupational therapist has a role in helping the individual restructure time in terms of behaviour and activity balance and also in helping to resolve difficult conflicts and maturational crises. She may also have a role offering help with anxiety and assertiveness problems that may emerge in the post-acute phase.

CRISIS INTERVENTION

WHAT IS CRISIS?

Crisis has already been defined as a turning point and a time of danger and suspense. The Chinese character representing crisis has two components, danger and opportunity. This apparent paradox is acknowledged in many schools of thought and philosophy. Bitter self-doubt and distrust (the danger) may lead to the dissolution of calcified patterns of feeling and reaction (the opportunity for change).

Someone in a state of crisis stands at a turning point. The insecurity, doubt and stress caused by this position may be profound. Existing coping mechanisms do not seem to apply to the current situation. Fear, worry and tension may make the individual feel less able to change, yet he may have no option but to face what underlies appearances. Finding a new set of solutions may seem impossible, engendering feelings of helplessness.

CASE EXAMPLE 18.10

Chris, a man in his thirties, was admitted to hospital following arrest by the police. He had been found wandering in a seaside town 50 miles from home, apparently in a state of fugue; a loss of awareness of one's identity, often coupled with disappearance from one's usual environment. His business had collapsed a short while previously and was declared bankrupt, and he was experiencing financial difficulty. His wife was expecting their third child. Chris had to live in separate accommodation temporarily as the family were waiting to be rehoused, following the repossession of their home.

After initially interviewing Chris, the therapist felt that he had come to a position of self-doubt and mistrust of himself and the world in general following a series of undesired changes which, for him, were catastrophic. He had lost a number of roles, particularly that of self-employed worker, and had been used to working from 7 a.m. to 7 p.m. daily. Most people would experience anger, fear, anxiety and a degree of depression after such life events, however, Chris evidently could not express his feelings or seek help. His emotions and thoughts had continued unknown to his family and unexpressed until his disappearance and discovery by the police.

During sessions with the therapist it emerged that Chris had employed this strategy for dealing with feelings and crises since the age of 11, when his father had suddenly died and he had been left to cope with emotions, feeling that the world was indeed an untrustworthy place. He felt he had never been able to grieve for his father fully. One task for the therapist was to encourage Chris to explore his present feelings, to share information and express himself with the hospital team and his family.

The crisis provided the opportunity to change patterns of feeling and reaction that were deep-rooted and had for many years remained undisclosed. Although Chris recovered from his loss of memory and subsequent depression he still found it hard to express himself. One year following his first admission he disappeared once again and experienced a state of fugue, following his wife's decision to end the marriage.

At this point the individual is unlikely to be able to strive alone for a resolution to his problem. He may question his former beliefs about himself and his world. On finding that his beliefs no longer accommodate present circumstances he is likely to develop an increasing feeling of low self-worth since he doubts his fundamental perceptions and understanding of his environment.

The individual requires immediate help; someone with whom to share the problem, test perceptions and develop effective coping strategies. He may also need help to reaffirm or rebuild his beliefs-structure around a new set of perceptions about himself in his environment, rather like experiencing a personal 'earthquake', in which the primary structures and supports are tested and may crumble.

CRISIS INTERVENTION AS TREATMENT

Kahn and Earle (1982) state, 'Crisis intervention which is described in its own literature as an independent process should be looked upon as the utilization of one particular frame of reference'. Mosey (1986) calls crisis intervention an aspect of preventative work. In crisis there are a number of commonly disrupted areas of life that are domains of concern for the occupational therapist:

- values
- occupational skills
- coping mechanisms
- communication
- fear
- anxiety
- other overwhelming feelings
- the environment.

The therapist interacts with client and treatment team, using highly developed interpersonal skills to prevent the breakdown of communication. Overall, her task in this area is to assist the client in achieving a state of equilibrium through growth and adaptation. Where poor adaptation and resolution occurs, problems and similar crises are likely to arise in the future.

Crisis intervention as a distinct therapy is a relatively new branch of psychiatry. There appears to be an increased need for formalised professional help when people become troubled in crisis. Historically, people lived in close-knit groups, for example, villages or large families living in proximity

in towns. Transport was limited and new offshoots tended to stay close to the nucleus of the family. In general terms a large supportive network existed, able to absorb the crisis because of the large number able to help. A coordinating or strong figure might have been the family matriarch or patriarch, the village priest or holy person. Up to relatively modern times families congregated in numerous houses in neighbouring streets of large Northern towns.

CASE EXAMPLE 18.11

Mary was 53 and had been brought up in a close-knit community. She often mentioned how, in the past, the family would 'rally round' in times of stress. Mary had suffered severe depression, having helped care for her sister until she died of cancer. Mary had also lost her home, following litigation. Mary's children had moved away a few years previously.

Though she began to recover spontaneously and through the work done with the therapist, a significant turning point came when her children decided to move back locally where they could rejoin as a separated but close family once again.

Individuals may find themselves at a distance geographically, emotionally and economically from their family, which now tends to be smaller anyway and perhaps less able to offer support. The roots of the methodology of crisis intervention lie in such theories as those of Sigmund Freud and Erik Erikson. Although their theories differ, both are developmental, suggesting that characteristic experiences and preoccupations dominate specific phases of an individual's life. These require some form of resolution or experience before further development can be satisfactorily completed. Change or crisis is expected and occurs at the transitional stage of personal development. The individual is experiencing vulnerability at the time of attempting to change his maturational status to meet his current experience and domains of concern.

One who has never resolved an early crisis, for example, trust versus mistrust as described by Erikson (1977), may experience regular crises because he is unable to embark upon or sustain all kinds of relationships. Reciprocally, the oppor-

CASE EXAMPLE 18.12

Donald, a 23-year-old man, was admitted to an acute ward following a period of restlessness and aggression. He had strong beliefs about world peace and environmental issues when interviewed by the therapist. He tried very hard to persuade family and others to align their beliefs with his. He lived at home. The admission followed one the previous year when he had been assaulted by two youths while on holiday. He had been trying to persuade them to believe as he did. His diagnosis was manic-depressive illness. He appeared afraid while an inpatient and often behaved aggressively, particularly to the ward staff. Sometimes he acted in a childlike way, for example, by hiding the walking stick of an elderly resident and refusing to reveal its whereabouts.

Using her knowledge of Erikson's developmental theories and with a dynamic model of occupational therapy the therapist made an assessment with Don. His way of behaving and his activities seemed to correlate to the role of angry person. His behaviour overall was characteristic of one who is recapitulating a maturational crisis, namely identity versus role-confusion. Characteristically, Don appeared to appoint certain individuals to play the role of enemy, although they might be either neutral or well-meaning in reality. He viewed other people in the multidisciplinary team idealistically and as suitable role models. The therapist felt that Don was experimenting with different roles, models and choices and that his angry role was a form of explorative play. She felt the play was a precursor to the selection of more mature roles, which Don had not moved into during past periods of maturational crisis.

Once allowed the freedom to explore roles and without the 'firm-parenting' originally offered as a model by the multidisciplinary team Don became less afraid and angry. He eventually came to perceive people as a mixture of good and bad and accepted others' points of view. He declined longer term therapy and returned to his job.

tunity to work towards resolution of the crisis occurs at the same time, hence the significance of the therapist's attitude to the client, and the therapeutic relationship formed. Although vulnerable at the time of crisis, the individual is especially able to make use of outside help.

According to Kahn and Earle (1982) the individual who has coped with one crisis is much more likely to succeed in surviving subsequent maturational crises. Conversely, failure experienced at one transitional phase may lead to subsequent expectations and experiences of failure.

Crisis intervention is also used where the individual is struggling to deal with unexpected change. Examples are bereavement, disfigurement, amputation, stillbirth, violent and/or sexual attack, the death of a child. Crisis intervention employs particular individuals and methodology in this type of situation.

Intervention in unexpected crises will only be successful if there is good communication between all team members. If the individuals concerned do not communicate properly the crisis is unlikely to be averted.

There is an increased need to develop crisis-intervention work in a variety of clinical areas. An example is crisis in the home, especially with elderly people. More elderly people now live in the community and for longer. Kay et al (1964) researching in Newcastle found that 41% of elderly people at home had psychological abnormality. The services could not sustain such a large number of potential clients in hospitals and methods of crisis intervention must increasingly be employed.

These methods work best when the therapist is able to move to and from community and hospital, working within the significant environment for the client.

SPECIFIC OCCUPATIONAL THERAPY TASKS IN ACUTE INTERVENTION

THE PROBLEM-SOLVING APPROACH

A problem-solving approach is employed by many professions. For example, some nurses use

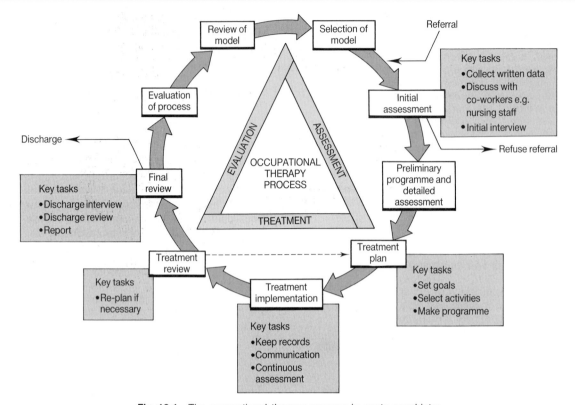

Fig. 18.1 The occupational therapy process in acute psychiatry.

problem-oriented medical records. Problem solving is a sequential process that may take place formally, being written down, or informally as therapist and client discuss ideas about possible solutions and means of change.

The problem-solving approach is the process used by occupational therapists (see Fig. 18.1). Evaluation is one formal part of the process and also forms a continuous part of all interactions, as the therapist attempts to find optimum conditions of treatment. Thus the occupational theraphy process offers a kind of ongoing quality assurance. It also means that the phases of treatment do not always follow one another, since there is the opportunity for repetition, rethinking, planning and revising.

Within an acute admissions unit the therapist may only have time for an assessment period prior to passing on a summary of problems identified by the client, and a profile of him, for example, an occupational role history. This may lead to dis-

satisfaction for the therapist who wishes to complete the whole process. In practice, some clients stay for a brief assessment period then go elsewhere, some are seen as outpatients by medical staff, some have much longer admissions, and some see the therapist as day patients and some as outpatients.

DATA COLLECTION

On receiving a referral the occupational therapist begins to collect information from and about the client to determine, first, whether the referral is desired or appropriate. Where admissions are brief it is important to collect the data quickly but carefully. Plenty of time should always be allowed for the initial interview with the client. Data can be obtained from:

● the referral card
● the nursing notes

- medical records
- verbal information given by nurses on the unit
- other colleagues who are also involved
- interviewing the client and/or his family.

Most therapists develop an individual style of interviewing. Because of potential constraints of time in acute psychiatry the data collection during the initial interview must be well designed so that it highlights specific areas of experience, need, strengths and problems. The therapist uses her skills to arrange an appropriate interview area. The criteria include:

- privacy
- sufficient undisturbed time, without telephone calls or other interruptions
- environmental considerations, such as lighting, heating, protection from noise and attention to aesthetics (the room should be clean, and pleasing to the eye), furniture should be comfortable with chairs of equal type and height.

The occupational therapist will arrange the furniture in a way that does not intimidate the client and encourages the sharing of information. The best position is often 3 to 4 feet apart and angled so that therapist and client are neither side by side nor directly opposite but so that both have a full facial view of the other.

A great deal of information may be collected during the interview and it is useful to allow at least 1 hour for talking. The time may not always be needed but it allows the therapist to feel relaxed and comfortable about the pace of the interview. This is invariably perceived by the client and assimilated as data about the environment. Some information is inferred from observation of the client. Other data is collected verbally.

Data gathered from observation

Manner of entering the room

Does the client seem:

- hesitant
- afraid
- nervous
- able to take the initiative?

Clothing and appearance

- Has the client put on his clothes correctly, for example, seams inside clothes, only one pair of trousers at a time unless it is very cold?
- Is the clothing cared for and coordinated according to the client's usual or past standards?
- Does the client appear to have groomed and cared for himself?

Posture

- Is the client slouched or upright?
- Is the client able to sit when invited?
- Does he sit forward or back?
- Does he hold up his head?
- Is there eye contact?

Gesture

- Does the client use gesture?
- Are the gestures matched to rate pitch and content of speech?
- Does the client use facial gesture?
- Do any gestures contradict the verbal information being given?
- Are the gestures closed or open, protective or relaxed?

Social skills

- Does the client have eye contact?
- If so, is the eye contact brief enough for the interviewer to feel she is not being stared at?
- Is it long enough to avoid seeming timid or furtive?

Tone of voice, pitch and rate of speech

- Do these seem appropriate to the content of speech?
- Does the client whisper so that it is a strain to hear him?
- Does he speak loudly or very quickly?

It is important to remain objective when observing a client. One cannot infer feelings from observed behaviour alone. However, much can be observed provided the therapist does not lose objectivity and respects the client's likes, dislikes and cultural practices. For example, it would be wrong for a therapist who dislikes Crimplene, for example, to infer that there is inappropriateness in an elderly client who chooses to wear a crimplene suit.

The therapist's observations are considered along with the verbal content of the interview.

Data gathered from verbal interaction

Cognitive process

This is a cortical process that involves the use of information for the purpose of thinking and problem solving. 'It is the process of perceiving, representing and organising sensory stimuli on the cortical level. It allows the individual to be oriented relative to dominant environmental features' (Mosey 1986). The following elements can be considered at the interview:

- attention
- memory
- orientation (to time, space, area)
- thought process
- conceptualisation
- factual knowledge
- ability to identity and solve problems.

The occupational therapist may wish to conduct more detailed assessments in each area, if the client agrees. For example:

- is the idea of occupational therapy familiar?
- if not, does the client want information?
- gathering the client's thoughts and opinions about the referral
- taking an occupational role history
- asking for an account of the client's environmental circumstances (past, present and future, if this has been considered by the client)
- expression of emotion

- opportunity to discuss recent life events
- does the client wish to participate in an occupational therapy programme?
- does the client have a positive or negative outlook?
- does he mention frankly depressed or psychotic ideas?

Following the collection of such data the therapist should have some idea whether the client is willing to continue towards an occupational therapy programme or not and will have explained the nature of occupational therapy and the process at an appropriate level for the client's current needs. She should also have some occupational and environmental history, yielding sufficient data to suggest areas of assessment.

ASSESSMENT

Assessment takes place over a period of time and within the parameters of a preliminary programme discussed and agreed with the client following the initial interview. Some reasons for using assessment in acute psychiatry are listed below:

- to allow client and therapist to recognise dysfunction
- to specify the parameters of the dysfunction
- to allow client and therapist to recognise areas of function and ability
- to identify a starting point for treatment
- to identify a baseline for future measurement of change
- to establish a deeper understanding of the client in the context of his environment, its culture, society and values
- to establish the client's desire and potential for change
- to help establish the appropriate model of occupational therapy
- to continue the establishment of rapport with the client.

Assessment may be planned and carried out by therapist and client in a wide variety of ways. It may be verbal, observed, and/or written. There needs to be a record of the assessment. Broadly, occupational therapy assessments measure development and social experience.

Some assessments are self-administered forms filled in by the client but the main means of assessment used will, of course, be activity. The skills of activity analysis are the therapist's key to formulating and understanding assessments carried out with the client. From detailed assessment, carried out over a period of time (from 1 day to about 6 weeks) the therapist gathers sufficient information to begin to formulate ideas about the model to be used, treatment and future evaluation. The evaluative process is constant, taking place throughout treatment sessions as well as in formal reviews, or standardised tests.

In acute psychiatry initial assessment may take place in small, low-key multi-activity groups of clients and therapists with problem identification being followed by the allocation of clients to other, more-specific groups. This gives the therapist the opportunity to observe and interact with the client in the context of a social group and through a variety of activities. This type of assessment often goes along with collecting a very detailed occupational role history, range of activities and balance of activity over time.

SETTING GOALS

The setting of goals is an important task for client and therapist, prior to the therapeutic intervention. In acute psychiatry the client needs consistent goals to work upon. Clients may be discharged quickly, sometimes without prior planning, yet require the means of continuing work begun in the unit. Goals may motivate the client, allowing him to impose his own framework upon what may be a personally chaotic situation. This may offer him the experience of locating control within himself rather than externally and will affirm his impact on his environment in their completion.

The goals may also represent a form of contract or agreement of work with the client. In practice there is often confusion between professionals, client and family about goals, aims and objectives. A goal is 'a written or spoken statement of intent by an individual or specified group of individuals with respect to their own performance and/or that of others' (Kushlik et al 1974). 'Objective' is another word for goal, often used in educational terminology. An aim is an overall statement concerning a hoped for outcome: a broadly based anticipated outcome that guides the formation of much more specific goals. Aims of treatment are arrived at during and following assessment, for example, helping Alison (Case example 18.3) overcome her anxiety about leaving the house.

A goal is much more specific and is useful for clarifying to all concerned who will do what with whom and how, when and over what period of time.

INTERVENTION

As with aims, and goals the intervention to be used is based upon the knowledge gained from assessment, together with the therapist's knowledge of activity and activity-analysis. Initial intervention may include both ongoing assessment and treatment. Very early stages may involve helping reduce symptoms prior to looking at underlying problems. A written treatment programme should be given to the client.

CASE EXAMPLE 18.13(A)

Janice, a 30-year-old woman in her 8th month of pregnancy, was married with a 3-year-old son. The diagnosis was anxiety and obsessive compulsive neurosis. The therapist met the client as an outpatient and the assessment took the form of:

- interviews
- taking an occupational role history
- extensive assessment of time structuring.

Time-structuring began as an assessment but swiftly became an important medium of treatment for Janice.

The initial intervention focussed on reducing anxiety using relaxation training, goal setting, confidence building and the promotion of a healthier and better-structured balance of activity.

EVALUATION

Regular formal and informal evaluation should take place throughout the occupational therapy process. Goals often involve some sort of time limit for reevaluation. This allows therapist and client to judge whether the goals were realistic, whether the overall aim has changed or not, which goals continue to require work and which, if any, new goals have emerged as the result of newly-gathered information.

CASE EXAMPLE 18.13(B)

Following the initial intervention, after 6 weeks, Janice was still experiencing anxiety and worries though they had lessened overall despite the stress of having a second child born shortly after the start of the treatment period.

Janice now felt more comfortable with her therapist and talked more deeply about her difficulties. There was, she felt, a lack of time structuring as a family. Further, she felt she was always criticised by one family member. This criticism made her obsessive preoccupations worse. This information broadened the scope of the therapy.

MOVING ON
New goals

Goals may be added or cancelled, completed or abandoned, when they have served their purpose.

CASE EXAMPLE 18.13(C)

For Janice, new goals emerged:

- spending time each week planning balanced activity along with her husband
- making her wishes known to her husband rather than concealing them.

She continued working on the goals of increasing confidence and practising techniques for reducing anxiety. The therapist became less involved as a teacher of anxiety-reduction methods and became a resource to help the couple with time structuring and balancing activity.

Continuing occupational therapy

For many clients, evaluation and new goals may involve the change back to living at home. This change may be an anxiety-provoking time where

they seek to test the ability to cope with a situation that may have contributed to their acute illness.

In continuing the treatment programme the therapist can be an important link, and guide. The client may come back as a day patient or an outpatient. Appointments may be daily, weekly or monthly depending on the clients needs. Because the therapist is concerned with the relevant environment for the clients, continuing treatment may take place at home or in the community. The therapist has an important role in affirming the client's confidence and sense of self as he reviews crisis, change and newly found equilibria over a period of time.

Referral to other agencies

The assessment, intervention and evaluation period may reveal that the client needs help from other specialist agencies.

CASE EXAMPLE 18.14

One anxious lady, Ruth, was the second wife of a widower whose teenage sons now lived with them. She was successfully engaged in an occupational therapy programme. Her confidence increased and she was able to focus on areas of her life other than symptoms. Once she came to make an assessment of her environment it became clear there was conflict in the family about parenting.

The client had not found this conflict distressing while she was anxious, nor had it been apparent to others in the family. Ruth became unhappy and unable to complete her programme and her bodily symptoms of anxiety began to recur. Her husband felt she needed something to 'cure' her. The therapist referred this client to a family therapy clinic, following discussions with the multidisciplinary team.

Any essential information should be passed on to the new agency. This will usually include a summary of the therapist's work. Referrals are frequently made following discussions with the team of professionals working together with the client.

Discharge

A discharge interview and evaluation are important for both client and therapist. By implication, discharge must be planned for and worked towards over the treatment period, however short or long. The occupational therapist uses the discharge interview to gather data about the efficacy of treatment ensuring quality of service for others in the future. The therapist may summarise the course of treatment, the client's achievements of strengths and areas of work which need to continue. There may also be a discussion of what is to be written in the discharge report. This report should be part of the client's medical and occupational therapy notes, and should be available to any relevant individual from other agencies to be involved after discharge. Lastly, the discharge interview forms a rite of passage; a formal ending of what may have been a significant therapeutic relationship. It may be a therapeutic tool for the therapist in making an ending an event of mutual regard and warmth, one not of rejection but of development for the client.

SUMMARY

The chapter began by defining terms and looking at the effects of admission on the client, going on to look at occupational therapy work in an acute setting.

Specific acute problems were then considered, and appropriate occupational therapy suggested for each condition, with Case examples to illustrate treatment methods. The chapter then looked at crisis intervention and how this can be used as treatment.

The final section covered the specific tasks of the occupational therapy process in the area of acute intervention, with sections on: data collection, assessment, goal setting, intervention, evaluation and discharge.

REFERENCES

Brooke et al 1980 Mental disorders: glossary and guide to their classification in accordance with the 9th revision of the International Classification of Diseases. WHO, Geneva
Chernin K 1985 The hungry self: women, eating and identity. Virago Press, London
Erikson E 1977 Childhood and society. Jonathon Cape, London
Kahn J, Earle E 1982 The cry for help and the professional response. Pergamon Press, Oxford
Kay D et al 1964 Old age mental disorders in Newcastle-upon-Tyne. British Journal of Psychiatry
Kushlik et al 1974 Goal setting. Open University, Milton Keynes
Mosey A C 1986 Psychosocial components of occupational therapy. Raven Press, New York
Reed K, Sanderson R 1980 Concepts of occupational therapy. Williams and Wilkins, Baltimore
Reilly M 1962 Occupational therapy can be one of the great ideas of 20th century medicine. American Journal of Occupational Therapy, 16(1)
Stafford-Clark D, Smith A C 1974 Psychiatry for students. George Allen and Unwin, London

FURTHER READING

French B 1987 Coping with bulimia. Thorson, Wellingborough
Goldberg D, Huxley P 1980 Mental illness in the community. Tavistock Press, London
Orbach S 1982 Fat is a feminist issue. Hamlyn, Middlesex
Storr A 1972 The dynamics of creation. Secker and Warburg, New York

19

Long stay

Tessa Durham

INTRODUCTION

Long, dingy corridors with tiled walls; huge, sparsely furnished day rooms with a characteristic odour; poorly dressed clients purposelessly shuffling and mumbling along; these are the images conjured up by reference to long-stay psychiatry. It is an area of psychiatry that often suffers from poor funding and poor staffing and that seems to offer little compensation for those who work there. Yet it is a field of practice which, while often difficult, is rarely without interest or challenge and to which occupational therapists have much to offer.

Bennett (1978) has written, 'Rehabilitation is the process of helping a physically or psychiatrically disabled person to make the best use of his residual abilities in order to function at an optimum level in as normal a social context as possible'. It is important that rehabilitation services should aim to provide good-quality continuing care for those who have only minimal chance of resettlement and this would include many of the long-stay population, as well as specific retraining for those able to return to community living. Rehabilitation for resettlement is discussed in Chapter 20. This chapter deals with the special needs of those clients who are less likely to be resettled. It describes who these clients are, explores their needs, offers suggestions as to how occupational therapy can help them and, finally, deals with some of the problems that may be encountered in long-stay psychiatry. Although this chapter focuses upon long-stay residents of institutional environments, the approach described has equal relevance to the range of alternative long-term care settings.

LONG-STAY CLIENTS

WHO ARE THE CLIENTS?

It is difficult to give an exact indication of the size of the long-term population, however, Wing estimated that some 420 per 210 000 of the general population are in receipt of, or in need of, psychiatric rehabilitation services (Wing and Morris 1981), although by no means all of them need long-term inpatient care. These chronic clients can be grouped, for purposes of description, into the following three categories, although these groupings are somewhat artificial and there are no clear-cut boundaries between them:

- old long-stay clients
- new long-stay clients
- new long-term clients.

Old long-stay clients

Twenty or more years ago British mental hospitals housed thousands of long-stay clients, many of whom were no longer in need of psychiatric care. Since the mid-1950s a policy community care and resettlement has placed many of these old long-stay clients into the mainstream of community life, with varying degrees of success. Those who remain in hospital are mainly frail, elderly and often physically disabled (Wing and Morris 1981). Resettlement away from an institutional setting is no longer feasible for most of these clients and, although their numbers are diminishing, they continue to constitute a considerable part of the inpatient population (Wing 1978).

New long-stay clients

These clients have more recently become long-stay residents in hospital and have received continuous inpatient care for a period longer than 1 year but less than 5 years. This group includes those who are chronically disturbed but relatively stable, as well as those who experience repeated acute disturbances with brief periods of remission (Mann & Cree 1976). Although they are in need of full-time psychiatric care at present, it is probable that at least some of these clients will be able to live more independently in the future.

New long-term clients

Both the old and new long-stay clients can be differentiated from a third group, the new long-term clients. These are people who have had repeated, extensive contacts with different aspects of the psychiatric service over a period of at least a year. These contacts may include admissions to acute or rehabilitation wards, day-care attendance, hostel or group home accommodation, etc. They can be seen to form part of a continuum between the acute admissions wards and the new long-stay client group (Wing 1982), and some of these clients may become the long-stay clients of the future. However, the focus of this chapter is on the current long-stay inpatient population.

CLIENT DISORDERS

It will be useful to explore the extent and nature of the handicap and disability experienced by long-stay clients. The very fact of their long-term residence in hospital gives some indication of the degree of disablement they face.

Multiple problems

Many long-stay clients have chronic psychiatric impairment that is either at a stable level or episodic in nature and that is only partially controlled by medication. They may have additional impairments, such as physical disability, sensory deficit, epilepsy or mental retardation, which considerably compound their disablement. In addition, the old long-stay clients are for the most part elderly and frail (Wing 1978). It is not uncommon for these clients to have had poor educational or employment records prior to admission and many have lost the family and social supports they once had. These factors conspire to make resettlement unlikely and often impossible.

Schizophrenia

Schizophrenia is the most common psychiatric disorder found among long-stay clients, so a description of the condition may be helpful. Schizophrenia is a psychotic disorder affecting approximately 1% of the general population, the onset occuring most frequently between the ages of 25–30 years. The causes of schizophrenia are not fully understood but it is thought that a combination of inherited predisposition and environmental stress are important, both at onset and relapse. Schizophrenia is not regarded as a single disease entity but rather as a syndrome characterised by clusters of symptoms affecting thought, behaviour and mood that are present in the absence of organic impairment or clouding of consciousness. Not all sufferers from schizophrenia will experience all of these symptoms, and only a minority will become long-stay clients.

Acute schizophrenia

Certain florid symptoms of schizophrenia most commonly, but not exclusively, occur during acute episodes, the presence of which is thought to be diagnostic. These were described by Schneider (1959) as 'symptoms of the first rank', among which he included:

- experiencing thoughts being put into or taken out of one's mind (thought insertion and withdrawal)
- believing that one's thoughts are known to others (thought broadcasting)
- hearing voices commenting on one's thoughts or actions (auditory hallucinations)
- hearing voices talking to each other (third person auditory hallucinations)
- feeling that bodily functions are interfered with by external agents (delusions of control)
- feeling that one's will or emotions or behaviour have been taken over by external agents (delusions of control)
- entertaining false beliefs that appear fully

formed and relate to normal events or objects, and that are not an attempt to explain other bizarre experiences such as hallucinations, for example, the client may feel that remarks heard on television refer to him personally, or that car number-plates have special significance for him (primary delusions).

Some symptoms that commonly occur during acute episodes of schizophrenia may also be present in other psychiatric disorders. They include auditory hallucinations, which are experienced as voices talking to the client, visual hallucinations, and delusional mood, in which familiar surroundings seem strange and there is an intense feeling of puzzlement. Another disorder of mood frequently seen in clients suffering from schizophrenia is flattening of affect, when facial expression is blank and wooden, voice tone is flat and expressionless, and emotional reactions seem blunted. Emotional incongruity may also be encountered, that is, the emotional expression is inappropriate for the circumstances, for example, laughter on receiving news of bereavement.

The behaviour of people suffering from schizophrenia is often disordered, sometimes in response to other symptoms, as when a client acts upon a delusion or 'converses' with an hallucinatory voice. Other disturbances of behaviour include:

- overactivity
- psychomotor retardation: slowness of thought and activity
- apathy and lethargy
- social withdrawal: difficulty in relating to others and preoccupation with own thoughts
- loss of social awareness: lack of sensitivity to others, sometimes leading to socially inappropriate behaviour.

Chronic schizophrenia

Although it is useful to think of chronic schizophrenia separately from the acute condition, in reality classification of clients is far from simple. The symptoms of chronic schizophrenia may be experienced as part of a florid episode and clients suffering from the chronic condition may have repeated episodes of acute psychosis.

A common feature of chronic schizophrenia is known as 'clinical poverty syndrome'. It is characterised by flattening of affect, underactivity, slowness of thought and movement, apathy, poverty of speech and social withdrawal (Wing 1978). A severely affected client may have little facial expression, very restricted conversation, a flat unmodulated voice, slow stiff movements, and poor posture and gait. Long-term clients suffering from schizophrenia often also exhibit thought disorder affecting verbal and non-verbal communication and leading to vagueness, distortion of perceptions and an inability to think purposefully. This causes an inability to pursue any activities other than relatively routine ones requiring little new thought. The resulting poor motivation and inertia present one of the biggest challenges to those working with long-stay clients.

Other psychiatric disorders

Other common problems, which are not confined to people suffering from schizophrenia, include odd, unacceptable, aggressive, self-destructive or unpredictable behaviours, and a lack of insight into the nature or extent of disability. Although schizophrenia is the most frequently occurring diagnosis it is not unusual to find clients suffering from manic-depressive psychosis, chronic severe neurosis, personality disorder, alcohol-related problems and pre-senile dementia among the long-stay groups.

Institutionalisation

The psychiatric impairment of these hospitalised clients makes it difficult for them to maintain positive social relationships in the family or the community. Clients become more and more socially isolated and suffer a corresponding loss of satisfactory life roles. This, in turn, leads to a weakened sense of personal identity and poor self-esteem. Many of these clients have had frequent and overwhelming experience of failure in their lives and this is sometimes exacerbated further, within the institutional setting, by a poor response to treatment programmes or by unsuccessful attempts at resettlement. The result is the development of excessive dependency on the institution. With repeated failure, the expectations of the client and of relatives and professional carers can spiral downwards, further lowering self-esteem and personal resourcefulness. Rather than developing positively through life-enhancing experiences, the long-stay client may become increasingly unmotivated, dependent and unable to exercise personal judgement and choice; in short, he can become institutionalised.

Institutionalisation, or institutional neurosis, is a condition that was first described by Barton (1976). The syndrome is not confined to the residents of psychiatric establishments but can also be found among long-term prisoners, monks and nuns (Goffman 1961). Institutionalisation gives rise to the following characteristics:

- apathy
- lack of initiative
- passivity and submissiveness
- loss of individuality
- narrowing of interest to the personal or the present
- deterioration in personal habits and hygiene
- acceptance of the status quo.

These features are not dissimilar from those of chronic schizophrenia and some arise from that cause but other factors were thought by Barton to be important in the causation of institutional neurosis. These include:

- loss of contact with the outside world
- enforced idleness
- brutality, browbeating and teasing by staff
- bossiness of staff
- loss of friends and personal possessions
- drug treatment
- lack of opportunity to leave the institution
- ward atmosphere.

It can therefore be seen that the institutional environment can have a marked effect upon its residents. Later in this chapter we shall look at ways in which the institutional climate can be changed or modified to prevent or remedy the institutionalisation process and thus enhance the quality of long-stay clients' lives.

THE LONG-STAY CLIENT

Case examples 19.1 and 19.2 illustrate the types of clients commonly encountered in long-stay psychiatry. The first is representative of the institutionalised established long-stay client, and second of the younger new long-stay group.

CASE EXAMPLE 19.1

Peter, in his mid-fifties and suffering from schizophrenia, was admitted to hospital in 1952 and has remained there since. His face is expressionless, his posture poor and his gait shuffling. He generally gives only monosyllabic answers to questions, never initiates conversation and rarely interacts with his peers except when asking for cigarettes, his main interest in life. He seems to accept his life in hospital passively and never deviates from the institutional routine. He takes no responsibility for himself and experiences great difficulty when faced with choice. He exhibits no thought disturbance and is not medicated. He has no contact with his family and rarely leaves hospital. An attempt at resettlement in the 1970s failed and Peter now lives in a long-stay ward.

CASE EXAMPLE 19.2

Patricia is much more active. She is in her early thirties but appears much younger. She is very overweight, rather grubbily and untidily dressed, with long straggly hair. She is talkative, often voluble, and can be charming and friendly. At other times she is grumpy and sullen, or even abusive.

She has spent the past 4 years in hospital but, prior to that, had drifted from foster home to hostel to living rough, with brief periods in acute admission wards. Her early life was chaotic and unstable and she has a history of self-destructive behaviour. She has fairly good independent-living skills but has had hardly any experience of success and her self-esteem is extremely low. She has become dependent on the hospital, which has provided her with the only continuity of care and support that she has known in years. She is a deeply unhappy person, suspicious of people, yet gullible. She remains extremely unpredictable and is prone to violent outbursts from time to time, especially if there is any hint of the possibility of resettlement.

GOALS OF LONG-TERM CARE

The references cited earlier (Mann & Cree, Wing) indicate that the new long-stay group continues to accumulate, even while the old long-stay population is gradually reducing in numbers. There continue to be clients who require extended periods of long-term care in sheltered, highly supervised environments because of the severity and chronicity of their mental illness. The need for asylum—a place of safety—remains for these clients. It is important that the current change in focus of health-care policy towards community-based services for the mentally ill encompasses this need. In some parts of the country large hospitals and institutions will continue to exist to provide for the long-stay and elderly mentally ill populations, while in other areas smaller units such as 'hospital hostels' are being built. Whatever the size of the long-term care setting, the highest possible quality of care should be available. This section focuses upon a philosophy of treatment that is relevant to all groups of staff and all care settings.

CURRENT CONCEPTS

In the past, people suffering from mental illness were locked away from society, and their opportunities for development were confined to learning how to become 'good' clients: conforming, passive, acquiescent, quiet. While this may still happen to some extent in long-stay wards, there has been a growing awareness among mental-health workers in the last decade of the need to change institutional practice, to enhance the quality of life of those who need long-term care, to prevent or remedy the effects of institutionalisation and to safeguard the integrity of the individual. These goals can be achieved partly through changes in the structure and organisation of the care environment, and partly through changes in approach and patterns of interaction with individual residents. Changes in societal attitudes towards those with mental illness, particularly those in need of long-term care, must also be fostered.

The principle of normalisation described by Wolfensberger (1972) and most frequently applied to the care of people with mental handicap, has much relevance to the improvement of the quality of life of mentally ill people. The normalisation principle implies allowing people opportunities and experiences, even within institutions, that equate as nearly as possible to those enjoyed by the 'normal', non-client population. It involves allowing individuals to make choices, to take risks, to make mistakes, to take the natural consequences of their own behaviour and to grow and develop. This principle is discussed in more detail in Chapter 23.

The environment

It is often difficult to know where to begin in attempting to change institutional patterns of care. The structural features of the hospital itself may offer little scope for improvement and, with limited resources, we often have to compromise on major capital expenditure but walls can be painted, pictures hung, windows curtained and the environment immediately becomes more friendly and home-like. The simplest changes often have a valuable impact, for example, different seating arrangements can actively encourage or discourage interpersonal interaction (Orford 1982).

Patterns of interaction with residents

Many of the institutional practices that most need to be changed are those that relate to patterns of interaction between staff and clients. These practices have been as commonly found in occupational therapy departments as in large back wards. Clients have often been subjected to an inflexible routine, with the use of both time and space being very rigidly structured. They have tended to be treated 'en masse' rather than as individuals, for example:

- everyone gets up at 6.00 a.m.
- everyone has a bath twice a week, no more, no less
- everyone is given tea from the same sugared tea urn, etc.

In recent years the emphasis of care has begun to move away from the needs of the institution, for smooth running, tidiness, efficiency etc., to the needs of the individual resident. The first step here is in recognising and supporting each person's individuality, allowing him personal space and possessions (and a secure place in which to keep them), allowing him choice and responsibility, and allowing him privacy and opportunities to develop relationships (Durham 1985).

The quality and frequency of staff interactions with clients are an important aspect of long-term care, or indeed of any field of psychiatry. Those institutions that foster greater individuality and independence among their residents also tend to have reduced social distance between staff and residents. Social distance can be measured in terms of wearing of uniforms, use of titles, separate toilet and sitting-room facilities for staff, etc. Generally speaking, the greater the social distance, the less opportunity there is for therapeutic interaction between staff and clients. Drawing together research into a variety of modes of intervention, Shepherd (1985) concludes that three key ingredients of therapeutic interactions between staff and clients are likely to bring about improvement in client functioning. These are:

- consistent, high but realistic expectations of behaviour, which are communicated clearly to clients
- specific feedback that is contingent on performance, and is given sensitively and combined with social approval
- recognition that few interventions or management programmes result in permanent change that continues after the programme stops, and that therapeutic involvement with clients must therefore continue on a long-term basis.

The philosophy of care

Occupational therapists and other staff are often accustomed to working within a framework based on the medical model, incorporating diagnosis—treatment—cure—discharge, which takes place within a relatively brief timeframe. The application of this approach to long-stay psychiatry quickly ends in frustration and a sense of failure, when the 'cure' and discharge never come. It is perhaps this lack of tangible results that discourages many occupational therapists from seeking jobs in this field.

The rehabilitation approach, on the other hand, attempts interventions that aim to maximise independence and quality of life within the limitations set by the client's disability (see Chapter 20). It implies a long-term commitment to the client, and with long-stay clients it means thorough assessment of the problems of the individual and careful management planning. As Shepherd (1984) so succinctly puts it, 'Rehabilitation is what you do when treatment fails.'

Management plans

The rehabilitation team is responsible for the second step towards meeting the needs of the individual, development of a management plan for each client. This is geared to helping him maintain the best level of functioning possible, despite his disabilities. In the plan, intervention must be scaled down and slowed down, so that small steps forward can be made.

The management plan should be designed to do the following:

- assist the individual to normalise his behaviour by learning to control inappropriate behaviour
- assist in the development of a more socially acceptable repertoire of behaviour
- help the individual to adjust to and cope with his residual disability
- maintain his current level of functioning and prevent further deterioration in his mental state
- offer opportunities and experiences that encourage personal growth and help the individual attain his full personal potential.

The management plan should be conceived as a means of drawing together a variety of therapeutic techniques and the skills of the different professions involved, to address the problems the client faces. Further, drawing up the plan should be a collaborative exercise between the client and the treatment team and should form a type of contract between them.

A wide range of interventions may be incorporated into the management of long-stay clients. Medication is obviously of great importance in controlling the primary impairment (the psychiatric symptoms) and psychological techniques based on learning theory are widely used. Behaviour modification techniques have application both in helping clients to control maladaptive or unacceptable behaviours and in maintaining desirable behaviours, and these are used both in individualised programmes and in the organisation of entire ward-management structures, for example, in token economies. Skills acquisition programmes, such as that described by Goldstein et al (1976), are of value in helping clients to increase their behavioural repertoire and here modelling, practice and clear constructive feedback are important. Behaviour therapy approaches have been described at length in Chapter 12 and their application to long-stay psychiatry has been discussed by Drouet (1986).

OCCUPATIONAL THERAPY WITH LONG-STAY CLIENTS

The rehabilitation approach, as we have seen, is to assist the individual to attain his optimum level of functioning in all aspects of his life, which is essentially the same as the general remit of the occupational therapist. Indeed, in long-stay psychiatry, the overall aims of the occupational therapist's intervention will be identical to those outlined for the management plan above. What, then, does the occupational therapist bring to client care in this field that is special, different, or of particular therapeutic value?

Occupational therapists are the members of the treatment team whose training is primarily and specifically focused upon the rehabilitation approach (Sims 1981). They are not employed to take care of clients nor to encourage them to adopt the 'sick role' but rather are concerned to establish a collaborative relationship with clients, through which they can be assisted to develop and adapt. Occupational therapists are always interested in the person as a whole and endeavour to facilitate the client's development in all aspects of his life, through the use of purposeful, meaningful and age-appropriate activities (Clark 1979).

Occupational therapy offers long-stay clients opportunities to engage in a wide range of activities of daily living, including domestic, social and work-related occupations, of which they might otherwise have little experience. It allows clients opportunities to experiment, to explore and to take risks, thus enhancing the quality of their lives and affording them the potential for growth and development of personal identity, self-esteem and increasing independence (Mosey 1973).

In the management plan outlined above, general aims for therapeutic intervention were outlined. We now need to move from the general to the specific: to the development of occupational therapy programmes and the use of specific therapeutic activities.

ASSESSMENT

The development of therapeutic aims and treatment plans must be based upon a clear knowledge of each individual's strengths as well as his deficits. The purpose of assessment is to determine the client's current level of functioning and his abilities, assets and weaknesses across the occupational spectrum (Willson 1984). In this section we will explore some ways of achieving this purpose.

Validity of assessment

Much of our assessment of clients will be based upon behavioural observation, therefore it is important to ensure that our observations are as accurate and objective as possible. Assessment has much greater validity if the observations are made of client performance in the criterion setting, that is, in the setting in which the activity would usually occur or as close a simulation as possible. (See Ch. 12 for a discussion of the value of simulation.) Thus if one wished to assess, for

example, ability to use a public telephone, one would need first of all to take the client to a telephone box. This may seem obvious, yet often assumptions or predictions about clients are made, based on little or no direct evidence, which may prevent the person being given opportunities for further development. For example, a client's reputation for being unable to handle his own money may precede him when he changes wards, and a decision may be made, based on this 'knowledge' of the client, that all his financial affairs must be managed for him, thus denying him choice, personal responsibility and independence. Of course, in some cases this decision may be justified, for example, if the client gives all his money away as soon as he receives it, but the decision must be based on firm evidence that it will be of benefit to the individual concerned.

Methods of assessment

Some occupational therapists will wish to develop their own assessment measures but a number have been specifically developed for use with the long-stay population. The two scales described in Boxes 19.1 and 19.2 are good examples of available assessment materials; Box 19.1 providing a general client profile and Box 19.2 an extremely detailed comprehensive assessment of clients' functioning.

What and when to assess

It is very often the case in long-stay psychiatry that clients have not been adequately assessed in the past and that they have therefore not been treated as individuals with differing needs. A full and comprehensive assessment of the clients, such as in Box 19.2, is well worth carrying out to provide a baseline for monitoring change and a foundation for therapeutic intervention. Such an assessment may well be carried out as a collaborative effort by all members of the treatment team and the information thus gained shared among them and used as a common basis for treatment. Assessment findings must be updated at regular intervals, probably every 6 months, and for this purpose a simpler and more readily administered assessment procedure, such as REHAB, will be more appropriate.

Box 19.1

The Rehabilitation Evaluation Hall and Baker (REHAB) was developed in the 1970s and published in its final form in 1983. This is a rating scale that has been extensively researched to ensure its reliability and validity. It is designed to give a broad overview of the client's behaviour in the hospital and community. The first part of the scale measures seven types of deviant behaviour, that is, behaviours that would be embarrassing if they were to occur in public. These include item such as incontinence, shouting, self-destructiveness and sexual offensiveness. In the second part of the scale the rater is asked to observe the client's general behaviour. Sixteen items are included, covering such behaviours as social interaction, time structuring, speech disorder and personal care. REHAB is designed to be completed by any member of staff who has been able to observe the patient closely for a period of one week, and is useful for compiling a broad general screening profile of each of a group of patients and for monitoring change. REHAB was adapted during its development by Hall et al (1981) to assess the social functioning of long-stay clients attending occupational therapy departments. This adapted scale, together with the original scale which is used on the wards and current status information sheets, constitutes the basis for a regular biannual review of long-stay clients at Whitchurch Hospital, Cardiff. Staff there found that consistency among assessment procedures used by different disciplines was helpful in encouraging effective team work, and that the regular and clear identification of clients' problems and needs helped them to define their treatment aims more clearly.

Box 19.2

The second example of an assessment package specifically for use with long-stay clients is that developed at Park Prewett Hospital by occupational therapy and nursing staff (Bartlett et al 1985). This was designed as a survey instrument upon which to base an entire hospital rehabilitation programme but also has application as an assessment measure for individuals. This assessment, in contrast to REHAB, which is very quickly and easily administered, is very detailed and comprehensive and correspondingly time consuming to complete. Each assessment must be carried out in its entirety by the same staff member, and takes approximately five sessions for one client. The resulting client profile includes details of his current physical and mental health, personal care, social and domestic skills and community-living skills. As such it provides a very sound foundation upon which to develop a treatment plan and is particularly useful for grouping clients within the rehabilitation service, for example, into those who could move into a hostel ward, and those needing a greater degree of supervision and observation.

These broad, general assessment data can then be supplemented by more-detailed and specific measures used by different members of the team, usually with a particular purpose in mind. The areas that are especially relevant to the development of an occupational therapy programme, and which the occupational therapist may want to examine in greater detail, would include occupational performance, social skills and daily living skills.

The commencement of a new group is a good example of an occasion that may lead to closer scrutiny of certain aspects of clients' functioning. The author and a psychologist colleague were running a weekly social group for long-stay clients, into which it was decided to incorporate some simple social and life-skills training. The members were all elderly clients who were highly unlikely to leave hospital but, it was hoped, could become less dependent on the institution. An assessment of hospital living skills was therefore drawn up, including items such as writing letters, handling small amounts of money, using the canteen, telling the time, leisure pursuits, etc. The assessment was in two parts: a yes/no inventory to be completed by a member of the nursing staff who knew the client very well, and an interview schedule, including many practical tasks, for use with each group member. From the results, a skills training curriculum was drawn up and was incorporated into the weekly group meetings.

When assessing clients it is important to ensure that the content of the assessment is relevant but to avoid prejudging a client's abilities and therefore precluding certain aspects of his life. For example, it may be totally inappropriate to carry out a detailed prevocational assessment on a 68-year-old long-stay client who has spent the past 33 years in hospital but this does not mean that the work performance of long-stay clients should never be assessed. Assessment measures, then, can vary greatly in their depth, specificity and usefulness. It is important therefore that the therapist chooses assessment materials carefully, ensuring they are appropriate for her purpose.

Recording assessment data

The information gained from assessment must be recorded in a way that is meaningful to others; a collection of numbers or scribbled notes on an odd scrap of paper is of little value. It is likely that most assessments will be based on a form of some type, such as a checklist, questionnaire or rating scale, which is usually kept by the assessor. The information contained therein should be clearly and succinctly summarised and communicated to other members of the care team. Assessment reports will normally include some recommendations for therapy. (See Ch. 5 on assessment.)

THERAPEUTIC INTERVENTION

Engagement in purposeful activity is crucial for the prevention of deterioration in the long-term mentally ill. The most important single factor influencing the extent to which long-stay clients exhibited acute psychotic symptoms was found by Wing and Brown (1970) to be the time they spent doing nothing; surely one of the clearest possible justifications for the provision of an activity-based therapeutic approach to this group. Our interest in a holistic approach to client care makes occupational therapists concerned with all aspects of a client's life and his physical well-being, social involvement, personal identity and self-image are of equal importance in the establishment of a comprehensive programme (Willson 1984). In this section the variety of therapeutic activities that form the occupational-therapy programme will be discussed.

Physical well-being

Long-stay psychiatric clients often suffer from a number of physical problems. The therapist must be particularly sensitive to the problems of frailty and physical disability that have already been mentioned and here the dual training of occupational therapists is an advantage. In addition, long-stay clients frequently have poor posture and gait, difficulties that are related to the apathy and loss of self-esteem of many clients and that are made worse by the effects of institutionalisation in some clients. Long-term treatment with phenothiazine medication, too, can give rise to some unpleasant, and sometimes irreversible, physical side effects, for example, tardive dyskinesia in which involuntary movements are present, particularly in the mouth and tongue but also the limbs and other parts of the body. The patient rarely experiences physical well-being.

A gentle programme of physical exercise may be beneficial here and should be pursued regularly and consistently, daily if possible. Social activities involving general physical exercise are also helpful and these may include walking, dancing and games such as bowls, skittles, deck quoits or floor draughts. Many clients are extremely reluctant to participate in physical activities and may take more than a little persuasion but, with time, new activities do come to be accepted. The guiding principle, as with all activities with this client group, is to take things slowly, gently and gradually.

Appearance is an important aspect of physical well-being and care of one's appearance does help to lift mood and enhance self-esteem. Normally the personal hygiene and clothing of clients is the responsibility of ward staff but, if patients are inappropriately dressed, smelly or unkempt, then both the client and the staff should be told. Within occupational therapy, beauty-care sessions may be enjoyed by some residents, although the emphasis should be on encouraging self-help rather than providing a free hairdo. Clients can be taught how to do simple mending of buttons and torn hems, how to clean shoes, and why hygiene is important. Modelling of acceptable appearance is very useful here, with staff frequently being the only models available to clients. If nursing staff continue to wear uniforms, it may mean that occupational therapists, social workers and doctors are the only people in everyday dress seen by clients. Staff should then be tidily dressed, in a manner that reflects their own personalities, but should be careful to avoid extremes.

Daily living skills

Although requiring long-term care, many long-stay clients are able, with encouragement, to do more for themselves than they normally do. Occupational therapists can foster independence in a wide range of activities within the institution, which should help to improve the quality of life and enhance the sense of personal identity of many clients. For example, clients can be encouraged to send Christmas or birthday cards to members of their family or to fellow clients, helped to make use of library facilities or newspapers within the hospital and taught to recognise coins and make small purchases at the hospital or local shop. Within occupational therapy departments it is often possible for clients to gain experience of other aspects of daily living, for example, cooking their own lunch, doing some personal washing or caring for a plant. Sometimes such activities can be incorporated into the overall pattern of care, as when long-stay clients live in hospital-hostel accommodation and are encouraged to take as much responsibility for themselves as they are able to manage (Bennett 1980).

Social activities

Long-stay clients tend to be extremely disabled in their social functioning. One of the most noticeable features of the clinical poverty syndrome is the individual's social withdrawal and isolation. This is combined with limited opportunities for social intercourse and a limited range of companions with whom to mix. Social withdrawal may be so severe that the client becomes mute but more typically monosyllabic responses to questions are given. The majority of clients are able to make simple conversation when approached by other people but have a great deal of difficulty initiating social contact, for example, one client had not found out the name of the person in the next bed, although they had been sleeping side-by-side for 4 years.

Warm-up exercises taken from remedial drama are often enjoyed by long-stay clients and can prove surprisingly effective at helping to create social links between them (Langley 1983). These exercises can be combined with more-familiar social pursuits, such as table games, quizzes or recreational activities. It is important for long-stay clients to have opportunities to socialise in settings other than those found in hospital and social outings to the community to shop or to visit cafes or pubs are useful. Indeed, it is often a revelation how well clients are able to control some of their bizarre behaviours when they are taken into normal social settings but it is important that these outings are not in themselves institutionalising. If clients are taken into the community in large groups, obviously shepherded by staff, and travel in an ambulance or coach with the name of the hospital on the side, the therapeutic value of the outing will be considerably diminished. In such circumstances, opportunities for interaction with the general public will largely disappear.

Social skills training

Formal social skills training is sometimes made available to long-stay clients. To be really useful, it needs to be as realistic and relevant as possible and combined with community experience (Durham 1983). Social skills training is sometimes concerned with the performance of 'micro' skills, such as good eye contact or speech volume, but these have little significance in relation to overall social adjustment and improvements attained in training sessions often do not generalise to everyday life once the reinforcement schedule applied in training discontinues. Shepherd (1980) has concluded that it is probably more useful to provide a context where normal social skills will be encouraged than to spend time training clients in the minutiae of social behaviour.

Many clients will exhibit behaviour that is socially unacceptable or bizarre, and helping them to develop control of this tendency must often precede the establishment of more-normal social responses. Behaviour modification techniques are often useful in extinguishing such behaviour and clear indications of what is acceptable must be consistently communicated by all staff. This often presents problems in institutions where staff and clients have known each other for many years and have become accustomed to behaviour that would not be tolerated elsewhere. Staff sometimes actively encourage inappropriate behaviour, perhaps unwittingly. Georgina, a very large young woman with a personality disorder and borderline mental handicap, habitually bear-hugged everyone with whom she came into contact, nearly suffocating them. Many staff reinforced this, laughing and asking for 'cuddles', rather than interacting with her in a normal, adult fashion.

Some long-stay clients need to relearn what behaviour is normal in society and some have become seriously disinhibited. Inappropriate sexual expression may be the result and clients who expose themselves or masturbate in public must be given clear feedback but also taught acceptable alternatives. Long-stay clients need close friendships and intimate relationships just as other people do, therefore normal means of sexual expression need not be discouraged if no-one is being harmed. Some long-stay clients with especially poor self-esteem are easy targets for sexual exploitation, often by other clients, and this must be discouraged. Discussion of personal sexual responsibility may be helpful.

Social interaction is a component of most activities that take place within occupational therapy (Willson 1984), and its promotion must always be given consideration in planning and implementing therapy programmes for long-stay clients.

Creative activities

Another aspect of occupational-therapy intervention is the use of creative activities such as art, music (Fig. 19.1) and crafts, which provide opportunities for emotional expression through doing, as well as through speech. Creativity is an essential

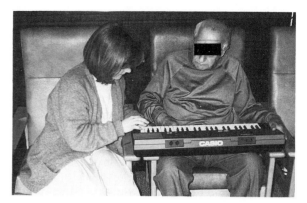

Fig. 19.1 Music is a creative activity that can be enjoyable and beneficial to long-stay clients. (Source: Sheena Blair)

feature of human beings and fulfillment of the creative urge is an important facet of self-actualisation. Long-stay residents of institutions also need to be able to express themselves and to experience the sense of achievement that comes from making things. Many long-stay clients are not able to express their feelings easily; for some, their affect is very flattened and their emotional tone very neutral, for others their emotions oscillate from one extreme to another and their expression of feeling is frequently inappropriate. It is also quite common for clients to have difficulty interpreting the emotional expressions of others, either from facial expression or from voice tone. Activities that are used projectively in other settings may be useful tools for exploring emotional expression, although the exploration of personal feelings would, of necessity, be more superficial than in other fields of practice. Emotional exploration with long-stay clients is essentially an educational/developmental process, which can be combined with supportive psychotherapy and social skills training. Videotape feedback can often be rewarding, if it is available, in encouraging clients to think about how they present themselves to others, to become aware of their own emotional expression or lack of it and to assist them in their perception of others' feelings (Durham 1983).

Craft activities

Craft activities are traditionally used in occu-

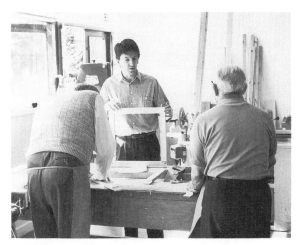

Fig. 19.2 Woodwork can be a rewarding activity.
(Source: Sheena Blair)

pational therapy as an outlet for the creative urge. The use of craft activities in psychiatry has declined in the past decade but they can often be useful in long-stay work. Sometimes clients have a long-dormant hobby, interest in which can be reawakened, and for others opportunities to pursue new leisure interests can be part of the normalisation process. Some of these interests can be taken up during evenings and weekends, further enhancing individuality and quality of life. One problem with the use of craft-work in this field of occupational therapy is that it is often difficult to find suitable activities that are age appropriate, reasonably interesting and worthwhile, yet simple enough for clients to be able to do. How often we see long-term clients restricted to threading chamois scraps or knitting dishcloths. More rewarding activities can be found and more complex tasks can often be adapted and simplified, although a certain amount of creative thinking on the part of the occupational therapist is required. Weaving, woodwork, cookery, art, pottery and needlework are among the many possibilities (Fig. 19.2).

Industrial work

Industrial tasks often form a part of the activity programme for clients in hospitals. Industrial work can be useful in providing a formal structure for clients, in offering them an opportunity to experience a simulated work environment, to take part in productive activities that are valued by others and to receive some remuneration for their efforts (Fig. 19.3), although unfortunately this last is often pitifully small.

As was stated earlier (p. 322), engagement in purposeful activity is crucial in the prevention of deterioration of the long-term mentally ill. For this reason many long-stay clients have been expected to spend their days in industrial therapy units or industrial workshops in occupational therapy departments. However, these large-scale workshops were generally established in the 1950s and 60s, when the long-stay population was much larger, and tended to be incorporated into the inflexible institutional regime. In the past, industrial work has often been provided to the exclusion of other activities but it is rarely appropriate today for full-time occupation. Many of the old long-stay client group are so elderly or frail that it is unreasonable and unfair to expect them to continue in such a structured work routine. If aspiring to a normal atmosphere is to be one of our goals, then we should remember that retirement at 60 or 65 is the norm, and therefore other activities may be more suitable for older clients. Clients from the recent long-stay group are often suffering from very severe chronic impairment, and find it difficult to concentrate on even simple repetitive tasks. They are often not able to perform an activity for extended periods of time, let alone full-time. While industrial contract work or other simple repetitive tasks continue to have a place in the therapy programme, such activities must be used judiciously, and the length of time to which people are exposed to them must be carefully monitored and graded.

STRUCTURING THERAPY
A therapeutic environment

The environment in which these activities occur is most important. One of the features of total institutions described by Goffman (1961) is that all daily living activities tend to be conducted in the same place, with the same people and under the same authority, whereas the norm in our society is

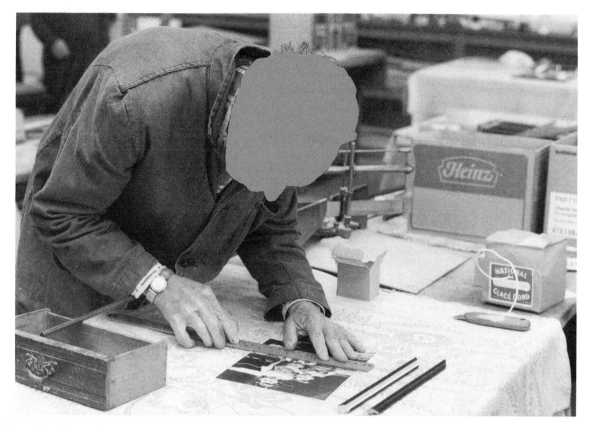

Fig. 19.3 Modern forms of industrial work are more rewarding than the repetitive work and long hours of the past. (Source: Lothian Health Board)

for people to work in a different location from that in which they live and sleep, and different again from that in which they pursue their social life. Leaving the ward for daily attendance at the occupational therapy department can therefore have a normalising effect on the client. The change of environment can in itself be stimulating, especially when accompanied by a change in companions.

Within the occupational-therapy department, it is common to find specific rooms for specific purposes, for example, kitchens or training flats for domestic work, small sitting rooms for social activities, and workshops for work-related activity. These approximate more close to real-life settings than does the ward environment and increase the clients breadth of opportunity. It is therefore recommended that occupational therapy programmes should take place away from the ward, if at

all possible. Of course, even the most modern and well-equipped occupational therapy department only begins to approximate to a realistic occupational setting and client should, whenever possible, be given opportunities to experience reality: to carry out activities in their normal setting.

Using groups

Having selected the environment in which to carry out the chosen activity, should the therapist work with individuals, or small or large groups? For the most part, small group work is the approach of choice with this client population, and the majority of activities we have considered can be applied in this way. The size of the group is important; between six and 10 members seems to work well. Bringing clients together in groups enables the therapist to draw upon the strengths and experiences of all the members. Social aspects of therapy can be fostered, and members can act as role models for each other within the group context. It encourages clients to share and cooperate with each other, while at the same time facilitating mutual respect and individuality.

There are some clients for whom group work is very difficult, either because they are threatened by being in the group or because they have poor self-control and concentration and tend to be highly disruptive. It is therefore appropriate to work individually with these clients and to integrate them into suitable groups gradually, as they become able to cope. Certain of the group activities may also be supplemented by individualised skill training, although this, too, can often be carried out effectively in a group setting.

Staffing

For a group of the suggested size it is ideal to have two members of staff working as co-therapists. This makes the implementation of activities far more successful and is very beneficial to the social interaction of the group. This may sound an expensive use of limited resources but is justified if the quality of the therapy is higher. Co-therapists are also able to offer each other mutual support and feedback and are likely to be able to sustain involvement with a group over a much longer period of time than when working individually. Finally, the commitment of two members of staff, who may be an occupational therapist and helper or an occupational therapist and nurse, for example, allows much greater continuity in group meetings, so that small gains made by clients are not lost through holidays or staff sickness.

Duration and frequency of activities

The duration and frequency of the group must also be considered. How often the group meets depends upon the activity in question. It may be best to do craft or industrial work or physical activities daily, while recreational or domestic activities can happen more intermittently. Available resources will have a bearing on this and it is likely that if a large number of clients are involved in the programme then a rota system will have to be operated. Long-stay clients find it difficult to sustain their concentration or level of engagement in any task for very long periods, therefore it is suggested that each session of therapy be confined to about 1 hour, with a short break in the middle. Three or four blocks of activity can thus be fitted into each day. Therapists should, however, be prepared for some flexibility in timing groups. If an activity is progressing extremely well, then why not let things continue a little longer, but if the session is unsuccessful, the clients unresponsive and the group leader jaded, it is better to conclude the session early, and start afresh next time.

It is probable that a diverse programme of activity will be drawn up for the long-stay clients attending the occupational therapy department, and that individual needs will be met by slotting clients into appropriate activities. It is essential, however, that the maintenance of the programme does not assume a greater importance than the needs of individual clients who should not be pursuing activities just because they happen to be there. Rather, the programme must be organised around specific aims of treatment for individuals or small groups of individuals, and both the treatment aims and the programme designed to achieve them should be regularly reviewed.

RECORD KEEPING AND EVALUATION

These topics are discussed at length in chapters 7 and 28. It has sometimes been assumed that long-stay clients change hardly at all, and that there is little point in keeping records as nothing of significance would be set down. This is patently not the case, and record keeping has as much value in long-stay psychiatry as in other areas of practice. While it is probably true that daily progress notes are not warranted, it is very important to monitor clients' performance regularly, as it is the very lack of documentation that can lead to the often erroneous impression of stagnancy. Repeated assessment measures such as simple rating scales can be a quick and efficient way of recording change.

PROBLEMS OF WORKING IN LONG-STAY PSYCHIATRY

Long-stay psychiatry is a demanding and challenging field of practice, which necessitates a high level of personal and professional skill and resourcefulness. Clients often respond only very slowly to treatment, there are many difficulties inherent in the institutional system, communications between staff are often poor, and morale can fall alarmingly low. Yet it is possible for these problems to be tackled, enabling the therapist to be more effective. This section first examines some of these difficulties and then offers some suggestions for improvements.

THE PROBLEMS
Slow progress

Although we have said that long-stay clients do change over time, this is not always obvious to the casual observer, nor is it always in a positive direction. Improvements that do occur tend to happen very slowly and to a very small degree. It can be difficult for staff to come to terms with this, particularly when they have expended great energy and effort in trying to help clients. The old long-stay group of clients are, by virtue of their age, going to deteriorate over time rather than improve, their abilities lessening with age and their problems compounded by increasing physical ill-health or disability. The new long-stay clients, on the other hand, tend to have repeated episodes of acute disturbance, so that a feeling of 'one step forward, two steps back' is common.

The nature of the institution

Other problems are inherent in the system itself. In long-stay psychiatry, there are often shortages of staff, so staff have insufficient time to do their jobs properly. There is often a feeling of being undervalued and unsupported. It is frequently the case that unqualified staff are given insufficient guidance and supervision. Coordination of resources and communication between team members is often poor. Sometimes staff themselves have become institutionalised and are overly dependent upon a rigid hierarchical structure.

An occupational therapist coming into this environment can very quickly feel swamped and lose motivation to try to promote change. 'Burnout' among staff is common in long-stay psychiatry, when staff members feel drained and unenthusiastic over a sustained period of time; they feel ineffective, unappreciated and disillusioned, and approach their work in a routine and mechanical way (Murgatroyd 1985).

OVERCOMING THE PROBLEMS
Changing the institutional climate

The atmosphere described above is not conducive to improving the quality of life for the residents who must try to survive within it. The environment in which they live loses its therapeutic value and passive acceptance of the way things are becomes the prevailing attitude of both residents and staff. The improvement of the institutional climate is as important for the raising of staff morale, changing attitudes and increasing their ability to sustain therapeutic intervention over time as it is for the effect on individual clients. Some aspects of improving institutional climate have already been touched upon, namely changing physical features of the environment, changing the emphasis of programme planning, reducing social distance, and changing the style of client–staff interaction. Other factors, such as improving communications, having clear aims and objectives, and concentrating upon quality rather than quantity in treatment planning, are also of value in overcoming problem areas.

Improved communication and coordination

Efforts to improve communication and coordination between staff are worthwhile. It is often the case that occupational therapists liaise with medical and nursing staff by attending meetings, writing reports, and so on, and that occupational therapy helpers, who are often in most contact with clients, are isolated from contact with other staff. In some units, staff meetings for all care personnel are a regular occurrence, while in other units, ward staff can be encouraged to visit the occupational therapy department or vice versa.

The occupational therapist must always make efforts to ensure that helpers are kept fully informed about what is happening on the ward, what decisions have been taken about clients and about services, and what the implications of these decisions are. Whenever possible, all staff should be involved in decision making and should be made to feel that their contribution is valued and respected. Regular meetings of occupational therapy staff working with long-stay clients can help to establish an atmosphere of mutual support, where difficulties can be aired and possible solutions discussed. All staff need to feel that what they do does not go unnoticed; they need feedback on their work and interactions with clients and guidance on how to improve them. Reinforcement of the positive aspects of their performance is, of course, just as important as criticism. Staff, as well as clients, need opportunities for learning and personal development, and in-service training sessions in conjunction with regular meetings can help to provide them.

Clear objectives

When looking at occupational therapy with individual clients, it is important that aims of treatment are communicated to all staff. Occupational therapy records should be accessible to everyone involved, although this may not be the case with confidential information from a client's medical history. What is expected from the client and from staff interaction with him should be made very clear. Achievable treatment goals should be part of each individual's occupational therapy plan. It may be necessary to set very limited objectives; what is important is that both staff and client should be able to experience some success (Lamb 1979).

Often, it is small indications of change that bring rewards, when an individual is able to make a choice for the first time, perhaps only choosing between two colours in an art activity, or is able to buy a coffee in a cafe, or knows the day

of the week. Such small steps are all indicators of growth and tell us that the client is responding to treatment and that his life is better than it used to be. Sometimes these rewards come as surprises, when clients respond to treatment programmes to a far greater degree than was ever expected and are able to move from long-term care to resettlement training and eventual discharge.

Personal relationships

It is easy, and perhaps tempting, to think of these clients as a group of very similar people with similar needs, experiences and interests but, in reality, each has his own personality and his own way of being. There will be those we like, those who amuse us, those whom we find irritating or frustrating and those whom we cannot help actively disliking. Relationships with these clients can, however, be very positive and often individual members of staff will develop a special, close relationship with one or two clients, for whom they become confidante and friend. Whatever their individual qualities and quirks, they can be encouraged to grow and develop, to achieve a degree of personal autonomy, and occupational therapists are, I believe, ideally placed to help them to do so.

A small but effective service

Shortages of staff have often led to occupational therapy departments having few qualified staff and large numbers of poorly supervised helpers, who have been required to provide activity for large numbers of clients on a full-time basis. Such dilution of the occupational therapy service, while no fault of the helpers concerned, does nothing to enhance its professional standing but merely fosters the attitude that occupational therapy is there to keep people occupied and out of the nursing staff's way for a guaranteed period each day. Helpers working in such circumstances can hardly be expected to have a good understanding of the therapeutic process and almost inevitably become disillusioned and stale. Such use of occupational-therapy resources is counterproductive and, where staff are scarce, it is far better to limit occupational therapy intervention to a selected small group of clients but to make that intervention effective and well documented: a fully professional service.

SUMMARY

Psychiatric clients in receipt of long-term residential care have been the focus of this chapter, which has looked at their characteristics and their needs, and considered how they can be helped. A philosophy of care, the rehabilitation approach, has been described, and can be applied to treatment by all members of the care team. This philosophy has implications for the care environment and the ways in which the institutional climate can be improved to enhance the quality of life of its residents have been discussed. Consideration of factors in the care setting that encourage or impede personal growth and development is of as much importance in small, community-based. units as in ancient hospital buildings.

This chapter has shown the many ways in which occupational therapists can be involved in the treatment of long-stay clients. By offering clients opportunities to engage in a wide range of 'normal' activities, both occupational and recreational, occupational therapists are facilitating personal development and allowing breadth of experience. The importance of involvement in a structured programme of purposeful activity for the prevention of deterioration of mental and physical health cannot be emphasised enough. Whether working with the residents of large institutions or small new hostels in the community, occupational therapists have, and will continue to have, a crucial, demanding yet rewarding role in long-stay psychiatry.

REFERENCES

Baker R, Hall J N 1983 REHAB: Rehabilitation Evaluation Hall and Baker. Vine Publishing, Aberdeen

Bartlett S et al 1985 Rehabilitation survey of long-stay clients at Park Prewett Hospital, Basingstoke, 1984, British Journal of Occupational Therapy 48(6)

Barton R 1976 Institutional neurosis, 3rd edn. John Wright, Bristol

Bennett D H 1978 Social forms of psychiatric treatment. In:Wing J K (ed) Shizophrenia: towards a new synthesis. Academic Press, London

Bennett D H 1980 The chronic psychiatric patient today. Journal of the Royal society of Medicine 73: 301–3

Clark P N 1979 Human development through occupation: a philosophy and conceptual model for practice, part two. American Journal of Occupational Therapy 33(9)

Drouet V M 1986 Individual behavioural programme planning with long-stay schizophrenic patients. British Journal of Occupational Therapy 49(7)

Durham R C 1983 Long-stay patients in hospital. In: Spence S, Shepherd G (eds) Developments in social skills training. Academic Press, London

Durham R C 1985 Creating therapeutic environments. In:Barker P, Fraser D (eds) The nurse as therapist: a behavioural model. Croom Helm, London

Goffman E 1961 Asylums: essays on the social situation of mental patients and other inmates. Anchor, New York

Goldstein A P et al 1976 Skill training for community living: applied structured learning therapy. Pergamon Press, New York

Hall J N et al 1981 Assessing long-stay patients in occupational therapy. British Journal of Occupational Therapy 44(6)

Lamb R 1979 Staff burnout in work with long-term patients. Hospital and Community Psychiatry 30(6)

Langley D M 1983 Dramatherapy and psychiatry. Croom Helm, London

Mann S A, Cree W 1976 'New' long stay psychiatric patients: a national sample survey of 15 mental hospitals in England and Wales 1972/3. Psychological Medicine 6: 603–616

Mosey A C 1973 Acitivities therapy. Raven Press, New York

Murgatroyd S 1985 Counselling and helping. British Psychological Society and Methuen, London

Orford J 1982 Institutional climates. In: Fransella F (ed) Psychology for occupational therapists. British Psychological Society and Macmillan Press, London

Schneider K 1959 Clinical psychopathology. Grune and Stratton, New York

Shepherd G 1980 The treatment of social difficulties in special environments. In: Feldman P, Orford J (eds) Psychological problems: the personal context. Wiley, Chichester

Shepherd G 1984 Institutional care and rehabilitation. Longman, London

Shepherd G 1985 Rehabilitation. In: Bradley B P, Thompson C (eds) Psychological applications in psychiatry. Wiley, Chichester

Sims A 1981 The staff and their training. In: Wing J K, Morris B (eds) Handbook of psychiatric rehabilitation practice. Oxford University Press, Oxford

Willson M 1984 Occupational therapy in long-term psychiatry. Churchill Livingstone, Edinburgh

Wing J K (ed) 1978 Schizophrenia: towards a new synthesis. Academic Press, London

Wing J K 1982 Long-term community care: experience in a London borough. Psychological Medicine Monograph Supplement 2. Cambridge University Press, Cambridge

Wing J K, Brown G W 1970 Institutionalism and schizophrenia. Cambridge University Press, London

Wing J K, Morris B (eds) 1981 Handbook of psychiatric rehabilitation practice. Oxford University Press, Oxford

Wolfensberger W 1972 The principle of normalisation in human services. National Institute on Mental Retardation and Leonard Crainford, Toronto

FURTHER READING

Hume C, Pullen I 1986 Rehabilitation in psychiatry: an introductory handbook. Churchill Livingstone, Edinburgh

Rollin H R (ed) 1980 Coping with schizophrenia. National Schizophrenia Fellowship and Burnett, London

Watts F, Bennett D (eds) 1981 Principles of psychiatric rehabilitation. Wiley, Chichester

20

Rehabilitation

Clephane A. Hume

INTRODUCTION

Since the introduction in the 1960s of phenothiazines to control psychotic symptoms, the rehabilitation and discharge of many long-term clients has become an accepted aspect of work in psychiatric hospitals. The recent increase in the number of hospital closures also means that adequate preparation of clients for discharge has assumed greater importance than in the past. It is equally important to focus on the use of the rehabilitative approach when working with clients in the community.

This chapter provides an introduction to the rehabilitative model of treatment as it is used in psychiatric practice. The theoretical basis is outlined, the context of practice is described and areas that will be most relevant to occupational therapy are discussed. No treatment plan can be devised in isolation and therefore relationships with team colleagues are also dealt with.

Needs and opportunities for education are covered and last, but not least, attention is given to some of the problems and constraints that concern the rehabilitation team.

WHAT IS REHABILITATION?

What do we mean by rehabilitation? Definitions are usually phrased in terms such as the following: enabling the individual to reach his/her maximum level of independence, physically, psychologically, economically and socially.

The World Health Organization describes the rehabilitation process as 'all means aimed at reducing the impact of disabling and handicapping conditions in individuals and enabling them to achieve maximum integration into the community'. Although this statement is geared to rehabilitation assistants working with the physically disabled, it is a philosophy with which occupational therapists can identify. Varied activities, techniques and methods are used to enable the client to develop competence in the skills necessary for leading as full a life as possible. Rehabilitation thus involves helping the client to compensate for any disabilities and to learn coping strategies. It is not appropriate to define general standards of independent function since the needs of individuals vary to such as great extent. What is a realistic aim for one person may be totally unattainable for the next.

Clark (1984) reminds us that rehabilitation is not all about protecting clients, rather it is enabling them to have the experience of success and thus the motivation to aim towards greater things.

It is necessary to consider rehabilitation in the context of psychiatric illness and consequent disability and handicap. Caplan (1961) suggests that handicap associated with mental illness is superimposed on the actual illness and is both treatable and preventable.

Disability does not mean that the person is handicapped. Someone who suffers from hallucinations may be able to adjust to hearing voices and learn to carry on living an effective life so that he is not handicapped in his day-to-day existence.

Active intervention is required if the handicapping effects of, for example, a schizophrenic illness are to be minimised. In this instance, the balance between stimulation and overstimulation of the individual is a fine one, which cannot be clearly defined. Too much pressure creates stress and precipitates retreat into psychotic behaviour.

Wing and Morris (1981) describe three factors that contribute to handicap:

- psychiatric disabilities arising from the symptoms and illness process
- social disadvantages such as poverty or unemployment
- adverse personal reaction to illness.

Although the focus of intervention is the individual patient, it is important to remember that family and friends, employers, fellow clients and staff all play a significant part in the rehabilitation process and in the degree of handicap experienced. Rehabilitation is not confined to the hospital and both hospital and community resources will be involved.

Other approaches to treatment may be used within rehabilitation, for example, the behavioural approach for social skills training and the humanistic approach to develop self-esteem.

The rehabilitation process consists of three stages:

1. preparation for resettlement
2. actual resettlement in the community
3. follow-up support as required by the individual.

Increasingly, the rehabilitative approach is being used to maintain clients in the community, possibly without any recourse to admission. The process then includes:

- identification of problems
- possible intervention
- follow-up support as required.

It should be recognised that progress in rehalibitation may be slow, often over a period of years, and will represent much hard work on the part of both clients and staff.

THE DIFFERENCES BETWEEN REHABILITATION AND LONG-TERM CARE

Many long-term wards are described as using a rehabilitative approach and this may, indeed, be the case. However, it is not helpful for wards to claim to be rehabilitation units when they are, in fact, providing continuing care. Euphemistic labelling helps neither staff nor clients and leads to false expectations. Consequently, there may be a feeling of failure when unrealistic goals are not achieved.

The long-term care ward aims to provide continuing care (very often permanent or lifelong) for clients with severe handicap. Such people may have an ongoing illness, such as schizophrenia, or a chronic condition such as Korsakoff' psychosis, and require shelter from the demands of everyday community life. The focus is on support through fluctuating periods of illness.

In a ward providing continuing care aimed at improving, or at least maintaining, clients' quality of life, staff can still use the rehabilitative approach to treatment. The aim of rehabilitation in this situation is to enable the client to gain a higher level of personal independence in the expectation that he will eventually move to an environment that allows him to be more independent.

Much of the difference lies in the team's attitude and approach to clients and this will be discussed later (see p. 344). Differences will also be evident in the environment and the daily routine of the wards.

The rehabilitative approach places more responsibility upon the client. For example, if he is going out somewhere, he will be expected to tell staff where he is going and when he is likely to return, whereas in the long-term ward he will be told to come back at a specific time. This difference in emphasis is subtle but, nevertheless, significant and may be quite threatening to people moving from one ward to another with a less structured approach.

Long-term care can seem to be under-resourced area, with consequent poor morale among staff. It is useful to bear in mind some of the positive aspects of long-term care for the client, such as social contacts, the use of facilities and the supportive structure that the hospital provides.

Wing (1971) has said that even the most intractable client retains the power to surprise the persistent therapist and, over a long period of time, clients may move from a long-term ward to a rehabilitation facility. Providing a high standard of care for long-term clients is, in itself, a laudable aim that should be encouraged and not neglected in the face of pressures for discharge to community care.

PRINCIPLES OF REHABILITATION

GENERAL GUIDELINES

What are some of the principles by which we should be guided in planning treatment programmes for people in rehabilitation units?

The rehabilitative approach has been described by Hume and Pullen (1986) as follows:

- listen to the client
- know the community
- pay attention to detail
- remember how the world has changed.

Using these principles as a general guideline, it is possible to devise individual programmes.

Listen to the client

All therapists listen to their clients but it may take a considerable amount of time to unravel their problems. Clients may, themselves, be unaware of what their real difficulties are and it becomes a shared process of discovery to identify the principal problems. The therapist must know the individual and be sensitive to verbal and non-verbal cues. It is also desirable to involve other people, for example, the family, who know the client well and can therefore identify problems that the individual himself may not recognise.

Know the community

The therapist must also be aware of what resources and facilities the community to which the client is to be discharged has to offer. It is simply not possible to prepare a client adequately for discharge if the therapist is unacquainted with the area to which he is going. It is necessary to know the cultural norms for the area so that clients can be given social skills training, if required. The occupational therapist does not know everything herself; knowing where to obtain the information is the crucial factor.

Pay attention to detail

It is easy to overlook apparently trivial factors that

may prove to be enormous obstacles for a particular individual. Inability to cope with what seems an easy everyday task may produce feelings of inadequacy and incompetence. Attempts to compensate for deficiencies may exacerbate any social stigma that the person is experiencing.

Another potential pitfall is to assume that skills will generalise, that is, be transferred to another similar behaviour. Ability in some aspects of activities of daily living, for example, does not imply competence in the others. It is necessary to be comprehensive in carrying out relevant assessments.

Remember how the world has changed

Awareness of the changes that have occurred in the world outside hospital is obviously of more significance to longer-term clients but this does not mean that others will not come across unexpected differences. Even a brief stay in hospital can inspire a feeling of being a stranger in your own home, let alone the wider community. Clients who are moving from one culture to another will obviously need considerable help in learning about their new locality. (see Ch. 25).

Other principles

Further principles, such as the following, can also be incorporated into the rehabilitative approach. Some of these are very familiar to the occupational therapist.

- The need for graded programmes—staged treatment goals that enable the client to build up to the ultimate goal. This is closely linked to activity analysis.
- Clients may need to be taught skills that they have never had the opportunity to learn or they may need to improve on skills that have not been used much during a period of hospitalisation. This includes an element of re-orientation to the everyday world.
- The therapist must bear in mind the proposed ultimate goal for each client. If someone is to be discharged to a hostel where all meals are provided it is less important to focus on meal

preparation than it would be for someone who will need to be self-sufficient in a group home.

ATTITUDES AND APPROACH

Attitudes are of paramount importance in carrying out rehabilitation programmes. Clients have a need for a consistent approach from staff. Rigid imposition of rules one day cannot be followed by a casual approach the next if clients—or staff—are to have any sense of security. Clients require an approach that can be compared to good parenting, that is, one that allows them to feel it is safe and natural to fail. We all learn from our mistakes and the subsequent encouragement to try again. Sometimes, of course, people need to fail to learn the extent of their limitations.

The client's attitudes must also be taken into consideration. What are his hopes and expectations? How realistic are these? How do his ambitions relate to the ideas of his family and friends? Are they at variance?

Another important factor is attitude towards medication. This is not the prime concern of the occupational therapist but it is worthy of consideration.

Clients may want to discuss their feelings about the need to take medication on a long-term basis, often a contentious issue.

If unexplained changes in behaviour occur, it is worth enquiring whether the person is failing to take medication as prescribed. It is easy to forget to take pills, especially when you do not feel ill. The use of long-acting depot preparations may help, as they are given by injection every 2 to 3 weeks. There is, therefore, no need to remember to take tablets other than to counteract the side effects.

Some clients may learn to adjust their own medication according to changes in symptoms.

BRIDGING THE GAP BETWEEN HOSPITAL AND COMMUNITY

Much of the rehabilitation process can be seen to be geared towards educating and reeducating clients for living outside hospital. Clients need to have information about local resources and support services; an important part of the preparation required before moving from hospital into the community.

Rehabilitation, however, as Caplan (1964) indicates, does not end with discharge and people require continuing support to enable them to integrate successfully into the community. With the increased emphasis on community care in Britain, adequate ways of providing such support are likely to remain problematic in the 1990s.

Ways in which community integration may be achieved will vary considerably according to the skills of the individual and the support services existing in a particular locality. Each rehabilitation team must devise its own system for ensuring that clients are not forgotten after discharge. It may be the task of the community nurse, the social worker or the occupational therapist to provide ongoing support. Some teams operate a key worker system which facilitates coordination of the people and resources involved. It may be that care is transferred to a voluntary organisation with overall medical supervision from the parent hospital or primary care team.

Whatever the system, one important consideration is to prepare the ground for the individual at the point of discharge. Are community support services ready to become involved? Have workers made contact with the client already? This is highly desirable (although sometimes impracticable), so that a known and trusted person can reduce the stress of change involved in moving to a new environment.

Is the individual familiar with the locality? With all good intentions, and despite all the team's efforts, this may not be the case if accommodation suddenly becomes available.

CONTINUED SUPPORT

As indicated above, the team should have decided, well in advance of discharge, how follow-up support is to be provided.

Health service and local authority staff may be involved or there may be assistance from voluntary and self-help organisations. In the latter case, it may still be necessary for the rehabilitation team to retain a monitoring role for a period of time, to ensure that the stress of community living does not precipitate any relapse. This may be achieved by providing support to the organization or maintaining contact with the individual so that prompt intervention can take place, if required.

It may be in the interests of the individual to maintain contact with the hospital as a day patient or referral to a day centre may be appropriate. For others, follow up outpatient appointments or attendance at a medication clinic may be all that is necessary.

CONTEXT

The theoretical principles of rehabilitation can be applied in any setting, including the client's own home. 'Rehabilitation begins with diagnosis'. (Caplan 1961). From the occupational therapist's point of view this does not necessarily mean a medical label, although it does indicate some of the common symptoms and problems that may be anticipated. Remember, however, that labels may be misleading (Hume and Pullen 1986). The therapist should base her identification of the individual's difficulties on her own assessment. (see Ch. 6).

There are considerations that should be observed according to the location of treatment, some of which will be described here.

ACUTE ADMISSION WARD

It may not be possible to transfer a client out of an admission ward once the acute phase of illness is over. Beds in slower-moving wards will not always be available when most appropriate for the individual's needs.

The nature of the acute ward means there are difficulties in attempting to introduce a rehabilitative approach for appropriate clients. Staff must focus their attention on clients whose immediate needs are most urgent. The person who is independent and not at risk will inevitably take second place and may not receive the support he requires to make further progress. Staff must be aware of this as a potential problem.

Admission to hospital provides support, in that the person is relieved of the responsibility of everyday tasks. It is nevertheless desirable to prevent people becoming institutionalised by preserving as high a degree of personal independence as is consistent with their illness.

Goals should be drawn up for the individual, following discussion by the client and the medical team. It is important not to keep the person in hospital, away from the realities of everyday life, for any longer than necessary, and some admissions may be of only a few days' duration. A programme that provides the client with his own specific goals must therefore be initiated as soon as possible. After discharge, such a programme can be continued in the community, possibly with outpatient follow up.

If the person is to be transferred to a rehabilitation unit, staff can ensure that he becomes independent in everyday matters such as personal hygiene and clothes care and takes responsibility for his bedroom and routine chores around the ward. This can facilitate the move to a unit where he will be expected to be independent in particular tasks. This is obviously best done in consultation with staff in the rehabilitation unit. Both groups should ensure that the team on the acute unit understands the philosophy of the rehabilitation unit.

REHABILITATION UNIT

As the name suggests, this is the best location for the rehabilitative approach. The entire programme will be geared towards promoting independence and the environment should also be structured towards this end (Hume and Pullen 1986).

Although difference in emphasis may be subtle, it represents a definite, potentially threatening change in personal responsibility for clients. From having been given 'safe' boundaries within which to operate, the client now finds that he has a greater degree of freedom and is expected to set his own limits, even though initially this is in relation to simple, undemanding tasks.

Sometimes the rehabilitation unit may be classed as a mid-term or medium-stay unit, where people may spend time after the acute phase of their illness, regaining confidence and practising skills, as well as learning new ways of coping. This will include any adjustments to their disability that need to be made. Such a unit may have a mixture of referral sources, including the acute unit, long-terms wards or direct admissions from the community. Most clients will not be experiencing acute symptoms and there is time to focus on the practicalities of daily life.

TRANSITIONAL CARE

This begins in the rehabilitation unit and then covers the period during which the client moves from hospital into the community. Depending upon local resources there may be a gradual progression from the rehabilitation unit to the hospital hostel or ward in the community and then discharge to a group home. Some hospitals have half-way houses or rehabilitation flats to prepare clients for living in small groups prior to discharge.

As the client becomes more capable of handling responsibilities for himself, supervision is gradually reduced.

Hostel or ward in the community

Hospital hostels provide an environment in which clients can live with minimal supervision. Usually such units are large houses, sometimes former staff accommodation, situated outwith the hospital grounds. The term 'ward in the community' has come into use to describe the role of units in which long-term clients are cared for in houses in ordinary residential areas. The two terms tend to be used synonymously, actual use being determined by local preference, although the term 'hostel' usually implies a greater degree of independence. For convenience, the word 'hostel' will be used here.

Staff may only be present during the day, night cover being on an on-call basis. On the other hand much valuable work can be done by night staff during the late evenings, when clients who are out during the day are actually on the premises.

As in any hostel, residents assume a high level

of personal responsibility, for instance, individuals may have front-door keys. Personal differences are sorted out by the residents, with minimal staff intervention, and domestic matters such as chore rotas are also tackled by the group. Clients have responsibility for their own decision making and the organisation of their day.

Preparation of meals may not be required of clients in a hospital hostel and this should be balanced according to the ultimate proposed accommodation for the majority. If most clients will eventually move on to hostels run by outside organisations, where meals are provided, it is not essential for them to be able to cook for themselves. In such cases, clients can develop their skills on an individual basis rather than as a group.

Services such as laundry and cleaning may be arranged on an individual or joint basis.

The occupational therapist may find her role in a hostel becoming more of a consultative one, with specific group sessions, rather than that of a permanent staff member, especially if clients are in work placements during the day.

Where hospital-based occupational therapists are responsible for community psychiatric services, the therapist will extend this consultative role to community hostels for discharged clients.

Group homes

These are the community side of transitional care. They are small houses or flats obtained through a variety of sources, ranging from district housing authorities and local mental health associations to individual enterprises.

At the stage of moving out of hospital and into the community, clients obviously cease to be inpatients and if they have not already been referred to as 'residents', this is the time to start adjusting them to their roles as ordinary members of society.

Group homes will be supervised in a variety of ways according to local custom and practice. Community psychiatric nurses or social workers may visit or, if the home is one among many organised by a large body, there may be a warden in overall charge. Often, volunteers may be involved.

The role of the occupational therapist may be minimal or she may be a key worker for a group of residents. Community-based therapists may be highly involved in giving follow-up support for group home residents or this may be provided on a day-patient basis.

Whichever system operates in an area, it is essential to remember that, however good the pre-discharge preparation programme has been, difficulties will always arise as a consequence of moving to a new environment. There is a great difference between a hospital half-way house and a real home in the community, even if the physical surroundings seem comparable.

OCCUPATIONAL THERAPY IN REHABILITATION

REALISTIC GOALS

Setting realistic goals within the context of rehabilitation may be a frustrating process. Scarcity of resources may preclude desired aims, although lack of resources should never be an excuse for omitting particular targets. Constraints may nevertheless operate and it is important that clients learn to cope with the realities.

As already indicated, clients' and relatives' expectations may not be realistic and the therapist must also beware of projecting her own hopes onto the client. An objective approach is essential.

Design of programmes relevant to individual needs is the crux of rehabilitation. (See also Problems and constraints, page 346). Any programme encompasses many aspects of the client's life and it is impossible to separate out any one aspect in actual practice. The main focus is likely to be on activities of daily living (ADL) but, for the sake of simplicity, aspects of care are here divided into four main areas:

● personal independence and social skills
● domestic skills
● leisure
● work.

Ideally, each aspect should be assessed using standardised assessment schedules or checklists (see Ch. 5). The tendency is for each department to have its own system for tackling these aspects of care. Examples of programmes and forms are to be found in occupational therapy journals, so only a few topics will be highlighted here.

PERSONAL INDEPENDENCE AND SOCIAL SKILLS

Included under this heading are self-care, interpersonal relationships and the social skills related to competence in both these areas. Decision making, day-to-day personal organisation and management of time (temporal adaptation) are also relevant (Fig. 20.1).

Self-care, in the sense of personal hygiene, will probably be largely the responsibility of nursing staff but there are opportunities for the occupational therapist to reinforce socially acceptable levels of hygiene. Use of make-up, facial care (for both men and women), and hand care, can all be included in self-care groups. The importance of discussion about other aspects of self-care, such as use of deodorants, menstrual hygiene and foot care, should not be overlooked as these areas may have been neglected. Hair care and clothes selection may also need attention.

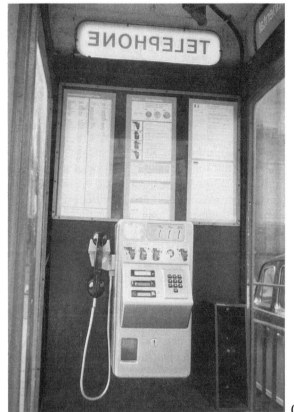

(b)

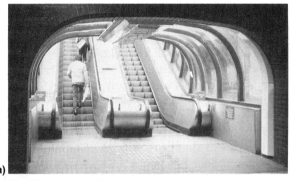

(a)

Fig. 20.1 Personal independence can be promoted by familiarising clients with different aspects of life in the community.
(a) Using escalators.
(b) Using a pay phone and promoting appropriate social skills.
(c) Traffic signals and general road safety.

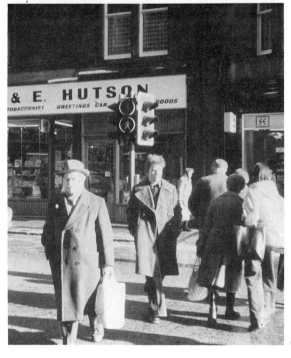

(c)

CASE EXAMPLE 20.1

Annie, a rather large lady, had visited the local charity shop where a bright red dress caught her eye. Although it was the correct size, the shortness of the skirt clearly identified it as being out of fashion and was, in fact, very unflattering, as well as inappropriate to her age. Some adverse comments about her appearance were made, although not directly to her, and the rehabilitation team felt that some intervention was required.

It took a fair amount of group discussion about choice of clothes enhancing personal appearance and tactful individual comments from a nurse with whom she had a good relationship to persuade Annie to exchange the dress for a pair of red trousers. Although almost equally bright, these covered her knees and did considerably more for her appearance. Subsequent positive comments from clients and staff reinforced the wisdom of her choice.

In the context of psychiatric rehabilitation, personal care also includes taking medication. This, too, will be supervised by nursing staff and it is essential that clients learn to administer their own medication well in advance of discharge. For those who are to attend a depot medication clinic it may be possible to arrange a visit to establish contact prior to leaving hospital. The occupational therapist may find that clients want to discuss this aspect of care along with other personal matters.

Competence in personal relationships must be considered and this is an area where social skills training may be required (see Ch. 15). Very basic skills may need rehearsal and clients who are withdrawn, particularly, should practise asking for information and making their needs known to others.

Assertive behaviour may be an area of difficulty for certain groups, for example, those who have been in hospital for long periods or tend to be self-effacing. Others may be inclined to aggressive outbursts and require to learn the difference between aggressive, assertive and passive behaviour in order to gain confidence and self-control.

Sharing a meal with a group of clients provides a realistic opportunity to assess and improve social skills. Such refinements as passing salt and pepper may be lacking and conversation totally absent.

More sophisticated social skills include sexual relationships and it may be appropriate to discuss responsibility for contraception and safe sexual practice.

Any individual deficiencies in social skills, or problem areas related to specific conditions, should be dealt with as relevant. For example, someone who has alcohol-related problems may need to learn and practise how to refuse a drink that has already been poured and is being handed to him, before encountering the real situation.

DOMESTIC SKILLS

The practicalities of daily life are often seen as one of the occupational therapist's major contributions to rehabilitation. Certainly, domestic skills, including cooking and household management, are crucial in any programme. Clothes care and awareness of general safety and security should also be part of any programme. Ideally, household skills should be practised in an assessment flat where the client has a weekly allowance and learns to budget for food, heating and lighting.

It is tempting to try to cover all aspects of domestic skills, sometimes to a degree of competence well above that of the average citizen. Not all of us can change a fuse, replace a zip or repair broken glasses, but we know where to obtain the necessary assistance.

Goals must be geared to the future. If the person is to live in a hostel where meals are provided, cooking a meal is of relatively minor importance. If using a launderette will be required, then learning to use the washing machine in the occupational therapy department or the ward is not necessarily helpful; focus on ironing instead and discuss the meaning of some of the more obscure laundry labels so that 'dry-clean only' clothes do not find their way into the wash.

Cooking may be a matter of refining existing skills in supportive surroundings, learning (if relevant) to use modern gadgets such as microwave ovens, or of covering the whole range of menu planning, budgetting and shopping, meal preparation and cleaning up. Hygiene and safety can readily be incorporated into kitchen activities, as can nutritional education. It is worth stressing that, although one kitchen assessment will demonstrate the individual's ability to produce a meal on that occasion, it does not ensure the motivation to do so in future nor the ability to cope with day-by-day economic menu planning.

The rest of the home must be remembered, perhaps by shopping for bed-linen, furniture or any other necessities for setting up home. Advertisers would have us believe that we require numerous gadgets and substances for efficient living. The realities need to be discussed.

Finally, remember that most rehabilitation units have an ever-open door and clients will need to consider security, keys and answering the doorbell when there is no member of staff to answer it. Practice of these latter skills is desirable before people move into their own accommodation.

LEISURE

The value of leisure in maintaining a balanced and healthy life–style is often overlooked and discussion about the benefits of leisure may be required. Hospital life often provides a structured day of work and, to a greater or lesser extent, a range of leisure activities. For many clients, the evenings and weekends may be a time of boredom and apathy and one of the important aims of the rehabilitation programme is to encourage them to use their free time. Clients should learn to pursue their own interests rather than to rely on things being organised for them because this will be their own responsibility once they leave hospital. Again, remember normality. We do not have to follow a hectic round of social activities to have a satisfying life. A balance between relaxation and activity needs to be learned.

The use of a leisure inventory (Fidler 1984), can be a useful way of introducing ideas, discovering preferences and fostering time-structuring habits. Identification of community resources for recreation and hobbies can also make clients aware of the range of opportunities available.

Sharing of information about individual interests may serve as an introduction to pursuits that may be continued on a long-term basis. Those clients who wish to do so can be encouraged to use special social resources within the locality, such as clubs

run by local mental-health associations. Support from a member of staff, a volunteer or another client may be necessary during the first visit. It is important that clients understand that other people will be sizing them up and that their welcome may not be all they had hoped for on the first occasion.

The cost of leisure activities is something that most people see as a potential barrier. Discovering resources that are free, or offer reduced rates to those on pensions or unemployment benefit is part of the activity-identification process.

For most of us, visiting friends is a key leisure activity and one which may be denied to clients who have lost contact with family or friends. Volunteers may help by befriending individuals, inviting clients to their homes or arranging outings. Clients can be encouraged to return hospitality, thereby developing hostess skills for the time when they can entertain others in their own home. (Social skills for dealing with unwanted visitors might also be contemplated.)

Physical health may be promoted through sports and more energetic pursuits. Current research indicates that such activity may also be psychologically beneficial (see Ch. 10).

WORK

In the current economic climate, what is the role of the occupational therapist in work rehabilitation? This question has been widely considered in the field of psychiatric rehabilitation. Monteath (1983) stresses that assessment and preparation for work are a key function of occupational therapy and that this includes work in the widest sense, paid or unpaid. On the other hand, recognition that clients may require preparation for unemployment is a reality. As the proportion of the general public that is unemployed rises, so the stigma for clients who cannot find a job falls, but this does not negate the value of work programmes as a useful aspect of rehabilitation (Dyer 1988).

'Work' may mean different things to different people so it is helpful to establish a definition of work, whether full- or part-time, paid, voluntary, sheltered or open employment, or housework, so that a relevant programme can be devised. The therapist should have contact with Department of

Employment staff and be aware of local resources, including training opportunities. Knowledge of local schemes designed to meet the needs of those seeking alternatives to remunerative employment should also be acquired.

For clients who are able to return to an existing job or similar work, development of general work habits is an obvious requirement and a full-time simulated work programme may be indicated in order to develop work tolerance (Fig. 20.2).

Many clients experience difficulties at work because of social withdrawal, rather than the actual job. Assessment of associated social skills should therefore encompass not only working relationships at different levels but also informal conversational situations, such as coffee breaks.

Pre-work groups, such as those described by Kramer (1984) are an excellent way of sharing knowledge, practising job-seeking skills and providing support to those undergoing interviews,

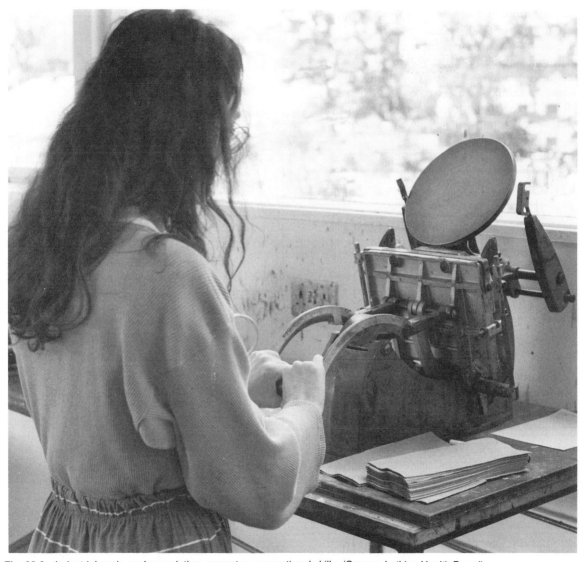

Fig. 20.2 Industrial work, such as printing, promotes occupational skills. (Source: Lothian Health Board)

particular those which are unsuccessful. The opportunity to discuss the 'Do I tell them I've been in a psychiatric hospital?' dilemma gives people a chance to make up their own minds about how to tackle this issue for themselves.

Pre-vocational assessment may be carried out if an individual wishes to try out various types of work prior to determining priorities for job choice. If a change of job is indicated, further training may be organised. In either case, attendance at an Employment Rehabilitation Centre (ERC) may be arranged. The possibility of gaining work experience through placements with local employers can also be investigated.

Liaison with voluntary agencies may provide work opportunities and the possibility of a reference for future job applications. Attitudes towards volunteers should be assessed as the expectations of the agency may not match those of the worker, in terms of commitment or task allocations.

PERSONNEL

One of the myths of rehabilitation is that it is an area in which high levels of staffing are not required. In fact, in order to carry out the necessary activities on an individual or small group basis, the reverse is true.

In a study of rehabilitation resources in Scotland, McCreadie, Affleck and Robinson (1985) investigated staffing in long-term wards, rehabilitation units and day-care facilities. They reported that occupational therapy helpers devoted more time to long-term wards than any other staff group, while qualified therapists tended to work in specific rehabilitation units or day units. (The study did not include students.) Although few in number, occupational therapy staff seem to be the most committed to hospital-based rehabilitation services.

THE MULTIDISCIPLINARY TEAM

The multidisciplinary team in the rehabilitation setting will have the same membership as in any other unit, depending upon local availability of staff. In addition to this core team, are the extended team and the community team (Hume and Pullen 1986). The composition of these will vary but may be as follows.

- Core team:
  - medical staff
  - nurses
  - clinical psychologist
  - social worker
  - occupational therapist.
- Extended team:
  - administrator
  - chaplain
  - catering staff
  - ancillary staff
  - volunteers.
- Community team:
  - community nurse
  - primary-health-care staff
  - community workers
  - volunteers.

STAFF TRAINING

Inevitably, members of the treatment team are trained according to the philosophy of their own profession. Individuals may have experience in a rehabilitation context during their initial education or not until postgraduate study, as is often the case with medical staff.

In order for the team to have a cohesive approach, there is a need for in-service education. This may be done partly on an informal basis, with individuals explaining their treatment objectives and the contribution they feel they can best make. Such sharing may help to iron out inter-professional differences and will also highlight individual areas of expertise. Staff can discuss attitudes and approach, for example, the difficulties of one professional standpoint being different from another or when medical and social models of treatment result in conflicting aims. Alternatively, one team member may be concerned about the demands being placed on an individual client.

Formal training is being established for professional groups, ranging from rehabilitation nursing courses to study days, on a multidisciplinary basis. Interest groups and organisations such as the

Scottish Psychiatric Rehabilitation Interest Group (SPRIG) or the World Associates for Psychological Rehabilitation (WAPR) can extend contacts on a wider basis through study days and conferences. Though the latter cannot strictly be regarded as training, the educational component is valuable.

Staff in rehabilitation units have a responsibility to educate their colleagues in other units. This is partly public relations but it also leads to more realistic referrals and expectations.

THE ROLE OF RELATIVES

Often there is no next of kin because of estrangement or death. Where relatives and significant others are involved, their contribution is crucial to the rehabilitation process. They may have their own specific needs for support in the situation.

Relatives will have contact with the staff team, particularly nurses, during visits and this should be extended to more formal contact in interviews with other staff. The occupational therapist may become involved, and many would say *should* become involved!

Initially reassurance about the nature of the illness and the possible outcome may be wanted. Although this should have been given at an earlier stage of the illness, initial worries may well inhibit understanding and the opportunity for further discussion should be offered.

Treatment planning requires the involvement of key people as soon as is practicable. Parents, spouses, employers and friends all have a part to play. Those most significant for the individual should be invited to discuss goals and aims. Their support and cooperation is vital; without it, it may be impossible to achieve particular aims.

Joint interviews may be arranged to deal with emotionally loaded topics such as possible separation or desirable changes in behaviour patterns. Interviews may also focus on situations where conflicts in parental behaviour are creating problems for the client.

The work of Vaughn and Leff (1976) regarding emotional expression has made it possible to assess family groups in order to identify the levels of emotional interaction. Patterns of interaction such as high incidence of critical comments or other emotionally demanding statements are referred to

CASE EXAMPLE 20.2

Linda, 26, had a diagnosis of schizophrenia with a history of several relatively short admissions to hospital.

She lived with her mother but relations between them were somewhat strained. Linda had had several periods of brief employment, mostly of a clerical nature. She was referred to the rehabilitation unit with a view to eventual discharge to alternative accommodation.

The team wanted Linda to become independent in various self-care skills and she said she was keen to learn to do things for herself. She already had an interest in cooking and demonstrated that she was able to prepare a meal for herself with minimal guidance. As Linda took an interest in her personal appearance it was decided that clothes care would be a good starting point.

A meeting was arranged with her mother, with the object of discussing plans for Linda to do her own laundry, including learning to use the local laundrette. Linda's mother declared this to be totally unnecessary since she had a perfectly good washing machine. No amount of discussion would persuade her to alter her viewpoint. Even if Linda was living somewhere else, she could still bring her washing home. (It is relevant to understand that this was one thing which she felt she could still do for her daughter and it also ensured that a degree of contact would be maintained).

The team had to agree that this objective should be put in abeyance and that Linda's other domestic skills could be developed. The mother was in full support of this idea since sharing chores in the house was something she had long tried to foster. Linda was keen to move from hospital and said that she would be interested in household management in a place of her own.

The mother joined a support group for relatives, where she discovered that other parents shared her fears about their children leaving home but were, nevertheless, able to encourage them towards independence.

After several months Linda developed her skills to a stage at which she was able to move into a bedsitter in a supported housing scheme and maintained contact with her mother. The quality of their relationship was much improved by living apart.

as 'high expressed emotion'. Once identified, such patterns of behaviour may be modified as families are taught how to respond. Reinforcing the content of delusions by agreeing with the person's statements is not helpful in promoting contact with reality.

Relatives can be helped to understand that the client's experience is real for him and that they should not dismiss bizarre statements as nonsense. Changing the subject or some other diversionary tactic may serve to defuse a potentially difficult situation and families can gain much by the use of such strategies.

Learning to set limits on unacceptable behaviour will not necessarily be easy. Families for whom the client's illness is a source of long-term stress may be supported through relatives' groups. The sharing of practical information and coping strategies, or the ventilation of the stresses of dealing with difficult behaviour, may relieve some of the feelings of anxiety or guilt.

LIAISON WITH OUTSIDE AGENCIES

Rehabilitation cannot take place solely within the confines of the hospital. Knowledge of community resources has already been emphasised as essential for members of the rehabilitation team. Every attempt should be made to initiate contact with outside agencies that can contribute to the rehabilitation process. Such agencies are many and varied, although they are most evident in urban areas. Local councils of social services or coordinating groups for services for the disabled will be able to provide information about local resources, as will social work information officers and local mental health associates. These bodies may be most concerned with specialised resources for people with particular needs.

Staff will have to be selective, or liaison can become a full-time job. Contact with self-help groups serves to provide clients with information about potential sources of help. Occasionally, staff might be involved in attending such a group for the purpose of giving information. Voluntary organisations such as the National Schizophrenia Fellowship welcome contact from staff and this is mutually beneficial.

Other agencies provide services for the community as a whole, for example, church lunch clubs and community centres, and clients can be encouraged to become involved in these during the transitional phase of rehabilitation. Occasional consultative visits from staff are usually appreciated by these groups and provide the opportunity for discussion of various concerns.

Education, leisure and employment resources should also be considered. No one member of the team can possibly be aware of everything but, if each member establishes contact with agencies most relevant to his work, the result will be a fairly wide-ranging body of knowledge that should be recorded in a place accessible to all.

PROBLEMS AND CONSTRAINTS

It is a frequent complaint that resources are inadequate and money is not available to improve the situation but what are the other difficulties which the rehabilitation team has to face? A selection will illustrate some.

ROLE CONFLICTS

Perhaps one of the biggest problems for individual staff lies in the fact that the therapist works in a team, rather than in her profession. Role blurring may lead to professional identity crises and the sole representative of a profession can feel very isolated within the team, hence the need for sharing and support.

Many health-care workers have been trained to care for clients rather than to let them do things for themselves. Learning to 'be cruel to be kind' can cause conflicts at a personal and interpersonal level.

RISK TAKING

Some of the tasks within the rehabilitation process carry with them an element of risk-taking behaviour, which can create tension and anxiety for the staff who feel, and are, responsible for their clients. Having clients climb stepladders or use potentially dangerous electrical appliances may be a necessary part of the skills they need to master and staff should be able to discuss their apprehensions in a supportive context.

MOTIVATION AND INTEREST

In many hospitals, staff are allocated to particular units, rather than being able to choose where they work. This can mean that people may be sent to work in wards that are not their principal area of interest. Rehabilitation is no exception to this and the subject must be dealt with openly to prevent undercurrents and dissatisfaction.

EXTERNAL CONSTRAINTS

Not all difficulties originate within the unit itself, although there may be a knock-on effect. After several months' work with an individual destined for a group home, there may be no suitable place available at the time when he is ready to move and it is difficult to maintain momentum in these circumstances. Equally, sudden availability of accommodation may lead to a precipitate discharge and feelings of incomplete preparation, which raise staff anxieties.

BURNOUT

A final difficulty, which is not peculiar to the rehabilitation team, is that of burnout. Working with the same clients over long periods of time can lead to feelings of disillusionment and rigidity. Greater awareness of this has prompted investigation and preventive measures can now be identified and implemented (Hume and Pullen 1986).

Innovation should be encouraged rather than rejected and attempts can be made to avoid becoming static. It must be recognised that change can be difficult and may be felt to be negating the value of current programmes.

Fidler (1984) outlines ways in which changes can be implemented to facilitate maximum acceptance of the new ideas by those who will be responsible for implementing them.

SUMMARY

The therapist has the responsibility for continually evaluating treatment and for introducing techniques and methods appropriate to the current needs of patients and society. The work is anything but static! Research is in its infancy but is much needed. The scope of rehabilitation is unlimited and it can be one of the most exciting areas of psychiatric practice.

This chapter has considered the following points:

- what rehabilitation is
- the principles of rehabilitation
- transition from hospital to community
- use of the rehabilitation approach in different contexts
- the role of the occupational therapist in rehabilitation
- personal independence and social skills
- domestic skills
- leisure
- work
- the multidisciplinary team
- staff training
- role of the family in rehabilitation
- liaison with other bodies
- problems encountered in rehabilitation.

REFERENCES

Caplan G 1961 An approach to community mental health. Tavistock, London
Caplan G 1964 Principles of preventive psychiatry. Basic Books, New York
Clark D H 1984 The development of a psychiatric rehabilitation service. Lancet 2: 625–627

Dyer J A T D 1988 Psychiatric rehabilitation. In: Kendell R, Zealley A (eds) Companion to psychiatric studies. 4th ed. Churchill Livingstone, Edinburgh, Ch 41
Fidler G S 1984 Design of rehabilitation services in psychiatric hospital settings. RAMSCO, Maryland
Hume C, Pullen I 1986 Rehabilitation in psychiatry.

Churchill Livingstone, Edinburgh

Kramer L 1984 SCORE: Solving community obstacles and restoring employment. Haworth Press, New York

McCreadie R, Affleck J W, Robinson A D, 1985 The Scottish survey of psychiatric rehabilitation and support services. British Journal of Psychiatry 147: 289–294

Monteath H G 1983 Work rehabilitation in the current economic climate. British Journal of Occupational Therapy 46: 8

Vaughn C, Leff J 1976 The influence of family and social factors on the course of psychiatric illness. British Journal of Psychiatry 129: 125–137

Wing J K, Brown G W 1971 Institutionalism and schizophrenia. Cambridge University Press, Cambridge

Wing J K, Morris B (eds) 1981 Handbook of psychiatric rehabilitation. Oxford University Press, Oxford

21

The elderly

Sheena Blair

INTRODUCTION

Few occupational therapists will pursue a career in psychiatry without encountering elderly clients suffering from multiple social and psychiatric difficulties, in physical, psychiatric and community settings. This client group requires of the therapist a complete integration of knowledge from the behavioural and medical sciences. The education of occupational therapists, with its broad range of subjects and emphasis on a holistic approach, comprehensively equips clinicians for work in this field.

Demographic studies show rising numbers of old people in the population, particularly the very old. Happily, the majority of people grow old without losing their independence but the average human life cycle leads to an expanding incidence of age-related problems.

Occupational therapists in psychiatric settings will be involved in working with functional and organic illnesses associated with or compounded by old age. The type of care offered within the National Health Service covers the day hospital, which provides regular treatment and support on specific days; clients living in the community; in-patient provision for the more acutely ill; and those with long-term problems requiring continuous care. Respite care is usually offered for 2 or 3 weeks at a time to assist relatives to provide their own long-term care at home. There is also an emerging role in counselling relatives and in examining the possibilities of prevention and mental health promotion in the elderly.

This chapter will briefly discuss theories of normal ageing, including developmental theories, disengagement theory, activity theory and biological theories, and some of the problems of normal ageing. A section is then given on psychiatric disorders of the elderly, covering organic and functional disorders. A section on working with the elderly discusses attitudes to ageing and the multidisciplinary team. The occupational therapy process is then described, from choice of treatment model through assessment procedures to the use and value of activity with the elderly. Details are given of the wide range of media available, including activities to facilitate personal adjustment, activities to promote independence, and activities for social and recreational needs. In conclusion, the chapter looks at the need for further research in this field.

AGEING

Before exploring some of the theories of ageing it is useful to gather a background of facts. Although the vast improvement in medical science over the century has undoubtedly played a part in increasing the average life expectancy, other factors are known to have had an even greater significance.

Demographics show that the biggest single factor has been improved social conditions at the turn of the century, in particular, better nutrition and sanitation, which were responsible for reducing the alarmingly high rate of infant mortality. This trend, in addition to a reduced birth rate over the past three decades, is not peculiar to Britain, but is repeated in other industrialised countries where the elderly now account for at least 15% of the total population (Table 21.1).

THEORIES OF AGEING

The study of normal ageing is vital to our understanding of psychiatric illness in the elderly. Psychologists, sociologists and biologists have produced theories that explain the processes involved in ageing. Occupational therapists have incorporated some of these theories into the

Table 21.1 The rising elderly population over the present century, shown in millions. (DHSS, 1982, Social Trends No 12, HMSO, London)

Year	Age 65–74	75–84	85+[†]
1901	1.3	0.5	0.5
1971	4.7	2.1	0.5
1980	5.2*	2.6	0.6
1991	4.9	2.9*	0.8
2001	4.5	2.8	0.9

* Peak levels   [†]85+ continues to rise

knowledge base of the profession in order to improve their understanding of the functioning of their elderly clients.

Birren and Renner (1980) examine some of the psychological factors promoting good adjustment in the elderly, for example, the ability to take advantage of opportunities to make effective interpersonal relationships. Developing these factors is frequently the goal of occupational therapy, in which psychological and practical adjustment are of equal importance in rehabilitation of the elderly. A perspective of the total lifespan of the individual, taking account of life-long coping strategies, is therefore necessary.

Clinical judgement, effective treatment and informed prognosis can only be based upon awareness of how someone is ageing, alongside our assessment of psychology.

Developmental theories of ageing

Lewis (1979) examines the developmental theories of Piaget (1950), Erikson (1959) and Kohlberg (1967) and outlines a way of understanding the behaviour of an elderly person and its implications for treatment. For example, childlike responses, such as compliance and quietness, occur when institutional life imposes rigid norms of behaviour.

Zemke and Gratz (1982) describe occupational therapy intervention as crisis resolution in the sense of Erikson's eight developmental crises. In the final crisis, the crisis of old age, the search for meaning and relevance in one's life may be facilitated through techniques such as reminiscence and life review.

Table 21.2 Developmental phases

Ages	Shakespeare's 'Seven Ages of Man'	Freud's classical libido theory	Erikson's eight stages of psychosocial development	Brown & Pedder
0–1	At first the infant mewling and puking in the nurse's arms	Oral	Trust v mistrust	Dependence (two-person)
1–3		Anal	Autonomy v shame and doubt	Separation—individuation
3–5		Phallic Oedipal	Initiative v guilt	Rivalry (Oedipal three person)
6–Puberty	The whining schoolboy unwillingly to school	Latency	Industry v inferiority	Psycho-sexual moratorium
Adolescence	The lover, sighing like a furnace	Puberty	Identity v identity diffusion	Psycho-social moratorium
Early adulthood	A soldier, full of strange oaths	Genitality and later stages of individuation emphasised by Jung	Intimacy v isolation	Marriage
Middle adulthood	The justice, full of wise saws		Generativity v self-absorption	Parenthood
Later adulthood	Lean and slipper'd pantaloon		Integrity v despair	Involution
	Sans everything			

Developmental phases have fascinated men of literature and science throughout the centuries. Table 21.2 shows some of the better-known conceptualisations.

Disengagement theory

Cummings and Henry (1961) believe that elderly people progressively disengage from life. They define this as 'an inevitable process in which many of the relationships between a person and other members of society are severed and those remaining are altered in quality'. This is not an entirely negative process but one in which alternative activities can be undertaken.

The therapist needs to distinguish between disengagement as a genuine choice or as the result of events such as retirement, bereavement or ill-health.

Activity theory

The activity theory of ageing (Maddox 1963, Lemon et al 1972) suggests that the same level of activity may be maintained in the elderly if appropriate facilities and encouragement are supplied. Support seems to be the key factor in this approach. Satisfactory adjustment to growing old is seen to depend upon continued involvement in some task or activity that gives a sense of purpose and fosters self-esteem.

Biological theories

Biological theories of ageing have been listed by

Lewis (1979). While a deep understanding of genetic and cellular structures may not be necessary for the occupational therapist, an awareness of physical changes and associated psychological factors is very important in individual assessment.

PROBLEMS OF NORMAL AGEING

The equilibrium of any person is shaken by ill-health, the death of a spouse or close relative, or a reduction in income, all of which life events become more common as we grow older. Often, a combination of losses and problems imposes strains that can temporarily or permanently conquer the ability to cope independently.

The foundation for successful ageing is laid in the adult years. Frequently, it can be observed that a client in adult or mid-life is surrounded by difficulties that do not augur well for a mentally healthy old age.

The term 'unhealthy life style' can include such elements as neglected health problems, poor nutrition, addictive disorders and factors stemming from poverty, unemployment, stress, and a lack of a regular and healthy balance of activity.

Dying, death, bereavement and grief

Because of the inevitability of death with advancing years, it is often assumed that elderly spouses are suitably equipped to cope with the experience of bereavement and the ending of a long relationship, which has usually spanned the whole of adult life. Society generally offers less sympathy for the relatives of those who have 'lived their lives', an attitude that can deny the expression of grief to a surviving elderly spouse. It is much more difficult to ask for help in coping with a grief that is expected to be silent or even absent.

The process of death can be very protracted and, for the dying, who find themselves unprepared and trapped within this process, there is also the need to grieve. Once more, grief can frequently be denied expression, either by carers who prefer to withhold from the dying the simple but perhaps painful truth about their condition, or by the dying themselves attempting to spare their rela-

tives the burden of their own anguish. Feelings often remain unexpressed and the survivors are left feeling ashamed and guilty.

PSYCHIATRIC DISORDERS OF THE ELDERLY

The elderly are susceptible to the same range of psychiatric disorders as younger people, including personality disorders, neuroses, psychoses and organic conditions. Kay et al (1964) discovered that neurosis and personality disorder accounted for the greatest number of diagnoses. Among many old people there is a generalised anxiety that stems from feeling vulnerable. Frequently, no clear psychiatric disorder will be present but a combination of handicaps, for example, deafness, combined with arthritis and with loneliness, produces isolation. This in turn nurtures suspicion and increases social withdrawal.

Health visitors, district nurses, family doctors and home helps frequently play a major role in giving support and allaying anxiety.

DIFFERENTIAL DIAGNOSIS

Careful examination of the onset of problems, home circumstances and physical health, together with a consideration of pre-morbid personality, are essential components to the forming of an accurate diagnosis. Occupational therapists are subsequently able to provide useful information on functional abilities gleaned from observing and working with the elderly client in a number of settings throughout the period of assessment.

The most common psychiatric conditions are briefly described here but it should be noted that many elderly clients present with a combination of symptoms that requires very careful multidisciplinary analysis.

ORGANIC DISORDERS

A number of dysfunctions, some of which are shown in Table 21.3, comprise dementia. Behaviour can be misinterpreted unless carefully

Table 21.3 Neuropsychological deficits, and simple detection tests (Source: Holden and Woods 1982)

Neuropsychological deficits	Effects	Simple tests
Language problems Expressive dysphasia	Difficulty in conversation	Listen. Word finding, odd words and sentences, little speech, or complete rubbish
Receptive dysphasia	Comprehension difficulty	Lack of appropriate response to questions
Agraphia	Writing difficulty	Write a simple sentence
Acalculia	Difficulty with numbers	Write numbers, add, subtract, multiply and divide simple sums
Alexia	Reading difficulty	Read notice on ward, on TV or from a magazine
Apraxia Constructional	Difficulty in putting things together to make a whole	Use matchsticks to make a star. Draw a star or a cube. Also use model for copying
Ideomotor	Difficulty in making a single gesture	Ask to be shown hair brushing, waving, clenching teeth, etc.
Ideational	Difficulty in making complex gesture	Pretend to get out a cigarette, light it and start smoking.
Dressing	Difficulty in dressing	Put on a coat, button it and take it off again
Agnosias Visual	Difficulty in appreciating meaning of objects	Use a letter or a number made up of other letters or numbers, e.g. a large 2 made of tiny 4s and see both are recognised
Colour	Difficulty in appreciating colour	Naming, matching and association
Spatial	Difficulty in finding the way. Unable to understand maps	Draw a plan of home
Autopagnosia	Difficulty in recognising parts of own body, or another's	Point to parts of own body, and that of examiner's
Anosognosia	Neglect of one side of body	Watch dinner plate. Draw clock face or house
Astereognosis	Difficulty in recognising objects by touch	Name a selection of coins by touch alone
Prosopagnosia	Difficulty in recognising faces	Naming familiar and unfamiliar faces from photographs
Simultanagnosia	Difficulty in perceiving a whole	Name a picture with something suitable to describe its content
Frontal involvement	Personality change. Euphoria or apathy. Disinhibition. Lack of initiative. Perseveration. Inability to plan	Watch. Ask relatives about previous personality. Use sequence of shapes or figures. Watch how games such as cards are played

monitored and this has a major effect on management. Some of the distinguishing features of the more common dementias are given here.

Alzheimer's disease

This is the most common form of dementia and was named after a German neurologist, who first described the disease in 1907. It is characterised by a progressive loss of function affecting thinking, understanding, memory and all aspects of personality. It is an isolating condition for both sufferer and carer and this intensifies as it becomes more difficult to communicate with the individual.

The Alzheimer's Society has subdivided the condition into phases of mild, moderate and severe dementia. These categories, with their respective levels of dependence, carry important implications for management, although it must be added that the ease of handling a particular sufferer often bears no correlation to the disease process itself. Every sufferer is unique and should be treated as such.

The disease will manifest in a variety of ways depending upon which part of the brain is affected and the implications that will have. When language is impaired, the likelihood is that there is damage in the lower temporal lobe, whereas problems with sense of direction may indicate that the posterior part of the brain is affected.

Management is aimed at maintaining function, minimising stress and manipulating the environment to make it more comprehensible or safe. In essence, the approach is mainly occupational, psychological and social, with medication used in some cases of disinhibition, depression, anxiety or aggression.

Multi-infarct dementia

This is the second most common form of dementia. It is caused by disruption of blood supply to areas of the brain, causing death of the brain cells in those areas. The condition is most likely to occur in people who have general vascular problems. Clinical features include:

- a rapid, but earlier, onset than Alzheimer's disease

- a greater prevalence in men than women
- an awareness of change in the client himself, producing anxiety or depression.

Pitt (1982) offers a very clear comparison between the features of Alzheimer's disease and multi-infarct or arterio-sclerotic dementia.

Pick's disease

This form of brain failure is fortunately more rare as it affects a younger age group. It affects mainly the frontal and temporal lobes of the brain and is mentioned here because there is a tendency to treat its sufferers within elderly care units, although most are in the fourth and fifth decades.

Other organic conditions

Other conditions that must be considered during assessment include:

- Korsakoff's psychosis, stemming from chronic alcoholism in the main, although not exclusively
- acute toxic reactions to bacteria or medication
- tumours
- vitamin and nutritional deficiencies.

The therapist needs to be aware of the overlap that exists between physical and psychiatric disorder (Table 21.4).

FUNCTIONAL DISORDERS

It is necessary to distinguish between organic and functional disorders in the elderly because the management will be very different. Some of the more common functional illnesses are briefly described here.

Reactive depression

The most common causes of reactive depression have been identified by Shaw (1984) and described as the 'lack syndrome', which encompasses the many losses experienced by the elderly. This is shown in a pessimistic outlook and a retreat into helplessness, hypochondriasis and depression.

Table 21.4 Physical conditions producing psychiatric symptoms. *(Source: Hume: 1986)*

Physical condition		Psychiatric symptoms
Endocrine	Thyrotoxicosis	Anxiety, overactivity
	Myxoedema	depression, dementia
	Pituitary	euphoria, depression
	Diabetes	confusion
Infections	Virus e.g. influenza and mononucleosis (glandular fever)	depression (may be profound)
	Infection causing high temperature	confusion (delirium)
Nervous system	Tumour	confusion
	Multiple sclerosis	euphoria, depression
	Head injury	personality change, dementia
Cardiovascular	Heart failure	confusion, paranoia, memory disturbance
Drugs and alcohol	Alcohol withdrawal	DTs (confusion)
	Alcohol addiction	dementia, recent memory disturbance
Prescribed drugs	Methyl dopa	profound depression
	Steroids	euphoria, confusion, paranoia
Illegal drugs		psychosis, withdrawal, confusion

Endogenous depression

Psychogeriatric assessment wards tend to have a high proportion of clients suffering from endogenous or psychotic depression. The most common symptom of psychotic depression is the presence of delusions of persecution, guilt, poverty or nihilism, as described by Pullen (1986).

Murphy (1983) described a 1-year study of 124 elderly clients presenting with depression for the first time. Of the original sample, 40% were considered to be suffering from psychotic depression and 60% from reactive depression.

The following points about depression in the elderly are significant:

- the suicide rate is high amongst the elderly
- atypical presentation, for example, cloaked under a variety of physical symptoms, coupled with agitation, is often mistaken for dementia
- it is amenable to treatment, which can be spectacularly effective.

Hypomania

The opposite spectrum of mood disorder is less commonly met and relatively few cases of florid hypomanic illness will be encountered by the occupational therapist. Symptoms of excitability, over-activity, disinhibition or aggression in the elderly are more likely to be associated with organic changes and the possibility of the onset of dementia.

Paraphrenia

This condition is characterised by a range of paranoid symptoms from suspiciousness to florid delusions of persecution. Auditory hallucinations are common, particularly so in sufferers who also have a hearing impairment, and a combination of symptoms produces a picture of a preoccupied, often verbally aggressive, elderly person. These clients are understandably not easy to engage in any relationship or to involve in group work. Yet, where aggression is absent and suspicion is clearly directed rather than diffuse, the sufferer can often encapsulate his delusions so that they have relatively little bearing on other aspects of his life. Once acute symptoms are modified by medication, relationships may be formed but independent living may be hindered by the client being unwilling to move a step further to allow the additional forms of support that make this possible. Paranoid behaviour can impose considerable strain on relatives, neighbours or home helps. Fortunately, the condition is often very treatable, at times leaving no residual symptoms or even any clear recollection by the sufferer of having passed through such an acutely disturbing episode.

Alcohol abuse

Drinking may be a resort to alleviate loneliness and unhappiness. However, many clients have long-standing alcohol addiction and show signs of organic deterioration. Age Concern, in conjunction with alcohol advisory services throughout the country, have produced a simple but useful series of leaflets on older people and alcohol addiction.

WORKING WITH THE ELDERLY

Anxiety and depression occur in almost 11% of men and 13% of women. The likelihood of dementia increases with age, occurring in only 3% of those between 65 and 70 years, but rising to 20% in those of 80 and over.

These figures are almost certainly artificially low since anxiety and depression, except in extreme form, are often dismissed in the elderly or regarded as accepted components of loneliness, or inevitable accompaniments of chronic physical illness and handicap. Dementia can equally go unnoticed when it is handled and contained by the devoted care of spouses and children, who often seek to conceal its presence within their families. The death of a caring spouse can sometimes reveal a surviving partner suffering from a marked degree of dementia and requiring help from the caring agencies for the first time in the illness.

ATTITUDES TO AGEING

Professionals have always viewed working with the elderly with ambivalence. Comfort (1967) gave a forthright description of stereotyped attitudes held by the medical profession. Butler (1969) wrote about 'ageism' as a form of bigotry. Pitt (1982) described a range of three negative attitudes that may be present when working with the elderly, all of which are attempts to defend against the personal stress aroused:

- defeatism
- domination
- insularity.

Such attitudes can lead to stereotyping of both clients, for example, 'the attention-seeking old lady', and staff, such as 'the well-intentioned but unrealistic occupational therapist'.

Maurice Chevalier is quoted as saying that he 'preferred old age to the alternative'. However, death is still a taboo subject in Western culture and staff may defend against the feelings it evokes by using many mental mechanisms including counter-transference, avoidance and denial. Although attitudes towards the elderly appear to be changing, staff still express feelings of ambivalence and being threatened, as identified by the Group for the Advancement of Psychiatry (1971). Kastenbaum (1979) suggested that conscious analysis of one's attitude should be built into the training of all those who work with the elderly and that skilled supervision is essential. Supervision may be individual or in multidisciplinary staff groups where the possibility of interdisciplinary learning is heightened.

The Royal College of Psychiatrists have devoted a subsection to the specialty of psychogeriatrics and many special-interest groups exist in the paramedical professions for those working with the elderly. This should result in improved standards of education and practice. Some forward-thinking schools incorporate the study of ageing within the community studies curriculum, and imaginative links between youth and age have been pioneered by schools and health-care staff.

Many client groups engender personal conflict in the therapist, who requires wise supervision and support, but with the elderly the question of working through these stresses has not been fully accepted within the health services. Some of the most common concerns for occupational therapists are:

- a sense of impotence at being unable to effect change in the elderly client or at least having to set limited goals and be content with very limited change
- projection onto the client of the therapist's conflict with her own elderly relatives
- lack of understanding by other staff of the reasons for an activity. With negative, defeatist and even hostile attitudes around her, the therapist may be seen as 'getting all the pleasant or easy jobs'
- no continuity of approach between staff, so that the therapist constantly has to struggle to sustain the client's motivation
- low self-esteem and apathy among staff saps effort and initiative.

THE MULTIDISCIPLINARY TEAM

There is always a risk of low morale when the client group is long-stay and dependent. The 'burnout' syndrome has been well documented with its list of symptoms arising from the state of exhaustion that can result from working for long periods with the most challenging of client groups. However, much of this can be counteracted by a multidisciplinary approach to the care of those with multiple problems. Each person in the team has a responsibility towards the quality of care and towards a shared philosophy. Boyd & Robinson (1983) outline numerous benefits of the multidis-

ciplinary team including therapeutic, educational and research advantages. Pollock (1986) specifies the benefits of teamwork in psychiatric rehabilitation to improve communication, provide consistency of approach, maintain continuity of care and allow a broader perspective in care provision.

Those confronting the problems of the elderly may feel a sense of impotence regarding change within a system. While acknowledging the difficulty of creating change in mental-health services, positive attitudes and a healthy atmosphere are created in those units concerned with the elderly if certain requirements are acknowledged and met.

- The need for a common philosophy of care of the elderly held by permanent staff, including a sense of optimism.
- Provision of in-service training for all staff. This is especially important because the majority of staff who work with the elderly are likely to be untrained.
- Learning resources need to be readily available.
- Direct involvement with clients in the form of a key-worker system to include appropriate back-up arrangements when holidays and sick leave intervene.
- Contact with relatives or carers.
- Supervision for staff, not only for those involved in counselling or psychotherapy, but also to identify emerging negative attitudes or low morale, generally.

Leadership of the multidisciplinary team has historically rested with the consultant, however, it can equally be invested in the senior nurse or any other professional who is enthusiastic, committed and sensitive to the pressures on staff.

Team membership

No profession formally teaches effective team membership roles. Effective collaboration may depend upon native wit, professional confidence or the length of time spent on the unit, which allows an understanding of norms, dynamics and procedures. The elderly are particularly dependent upon harmonious staff relationships, which help to create healthy surroundings. Shaw (1984) lists a variety of desirable qualities in team members, accentuating flexibility in attitude and approach.

THE OCCUPATIONAL THERAPY PROCESS AND THE ELDERLY

The occupational therapist may find her role and priorities determined by the setting and culture of the area in which she is working. Assessment units have a different ethos from day hospitals and continuing care units.

In continuing care units, the syndrome of 'social death' may be apparent. Staff feel they cannot communicate or influence events, therefore they pass on their sense of alienation by dehumanising the residents. Moving to residential care can be traumatic for many elderly people, who feel they are sacrificing independent life.

Staff in day hospitals need to be aware of the needs of carers of the confused elderly person who experience a multitude of conflicting feelings about their relative. They grieve for the person they once knew and this needs to be recognised by staff and support or counselling offered.

Occupational therapists working with a group who have a relatively high mortality rate need to:

- realise that clients need to be able to discuss painful feelings, in confidence
- recognise signs of grieving in the client
- be aware of the need to reminisce
- be sensitive to those who are fearful about their own death.

Johnson (1983) reminds us that in the USA the role of assistant or helper has expanded rapidly, especially in work with the elderly. This may mean that the therapist is also responsible for the education and supervision of untrained staff.

The occupational therapy process with the elderly follows the same pattern as with other client groups:

- selecting a model
- assessment
- treatment planning and implementation
- quality assurance.

SELECTING A MODEL

Lewis's developmental theories (1979) offer the occupational therapist a credible frame of reference from which to organise views about ageing, and this in turn enables the clinician to:

- recognise patterns of behaviour and analyse their significance
- establish treatment plans that respond to the unique development and maturation of the elderly person.

Erikson (1959) describes the final developmental stage of life as ego integrity versus despair and this provides an excellent model of the mental state of many clients. Despair is not difficult to find, as well as anxiety, depression or confusion in the elderly.

Much time within treatment programmes is concerned with supporting the ego through involvement in familiar activities and those in which self-esteem will be bolstered. Maintenance of self-esteem is considered by many clinicians to be the best indicator of successful outcome and considered by some to be the lynchpin of adjustment. Markson (1973) highlights the significance of the time element in relation to healthy integration in the elderly. The following factors can usefully be noted:

- the structure of time for people in hospital must be carefully considered
- elderly people, particularly at their first contact with psychiatric care, need skilled support to reorientate themselves towards optimum adjustment to time
- any therapeutic intervention needs to include a balance between attention to the future, in terms of rehabilitation, and attention to the past in terms of reintegration of past experiences.

ASSESSMENT

Assessment is a collaborative event when working with the elderly suffering from psychiatric disorder. It is a complex, conceptual process (see Chapter 5) dependent upon an awareness of the client's premorbid personality, the effect of ageing on the person, both physical and psychological, any emotional or environmental pressures and accurate identification of the illness.

The assessment process can be subdivided into: preliminary, intermediate and predischarge. See Table 21.5

Occupational therapists are usually asked to provide the team with specific information about basic living skills. The methods by which information is gleaned are through accurate observation, interview or the use of checklists. Standardised tests, such as rating scales, indicate the level of severity of the illness and its possible management. These have tended to be the domain of the psychologist, although occupational therapists are now developing more standardised tests. A range of rating scales in frequent use with the elderly is described by Boyd & Robinson (1983).

From the great preponderance of tests and procedures it is useful to identify one which carries broad multidisciplinary respect.

The Clifton Assessment Procedures for the Elderly (CAPE) is particularly valuable in any setting, and can be used in its entirety or in part only. It provides a dependency rating, ranging from A (independent) to E (maximum dependency), which is useful for treatment planning and the resettlement of clients into care appropriate to their individual needs. The test is published with a manual on its exact use and administration and is available to all qualified staff working with the elderly.

Table 21.5 Assessment within occupational therapy

Preliminary	Intermediate	Predischarge
When Within first week of contact for inpatient or day patient	When all recommended physical and psychological treatments have had time to take effect	Prior to discharge to home, day care or residential care
Method Interview Observation in a wide spectrum of activities Standardised tests	Specifically recommended assessment: home, safety, self-care, money management. Home visits, public transport. Continued observation during activities	Activity carried out in the home Performance checks
Goals Formation of therapeutic relationship Analysis of performance Identification of problems Mental state assessment	Identification of nature and degree of functional capacities Potential effects of problems Assets and intact functional areas	To measure response to treatment and indicate areas for continued help
Reported: Continuous feedback to ward team Recorded: In occupational therapy records Kardex	Continuous feedback to team Occupational therapy records Kardex Case notes	Continuous feedback to team plus report to GP Case notes

Specific functional assessment

If the team requires an assessment of general ability in daily living activities, the occupational therapist may design an assessment schedule of several activities that incorporate cognitive abilities and orientation, diet and nutrition, money management and road safety. This information is often required for Social Services case conferences when a client is being considered for extra day support or re-housing.

CASE EXAMPLE 21.1

Mrs Bain was perplexed about paying for goods, unless she had £1 note to offer. She was confused about newer coins, particularly the £1 coin and 20p coin. It was proposed that an initial assessment should be conducted to determine if this was lack of confidence, fear of making mistakes or whether there were signs of organic changes.

A box of groceries was used by the therapist, who asked Mrs Bain to exchange the correct money for various goods. This required addition, calculating change and discussion of prices.

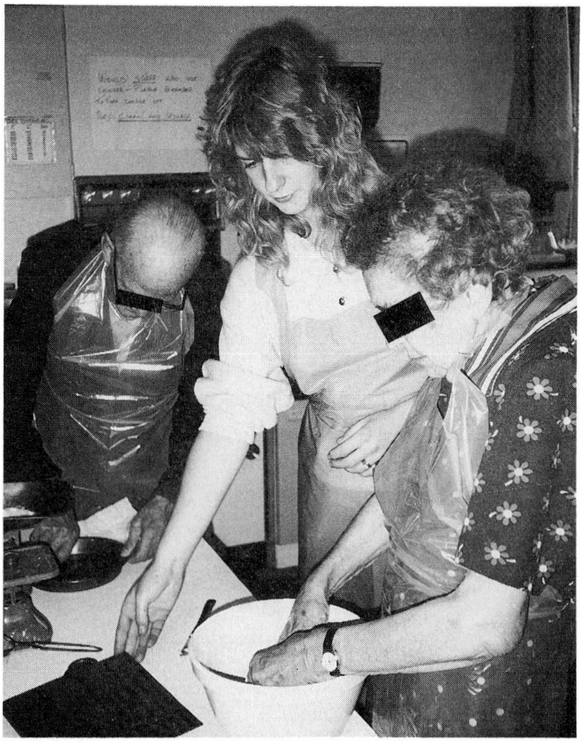

Fig. 21.1 Cooking skills are an important aspect of domestic assessment.

Domestic assessment

Very often a domestic assessment is required to ascertain basic safety, nutrition and awareness of kitchen procedures (Fig. 21.1). In many psychiatric illnesses, for example, depressive, paranoid or organic conditions, the elderly exhibit difficulties with such routine habits. A checklist is used to ensure a standard approach covering:

- preparation of the task
- method, including routines, sequence, timing
- safety in the kitchen
- interest in diet, food or appetite
- hygiene.

Home assessment

It is sensible to carry out an assessment in the familiar surroundings of the client's own home whenever possible. Although it provides the most accurate information about how the person is functioning, a home visit can be stressful, particularly if it has been long awaited and much is seen to depend on the outcome. The therapist has to be sensitive to these stresses and tolerant of life-long domestic routines.

During the visit the therapist must be vigilant for signs of forgetfulness, such as burnt pans and singed tea towels, or other more incongruous phenomena, such as cupboards full of paper or fridges filled with clothes, which indicate confusion and disorientation.

A home visit may be carried out several times as improvement occurs and the client becomes progressively more confident.

TREATMENT PLANNING AND IMPLEMENTATION

Activity as treatment for the elderly is the focus of this chapter for three reasons:

1. it is the tool and hallmark of occupational therapy
2. some studies suggest that life satisfaction is related to social action or occupation (Lehr & Rudinger 1969, Neurgarten 1977, Maguire 1984)
3. function and competence can be increased through meaningful activities.

The use of activity to increase competence is emphasised by Clark (1979), in her outline of a conceptual model for occupational therapy. In this model, she states the need for a balance of activity between self-maintenance, play and work. When working with the elderly there is often an imbalance in therapeutic activity biased towards basic self-maintenance. This is because low energy, low motivation, low confidence or low self-esteem cause the client to have poor self-care skills. It may be necessary to provide a wider range of activities in order to boost confidence and self-esteem before the client is ready to tackle self-care. There is a danger of treatment programmes being designed with a limited selection of activity, with minimal attention paid to the total range of human needs.

While Bromley (1971) realistically reminds us that the majority of well-adjusted old people lead lives that are fairly tranquil and revolve around routine personal activity, he, too, stresses the benefit of engagement in activities to prevent stagnation of interest and loss of mental and physical skills through disuse.

Treatment planning

With the elderly, it is particularly important to analyse activities into their physical, psychological and social components. The occupational therapist should also consider patterns of activities throughout the life span (Flowers and Kraiem 1982) and the relationship of those activities to well-being and life satisfaction (Maguire 1984).

Therapeutic success can be greatly enhanced by how much the client understands of the goals of treatment and to what extent the therapist can engage his motivation.

CASE EXAMPLE 21.2

Mr Sloan was an articulate, forthright man of 70, but unhappy, agitated and fearful about the future without his wife, who had died 6 months earlier. He had been in an admission unit for 4 weeks, in which time his aims in occupational therapy had included: training for domestic independence, anticipation and control of symptoms of anxiety, and investigation of local social groups. In discussion with the therapist he would accept the logic of the aims and seem to respond to encouragement, but would end conversations with the retort 'It's only words, my dear, only words'. Gradually, as the weeks passed, he began to take more initiative for what he would tackle in the kitchen and went willingly with the therapist to seek out possible church and hobbies groups. Significant progress was made when he discovered the work of the adult basic education unit and thought that he could help as a tutor in English.

When Mr Sloan began to accomplish tasks for himself and, more importantly, to find personal goals he felt more in control of his life and a part of someone else's. Although initially he understood the aims of treatment, the step of actually doing something was a vital part of his adjustment. Thus, the activities became goal-directed and meaningful for this man who, in the context of a therapeutic relationship, began to test out possible alternatives.

Goal planning

Goal planning is an approach to treatment of the elderly that can involve all members of the team, as well as the clients' families. It requires carers to acquire the skills to work out individual plans for elderly clients, based upon perceived needs and strengths identified by observation and assessment. All relevant obtainable information about an individual is considered in formulating a goal plan. The method allows staff to look at clients in a positive way instead of as 'behaviour problems' and, in so doing, challenges ingrained assumptions about the elderly by demonstrating their powers for constructive change.

The following steps are taken:

1. the assessment of an individual to identify strengths and needs

2. the selection of an important need upon which to concentrate
3. the formulation of the specific goal, using the individual's strengths
4. use of the list of strengths to develop approaches to meet the defined goal
5. breaking down the goal into intermediate steps that are achievable in the short term
6. assisting the client to practise each step the required number of times
7. the recording of progress on a chart written in a clear and exact way for the use of other staff or carers
8. the holding of a weekly meeting to monitor progress, discuss problems or difficulties, and reach an agreed method and criteria of success.

Working in groups with the elderly

Some of the earliest work recorded on the use of group approaches with the elderly was with senile patients (Silver 1950) and institutionalised senile women (Linden 1953). The emphasis was on participation and providing real, immediate social satisfaction. As literature on group approaches increased, the common theme was a supportive approach that often included reminiscence and life review. More explorative methods have been used by Berland and Poggi (1979), focussing upon dependency, loss and death. Leszcz et al (1985) described an elderly men's group in which some technical modifications were made, including a high level of participation by the therapists.

This is a familiar modification for occupational therapists who realise the potential and need for group work but have had to discover ways of encouraging verbalisation through activities. For example, participants can be asked to draw a life map and write significant milestones at appropriate points. This becomes a focus of discussion.

Groups may be organised around a practical task: recreation, leisure or orientation. The key elements are support, social and verbal interaction, and increased awareness. One of the most successful practical groups is the baking of a Christmas cake. The spices, tastes, smells and communal stirring stimulate the senses and encourage communication affecting the total ward atmosphere.

REALITY ORIENTATION

Reality orientation is a method of treatment that places great emphasis upon environmental factors in the approach to people suffering from memory impairment. It aims to improve orientation in time, place and person by using material designed to stimulate the individual through each of the senses and thereby helping him to improve and maintain contact with his surroundings.

The method may be practised either in intensive half-hour classroom sessions or throughout a 24-hour day of ward activity. To have real effect the approach must include all members of the treatment team and clients' relatives, where possible. The occupational therapist usually selects appropriate candidates for treatment, organises classroom groups and measures outcomes at appropriate intervals. On occasions, the clinical psychologist may be on hand to assist in constructing base lines and, from the use of predictive tests, identifying the individuals most likely to benefit.

Holden and Woods (1982), in their work on reality orientation, use the group setting as a vehicle for communication but stress that this approach is not solely intended for a group arena. They found that, even when working with very impaired and confused elderly people, who can seem like a collection of isolated individuals merely seated in a group, contact can be made using increased verbal activity or touch.

Prerequisites for working with the elderly in groups include:

- a sound knowledge of group processes
- awareness of how to adapt activities for maximum therapeutic potential
- supervision, if working in a psychotherapeutic manner.

Supervision is most beneficial when held regularly and the supervisior also has access to written records. The objective listener is able to elicit stereotypes about ageing, transference and counter-transference and recurring patterns of behaviour.

QUALITY ASSURANCE

Quality assurance has been defined as 'a process in which achievable and desirable levels of quality are described, the extent to which these levels are achieved and action taken to enable them to be reached is taken'. (Scottish Home and Health Dept 1989).

Quality assurance has been seen to relate to three broad areas of consideration, namely structure, process and outcome. In the context of this chapter it relates particularly to the outcome of the occupational therapy process. As the therapist returns to the treatment plan it will be apparent whether or not the desired result has been achieved. Complete cure or restoration of a particular function may not be possible.

It is important to consider carefully what the client expects or hopes to have achieved. Expectation is frequently low in this client group when illness is often thought to be the inevitable accompaniment to advanced age. It is an important part of the therapist's role not to lend weight to this theory. By helping to raise levels of expectation in the elderly, and encouraging relatives to allow their elderly to use and continue to practise their old skills, the therapist can do much to form educated attitudes to avoiding undue dependence in this client group.

In the absence of cure the therapist needs to be aware of the helps and support systems available to her clients and to those who care for them in the institutional or community setting.

ACTIVITIES FOR THE ELDERLY

TREATMENT MEDIA AND RESOURCES

The range of activities and techniques that can be used with the elderly is limited only by the resources available. The analysis and selection of activities according to priorities and needs depends on the clinical skill of the occupational therapist.

Flowers and Kraiem (1982) make the distinction between a task and an activity and urge occupational therapists to understand that people view these differently. Also, a task at one age may be considered as an activity at another. Basic living skills are common to most ages and remain essential for independence.

Kassel (1963) believed that we all require to divide our activities between those related to work and earning a living, those involving physical activity, those concerning leisure and, most importantly, those involving continued learning. Of all Open University students, 15% are aged between 60 and 65 and are amongst the most motivated and consistent.

Leisure activities offer an enormous range of possibilities, which can involve volunteers and specialists from outside the hospital, making it possible to provide choice and provide a comprehensive activities programme. Imaginative schemes like this have been described by Wheeler (1986). Methodology and resource material for reality orientation and reminiscence with sensory stimulation is plentiful, from Holden and Woods (1982) onwards.

The life-review approach can be used to explore and examine unresolved conflicts. In this context, listening, as shown by Lewis (1979), is of equal therapeutic importance to more action-orientated techniques. Age should not prove an exemption from the psychotherapeutic approach as shown by Hildebrand (1982). There is much scope for counselling, particularly involving issues of loss, and where confidence in self-expression, describing feelings and interacting with others is low it is possible to use remedial drama.

Units based upon the therapeutic community model lay emphasis on the social factors contributing to mental health. Occupational therapists, with their skills in group leadership, may help to create a sense of belonging. Activities that involve caring for the environment, sharing in group projects, either simple chores or more ambitious joint efforts for relief agencies, all encourage this philosophy.

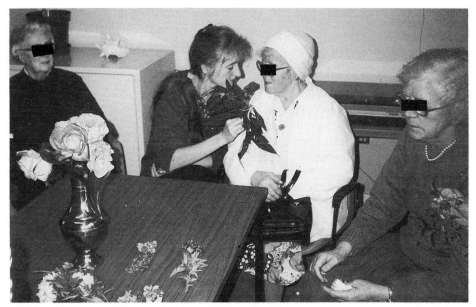

Fig. 21.2 Sensory stimulation as part of reminiscence work

The environment and tone of the unit has an enormous effect on both clients and staff, in connection with the elderly. Occupational therapists are frequently responsible for the conversation 'props' in a unit, such as the wall hangings, reality orientation materials or craft work, that may decorate a building. This should be well presented to avoid giving a kindergarten impression.

The range of activities available includes:

- activities to facilitate personal adjustment
- activities related to independence
- activities related to social and recreational needs.

Personal adjustment

Activities under this heading can be of equal benefit to those with organic and with functional illness but different emphasis is put on approach and technique. For example, while reminiscence may be actively encouraged with Alzheimer's sufferers as a means of communication, the same technique may be used with a depressed woman to put past conflicts into perspective and achieve a more-secure personal identity.

Reminiscence

Reminiscing and life review are adaptive tasks of ageing and the leader of the group can become the learner about events, attitudes and situations of years past (Kiernat 1979).

Some of the materials available include:

- slides
- videos; many are commercially available from 'Help the Aged'
- photographs
- music—listening, singing or making music
- poetry, story-telling, jokes
- visits to museums and places of interest
- looking at antiques, mementoes, scrapbooks, photographs, albums, life maps
- smells, tastes (Fig. 21.2)
- homecrafts, old-fashioned shop signs or goods
- coins, old toys, traditional cards, souvenirs, clothes (See Fig. 21.3).

Langley and Langley (1983) offer a helpful literature review of work done on reminiscence and describe the claimed effects and possible contraindications. The therapist must guard against stereotyping the elderly as being totally preoccupied with past events. Healthy old people are

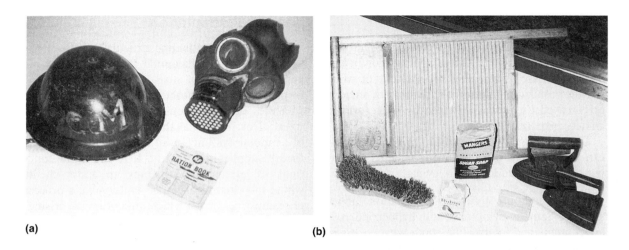

(a)

(b)

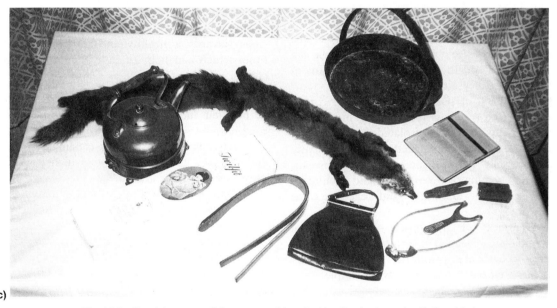

(c)

Fig. 21.3 Reminiscence articles can provide valuable stimulus in work with the elderly.

primarily concerned with the present and future, in common with other age groups.

Reality orientation

Reality orientation (RO) is based upon the assumption that repeated basic information can reinforce memory and ameliorate confusion and disorientation. It may precede or permeate many activities. Occupational therapists usually select a theme for a session and prepare associated conversational aids, so that association enables recall.

It is considered more beneficial if the approach is adopted by the whole team and is supplemented by memory aids and short, structured sessions. Holden and Woods (1982) offer an explicit and comprehensive account of reality orientation and also emphasise the need for adequate staff training.

Anxiety management

Preoccupation and fearfulness often surround the elderly person. Disorientation, which accompanies organic disease, is often the main source of panic but the vulnerability felt by the depressed, anxious or bereaved client can be helped by some form of anxiety management.

The training schedule outlined by Cullen (1984) can be used with inpatients, day patients or outpatients, and includes the following.

- Provision of accurate information about anxiety. Somatic symptoms and hypochondriasis are common and information about what occurs in the body when under stress can be shared. Visual aids are helpful and also recognition of the positive features of anxiety.
- Recognition of negative attitudes. The chronic low self-esteem of many elderly people can be highlighted and the loss of role and origins of low self-confidence aired.
- Acquisition of positive attitudes and coping strategies. The accent is on planning in this session, as many elderly are isolated due to fear of being hurt, robbed or mugged and consequently lead a socially impoverished existence. Investigation of community resources and volunteer groups can be discussed and even set as homework.
- Awareness of the onset of physiological symptoms and rehearsal of simple relaxation techniques. (There are a number of commercially available relaxation tapes, for example, the Mitchell method.)
- Acquisition of relaxation skills; a practical session.
- Application of relaxation as an approach to everyday living.
- Acquisition of coping skills, role play and visits to anxiety provoking situations can be undertaken.
- Confrontation of alarming situations.

Reinforcement of earlier work and practice are the key ingredients of these sessions.

Temporal adaptation

This is also known as time structuring. Mosey has described temporal adaption as 'the ability to organise one's time in such a way as to fulfill the responsibilities adequately and to enjoy the pleasures of one's required and/or desired social roles'. Developmental theory explains the causes of temporal dysfunction in the elderly and activity theory supplies the remedy. It is one of the functions of occupational therapy to assist clients whose life circumstances are undergoing a process of readjustment from which difficulties are arising. This intervention will focus on an exploration of clients' needs, interests, values and expectations set against their physical, mental and financial resources.

Mosey has neatly identified a series of practical steps towards a healthy and purposeful use of time, which can help an individual to manage a change of role. These are as follows.

1. *Fact finding* This involves taking a close look at how an individual's time is currently being used.

2. *Assessment* Each activity is looked at singly and analysed for the extent to which it fulfils a purpose or satisfies a need.

3. *Option search* A whole variety of activities can be explored and considered for their possible value to the individual.

4. *Selection of options and planning strategies* The decision-making process of how to implement desired options, taking a step at a time, takes place.

5. *Implementation* The changes start to happen in the life of the individual, with the continued support of the therapist if needed.

Promoting independence

Self-care may be neglected due to grief, depression, eccentricity or delusions. Basic life skills are similarly affected, with the additional complication of safety hazards. Forgetfulness means that cookers, fires and other electrical or gas appliances may be inappropriately used or left on. In the

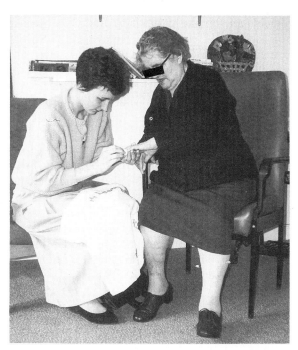

Fig. 21.4 Hygiene and self-care should not be neglected in the elderly.

course of assessment, specific problems may appear in:

- dressing and self-care, including hygiene (Fig. 21.4)
- kitchen work, budgetting, cooking and menu planning
- money management
- familiarity with traffic, supermarkets and community resources.

Individual treatment plans are formulated according to individual needs and retraining commences. Attention must be paid to sensory deficits, such as poor hearing, that reduce independence. Small adjustments can bring large benefits to the lives of the elderly, without which maximum potential will never be achieved. These include spectacles, hearing aids, dentures, appropriate nutrition, footwear and walking aids. Similarly the environment can also be adapted to improve functional performance with the aids to daily living that are familiar to all occupational

therapists, together with more unusual resources such as telephone amplifiers, talking books and large-print books, which local libraries supply.

For those in continuous care it is necessary to be sensitive to the smallest signs of independence. Social models of care that aim to counteract institutionalising attitudes and routines encourage staff to have positive attitudes towards residents.

Bayne (1971) describes how difficult it is for staff to relinquish a dominant role and allow clients to take responsibility for themselves.

Social and recreational needs

Occupational therapists need to study this area very carefully, as recreation can be used to meet many needs, especially for people who are deprived of a range of normal outlets through hospitalisation.

Nystrom (1974) divided activity patterns and leisure concepts among the elderly into:

- *passive*, where the participant brings the world to him, for example, reading, watching television, caring for plants, listening to the radio
- *active*, going to the world by visiting relatives, attending clubs, going to church or entertaining friends.

He saw the need for options and choices of activity so that, if one activity was restricted due to physical ill-health or other factors, an alternative could be sought. The need for leisure education amongst adult populations was also a priority.

Ravetz (1984) also reviewed participation in leisure throughout the life cycle and discussed various roles that the therapist might undertake within leisure rehabilitation.

Further learning

Perhaps this is an area of leisure that is underused by occupational therapists, but Lewis (1979) firmly believes in encouraging the elderly to continue learning. The University of the Third Age covers all kinds of educational, creative and leisure activities and its members organise their own pursuits. Voluntary agencies can initiate such schemes in consultation with the therapist.

Other leisure options

Treatment resources can be extended by the contribution of helpers who adapt recreational equipment or design remedial games for the elderly (Fig. 21.5). Horticulture provides an extensive range of activity for both indoor and outdoor work, and raised gardens can be designed for comfort (Fig. 21.6).

The contribution of exercise programmes to physical health and well-being is widely recognised. Never before have sporting activities and fitness clubs enjoyed such popularity. The elderly should not, on the grounds of frailty, be denied this source of cooperative enjoyment, with its benefits to respiration, circulation, balance and mobility. If necessary, it is possible to exercise all parts of the body from the safety of a chair to a musical accompaniment, which may also be a warming-up for a sing-song or quiz, without the need to move places.

Lewis (1979) discussed the advantages of exercise programmes for the elderly and illustrated this with the work of the Senior Actualisation and Growth Exploration Group (SAGE) in the USA which has been particularly helpful for depressed older people. In Britain, exercises specifically for the elderly have been designed by the EXTEND group, who will provide training for interested professionals and volunteers.

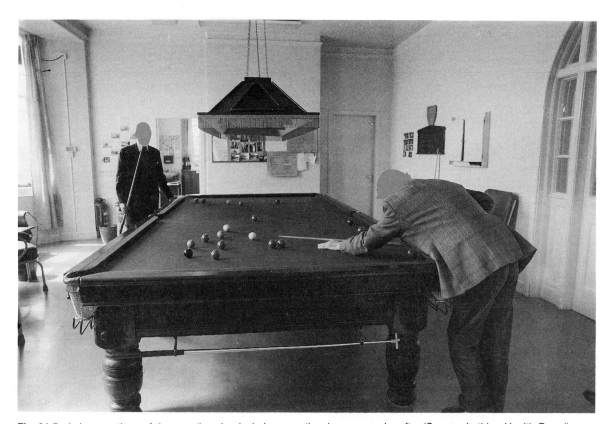

Fig. 21.5 Leisure options of therapeutic value include recreational games and crafts. (Source: Lothian Health Board)

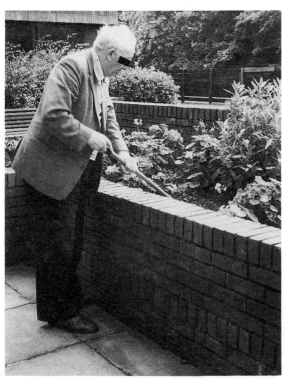

Fig. 21.6 A raised garden makes horticulture more comfortable for the elderly.

RESEARCH

Occupational therapists need to be aware of current research on the elderly with psychiatric disorder as it has implications both for clinical approach and for deployment of staff.

Of the 21% of individuals aged 65 and over with mental disorders, approximately two thirds are suffering from benign illnesses that are amenable to treatment (Richter 1984). This highlights the need for accurate assessment and diagnosis.

From an occupational therapy perspective, research is in its infancy. Most studies are from the USA and examine activity patterns and leisure concepts among the elderly (Nsytrom 1974, Flowers & Kraeim 1982) or study the effectiveness of a particular technique.

The elderly constitute a large group of our clients and numerous questions about the efficacy of our involvement are raised in the minds of staff and students alike. For example, who are occupational therapy's clients and what characteristics of these people are pertinent to the goals and philosophy of occupational therapy (Yerxa 1983)?

While clinicians observe well and record data from their involvement, the next stage towards research is to learn how to test and document results. This needs investment of time and money to create research posts and to provide the necessary supervision.

Occupational therapy is still based on tradition and untested hypothesis. As the elderly constitute the largest group of clients with whom occupational therapists work, this seems a fertile field for research.

SUMMARY

This chapter has looked at theories of ageing and the normal ageing process, as a prerequisite for understanding the functioning of elderly clients. Both organic and functional psychiatric disorders of the elderly were then considered, with sections on the most commonly occurring disorders.

A section on working with the elderly led into consideration of the particular application of the occupational therapy process to this client group.

Specific treatment media and resources for use with elderly were then detailed and, finally, potential research areas were considered.

This account has provided a general introduction to the work of the occupational therapist with the elderly mentally ill. The breadth and scope of the work is enormous, so much so that the therapist might have difficulty in identifying the priorities. These are just some of the questions that need to be seriously considered:

- where should the effort be concentrated?
- which techniques can be seen to produce the best results?
- which areas can be tackled by support staff and volunteers?

- how is it possible to recruit and retain staff in a field thought to lack appeal?
- which factors ensure quality of life for client groups requiring custodial care after losing the mental ability to maintain and support their lives?

- how do occupational therapists assure the quality of the service they offer to this most vulnerable and dependent of their client groups?

REFERENCES

Bayne J R D 1971 Environment modification for older persons. Gerontologist 11

Berland D I, Poggi R 1979 Expressive group psychotherapy with the ageing. International Journal of Group Psychotherapy 29

Birren J E, Kenner V J 1980 In: Birren J E, Sloan R B (eds) Handbook of mental health and ageing. Prentice Hall, New Jersey

Boyd W, Robinson S 1983 Psychiatry of old age. In: Kendall R, Zealley A (eds) Companion to psychiatric studies. Churchill Livingstone, Edinburgh

Bromley D B 1971 The psychology of human ageing. Pelican books, Harmondsworth

Butler R N 1969 Ageism, another form of bigotry. Gerontologist 9

Clark P 1979 Human development through occupation: theoretical frameworks in contemporary occupational therapy, Part 1. American Journal of Occupational Therapy 33(8)

Clifton assessment procedures for the elderly 1984 Hodder & Stoughton, Essex

Comfort A 1967 On gerontophobia. Medical Opinion Review, September

Cummings E, Henry W 1961 Growing old: the process of disengagement. Basic Books, New York

Erikson E H 1959 Identity and the life cycle: selected papers. Psychological issues (monograph). International Universities Press, New York

Flowers Y, Kraeim R 1982 Patterns of activities throughout the life span. Proceedings of the 8th International Congress of the World Federation of Occupational Therapists, Hamburg

Group for the Advancement of Psychiatry 1971 The aged and community mental health 8. vol 8 report 81, November

Hildebrand P 1982 Psychotherapy with older patients. British Journal of Medical Psychology 55

Holden Y, Woods R 1982 Reality orientation. Churchill Livingstone, Edinburgh

Kassel V 1963 Continuing education for the elderly. Geriatrics July

Kastenbaum R 1979 Growing old. Harper & Row, London

Kiernat J M 1979 The use of life review with confused nursing home residents. American Journal of Occupational Therapy 33(5)

Kay D W K et al 1964 Old age: mental disorders in Newcastle-Upon-Tyne. A study in prevalence. British Journal of Psychiatry 110

Langley D M, Langley G E 1983 Dramatherapy and psychiatry. Croom Helm, London

Lehr U, Rudinger G 1969 Consistency and change in social participation in old age. Human Development 12

Lemon B et al 1972 An exploration of the activity theory of aging: activity types and life satisfaction among in-movers to a retirement community. Journal of Gerontology 27

Leszcz M et al 1985 A men's group: psychotherapy of elderly men. International Journal of Group Psychotherapy 35(2)

Lewis S C 1979 The mature years: A geriatric occupational therapy text. Slack, New Jersey

Linden M S 1953 Group psychotherapy with institutionalised senile women. International Journal of Group Psychotherapy 3

Maddox G L 1963 Activity and morale: a longitudinal study of selected elderly subjects. Social Forces 43

Maguire G H 1984 An exploratory study of the relationship of valued activities to the life satisfaction of elderly persons. The Occupational Therapy Journal of Research 3(3)

Markson E W 1973 Readjustment to time in old age. Psychiatry 36, February

Mosey A C 1973 Activities therapy. Raven Press, New York

Mosey A C 1986 Psychosocial components of occupational therapy. Raven Press, New York

Murphy E 1983 The prognosis of depression in old age. British Journal of Psychiatry 143

Neurgarten B L 1977 Personality and aging. In: Birren J E (ed) Handbook of the psychology of aging. Van Nostrand, New York

Nystrom E P 1974 Activity patterns and leisure concepts among the elderly. American Journal of Occupational Therapy 25(6)

Pitt B 1982 An introduction to the psychiatry of old age. Churchill Livingstone, Edinburgh

Pollock L 1986 The multi-disciplinary team. In: Hume C, Pullen I (eds) Rehabilitation in psychiatry. Churchill Livingstone, Edinburgh

Pullen I 1986 Rehabilitation and the elderly. In: Hume C, Pullen I (eds) Rehabilitation in psychiatry. Churchill Livingstone, Edinburgh

Ravetz C 1984 Leisure in occupational therapy. In: Willson M (ed) Occupational therapy in short term psychiatry. Churchill Livingstone, Edinburgh

Richter D 1984 Research in mental illness. Heinemann, London

Shaw M W 1984 The challenge of ageing. Churchill Livingstone, Edinburg

Silver A 1950 Group psychotherapy with senile psychotic patients. Geriatrics 5

Wheeler N 1986 Dignity through social activities. Therapy Weekly 7 August

Zemke R, Gratz R 1982 The role of theory: Erikson and occupational therapy. Journal of Occupational Therapy in Mental Health 2(3) Fall

22

Child and family

Lesley Lougher

INTRODUCTION

This chapter will describe a family approach to child psychiatry and an occupational therapist's role in that service. This will be further developed by an examination of the life cycle of the family, showing the changes required at each stage and the problems that ensue if the stage is not adequately negotiated. The therapeutic interventions will be discussed briefly at this point but explained more fully in the final section. Special mention will be given here to family and women's therapy and readers are also referred to the Chapters 13–16 on the use of group psychotherapy, drama, social skills training and play therapy.

DEFINING THE FAMILY APPROACH

The notion of treating an individual as a whole person rather than looking at the sick components has always been an important one for occupational therapists. A systems approach to therapy places the individual within the social systems of which he is a member, the most important of which may be said to be the family. Other systems have varying degrees of importance during the life cycle, such as school, work, friendship and recreational groups. There is no doubt that dysfunctions in any of these systems will have an effect on the individual. Life events such as divorce, moving house, or change of job have been shown to affect health and happiness, as have social circumstances and employment (Brown et al 1978). Just as occupational therapists learn to encourage the functioning of the whole person, so we also need to understand the functioning of the person within his social system.

This systems approach to treatment is generally known as 'Family Therapy', although practitioners need to be aware that the family is not necessarily the only significant system in an individual's life. It is perhaps not surprising that some of the pioneers in family therapy were working in Child Guidance Clinics or Child Psychiatric Units (Walrond-Skinner 1981), as a child is usually brought into treatment by a member of the family or referred from school. It was and still is common practice to interview mother and/or father to assess the child's problems so that it becomes a logical development to involve the whole family and, perhaps, the school in therapy.

Although the term 'family' is used, a more accurate description would be the 'household in which the child lives'. This may include several adults and children who are not relatives but who constitute the child's 'family' at the time. Other people outside the household may also be invited to therapy sessions, such as divorced fathers or baby-minding grandmothers.

THE FAMILY-BASED CHILD PSYCHIATRIC UNIT

This is a child psychiatric service designed to assess and treat the child within the context of the family and the wider social group. The type of problems presented by children (enuresis, school phobia and anorexia) frequently show a reluctance on the part of the child to move on to the next stage of development. The child's problem may indicate reluctance by the family to allow him to grow or may be the child's way of clinging to a safer period of life in response to pressures either from the family or outside. The family's method of coping with the child's distress will then influence his ability to let go of the symptoms or to escalate them.

In order to enable the child to move on to the next stage of development, it is essential to intervene in the total system of interaction of which the child is a part, for example, a case of enuresis following the birth of a younger sibling. Many families will have experienced a previously dry toddler wetting the bed after the birth of the new baby. This is often solved by the family itself: father or grandmother notices the child is feeling left out by his mother's preoccupation with the new baby and spends more time with the toddler or takes over more household duties, freeing the mother to spend some time with the older child. The aim of family therapy is intervention in a family system experiencing problems to enable the family to draw on its own resources to resolve its difficulties (see Case example 22.1).

THE ROLE OF THE OCCUPATIONAL THERAPIST

Llorens (1970) defines occupational therapy as '. . . a problem-solving process involved with the treatment and training of the ill and disabled for the restoration of function and the interventions into the lives of the well and able for the prevention of disability and maintenance of health.'

This 'problem-solving process' equips occupational therapists with a philosophical approach that is akin to that needed for family therapy. Other health professionals are trained to treat illnesses and parts of people, whereas occupational therapists believe that the person is an interplay of functioning parts and is greater than the sum of those parts. The concept of treating a person within his family and environment is not new to occupational therapists. Llorens also suggests that occupational therapists look for disturbance of function in terms of the family rather than the individual but the approach is similar.

Family therapists tend to be health professionals employed as doctors, psychologists, social workers, occupational therapists and nurses, as there are few posts designated solely as family therapist, and each profession contributes its own style and expertise. A family therapist is more actively involved with the family than is usual in

CASE EXAMPLE 22.1 FAMILY THERAPY

Problem

A 5-year-old boy, Dean Smith, is referred by his general practitioner, who writes that the mother can no longer cope with the boy's destructive behaviour. On initial interview, the therapist discovers that the boy's father is largely absent due to his job as a long-distance lorry driver. The boy's mother feels tired and weary, unsupported by her husband and angry with her mother, who visits briefly to criticise her daughter's handling of the grandson.

Dean is a bright, lively child, who prefers to leap around the furniture rather than sit down and watch television quietly, and is reluctant to go to bed before 10.00 p.m. He is also likely to throw a temper tantrum in a shop when thwarted in his desire for a third ice-cream.

Mr Smith does not understand his wife's concerns about the boy: he is proud of his mischievous son and suggests that his wife is not firm enough. Mr Smith enjoys playing darts at the local pub; he would like his wife to accompany him as she was also a good player but she refuses, saying that no babysitter could cope with Dean.

Mrs Smith is lonely and isolated, she dreads going out because of Dean's bad behaviour. The more miserable she becomes, the less she is able to play with her son and direct his energies more productively. Dean is an active child and responds to his mother's lethargy by even more active behaviour, to provoke a response.

The relationship between Mr and Mrs Smith has become very strained and much of their little time together is spent in mutual criticism. Mrs Smith feels unable to ask her mother for any constructive help due to their previously poor relationship. A school report shows that Dean's behaviour is manageable but he has few friends and tends to be rather tired.

Aims of therapy

- To enable Mr and Mrs Smith to give Dean more controls so that he has sufficient sleep and becomes more acceptable to other children
- To suggest Mr and Mrs Smith define their relationship both as parents and as a marital couple
- To assist Mrs Smith to establish her own social networks.

Possible intervention

- *Behavioural programme*: Dean and Mrs Smith.
A star chart to reward Dean for going to bed when told. This would be administered by Mrs Smith.
- *Handling group*: Dean and Mrs Smith. Mrs Smith could discuss with other mothers and group leaders different tactics to use to control bad behaviour and encourage good.
- *Women's therapy group*: Mrs Smith. This would help Mrs Smith to reestablish contact with other mothers facing similar problems and give her an opportunity to work through her resentment of her own mother and the effect this may have on her own ability to mother.
- *Family or marital therapy*: This is considered but may be impossible owing to Mr Smith's job commitments. Mrs Smith and Dean have both received different types of therapy and, although Mr Smith has not been able to attend, he will be affected by the changes in his wife and son. This could result in him spending more time at home as the situation is more enjoyable. On the other hand, he may not be happy with his wife having more friendships and being less emotionally dependent on him.

An occupational therapist could have been a therapist in any of the sessions they attended.

Several members of staff from the multidisciplinary team are likely to be in contact with this family. The occupational therapist may work with a psychologist to draw up a behavioural programme. She may run a handling group with a teacher or nurse, in which she contributes her experience of role play or modelling. Occupational therapists usually have some training and experience in group-work skills and so may choose to run the women's group, possibly using some activity-based sessions. The occupational therapist may join with another member of staff for the family-therapy sessions.

other forms of psychotherapy, in that the family may be given tasks to perform within the session both as an assessment and as therapy. An occupational therapist is trained in the therapeutic use of activities and is well equipped to enable a family to work together to produce a family tree or to use role play, so that family members experience each other's positive attributes. She may suggest tasks and activities a family may perform between sessions that will aim to change entrenched patterns of relationships.

An occupational therapist in a family-based service may use play therapy with individual children, run psychodrama groups with adolescents, and lead relaxation groups with mothers. It is an area where many other professionals are also experimenting with more structured therapies, so that an occupational therapist working in this type of setting needs to be confident of her own abilities and is more likely to be the only occupational therapist working in a multidisciplinary team where there may be several members of other disciplines.

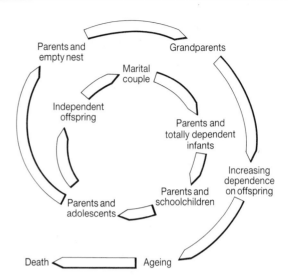

Fig. 22.1 The family life cycle. (Adapted from Evans 1973)

THE LIFE CYCLE OF A FAMILY

A theoretical approach using the life cycle of an individual has been suggested by Llorens (1976) as useful to occupational therapists. She describes the developmental life cycle longitudinally, over time, and horizontally; neurophysiological, physical, psychosocial, and psychodynamic growth and development in language and socio-cultural skills. The family has also a developmental cycle in which each individual member requires different skills to negotiate each stage of the cycle. Dysfunction in one family member may signal family difficulty in moving on to the next stage.

The stages in the family life cycle, as shown in Figure 22.1, overlap in that the generations are negotiating different stages simultaneously, that is, the birth of a new baby creates new parents and grandparents.

The stages are defined as marriage, parents and infants, parents and schoolchildren, parents with adolescents, parents alone and young adult.

Each stage requires the family to make certain changes. If these are not accomplished, the family or an individual within it shows symptoms of distress. The symptom-carrier may be the person who is most aware of the pressure to change and resists it on behalf of the family, even to protect the family. That the family continues as a system

is proof of its flexibility, since it must respond to internal and external changes and must be able to transform itself in ways that meet new circumstances without losing the continuity that provides a frame of reference for its members (Minuchin 1974).

MARRIAGE

A marriage signifies the birth of a new family but one that is heavily influenced by the families of the new couple. Marriage may be a smooth transition from one stage of the life cycle to the next or it may signify a desperate move on the part of one or both partners to bring wholeness to their lives. Skynner (1976) suggests 'Marriage is always an attempt at growth, at healing oneself and finding oneself again, however disastrously any particular attempt may fail for lack of sufficient understanding or external help'.

There is an interaction of unconscious forces, cultural choices and conscious values in the choice of a spouse which Dicks (1967) classified as three levels of bonds.

Changes

The transition from one stage of the life cycle to

the next always involves some change. On marriage, the partners separate from their families of origin and establish a new adult relationship. The marital relationship requires a negotiation of gender roles and the development of a sexual relationship.

There are three stages to be negotiated in a marriage (Skynner 1976).

1. *Falling in love*: the relationship is characterised by mutual admiration, even idealism, and excitement. There is a sense of fulfilment and belonging.

2. *Disappointment*: reality intrudes and the idealised other no longer exists as the partners get to know each other. There may even be a sense of loss, accompanied by a feeling of loneliness.

3. *Autonomy*: there is an acceptance of each other's qualities, both positive and negative. There is trust and commitment and a greater confidence in the relationship.

Problems

Difficulties may arise when these changes are not negotiated. One or both partners may not be able to separate sufficiently from their own parents. The degree of separation required may vary as in one marriage it may be acceptable that the woman maintains close emotional and supportive links with her mother, whereas in another this would be dysfunctional.

The allocation of gender roles within the marriage may differ from one or both families of origin. The couple decide who will be the main wage earner, who will organise the domestic duties, who does the gardening and who pays the bills. Either partner may feel anxious about being expected to perform a task she/he feels is in the province of the other sex.

Sexual problems may have their origins in gender insecurity, inability to express emotions physically, fear of losing control or technical ignorance.

Building and maintaining a marriage requires skill and persistence. Two people, possibly from very different types of family, have the task of creating a third family, which will be mutually satisfying and will provide a secure foundation for children if required.

Therapeutic interventions

While most couples negotiate the ups and downs of a new marriage by talking through the difficulties together and/or using their support networks of friends and relatives, some may need outside professional help. This may take the form of marital therapy or sexual counselling, or one person may need individual therapy to work through problems from childhood. An example is where one partner has been sexually abused as a child and finds old fears returning in this new, intimate relationship.

PARENTS AND INFANTS

Having begun to establish a marriage to their mutual satisfaction, the pair then has to change to incorporate a third. Pregnancy may provide some preparation as the couples begin to fantasise about the presence of the baby but few are fully prepared for the disruption in their lives.

Changes

Practical

One parent, usually the mother, may cease outside employment, thus depleting the income. This may also influence the allocation of domestic duties. The baby's presence dominates all activities; the daily timetable revolves around the child's pattern of needs. A baby demands 24-hour care and a mother may find herself having very little sleep and no privacy.

Emotional

The mother will, at least initially, develop close bonds to the child and will have less time and resources for her husband. The man usually has financial responsibility for two people and may be required to give more support than he receives. Both partners have the task of negotiating with their own parents the role of the new grandparents.

Problems

- Either or both partners may feel unsupported by the other.
- The man may be envious of the love and attention given to the baby by his wife. He may worry about the reduced family income.
- The mother may not love the baby as she and others expect. This may be a transitory phase due to the trauma of the labour and the physical demands of early motherhood, or may be an early indication of a long-term problem.
- The woman may miss her former independence and may have difficulty adjusting to the constant demands of motherhood. Oakley (1980) found that most women were less than satisfied with their new role and had mixed feelings about their babies.
- Whereas many new parents become closer to their own parents and feel supported by them, some feel either ignored or intruded upon.
- The act of parenting may remind either parent of their own childhood difficulties, particularly when they themselves were not adequately parented or even abused.

Therapeutic intervention

- Most parents at this stage are too busy coping with the day-to-day tasks involved in caring for a baby to seek other than practical assistance. Health visitors give advice on routine baby-care and may help to suggest techniques on coping with sleep problems.
- Looking after a difficult baby requires parents to agree on methods of coping, so that a session focusing on joint decision making may be helpful. A mother may put the child to bed before her partner arrives home, only to find that on return the father likes to wake the child up to play. The baby is then bright and alert and unwilling to sleep.
- Women who have been sexually abused in childhood sometimes begin to experience flashbacks and nightmares during pregnancy and after the birth, particularly of a daughter. It may not be advisable to offer intensive psychotherapy to a woman coping with a young baby but she may be reassured that what she is experiencing is not unusual.

PARENTS AND SCHOOLCHILDREN

This stage of development in the family life cycle requires yet more skills in parenting and a further change in the marital relationship.

Changes

- As the child becomes more independent, the mother has more time to develop her own interests, which may include returning to work.
- The child's increasing independence also requires the parents to develop methods of controlling the child's behaviour for his safety and to ensure the behaviour is socially acceptable.
- The children start school and begin to move into a world outside home, learning new skills, meeting people other than family, and will begin to bring in ideas and opinions from elsewhere.
- The woman's increasing independence from children enables her to resume her adult relationship with her partner. It is often suggested that parents need to 'remarry' at this stage (Schlicht 1984).
- Grandparents may take a more active interest in their grandchildren, sometimes gaining more enjoyment from them than they had from their own children.

Problems

It is at this stage of development that children may begin to show symptoms in their own right. Babies may be battered or respond to their parents' anxieties or depression but the behaviour of young children may show a level of distress. Typical parenting problems of pre-school children are 'hyperactivity', bed wetting, soiling and temper tantrums. School-age children may refuse to go to school or begin stealing. In some families, the children may be mentally, physically or sexually abused, or all three. Many of these problems may be a combination of the child's own personality and the parents' inability or difficulty in fulfilling their parental tasks. Some parents, having survived a difficult childhood themselves, find themselves reexperiencing past emotional pain when passing through the same stage of the family life cycle, as parents. In some families, the child's problem behaviour has the function of bringing into therapy parents who would otherwise be unable to ask for help.

Therapeutic intervention

- Behavioural programmes may be devised to reinforce children's positive behaviour rather than punishing the negatives. For instance, a star chart may be used to reward a child using the lavatory rather than drawing attention to the times he fails to do so. This may be used as a family task, as both parents may be asked to set up and monitor the chart, and possibly to devise a similar one for another child. The children are asked to illustrate their charts. The symptom that tended to divide the family may then become a focus to organise everyone around a common task.
- Some children's problems may be symptoms of family disharmony, so that the underlying problem may be worked in with family therapy.
- Child abuse may need several types of intervention, which will be dealt with in further detail later.

PARENTS AND ADOLESCENTS

Adolescence marks the transition from childhood to adulthood in both physical and emotional development. In the family, the parents need to mirror the child's development with their own ability to 'let go' and allow the new adult to emerge. The adolescent's identity crisis may coincide with the parents' mid-life crisis as they seek to come to terms with their own successes and failures. The grandparents' health may be failing and they may be becoming increasingly dependent on their children as the grandchildren move away.

Changes

- The adolescent becomes more involved in his peer group as a source of validation for his beliefs and opinions. Parental values may be scorned, at least temporarily.
- Having worked to keep the children within their control in previous stages, parents now have to relinquish some of this to allow their offspring to take more responsibility. Some limits are still needed so that the adolescent has freedom to rebel safely. An example of this could be the nightly curfew: if a time is set which is appropriate to the age of the child, the child may then argue about it, rebel occasionally by being late or put forward reasoned arguments for special considerations for particular occasions.
- Parents and grandparents may have to face making decisions as to whether the two households should combine if the grandparents are unable to cope alone.

Problems

- Parents may feel undermined and inadequate by the criticisms of their children, particularly if they lack confidence and have inadequate support systems of their own. This may result in an inability to set some limits on the child's behaviour so that the child becomes increasingly delinquent, in testing out non-existent limits.
- If the parental couple have had sexual problems, these may be highlighted in the emergent sexuality of the adolescent. There may even be envy of the child.
- The family may not wish to move on to the next stage, and the child shows this by developing a symptom such as anorexia nervosa or nocturnal enuresis which involves the parents in 'looking after' the child and the child is unable to move away.
- One or both parents may be anxious that the child will repeat their own mistakes, such as failure in education or unplanned pregnancy. In an attempt to prevent this happening, parents may unwittingly increase the likelihood by putting pressure on academic achievement and having unrealistically strict rules about boy- or girl-friends.
- Adolescence is a period when children experiment; some of these experiments may verge on being dangerous or illegal, such as delinquency and drug-taking. Parents have the constant

dilemma of how to balance firm controls with understanding and when to involve agencies outside the family: police, social workers or hospitals.

Therapeutic intervention

• Family therapy is often an important intervention at this stage in the development of the family. Adolescents are able to speak for themselves and work may focus on problems around generational boundaries. For instance, parents may need encouragement to maintain the role as lawmakers and endure the adolescent anger.

• An adolescent may require therapy for himself, either individually, in a group, or occasionally in a residential setting.

PARENTS ALONE AND YOUNG ADULT

In most families, children do decide to leave home and embark on an independent life. This may occur through education as the child leaves for college at around 18 years of age, or to work away from home. Others prefer to stay at home until they marry. The degree of separation between parents and children may depend on cultural beliefs and social values. The two generations may choose to remain in the same household or may live in separate households but geographically close so that there is frequent contact. In others, either by choice or circumstance, the children may move far away and there is little contact between family members. Maturity involves a degree of separation between parent and offspring that cannot be judged by physical distances.

Changes

• The parents become a couple again and may well have the house to themselves.

• Both parents and children begin to develop mutual respect for each other as adults, as they develop along their separate ways.

• The child takes on adult roles through work, sexuality and social life.

• The parents face retirement of the wage earner, with changes in the pattern of their lives and possible financial restrictions.

• The grandparents may become increasingly dependent or die.

Problems

• The parents may find they no longer wish to be a couple and may have to decide whether they want to stay together for their own sakes rather than a family ideal.

• The parent who has spent most time in childcare, usually the mother, may feel bereft and useless. The parent retiring from work may feel life is simply empty.

• The child may find it difficult to make the necessary sexual and social adjustments, and may become increasingly isolated, leading to attempts to resolve this through drug abuse, early pregnancy or even suicide attempts.

Therapeutic intervention

Some young people require assistance in negotiating the transition from adolescence to adulthood.

• Family therapy may be used to facilitate the change from an adult–child to an adult–adult relationship.

• Individual or group work may be offered for the young person to 'let go' of childhood, particularly where they have not received the security a child has a right to expect.

NON-NUCLEAR FAMILIES

With a divorce rate of one in three marriages, there are many types of households raising children. Many children now grow up having intermittent contact with one parent. Some contact with a non-custodial parent is usually preferable to none, however difficult the access arrangements may seem.

SINGLE-PARENT FAMILIES

These are more likely to be families headed by the mother but some fathers are also in this position.

The reasons for this type of family system will affect the changes to be negotiated and to some extent the problems that arise.

Changes

• Death of one parent may leave the other parent to cope with his/her bereavement, the children's loss and financial problems, while having to cope with the day-to-day tasks of running a family. The amount of support networks such as family, friends and child-care facilities will have an impact on the enormity of the task.

• Some families have always been single parents, either by choice or by circumstance, and again the amount of outside help will influence the situation.

• Divorce or separation accounts for many single-parent families. In some divorces, the parents agree to have joint custody so that the children may retain close contact with both parents. Another alternative is where one parent has care and custody of the children and other has regular access visits to which he adheres. Other families have this arrangement but the non-custodial parent is erratic in maintaining contact. In some families, the non-custodial parent ceases to see the children.

Problems

• As most single-parent families are headed by women, the family's income is generally reduced and they may require state benefits. However, in some families, this may mark an increase in their finances as the mother now has complete control of the income.

• A single parent has, at least initially, to meet all her children's needs with no-one else to fall back on. The separated parent may be supportive in the challenges of rearing children or he may be critical. Where there is a difference in perception, the children may still be caught in parental arguments.

• A single parent has very little time for herself. Babysitting, if affordable, may be difficult as many babysitters require transport home at night and this would involve either leaving the children alone or getting them up. It may be much more difficult for the single parent to make and maintain friendships. This is much improved where there are regular and reliable access arrangements.

• Many single parents feel stigmatised in a social life dominated by couples and feel they have let their children down by not providing a 'normal family'.

STEP FAMILIES

This is a term applied to families where there has been a remarriage with children involved. A typical example would be where a divorced woman with children remarries a divorced man with children. The new household will then consist of mother, stepfather, mother's children and father's children who visit at weekends.

Changes

• The role of the new partner as to his/her parenting responsibilities must be agreed.

• The children now have to share their mother with her new partner and have new step-siblings.

• The children may be in contact with father and step-father and three sets of grandparents.

• The customs and habits of two households have to be coordinated into one family.

Problems

• The natural parent is often unsure as to how much parental authority to accord to the new partner and over what time. If children are unsure about this, many will misbehave until the step-parent's position is clarified.

• Both partners and families, having experienced the breakdown of one relationship, may be unsure how much to trust this new one.

• Initially, at least, there will be rivalry between children and step-parent for the natural parent's affection. Step-siblings may also be jealous of each other.

• The children may be members, if only part-time, of two households, which will have some different rules. It may take time to adjust to this or may be exploited by insecure children.

• In families where there is no contact with the departing parent, children may need to grieve that parent and may take out their anger on the remaining parent.

Many of these problems relating to reconstituting families exist because this is a fairly new form of family structure for which no rules have evolved. Each family has to negotiate its own terms, most presumably managing to do this to their reasonable satisfaction, but it is perhaps not surprising that the divorce rates of second marriages are greater than first.

Therapeutic intervention

The interventions to be made in non-nuclear families are little different to those in a nuclear family. It is important to look for the positive strengths in these families rather than compare them unfavourably with families where both birth parents are present. A single mother may be working extremely hard to be a breadwinner, parent and homemaker, and this needs to be acknowledged before the therapist focuses on any problem resulting from the absence of a father.

Similarly, for all its difficulties, a step-family may provide the children with a far richer experience, with more adults caring for them, and encourage a tolerance for different ways of living.

Case example 22.2 describes a step-family that was helped by a variety of interventions. These methods are described in detail after the case history.

CASE EXAMPLE 22.2   A RECONSTITUTED FAMILY

The Moore family:
Jill Moore, aged 37
Jack Moore, aged 42   referred family
Mary Cross, aged 14
Gordon Cross, aged 12

John Cross, aged 40
Lisa Cross aged 25
Jason Cross, aged 12 months
Pat Moore, aged 42
Sharon Moore, aged 17
Tracey Moore, aged 14.

Jill Moore requested an appointment for her daughter, Mary Cross, at the local Department of Child Psychiatry. She explained to her general practitioner that Mary had a violent temper and refused to do anything her mother asked. She was particularly worried about her daughter's refusal to go to school. The Education Welfare Officer supported the referral as her interventions had helped Mary return to school 6 months ago but were now having no effect.

First session
Mrs Moore was asked to attend the department with her whole family to be seen by the psychologist and occupational therapist. She attended with Mary and Gordon, saying that her husband, Jack Moore, had difficulties getting time off work and that Mary and Gordon were her children from her previous marriage. Mrs Moore expressed her concern about Mary's behaviour and explained that Gordon was not a problem as he was rarely at home. Mary appeared angry and refused to speak. The therapists decided to spend the first session drawing a family tree in order to collect information on the family history and to involve both children in the process. Mary and Gordon both joined in drawing the genogram and asking their mother about their relatives.

In doing this, the therapists learned about the three households listed above. They discovered that Mary and Gordon saw little of their father, John. He lived in the same city but was evasive on the telephone about arranging meetings and, when he did so, he tended not to arrive as arranged. Gordon would cycle over and occasionally catch his father at home but Mary rarely saw him. Neither child had any contact now with the paternal grandparents, who lived 50 miles away. Sharon Moore would arrange to see her father occasionally at lunchtimes but Tracey was at present refusing to see her father following an acrimonious divorce where she placed her loyalties with her mother. It was also learned that Mrs Moore was very close to her own parents, respecting her father for his authority in the household and turning to her mother for emotional support.

The therapists suggested that Mr Moore was an important member of the household and that his attendance at the next session would be valuable. This elicited tears from Mary and threats not to return. However, Mrs Moore agreed to bring her husband.

Second Session: 2 weeks later, with the same therapists

Mr and Mrs Moore arrived with Mary and Gordon. Mary was quiet and tearful, refusing to speak. The therapists decided to focus on the issue of school refusal as both the adults were present. Mr Moore left home first at 8.00 a.m., at which time Gordon would be getting up and Mary was beginning the daily arguments. She would be reluctant to get up and dress and then refuse to go to school. Gordon would leave the house at 8.45 a.m. to go to school, and Mrs Moore would continue imploring Mary to go to school. By 9.00 a.m. Mrs Moore would be upset and exhausted and would have to go to work, leaving Mary alone in the house.

Mrs Moore worked in the mornings in a shop in the local shopping centre and was invariably late for work. When she returned at lunchtime, Mary would either have returned to her room or spent the morning doing housework. She rarely left the house. Mother and daughter would spend time discussing why Mary was refusing to go to school and was so unhappy. These discussions would end up with both in tears and no further understanding reached.

Mrs Moore became increasingly upset when speaking, saying she felt such a failure in being unable to help her daughter. Mary refused to speak, alternatively appearing angry or sad. Gordon said Mary did not get on with some girls in her class but could not understand why she hated school so much.

Mr Moore expressed his frustration at his inability to intervene. He was prepared to go into work late after taking Mary to school by force, if necessary, but Mrs Moore was reluctant to allow him to do this. Mr Moore felt his wife did not exert sufficient authority over her daughter and said he would never have allowed his daughters to treat their mother like that. There was then more discussion about the rules in Mr Moore's previous household and about Mary's feelings about her own father.

The therapists felt that there was a great deal of confusion in this family. It was unclear whether Mrs Moore wanted support from her husband in dealing with her daughter and, if so, what form this support should take. Mary felt let down by her own father and seemed to take out her resentment on her stepfather. Gordon spent

as little time as possible at home, having a full timetable of extra-school activities and going to friends' houses whenever possible. It was therefore decided to see Mr and Mrs Moore alone for the third session, to discuss how they wished to parent Mary and Gordon.

Third Session: 2 weeks later

Mrs Moore stated that she did need and want her husband's help in managing both children, particularly Mary. She was brought up in a household where the father took an active part in disciplining the children. However, she also felt sorry for Mary and felt responsible for not being able to keep the original family intact. She had difficulty in being firm with Mary, as she felt she herself was to blame for the situation and yet was worried that involving Mr Moore would alienate Mary still further. Mr and Mrs Moore rarely went out together as Mrs Moore was worried about leaving the children with Gran to babysit, as they always complained. Mr Moore said he frequently felt angry with Mary but always held back as he accepted his wife's reservations. He would also like to go out more with his wife but respected her concerns. He also missed his own daughters.

The therapists stated that, in their experience, children always benefited from clarity in a situation and that Mrs Moore should tell Mary that she expected her to go to school rather than spend hours searching for the reasons for Mary's misery. If Mrs Moore wanted her husband's support, then she should involve him without asking the children's permission. The couple were told they had every right to go out together as long as they had made appropriate arrangements for the children. They were also told that Mary's behaviour was likely to worsen initially in response to their united firmness.

Fourth Session

Mr and Mrs Moore were now closer, Mrs Moore feeling more supported by her husband. They had also managed one evening out together. Mary was, as expected, even more miserable and the therapists felt it was an appropriate time to consider admission to the inpatient adolescent unit. This was now possible as Mrs Moore felt stronger and supported by her husband, so could take the difficult decision to request admission and insist that Mary go.

Mary was admitted to the unit and stayed 6 months. She learnt to cooperate with her peer group, fulfilling her duties in rota commitments in

(Continued on p. 382.)

(Case example 22.2 continued.)
cooking and in tidying the unit. She was able to talk through her feelings of sadness and anger about losing contact with her father. After some hesitation, she overcame being bullied and emerged as a group leader. Towards the end of her admission, she returned part-time to school and was able to return full-time to school on discharge.

Meanwhile, Mr and Mrs Moore attended weekly multi-family groups, where the parents of the resident children met to discuss how the family had coped over the weekend (as the unit operated on a 5-day-week basis). In talking with other parents in similar situations, Mrs Moore was able to become much firmer with Mary, with her husband's backing.

On discharge, it was felt that the family had reorganised itself more appropriately. The power in the family was more evenly distributed, Mr and Mrs Moore could take parental authority and responsibility and Mary was able to invest more emotion in her peer group, having a full social life and experiencing success at school. The family were also able to choose to spend time together, Gordon no longer needing to absent himself. Both children began to value Mr Moore as a more consistent father-figure than they had previously experienced.

Summary
Initial assessment had shown this family to be controlled by the 14-year-old daughter, Mary. Her brother stayed out of the house, her mother was kept in and stepfather was kept on the fringe. The mother had allowed this situation to develop as she felt guilty about the break-up of her first marriage and was trying to make reparation to the children. The stepfather was ambivalent about his position, feeling sad about the minimal contact with his own daughters, angry with his stepdaughter and yet unable to resolve any of these problems.

The aim of therapy was to remove Mary from this position of power, which only served to imprison herself within the family. Two points of intervention were required to achieve this. The parental couple were given the task of deciding on their responsibilities and then acting upon them. The children were required to give a better balance of their lives, the brother to develop family contacts as well as his peer group and the girl to give up her power within the family and develop more appropriate peer relationships.

Mary Cross was identified as the person requiring treatment in this family and yet she would have had great difficulties in making any changes in her life unless the other members of the family were changing their positions simultaneously.

METHODS OF THERAPY

A child referred to a Department of Child and Family Psychiatry will be initially assessed within his family and any treatment offered will be seen within these family dynamics. There is a range of therapy available either to the whole family; a sub-system, mother–child, marital couple; or an individual, the child, the mother or the father. The treatments offered may be individual therapies such as psychotherapy, play therapy or behavioural therapy, or group therapy, such as, social skills, art, women's therapy and multi-family groups. These will be discussed in more detail later. Although these therapies may be directed at an individual, the effect of any change is seen in terms of the influence on the family system.

Many of the therapeutic interventions used in a family-based service are the same as used in an individual-centred service, the difference being that the interventions are monitored as to the effect they have on the whole family or network of relationships. The aim of therapy is to assist the family to reorganise itself in such a way that an individual no longer needs to present symptoms. In a child-psychiatric service, this entails helping the family to care more adequately for the child rather than replacing the parents by 'better parents', that is, therapists. A child-psychiatric service may offer therapy to the parents in order to support them in parenting as the most important need of children, particularly young children, is to be adequately parented. The child may require symptomatic treatment, for example, for bedwetting or school phobia, and adolescents may need time away from parents in order to deal with their own identity problems. Children who have been abused either physically or sexually or are generally neglected may also need long-term therapy.

This section will look in more detail at the different therapeutic interventions used to achieve these adjustments within the family system.

THE SYSTEMS APPROACH

Family therapy

The behaviour and emotions of a child are affected if not caused by the interaction between parent and child. All child psychiatric services spend some time with at least one parent, usually the mother, but in family therapy the whole family is seen. This includes mother, father and all the children and may involve grandparents or other significant relatives or friends.

There are three main approaches (Speed 1984) in family therapy, two of which developed in the USA. British and Australian practitioners tend to adapt these approaches according to the needs of their own service or person preferences.

THE STRUCTURAL APPROACH

This approach was developed by Salvador Minuchin in Philadelphia. The therapist looks for dysfunctions in the family's internal organisation, such as the lack of differentiation between parental and child responsibilities, leading to lack of parental authority. The therapist would seek to restructure the family's organisation with the result that the original symptom would no longer be necessary. Minuchin aims to achieve this within the sessions so that the family experiences these new ways of relating.

THE STRATEGIC APPROACH

The Brief Therapy Project at the Mental Research Institute (MRI) at Palo Alto, developed the strategic approach. This group looks for detailed explanations of the behaviour being presented and then examines the sequences following from this behaviour. Their concern is to tackle the presenting problem by changing the sequences of responses usually elicited by that behaviour. They are not aiming to change the family structure.

THE MILAN OR SYSTEMATIC APPROACH

This approach was developed by Palazzoli, Boscolo, Cecchin and Prata, working together in Italy until 1980. Therapists influenced by this approach take detailed information from each family member, often asking sister to speak for brother, father for mother so different members' interpretations of events and ideas are gathered. The aim is to gain a clear picture of the family's patterns of relating and to block or disrupt the dysfunctional ones in order to allow the family to develop new ones. This may consist of giving the family a message that they find provocative or ridiculous. For instance, a child may be told to continue to stay home to look after her mother, as the mother is unable to stay home alone since the death of her own mother, and that this then enables father to work the long hours he feels necessary. A message such as this is to jolt the parents into making more appropriate arrangements for their emotional support.

PRACTISING FAMILY THERAPY

Family therapists in Britain may use ideas from any or all of these schools of thought and may also be influenced by psychoanalytic theories, particularly object-relations theory, which concerns the learning of different relationships and the influence these early relationships have on later ones. This is frequently seen in patterns of mothering passed down from grandmother to daughter and granddaughter. Lieberman (1978) has also developed the use of the genogram or family tree in order to understand family patterns over generations.

Family therapists usually work in multidisciplinary teams, supervising and supporting each other by the use of co-therapy, video or one-way screens. Most are doctors, social workers, psychologists, nurses or occupational therapists. They may practise only family therapy or may integrate it into their other responsibilities. A family approach can be practised where only an individual is in therapy if the aim is treatment within the context of the family.

This approach to therapy is of particular interest to occupational therapists as it looks at the functioning of whole structure. The techniques used are often very active compared with traditional psychotherapy. The structural approach includes moving people from chair to chair to experience different degrees of closeness to family members and other techniques also used in dramatherapy. A family may be given a task to perform in the session to assess their patterns of organisation, such as a family meal for families of anorexic clients. The drawing of a family tree is a task that the therapist may use to involve all family members, including small children. An awareness of the individual's role in the family is crucial to so much of the occupational therapist's task in facilitating the client's return to that family.

Aims of intervention

By assessment of the child within the family, the context of the child's symptoms are understood. For instance, if there is marital disharmony a child's nightmares or failure to sleep may distract attention from parental arguments in bed. The aim of the family therapist is to enable the family to make the changes within itself that will allow the child to relinquish the symptoms.

NETWORK MEETINGS
Aims of intervention

Some families are in contact with many professionals simultaneously such as general practitioner, health visitor, social worker, NSPCC worker, teacher, psychologist and occupational therapist. The combined input of network of professionals may only result in the family staying exactly as it is. It may be important to have occasional meetings of the network to observe how the family use different members of the network and how the professionals involvement reflects this.

Common problems

Network meetings are more often required when the family has multiple problems that engage several agencies (Miller et al 1981). For example, the Grey family consists of Mr Grey, who is in prison for theft and Mrs Grey, who is having difficulty coping with the three children, aged 12, 8 and 2. The professional network could include:

- Probation officer: preparing for Mr Grey's release
- Social worker: child protection worker
- General practitioner: Mrs Grey's anxiety and depression
- Health visitor: care of 2-year-old
- Homestart: voluntary agency helping with young children
- School nurse: concerned about physical welfare of 8-year-old
- Teacher: 8-year-old
- Teacher: 12-year-old
- Occupational therapist: } working with Mrs Grey to gain more control over the children's behaviour.
- Psychologist:

MULTI-FAMILY GROUPS

Several families may be asked to meet together in a group to discuss the difficulties they encounter. This may also involve their children.

Aims of intervention

It is often reassuring for parents to realise other families are struggling with similar problems and they may be able to offer each other practical advice as well as moral support. These groups are often associated with residential units so can also be used for residential staff and parents to compare their handling of a child (Barker 1986).

Common problems

Families or households who do not conform to the accepted norm of mother, father and two children may be able to share their innovative methods of coping, for example, step families or single-parent families. Other families may have similar crises to overcome, for example, bereavement, child sexual abuse, or a member in prison.

THERAPY FOR ADULTS

Co-parenting

The problem in many families referred for treatment is that they have no previous experience in parenting and may not have had the opportunity to learn from relatives or friends. Others have very strong opinions on parenting, learnt in their families of origin, but these opinions may be conflicting.

Aims of intervention

The task in the first group is to teach the parents adequate parenting skills, which may involve behavioural tasks, for example, telling the child clearly what is expected of him and ensuring that he does as he is told, using appropriate punishments where necessary. The parents need to learn to be consistent over time so that the child learns when mummy says 'no' she means it and also that both parents mean 'no' so that if mother has said 'no' and father is appealed to, he will back up his wife. This will entail parents spending time together deciding on family rules and appropriate sanctions, which is likely to give greater security to the children and a feeling of mutual achievement for parents when they experience the success of their combined efforts.

Where there are conflicting opinions about styles of parenting, the couple may find it useful to compare their own experiences and expectations for their children and then to work out mutually acceptable compromises.

Common problems

- Inexperienced parents facing the toddler's first tantrums or baby's sleep disturbances.
- Relationships where one parent is frequently absent, such as lorry drivers or forces personnel.
- Divorced couples may require support to continue their parenting roles after the marital relationship has been dissolved.
- Couples whose relationship is strained may be more able to join together on parenting responsibilities. Success in achieving a common task may then enable them to discuss difficulties in the marital relationship.

MARITAL THERAPY

Aims of intervention

Occupational therapists may have little experience in this area of work, until working in a Child and Family treatment setting. Many of the approaches in family therapy may be used in couple therapy, as there is now more emphasis placed on interpersonal relationships than intra-psychic difficulties. Barker (1986) provides a useful introduction to different types of marital therapy and cites further references. A conciliation service may be offered to a couple during divorce to assist the parents to come to a relatively amicable arrangement about the custody of the children.

Some children may be showing behavioural disturbances because they are sensitive to the disharmony in their parents' marriage. The parents may no longer be able to take joint responsibility for parenting the children. One or both parents may be very sad or angry about their situation and the children may be called on to support one or another parent. Many couples recognise that the children are reflecting themselves.

Common problems

Children caught in the emotional cross-fire between parents may present with any range of problems. Particularly after a divorce, a child may struggle to bring his parents together again, and even feel to blame for the separation.

Group work

A range of groups may be offered to support parents who are struggling in the tasks of parenthood owing to their personal difficult experiences.

WOMEN'S PSYCHOTHERAPY GROUPS

Mothers of referred children are placed in a group to discuss the difficulties they experience in managing their children. We discovered that most women referred had also experienced some level of inadequate care in their own childhood. This may have been taking inappropriate responsibility for other siblings at an early age, a mother suffering psychotic episodes, or sexual abuse. The mothers require support in talking about their own childhood, receiving nurture and support from other group members and therapists before they are able to accept other forms of therapy offered for them and their child.

GROUPS FOR ADULTS ON CHILD SEXUAL ABUSE

Many agencies are now using group work for adults in this situation. Mother may be involved in groups running parallel to the children's groups (Damon and Waterman 1986).

Perpetrators (who may be fathers or stepfathers) are increasingly placed in groups run by probation officers in order to confront their behaviour. Foster parents or grandparents who may be caring for children following disclosure of abuse may also benefit from meeting others to discuss the difficulties of caring for children who may be showing very disturbed behaviour.

Occupational therapists often have more group-work experience than other professionals in the team, so may well be involved in the groups for mothers or caretakers.

Aims of intervention: mother's groups

- To assist mothers in talking about their feelings about the abuse of their child, which may include disbelief, anger, guilt, or self-blame.
- To help mothers protect their children from reabuse.
- To give support to mothers in whom memories of their own abuse has been triggered. The aims for the caretakers' group are similar to those of the mothers', particularly the second

point, but the caretakers may also need to ventilate their feelings about experiences of abuse.

THERAPY FOR CHILDREN

Individual play therapy

Young children are often unable to talk about their troubles but by the use of play materials may be able to enact their worries. The child's perception of family relationships can often be observed in their play with the dolls and doll's house. Investigation into possible sexual abuse frequently uses anatomically correct dolls. These are also used in therapy for the abused child. Play therapy is an area in which many occupational therapists are developing special skills (see Ch. 16).

Residential treatment

The situation in some families requires that the child be separated from the family and admitted to a children's or adolescent unit. This may be 7 days per week or may allow the child to return home at weekends.

Aims of intervention

- To provide a separation between parents and child where the situation is intolerable for either party and yet there is a desire to work out a solution.
- To allow the child time away from the family to talk about what may have been very difficult experiences, such as abusive or neglectful parenting.
- In a service where emphasis is placed on family relationships, admission does not mean parents give up responsibility for their children but are required to be actively involved in therapy, by attending multi-family groups and having the child home, possibly at weekends. It is felt that the service will be unable to help the child without the backing of the parents.

Common problems

The most frequent reasons for admission are where the parents are no longer able to control the child, where the child is at risk of abuse from the parent or, in the case of adolescents, where the family structure is such that it prevents the young person from becoming more independent or self-reliant.

The role of occupational therapists in child and adolescent units varies enormously. Many occupational therapists are becoming play-therapy specialists, others run groups for adolescents or parents, or may practise family therapy. It is worth noting that most units employ teachers for school-age children so there is frequently some overlap between therapists and teachers in the use of activities.

GROUP WORK WITH CHILDREN

Groups may be used with children of 5 years and above. The techniques used need to be appropriate to the developmental level of the child, so that young children will require media- and action-based therapy, whereas adolescents have the ability for verbal psychotherapy groups. Art and drama are appropriate for all age groups.

Aims of intervention

- Groups may be behavioural in approach to enable the child to learn different methods of reacting to situations. Role play, video filming, and task setting may all be used.
- Occupational therapists may run these groups in conjunction with psychologists or teachers.
- Group work with adolescents may enable them to share their difficulties in negotiation of an independent identity, exploring sexuality and making decisions about possible careers. Specific groups may be arranged for girls with eating problems or children coping with bereavement.
- Some psychotherapy groups enable children and adolescents to express their feelings about traumatic events in their lives, such as groups for survivors of sexual abuse. Survivors may need to explore their conflicting emotions about their parents, their fears of being damaged, coping with the stigma, and hopes for the future. These groups usually involve some action techniques, as these very powerful emotions may be difficult to put into words. Again, this is an area where occu-

pational therapists have much to contribute. It is also a very difficult area, and any therapist requires supervision and support from a team member experienced in sexual abuse work.

BEHAVIOUR THERAPY

Although behaviour therapy focuses on the child's actions, the parents are also required to learn different methods of coping with their children. Parents specify the behaviour they would like their child to change. The therapist then notes events leading up to the undesired behaviour, the behaviour itself and the parental response. It is also important to be aware of when the child behaves well, as the effectiveness of behaviour therapy is in the child learning to behave well for the rewards this brings. Ultimately these rewards are parental approval, respect and attention.

One method of achieving this is by use of a star chart. Child and parents make a chart to record the required behaviour. For instance, if a child wets the bed, he receives a star for each dry night. The first week he may receive a treat from the parents for two stars, the next week three stars, and so on, until the child no longer needs the chart. This will generally help the problem within the first few weeks if it is the appropriate tool.

Aims of intervention

- To change the problematic behaviour of the child by rewarding positive behaviour.
- To enable parents and children to define realistic goals.

Common problems

Specific behavioural problems such as bedwetting and soiling may respond to a change in the reward system. Temper tantrums may also be controlled where the precipitating factors can be defined, such as demanding sweets when shopping or refusal to go to bed.

SUMMARY

A family approach to individual problems represents a major shift from one professional working with one client. The aim of therapy is to enable the family to develop its own resources to heal itself, in contrast to a medical model of treatment where the doctor or professional heals the client. This requirement for the client to take an active role in his therapy is also part of the rehabilitation process that enables the client to resume his position in his family and social networks.

The role of an occupational therapist in this type of setting may be very varied so that an ability to define one's own role within a multidisciplinary team is essential. There may be only one occupational therapist on the team and so she needs to be able to take and give support and supervision from other disciplines.

Occupational therapists working in other areas of psychiatry, or indeed general medicine, may find an understanding of family dynamics useful in the rehabilitation process. Families caring for mentally handicapped members are necessarily involved in treatment and an awareness of family processes may aid an occupational therapist in working with the family. The attitudes of families to disability may also play a critical part in successful rehabilitation. Occupational therapists working with clients in groups in adult psychiatric settings may also enable the client to work with his family problems within the group.

A family approach is a relatively new area of psychiatry, which may gain some influence in outpatient treatment, and particularly in the development of community psychiatry where some contact with the family is inevitable, but the understanding gained from the theories behind it can be of value to occupational therapists working in many settings.

REFERENCES

Barker P 1986 Basic family therapy. Collins, London

Brown G H, Harris T 1978 Social origins of depression: a study of psychiatric disorders in women. Tavistock, London

Damon L, Waterman J 1986 Parallel group treatment of children and their mothers. In: Macfarlane K, Waterman J (eds) Sexual abuse of young children, Holt, Rinehart & Winston, London

Dicks H V 1967 Marital tensions, Routledge, Kegan & Paul, London

Gordon V 1981 A multi-resource approach. In: Miller et al (eds) Direct work with families. Bedford Square Press, London

Lieberman S 1978 Transgenerational family therapy. Croom Helm, Kent

Llorens L A 1970 Facilitating growth and development: the promise of occupational therapy. The American Journal of Occupational Therapy 14(2)

Miller et al 1981 Direct work with families. Bedford Square Press, London

Minuchin S 1974 Families and family therapy. Tavistock, London

Oakley A 1980 Women confined. Martin Robertson, Oxford

Schlicht J 1984 Personal communication

Speed B 1984 Family therapy: an update. Association of Child Psychology and Psychiatry Bulletin 6(1) January 1984

Skynner A C R 1976 One flesh — separate persons: principles of family and marital psychotherapy. Constable, London

Walrond-Skinner S (ed) 1981 Developments in family therapy: theories and application since 1948. Routledge, Kegan & Paul, London

FURTHER READING

Family therapy

Barker P 1986 Basic family therapy. Collins, London

Synner R, Cleese J 1983 Families and how to survive them. Methuen, London

Treacher A, Carpenter J 1984 Using family therapy. Basil Blackwell, Oxford

Jacques P 1987 Understanding children's problems: helping families to help themselves. Unwin, London

Women's therapy

Eichenbaum L, Orbach S 1983 Understanding women. Penguin, Harmondsworth

Lawrence M 1984 The anorexic experience. The Women's Press, London

Child sexual abuse

Elliott M 1985 Preventing child sexual assault: a practical guide to talking with children. Bedford Square Press, London

Macfarlene K, Waterman J 1986 Sexual abuse of young children. Holt, Rinehart and Winston, London

Sgroi S 1988 Handbook of clinical intervention in child sexual abuse, Lexington, Massachusetts

Glaser D, Frosh S 1988 Child sexual abuse. British Association of Social Workers. Macmillan, Basingstoke

Behaviour therapy

Westmacott E V S, Cameron R J 1981 Behaviour can change. Macmillan

USEFUL ADDRESSES

Association for Family Therapy (AFT): produces Journal of Family Therapy, has local branches and groups and organises an Annual Training Meeting.

Institute of Family Therapy (IFT)
43 New Cavendish Street
London W1
(Organises workshops and courses on Family Therapy.)

The Association for the Psychiatric Study of Adolescence
David Duff (Membership Secretary (APSA)
13 Bondly Drive
Edinburgh EH13 OEJ
(Produces the journal of Adolescence. Organises Annual Conference.)

Association for Child Psychology & Psychiatry (ACPP)
4 Southamptom Row
London WC1B 1AB
(Produces a newsletter and journal)

23

Mental handicap

Jennifer Creek

INTRODUCTION

Mental handicap refers to a failure to develop normal intellectual functioning, associated with impairment of adaptive behaviour. Approximately 3.7 per 1000 of the general population can be so described, although the incidence varies slightly in different countries due to environmental factors (Hall 1984). When normal development is delayed, the individual will have special difficulty in coping with life events, even minor ones, and may use maladaptive behaviours in order to reduce the anxiety generated by failure. These secondary handicaps are usually a greater problem than the primary mental handicap.

This chapter looks at how occupational therapy can help people with mental handicaps to overcome secondary handicaps and develop to their fullest potential through the use of appropriate activity. Traditional ways of classifying mental handicap and of caring for people with mental handicaps are outlined. The concept of deviance is then discussed, and this provides a background to examining changes in outlook now taking place. The concept and application of the principle of social role valorisation are described, highlighting how it has influenced new patterns of care. Occupational therapy is described in the context of this new approach. The process of assessment, setting aims, treatment planning and implementation and evaluation of outcomes is outlined using Case examples to illustrate treatment of different problem areas. Looking ahead to the closure of mental-handicap hospitals, the role of the occupational therapist in helping people through the transition from institution to community is examined. Finally, the variety of work undertaken by occupational therapists in the community is described, using case histories as illustrations.

WHAT IS MENTAL HANDICAP?

There are many ways of looking at mental handicap, for example, by level of intellectual skill (IQ), amount of care needed, functional ability or cause. Most classification systems include several factors, such as the four categories described by the World Health Organisation (WHO 1980):

1. Mild mental handicap (IQ 52–67) may only be a matter of delayed development. Children can be educated and adults can work in ordinary employment following training. They may lead independent lives and never be classified as being mentally handicapped.
2. Moderate mental handicap (IQ 36–51). Affected persons are obviously handicapped but may learn self-help skills and work in sheltered employment.
3. Severe mental handicap (IQ 20–35). There may be delayed development or failure to develop physical and communication skills. Often, affected people are also physically handicapped but they can still show limited independence.
4. Profound mental handicap (IQ 0–19). Affected people require 24-hour care for survival. Physical and sensory development may be grossly impaired, with physical handicap.

People with mild handicap make up approximately 89% of the total mentally handicapped population, those with a moderate handicap comprise 6%, those with a severe handicap 3.5% and those with a profound handicap 1.5% (Copeland et al 1976).

DEFINITION OF TERMS

WHO (1980) supplied the following definitions.

● *Impairment*: 'any loss or abnormality of psychological, physiological or anatomical structure or function'.

● *Disability*: 'any restriction or lack (resulting from an impairment) of ability to perform an activity in the manner or within the range considered normal for a human being'.

● *Handicap*: 'a disadvantage for an individual, resulting from an impairment or disability, that limits or prevents the fulfilment of a role that is normal (depending on age, sex and social and cultural factors) for that individual'.

CAUSES

Mental handicap may be caused by single or, more usually, multiple factors, both genetic and environmental. WHO divides causes into 10 groups:

0. following infection and intoxication
1. following trauma or physical agent
2. associated with disorder of metabolism, growth or nutrition
3. associated with gross brain disease (postnatal)
4. associated with diseases and conditions resulting from unknown prenatal influence.
5. chromosomal abnormality
6. associated with prematurity
7. following major psychiatric disorder
8. associated with psychosocial (environmental) deprivation
9. unspecified.

The cause of mental handicap is known only in just over half of the cases diagnosed. In the UK, genetic factors are thought to be the primary cause in about 37% of cases and environmental factors in about 20% of cases (Heaton-Ward 1975). Most causes of mental handicap are non-progressive.

PREVENTION

As the causes of mental handicap are discovered, measures can be taken to prevent handicapped children from being conceived or born. In the cases of genetic or chromosomal disorders, counselling can be given to parents, advising them of the risks. Health education and public health measures play an important role in preventing disease, malnutrition or poisoning through ignorance of the dangers to the unborn child. When an abnormality is suspected in the foetus, scans or amniocentesis are used to confirm a diagnosis so that abortion can be offered.

Some simple screening tests are used on all new-born babies to detect any obvious handicapping conditions, such as Down's Syndrome (a genetic defect) or phenylketonuria (a metabolic defect). Some diseases, such as phenylketonuria, can be controlled by a strict diet, which prevents the abnormal accumulation of metabolites in the body. In other cases, the emphasis is on family support and provision of appropriate stimulation so that the child's development proceeds as normally as possible in spite of the handicap.

Further developmental screening is offered at regular intervals for every pre-school child, and children falling behind their peers are assessed further to seek the cause.

However, it is likely that for the foreseeable future there will be a percentage of people born with some degree of mental handicap and, as Western medicine becomes more skilled in keeping very physically ill or disabled people alive, a greater proportion of them will have severe or profound handicaps.

CHANGING APPROACHES TO MENTAL HANDICAP

The majority of children and adults with a mental handicap live at home, this being seen as the ideal environment in most cases. For those whose families cannot cope, the main mode of care in Europe this century has been in institutions, segregating them from the general public. At its best, the institution is a true asylum, providing for all the needs of people who cannot cope with life in the open community. The main drawback of this type of care is that it does not encourage, or even allow for, change and growth in the individual, so that once admitted to the institution it is very hard for a person to develop the skills that will enable him to leave again.

The traditional view of mental handicap as inevitably disabling is gradually being superseded by a social model. Increasing knowledge about the causes and treatment of mental handicap and new methods of assessing and training handicapped people encourage the realisation that they can be helped to overcome their disadvantages.

In the UK, current government policy is to run down large institutions for people with mental handicaps and to resettle the residents in small hostels or houses scattered throughout the community. This is part of a move to take away the stigma of mental handicap and to allow people to live as normal a life as possible. The policy has been in operation for several years and large numbers of people have already been resettled. It is hoped that all large institutions will be closed by the end of the next decade.

In this section we look at both traditional care and at alternative ways of viewing mental handicap, with the new patterns of care these views have generated.

THE TRADITIONAL APPROACH

Community occupational therapy is a relatively recent innovation, and people living at home have not had access to the service unless they attended a day centre. The main role of occupational therapists has traditionally been in large institutions.

In a setting where people are seen as needing permanent care, the role of the occupational therapist becomes that of enhancer of the quality of institutional life. In 1948 Chorley described the role of the occupational therapist in the institution:

The fact must be faced that mental defectives are part of the community in which we all live. Sooner or later they will be segregated and sent into an institution, here to be dependent on those into whose care they have been sent to give them as much care and training as will make them happier and more useful citizens in the institutional life they have been forced to adopt, maybe for the rest of their lives. Work is a necessity to life. The types of patient that need the trained occupational therapist are those who would otherwise be sitting in the wards or aimlessly wandering around the closed-in gardens. They are sent to the handicraft room. They go to *work*. The joy it gives them to be at *work*, the added meaning it gives to their simple lives is worth any amount of time expended on them.

Basic physical and security needs are met at ward level, leaving higher needs, such as productivity and self-esteem, to be dealt with by activity programmes. The emphasis has traditionally been put on productive work that allows people to feel that they are contributing members of society in spite of being segregated from it, as emphasised by Chorley (1948).

Occupational therapists tend to work with large groups of clients and there is a high proportion of unqualified to qualified staff. The range of activities used must, to some extent, be dictated by heavy caseloads and low staffing levels.

Activities traditionally used include industrial work, woodwork, gardening, care of animals and crafts. Some training in self-care and domestic activities may be given to help people attain a degree of independence, although the success of such programmes is dependent on the attitude and involvement of ward staff. Recreational and social programmes are also seen as important for people whose whole life is to be spent within the institution. Activities used include sports, dancing, games, drama, concerts and outings. Most hospitals have their own bus, which is used for taking clients out, so that they are in a sense still within the institution while in the community.

NEW APPROACHES

We have looked at ways of classifying mental handicap by the cause or by the degree of disability the individual suffers. However, it is also possible to see handicap as socially defined. Each culture decides what constitutes a handicap and what is within normal limits. For example, in a rural area where the work is mostly physically demanding but routine and unvarying, intellectual ability is not as important as it would be in a fast-changing, highly mobile urban environment. Increasingly, handicap is being seen as the outcome of interaction between the individual and the environment rather than being the inevitable consequence of having an impairment (Hogg & Raynes 1987).

Mental handicap as deviance

Deviance means a significant difference from the cultural norm that is given a negative value. A deviant person is considered to be inferior to the rest of society in some important characteristic; for example, prostitutes are seen as socially unacceptable in Britain because of the way they earn money. A difference that is valued negatively in one culture may be positively valued in another, for example, homosexuality is condemned in some societies while in other it is considered normal, or even desirable, therefore deviance is socially defined.

When a person bears a visible difference, called a 'stigma', he is often perceived as being deviant not only in the visible negative characteristic but often as a whole person. The stigma becomes generalised to include his whole identity and other defects may be attributed to him because of it.

The process of giving a person a deviant status is called 'labelling', for example, someone who has difficulty controlling his drinking is labelled an alcoholic. Once a person is labelled, there are expectations that he should respond in a certain way, and all his behaviour may be seen as deviant, even behaviour that might be seen as normal in someone else.

In many cultures, people with a mental handicap are perceived as deviant and given low social status. The deviant individual learns that he bears a stigma from the responses that he evokes in social encounters. Many people eventually come to accept the label and status given to them. This then becomes a self-fulfilling prophecy; the individual conforms to the expectations placed on him (Goffman 1963, Mangen 1982).

Social management of deviance

Since deviant people, by definition, do not conform to the norms of society, society has to find ways of containing them, preferably in a way that will not disrupt others. Erikson (1967) suggests that deviants serve a stabilising function in society by marking the boundaries of acceptable social behaviour. By condemning deviant behaviour, society is confirming the acceptability of normal behaviour.

Deviance can be managed by removing deviant individuals from society or by reversing the deviant characteristic. Segregation is achieved by placing the deviant person outside society, for example, by siting institutions for the mentally handicapped in the country, away from population centres.

Reversal of deviance may be achieved by treatment or training to remove the stigma or, since deviance is socially defined, by social redefinition. Social redefinition of mental handicap, to avoid the negative value attached to it, would involve placing less positive value on intellectual achievement. Some sub-cultures, such as certain religious groups, do not place undue emphasis on intellect but the mainstream of society values intelligence highly. Even if people of low intelligence are accepted into the community, training is an essential precursor to discharge from an institution if they are to be enabled to remain there. Any serious evidence of deviance is likely to result in social rejection and resegregation.

The changing role of the occupational therapist

The traditional role of the occupational therapist, as described earlier in the chapter, is no longer applicable in the new type of service for people with handicaps. There are exciting new opportunities for becoming involved in all aspects of care, from facilitating the move out of institutions to improving the quality of life in the community.

In the field of mental handicap, above all others, the therapist works as part of a team. No one profession or individual member of staff can meet all the needs of the person with multiple handicaps: intellectual, emotional, social and possibly physical.

The multidisciplinary team usually consists of nurse, psychologist, occupational therapist, physiotherapist, psychiatrist, social worker and, perhaps, parent.

In many instances, team members work separately but maintain strong liaison and communication structures so that work is coordinated. However, multidisciplinary programmes may be developed, such as behaviour modification programmes, which require everyone to be involved in planning, implementing and evaluating the outcome. It can also be very beneficial to work together in joint-therapy sessions so that staff learn

from each other's skills, support each other in using techniques and generate new ideas (Creek et al 1987).

Occupational therapy has its own unique contribution to make from the occupational, holistic and developmental perspective of the profession. While acknowledging the core skills that all therapists have, it is useful to identify the special contribution of the occupational therapist in the three main areas of service provision:

1. developing new skills
2. helping people prepare to leave the institution
3. working with people living in the community.

DEVELOPING NEW SKILLS

After many years in an institution, most people will have learned skills for living comfortably within such an environment. A move to a totally different environment, such as a private house in the community, requires that the individual not only learns new skills but also unlearns some of his institutional behaviour. Occupational-therapy media and methods are designed to promote the development and maintenance of new skills for the performance of self-care, work and leisure activities.

THE PROCESS OF INTERVENTION

Intervention involves the client and therapist agreeing on an overall goal that is compatible with the goals of the multidisciplinary team. The overall goal is broken down into sub-goals, which are the steps the client will take, or skills that he will learn, on the way to the final goal. In practice, the life experiences of many handicapped people are so limited that they may not be able to visualise large changes and can only participate in planning small, short-term goals. However, the therapist and team will always have a final goal in mind, such as acquiring the skills necessary for successful resettlement in a group home.

The whole process of intervention, from assessment through goal setting, treatment planning and treatment implementation, is a collaborative exercise between client and therapist.

Assessment

Prior to attempting to set goals, the therapist assesses the client's skills and areas of skill deficit so that these can be measured against the anticipated demands of the future environment. Assessment results are for the benefit of the client as much as for the therapist, since he will more easily engage in treatment if he understands the aims.

Assessment is the process of collecting and organising data, in collaboration with the client, to use in making decisions about aspects of his life (Harvey 1986). The type of data that is required will be dependent on the model being used; for example, within a behavioural model the therapist will want to know how a client behaves in particular situations and under specified conditions. The model will also determine the method of data collection to be used, for example, the Role Checklist was developed for use within the model of human occupation (Kielhofner 1988).

Several different types of assessment methods are used with people who have a mental handicap:

- *Psychometric tests* designed to measure specific skills or abilities, such as intelligence and memory tests. These types of tests are not widely used by occupational therapists.
- *Developmental screening*, or norm-referenced tests, used to find out how someone is performing in relation to his peers.
- *Checklists and rating scales*, such as activities of daily living checklists. Some of these are comprehensive and very complex, building up a picture of the person's abilities and deficits over a wide range of skills.
- *Interviews*, including unstructured, semi-structured and structured interviews.
- *Observations*, including random observation during treatment, observation during structured activities and systematic observation using a sampling schedule. Observation is widely used by occupational therapists and can include the use of checklists to ensure that no important functions are missed.
- *Criterion-referenced tests* or behavioural train-

ing packages, such as the Bereweeke Skill-teaching System (Felce et al 1986). These packages include a checklist of the desired skills in the sequence in which they are to be learned and suggested activities for assessing each item.

Treatment planning

In some settings where the therapist works with people who have a mental handicap, the time-scale for intervention is relatively long, but in others there is a fixed date for the closure of the institution and the therapist must keep to a schedule of resettlement.

When a referral is received, the occupational therapist reviews any records available and discusses the client with staff who already know him, such as the nursing staff. She then meets the client and decides how to carry out her initial assessment. An interview is the usual way, if it is appropriate. At this stage, the therapist does a preliminary analysis of the information collected so far and identifies which areas of performance are most basic and need to be developed.

If the therapist does not feel that the client can benefit from intervention at this time, either because the necessary resources are not available or because his active cooperation cannot be engaged, then she may either decide to refuse the referral or to put the client into a programme of undemanding activities that give structure to his time.

If active intervention seems appropriate, the therapist and client collaborate to plan a preliminary programme for the threefold purpose of:

1. introducing the client to occupational therapy and engaging his interest
2. making further detailed assessment of the problem area identified
3. starting treatment.

The programme may be full-time or only a few sessions a week, depending on the client's need and the places available.

The preliminary programme may vary in length but 6 weeks to 3 months is probably a realistic time. At the end of this period, a meeting is held to review the data gathered and plan a full programme. At this stage agreement should be reached on the long-term goals of therapy but it should be remembered that these goals may change as more information emerges. The main considerations in setting goals are:

- the client's personal goals, for example, marriage
- the overall goals of the treatment team, for example, transfer to a group home
- the current level of functioning of the client, resources available for intervention and predicted outcome (this may be modified during the course of treatment).

CASE EXAMPLE 23.1   SETTING GOALS

James is a 53-year-old man who has spent most of his life in an institution. The hospital is now scheduled for closure and James will have to move to alternative accommodation. In setting goals for intervention the therapist considers:

- James's expressed desire to live alone and independently
- the local policy for transferring all residents into social-services-staffed group homes
- James's skills and deficits in the areas of self-care, communication, emotional stability, knowledge of community resources and social skills.

The long-term goals set in agreement with James are to:

- improve his self-care skills to a level at which he can look after his hygiene and dressing without assistance
- assist him to have a more realistic view of his abilities and needs so that he will accept help when necessary
- introduce him to community resources, particularly those he might be able to use without help
- improve his social skills to a level that will be acceptable in the community.

Long-term goals are broken down into steps that are used as short-term goals. These are planned in a hierarchy so that each goal achieved forms the basis for the next one. As each set of short-term goals is reached, a new set is agreed between the therapist and client. This can be done without calling a case review if the new goals are still within the agreed long-term plan. If the experience of working towards short-term goals suggests that the long-term goals need to be modified then a case review should be organised, including all the people who were involved in the original treatment plan.

Selecting activities for attaining goals is an essential part of treatment planning. The therapist can suggest activities she knows from her analysis will meet the client's needs but the client must make a commitment to engage in the activity or it will be of no value. Some clients are able to tolerate an activity they do not enjoy because they can see the benefit it will bring but most people with a mental handicap would have difficulty understanding how they can benefit from being uncomfortable and need to find the activity pleasurable.

Treatment implementation

Organising a department to cater for the varied needs of clients is not easy, especially when there are staff shortages and the buildings are unsuitable for small group or individual therapy. Activities must be selected to meet the needs of the client, not clients selected to join in preplanned activities. Each client will have an individual programme designed to meet his short-term goals. Ideally, this timetable will be written down so that the client and everyone else is aware of it. Even someone who cannot read may enjoy having his own programme, which symbolises his individuality and importance.

Fortunately, there are many activities which are known to be adaptable and to meet a range of needs (Creek & Wells 1988). These can be programmed into a basic weekly timetable so that new clients can be slotted into appropriate sessions according to their needs. The therapist's skills in activity analysis and synthesis can be used to tailor each session to the specific needs of the clients. The actual groups on offer at any one time will change as the needs of the client population change.

In addition to group work in the department there may also be daily work-orientated sessions, run by unqualified staff, and outings on a regular or occasional basis. There will also be time for working with clients individually and time for seeing new clients. There are always times in the working day when clients are not available for therapy, for example, because of transport or mealtimes, and these time can be used for non-client activities such as staff meetings, administration and writing notes.

Given the broad range of needs of people with mental handicaps, the shortage of qualified-occupational therapists in the field and the large numbers of people requiring intervention in any one treatment setting, the occupational therapist must have a clear picture of her role and priorities if she is to cope with her workload. Whether referrals are made individually or the therapist can select her clients from the total population, there are three options available:

1. To provide some kind of service for everyone who is referred for occupational therapy, usually with major input from unqualified staff. This type of service is likely to be geared to the group rather than to the individual. It has the advantages of pleasing other staff, who are freed to do more specific work with individuals, and satisfying the managers' requirements for large numbers of people to be 'treated'.

2. To select clients who are most likely to benefit from intervention, which does not necessarily mean the most able people, and work intensively with them until they are able to move on to other settings such as sheltered accommodation.

3. To provide a certain amount of input to everyone referred, even if it is only one or two sessions a week. Each person is given the quality of intervention he requires, although not the ideal quantity. This is a compromise between quality and quantity of intervention but is usually an acceptable one, given the constraints most therapist work under.

Usually, several skill areas will be developed simultaneously, which is how normal development occurs. For example, by engaging in an activity successfully the individual has the opportunity to:

● learn that he can affect his environment, thus changing his self-image

● discover that this activity exists and is available to him, thus extending his range of choices
● experience the process of carrying out the activity so that he is exposed to the need for a mental plan of action
● find out whether or not he enjoys the experience or finds it valuable, thus beginning to develop his own value system
● begin to learn the skills required for the performance of the activity, even if he is only performing at the playful/exploratory state of learning
● gain feedback from the environment to discover what his actions have achieved and how other people view his actions.

Intervention may involve blocking habits that have been developed within the institution in order to promote healthy new development. The process of redeveloping skills is facilitated by the removal of any barriers to successful performance, both intrinsic, such as maladaptive habits, and extrinsic, such as social isolation.

It is rarely possible to give each client the amount of time he appears to need but, if intervention is at an appropriate level and engages the client's interest, then he should be able to continue developing skills outside the treatment sessions. Occupational therapists merely offer the option of therapeutic activity, the client does the work of using occupation to make changes, therefore the therapeutic process is not dependent on the presence of the therapist.

ACTIVITIES TO FACILITATE THE DEVELOPMENT OF NEW SKILLS

Occupational therapy facilitates the development of new skills in three stages.

1. Giving people an opportunity to explore different options and see the choices open to them so that they can make genuine decisions for themselves. The first stage of learning is playful and client centred, not product centred.
2. Providing opportunities to practise skills in a variety of situations until a level of competence has been reached. If someone has a low cognitive level

then they may need many trials before they master a new skill.

3. Enabling clients to use skills to attain their own ends. Skills will fade if not used and people will only continue to use skills which bring about a desired result.

People with mental handicaps often have extra difficulty in learning new skills, particularly because within the institutional environment they have never had opportunities to be playful and have always been encouraged to 'act their age'. Part of the task of the therapist is to enable them to enter the explorative phase of learning in a playful and relaxed manner. A long time may be spent enabling playfulness before learning can begin.

As already stated, people normally develop several skills at the same time through activity but activities can be selected or adapted to facilitate the development of particular skills. The remainder of this section suggests activities that might be used to develop:

- physical skills
- cognitive skills
- intrapersonal skills
- interpersonal skills.

Case histories are used to illustrate how activities might be used to develop particular skill areas.

Physical skills

Physical activities may range from general keep-fit and sports sessions to programmes for developing specific skills in individuals, such as training hand–eye coordination. If possible, these sessions take place in community facilities so that the benefits of integration are achieved at the same time as the benefits of exercise. For example, the residents of one institution were taken horse-riding at the local stables and for gym at a local community centre (see Ch. 10, p. 155). Any contraindications to vigorous exercise should be observed and programmes should be coordinated with the work of the physiotherapists.

Examples of physical activities include:

- keep fit

- swimming
- dancing
- gardening
- sports
- crafts
- cookery.

CASE EXAMPLE 23.2 INTERVENTION IN THE AREA OF PHYSICAL SKILLS

John is a 42-year-old man with a profound mental handicap and spastic quadriplegia. He is doubly incontinent, has no speech and is not independently mobile. He has limited hand function and does not feed himself. However, he can recognise people he knows and reacts with smiles to people he likes.

John's cognitive ability is low and further development is hampered by his inability to explore the environment. He can focus his gaze on an object of interest, such as food or a face, and can reach a short way towards something he wants, but he has difficulty in visually following a moving object.

He is generally a contented man who loves being in company, watches and listens to people around him, responds joyfully to individual attention and tries to communicate. If left alone for too long he shouts until someone comes to him.

Although John has deficiencies in all four skill areas, it is clear that the most basic development is physical and that he needs intensive intervention to facilitate development in this area.

The physiotherapy department is working on improving his seating so that his posture is more upright, improving general mobility by hydrotherapy and trying to extend his reach. The occupational therapist is giving John a feeding programme and working on tracking a moving object and hand–eye coordination, using a range of art media. The speech therapist is also involved in this programme as she hopes John will learn to use a signing board when his reach improves and he can visually scan.

Cognitive functioning

Cognitive skills are an integral part of any purposeful activity and must be considered in activity analysis. Activities used by occupational therapists can vary in complexity from learning to make a

---

CASE EXAMPLE 23.3 INTERVENTION IN THE AREA OF COGNITIVE SKILLS

Fred is a 38-year-old man with Down's syndrome who has lived in an institution all his life. He is overweight but is physically active and particularly enjoys swimming and dancing. His vocabulary is very limited but he loves being in company and has a high level of social skills. He is usually very contented but hates any change in his routine and will react to change by becoming quiet and withdrawn for a while. He has several close friends.

Fred's main problem is his limited cognitive skills, although this is often masked by his excellent social skills. He performs well in routine, simple tasks that he is very familiar with but needs help to develop more concepts and make more sense of his world so that change becomes less threatening.

Fred has been attending for a full week of activities in the department for 3 years, mainly in the workshop. The decision is taken to introduce new activities gradually into his programme, giving him time to get used to each one before any more changes are made. To begin with, he is to be included in an art group once a week with three other people he knows well, to do painting and three-dimensional constructions. The group is client centred and participants are encouraged to carry out their own ideas. The other members have a higher cognitive level than Fred so they can act as role models for him.

Once Fred has been attending the art group happily for several weeks, he will be introduced to a small project group once a week. This group carries out projects of about 3 months' duration, including making and using puppets, making and using simple musical instruments, learning country dances, and doing a dance-drama of 'Peter and the Wolf.' Each of these projects involves using a range of cognitive skills and the therapist can reduce her input as the group becomes more confident and capable.

---

simple choice to learning how to budget and shop for food. A complex activity may be broken down into its component skills and each one taught by whatever method the occupational therapist favours, such as chaining. Simple skills may be learned as a whole.

Examples of activities to facilitate the development of cognitive skills include

- crafts
- community orientation programmes
- dance
- cookery
- discussion groups
- games
- drama.

Intrapersonal skills

The development of intrapersonal skills can be facilitated through the use of any activities that are appropriate to the present level of functioning of the client. The way in which an activity is presented and sequenced is more important in developing intrapersonal skills than the actual activity. Factors to consider include:

- need for appropriate level of individual attention or group interaction in order to develop a sense of being valued and valuable
- need for curiosity to be aroused by selecting an activity that is difficult enough to be challenging to the client without being so difficult as to cause frustration.
- need for success so that a sense of the self as being active and competent is developed (Burke 1977)
- need for new experiences and choices in order to develop the ability to identify personal needs, interests and values (Kielhofner & Burke 1980).

Interpersonal skills

All activities used by occupational therapists require some degree of interpersonal interaction, either one-to-one or in groups. The amount and quality of this interaction can be manipulated to help the individual to develop new skills. Specific skills can also be taught by whatever method seems most appropriate for the individual client, such as modelling or role-playing. The initial training may be carried out within the hospital but people who have been living in institutions for a long time can only learn appropriate skills for

CASE EXAMPLE 23.4 PROMOTING THE DEVELOPMENT OF INTRAPERSONAL SKILLS

Ernie is a 36-year-old single man who has been resident in hospital for 20 years. He has a moderate mental handicap.

Ernie's mother died when he was a small child. His father remarried but the stepmother did not like Ernie and he was sent to live with his grandmother. The stepmother eventually left the father, who remarried again and took Ernie back home. Ernie received little support or attention while at home and has had no visits from his family since his admission to hospital.

Ernie was admitted to hospital at the age of 16 because he reacted to emotional upsets at home by becoming verbally and physically aggressive. When frustrated he becomes verbally abusive and sometimes physically violent. He has a habit of 'collecting' any papers he finds and putting them in his sports bag.

He has no apparent problems with perceptual-motor skills. He is able to comprehend and follow instructions, except when angry. His vocabulary is wide enough for him to communicate without difficulty. He can read and write his own name. However, Ernie has very low frustration tolerance and is unable to control his own aggression. He does not seek the company of his fellow residents. His relationships with staff are those of a child to adults rather than of an equal. His stealing and collecting, and his constant demands for attention, suggest a need for security, which he obviously did not have in childhood.

Ernie has no serious physical or cognitive problems and his social isolation seems to be due to his limited emotional development. He needs to have the opportunity to make stable relationships with adults of both sexes who can give him some of the good parenting he lacked as a child. Within the context of good parental relationships he can begin to develop a positive self-image, frustration tolerance and acceptable ways of coping with strong feelings.

Within the occupational therapy department he has a programme of individual sessions with a male technical instructor and with a female art therapist. He has a good, trusting relationship with both these staff. He also attends two workshop sessions a week when he is expected to carry out his own tasks without disrupting other people's work. When Ernie is disruptive he is sent back to the ward until he calms down. The staff are consistent in their disapproval of such behaviour but Ernie is never denied their unconditional positive regard.

CASE EXAMPLE 23.5 INTERVENTION IN THE AREA OF INTERPERSONAL SKILLS

Sarah is a 42-year-old woman who lives in a group home with three other people. She is severely mentally handicapped but is physically fit and mobile. Her concentration is poor so she is under-occupied during most of the day, even at the day centre where she wanders around talking to people.

She is a happy person who rarely seems to be bored or in a bad mood. Although she is very distractable, she has an excellent memory for anything she is interested in, which is people. She approaches people she knows or strangers with equal enthusiasm, often hugging them and keeping up a constant barrage of questions, which she does not wait to have answered. She is particularly interested in young men and will follow one around if allowed to. She has no close friends but does occasionally take a dislike to a particular person. Otherwise she is friendly with everyone.

Sarah's way of approaching people is very off-putting, especially for people who do not know her. Her habits of talking all the time and of touching inappropriately make her company undesirable. She needs help to develop more acceptable social skills so that people she approaches make her welcome and encourage her to stay with them.

Sarah's occupational therapy programme is a variety of small group activities, such as cookery and country dancing. She also goes out with the therapist as often as possible to the local shops or cafe. When Sarah is engaged in activity she is given praise and attention but when her behaviour is inappropriate she is given social disapproval, such as a frown or a word of censure.

The programme is effective for the time that Sarah is in it but she needs a full daytime programme, including a variety of interesting activities, that is not available at the moment. Sarah illustrates the need of people with disturbing behaviour problems to have their needs met rather than merely having their behaviour controlled.

community living by going out into the community to practise.

Suitable community activities include:

- shopping
- eating in a cafe or restaurant
- going to a pub
- using the local swimming baths or sports centre
- using the public library
- going to the cinema.

PREPARATION FOR MOVING OUT OF AN INSTITUTION

The task of preparing people to move out of institutions and into the community is immense, requiring the coordinated efforts of all staff. The occupational therapist might become involved because she has been working with the client in hospital, or because she is part of a community-based mental handicap team. Any intervention must include close liaison with other staff in the hospital and in the agency who are to take major responsibility for the client after discharge, whether health service, local authority or a charitable organisation.

WHAT IS PREPARATION FOR DISCHARGE?

Living in an institution, perhaps for many years, means that a person's entire home, work and social life is contained within that structured environment. In moving into the community people must learn to adapt to many new places, social situations, responsibilities, roles and people. People who have always lived at home with their families are usually independently mobile and accepted in social situations by the time they reach their teens, so a person who has very few community experiences has a lot to catch up with.

Some of the areas of preparation that the occupational therapist might be involved with include:

- introducing the concept of community to people who have little or no experience of it
- assisting people to find compatible companions to live with
- helping in the choice of a suitable home.

Introducing the concept of community

Before people can begin to learn practical living skills they need to know what the community is, whether they want to live there, who they want to live with and how much support they would like if they choose to make the move.

One method of putting over accurate information in a way that can be understood by most clients is to run a regular informal discussion group. Topics for discussion are raised by those attending so that people's anxieties can be expressed and dealt with. People who cannot speak or who need information to be repeated or put forward in different ways are encouraged to attend until they have obviously begun to grasp the concept of leaving the hospital.

The most obvious way of introducing community life is to accompany people out of the hospital grounds to use vaious community resources such as shops, cafes, libraries or swimming pools.

Finding compatible living companions

Many considerations influence the choice of who to live with on leaving the institution. Co-habitees may be from the same institution or possibly from different districts, now moving back to their area of origin or to the area where the family are living. People are often considered as possible co-habitees because they share the same ward and have similar abilities and level of independent functioning. Some people have particular friends and communicate readily that they would like to share a home.

Therapy sessions can be a good time for all staff to take note of:

- who appears to interact with whom in a positive way

- what needs of one person complement the needs of another
- what level of support each potential couple or group might require.

If a possible grouping emerges from these observations then the matter can be discussed in detail with those people concerned and all other staff with whom they come into contact.

If the group is still considered a possibility at this stage, then a weekly occupational therapy session can be arranged in order to:

- further test out as far as possible the compatibility of group members
- give opportunities for the clients to experience working as a group
- encourage clients to think about moving out of hospital.

CASE EXAMPLE 23.6 ESTABLISHING A GROUP OF COMPATIBLE PEOPLE

Ian, a man in his late forties with a mild mental handicap and severe physical handicaps, regularly attended a pre-discharge discussion group. Also in the group were Alec, in his early forties and with a moderate mental handicap, and Joan, a lady in her later thirties, also with a moderate mental handicap. Alec and Joan both had slight physical disabilities. All three took an interest in the possibility of moving out of the hospital. They lived on separate wards and so the features that suggested they were a compatible group emerged primarily during the discussion group and their weekly lunch cookery session.

These features included their all being a similar age and all having a lively sense of humour. Alec easily became anxious with men but felt comfortable in the company of women. However, he could offer practical help and assistance to Ian and thus feel more comfortable with him. Ian enjoyed the fact that the other two people made him feel part of the group and included him in their conversations, despite his being unable to speak. Joan found it difficult not to be clumsy, for example in the kitchen, but did not feel embarrassed about this in the company of the men, who never criticised her but helped clear up and made a joke out of the issue. Finally, all three required assistance in daily living skills, therefore nobody would monopolise the attention of support staff at the expense of the others.

Choosing a home

Following the identification of a group who have chosen to live together, plans must be made for the type of house required, where it is to be situated, what facilities are required, and so on. Staff who know the clients well must be the key workers in assisting the client in this process. If the occupational therapist has been working with the client at the stage of choosing compatible partners then she will also be involved in the move out of the hospital, in order to make the transition as smooth as possible.

The occupational therapist may contribute her knowledge of the client's strengths and needs and abilities in daily living skills by suggesting what type of support each person needs from staff in home and how much help should be offered in each activity of daily living. When a person has specific physical needs, such as wheelchair access, the therapist can offer her skills and knowledge in this area.

The person's interests should also be considered, for example, one man enjoyed riding a bike but had not yet learnt sufficient road-safety skills to ride it on public highways. In choosing a home he looked at houses that would afford him the opportunity to ride his bike in comparative safety; the headmaster of a school across the road willingly agreed to let him use the school playground to bike ride after school hours.

The actual move will be a gradual process so that each person has time to adjust to the idea of moving, get to know his living companions, choose furniture, wall coverings, carpets and pictures for the new house, learn about the local resources in his new neighbourhood and establish a daytime routine for the future.

Daytime routine

The occupational therapist also has a contribution to make in ensuring that the person leaving hospital has a suitable daytime occupation or programme of activities. Provision varies in different areas, but there are two main options.

- To continue a programme of occupational therapy, art therapy, physiotherapy, speech therapy and any other activities established in the institution. This option is likely to be more appropriate for people with additional problems such as behaviour disorder, sensory deficits or severe physical handicap.

- To gradually withdraw from hospital services and make full use of existing community resources. These may be special day centres, sheltered work or open employment. This option is discussed in more detail in the following section, 'Community-based occupational therapy'.

Once the client is established in his own home, a decision must be made as to whether occupational therapy is still necessary and, if so, whether the hospital based or the community-based occupational therapist is the most appropriated person to continue. The deciding factors will be the availability of occupational therapy resources and local arrangements for people in their own homes.

COMMUNITY-BASED OCCUPATIONAL THERAPY

Some therapists work solely with adults, or solely with children, or with both, depending on local arrangements. An occupational therapist might be employed in work in a single day centre or residential facility. However, the majority of therapists working in the community in this field work as part of a community team. This section describes the work of the occupational therapist with adults living in the community who have mental handicaps.

IDENTIFYING THE PEOPLE WITH HANDICAPS IN THE COMMUNITY

Many people who have a mental handicap do not seek the help of voluntary or statutory mental handicap services. Some local authorities keep registers of people who have been given the label of 'mentally handicapped' in order to predict the type of services required in the present and future.

It has been suggested, however, that maintaining a register promotes the segregation of people with a mental handicap from others in society.

Integration needs to occur in the areas of living accommodation, workplace, social settings and use of community resources such as shops and health-care facilities.

Accommodation

There are many more people who have a mental handicap living in homes of their own, or with family or friends, than are living in hospital. These people are not necessarily more able than those living in hospital; social and other factors are also involved.

Other types of accommodation include private houses and residential facilities that exist specifically for people with a mental handicap, run either by local authorities, health authorities or charitable organisations. These are houses or hostels built or adapted to accommodate between 5 and 30 people supported by staff, usually on a 24-hour basis.

Many of these hostels or group homes are now reducing in size, and indeed some are closing, encouraging people to move into homes with just one or two of their friends in order to facilitate better community integration.

People who live in hostels or group homes have, by the nature of the establishment, limited opportunities to live as many other people in the community do. They have the status of 'residents', without the same permanence and acceptance by society as people who rent or own their own homes.

Daytime occupation

For many years, people who had mental handicaps were considered unsuitable for paid employment. Since it has been recognised that everybody has the potential to learn and contribute to the community in some way, given the right level of support, people with mental handicaps are being encouraged to prepare for and seek paid employment; a difficult task at a time of high unemployment.

Many attend day centres run by local authorities. These used to be called 'adult training centres' and provided repetitive industrial work for very little pay. Many of these centres still exist but now have a much broader spectrum of opportunities on offer, such as community living skills groups and leisure and recreational facilities.

Various full-time or part-time courses are on offer at local colleges specifically for people with learning difficulties, and some areas have befriending schemes that match non-handicapped people to those with handicaps for the purpose of attending ordinary adult education classes.

Some people who have mental handicaps have paid occupations; either gained through their own independent achievements or with help from disablement resettlement officers, Pathways officers or occupational therapists. This aspect is discussed in detail in the section on 'The role of the occupational therapist' on page 405.

Other people have very little in the way of purposeful daytime occupation and spend much of their lives at home. Unless they become a problem to their families, they are unlikely to be referred to an occupational therapist.

COMMUNITY MENTAL HANDICAP TEAMS (CMHTs)

CMHTs were set up in response to the document 'Better Services for the Mentally Handicapped' (HMSO 1976) which emphasised the need for a local community based service for people who have a mental handicap.

The constitution and policy of each team varies from area to area, depending on various factors including:

- the needs of the local population
- services already provided in the area
- ability to recruit staff, particularly paramedical staff.

A team will generally consist of an occupational therapist, a speech therapist, a physiotherapist, a psychologist, a social worker, a community nurse and a doctor. Some teams lack one or more of these professionals, usually because of the national shortage of, for example, occupational and speech therapists. The number of staff from each discipline varies also.

Acceptance of the principles of social role valorisation has made some teams consider whether they should be identified as specifically supporting people with a mental handicap, since this contributes to segregating them from other people. It may also be argued, however, that within any community certain groups of people are segregated so that services can be tailored specifically to their needs. Examples include Mother and Baby Sessions and Over Fifties Keep Fit Sessions.

The role of the occupational therapist

It is difficult to define the precise role of the occupational therapist in the CMHT when the staffing and structure of teams vary so greatly. The contribution that each occupational therapist makes depends upon personality, interests, previous training and experience, the needs of the client group and the skills of other team members. The essential attributes of the occupational therapist who is developing her role within a team are:

- a commitment to team work
- acceptance of some degree of role overlap
- skills that complement those of the other team members.

For example, a person may have been advised by the physiotherapist to swim regularly for specific physical benefits and may also be considering swimming as part of a constructive use of leisure time project with the occupational therapist. Either the physiotherapist or the occupational therapist may take the client swimming until he is able to go alone or with friends. The decision could depend upon which professional feels most comfortable in water, who has time, or other factors. One of the best ways for a new team member to develop a role within the team is to find out exactly how the other members work by, for example, spending a day or more with each of them.

Working together with other members of the team will ensure that the needs of the client and the family or carers are met. For example, a large part of the social worker's role involves communication with the family, whereas the occupational therapist works more specifically with the client, and this is where the social worker and therapist can work together to achieve mutual aims.

In order to illustrate ways the occupational therapist might intervene with people living in the community, three case studies have been selected to show three aspects of community work. The studies illustrate the variety of activities that can be used to meet the different needs of people, the different settings in which the therapist works and the close liaison between the therapist and others involved in provision of the service. A further example is given of an educational group run by an occupational service and a social worker.

CASE EXAMPLE 23.7 PREPARATION FOR THE FUTURE USING DOMESTIC ACTIVITIES

Brian is a 45-year-old man with a moderate mental handicap. He lives with his mother who is in her 80s. They have both lived in the same house in the same village for over 40 years. Brian's father died when Brian was very young and Brian has attended the local social centre since he was in his teens. He has many friends there, although he has no one particular friend. He spends most of the day in a workshop doing basic sanding, construction tasks and errands for the staff.

The community nurse has been involved with Brian and his mother for the past 2 years and asked the occupational therapist to become involved as she felt that Brian could do more around the home to help his mother.

The therapist began by visiting the home with the community nurse, who outlined to Brian and his mother her ideas for occupational therapy involvement. The therapist then arranged to meet Brian at the Centre where he could show her what he did during the day. This also gave her an opportunity to discuss with the staff their perception of Brian's needs and how they thought she might help.

It was agreed between Brian, his mother, the centre staff and the therapist that Brian would begin to assist his mother more around the home by helping to make tea twice a week. This plan was to be reviewed regularly. The aim was to prepare Brian for the time when his mother was no longer at home, either because of illness or in the event of her death. The goals which needed to be achieved included:

1. To encourage Brian to gain more insight into what is required in running a home, so that he can do more by himself and help his mother.
2. To help Brian's mother see that her son

has the ability to learn much more than he already knows and that through doing more for himself his self-image and confidence will improve.
3. To acquire some accurate knowledge of what support Brian will require in the future, depending upon whether he wishes to remain living in his current home or to move.

Brian's mother was anxious about how much responsibility she would allow her son to have with the gas cooker, hot pans and knives, and her anxiety quickly passed to Brian, lessening his confidence. The therapist asked Brian if they could meet at the Centre once a week to make part of the meal which could then be taken home, so that Brian had the opportunity to gain more confidence.

As Brian had never done much at home his perceptual skills, such as spatial relationships, shape and colour concepts, were not advanced enough to prove functional in cooking and other domestic tasks. His hand function was also shown to be restricted during the sessions at the Centre. Brian was able to work on developing these skills while preparing part of the evening meal.

To identify exactly what Brian could do at home to assist his mother, the preparation of the meal was analysed into a series of tasks. Each time the therapist visited the home, Brian and his mother marked on the analysis format which tasks Brian did independently, what he required help with and what his mother did. The aim was to encourage the mother to recognise how much more her son is able to do and to allow him to do it.

In future Brian may be asked if he would like to attend a weekly group of other people in a similar position to himself, to prepare him emotionally for the time when his mother is no longer living with him due to illness or death.

CASE EXAMPLE 23.8   ENCOURAGING THE DEVELOPMENT OF CONCENTRATION AND MOTIVATION

Richard is 21, with a moderate mental handicap, and lives with his mother and father. His mother copes with her son's handicap by treating him as a dependent child. He responds accordingly and shouts, swears and loses his temper in order to get his own way. Richard attends a day centre on a sporadic basis, only going when he chooses and preferring to go on outings with his parents. They are keen, however, for Richard to attend the centre regularly so that he can make new friends and they can have some time to themselves.

The occupational therapist was asked to become involved as Richard's parents were concerned that he would do little for himself, such as bathing and dressing, although they felt he had the ability to learn these skills. A home visit revealed the need for bath aids to assist Richard to bath himself, and the visit also gave the therapist an opportunity to talk to Richard and his parents.

Richard felt there was little to interest him at the centre, and yet he was also bored at home. He found it difficult to converse with people due to speech problem, for which the speech therapist had recommended plenty of conversation practice.

The occupational therapist felt that the most basic need was to help Richard enjoy learning to become more independent, and give him a positive self-image as an active person. She suggested working with Richard at the centre, to give more structure to his day there and to make use of the centre facilities. If the programme was successful, Richard would both be motivated to attend the centre and be less bored at home.

For one session per week, Richard and the therapist worked using books, photographs and the computer to improve Richard's concentration, eye contact and conversation skills. The subject matter always included a particular interest of Richard's, such as football or farming, and tried to introduce new interests, such as different sports that he might pursue himself and that would also contribute towards physical independence.

Once the programme was well established, the therapist then saw Richard at home on several occasions to assist him to develop further skills in personal care.

CASE EXAMPLE 23.9   GROUP WORK

A community mental handicap team was approached by staff from a local hostel where 30 young people with a mental handicap lived, requesting assistance in helping some of the residents to gain an understanding of their own sexuality and in giving basic sex education.

Some of the residents showed little understanding of what is considered appropriate sexual behaviour and generally lacked information on contraception, venereal diseases, sex and the law, conception, sexual intercourse, male and female anatomy and similar topics.

People with mental handicaps do not have access to even basic information on sex except on an individual basis following a crisis. The team felt that this request provided an ideal opportunity for interested team members to be involved in initiating a group for such adults.

The occupational therapist, who had experience of working in small groups, and the social worker, who had experience in one-to-one sexual counselling, volunteered to plan and run a group, later named 'You and your feelings about others'.

Preparation for the group included research into suitable resources and teaching materials to use with the group, attending courses on sexuality and mental handicap, talking to staff and parents to help them overcome their anxieties and, most important of all, assessing the needs of the group members.

The group was started on a regular weekly basis with six members. As most of the group members were out during the day, sessions were held in the evenings at the hostel. A different topic was discussed each week for 14 weeks, including:

- experience of relationships and which were valued
- how our bodies work
- the importance of using contraceptives
- sexual relationships
- responsibilities of parenthood.

During these sessions, people were able to learn a great deal about themselves and others, and to understand how to be a responsible adult with sexual needs like anyone else.

This first group was the starting point for many other groups in a variety of different establishments, involving people with varying needs and levels of ability. The occupational

(Continued on p. 408.)

(Case example 23.9 continued.)
therapist and social worker eventually developed their role in educating staff, carers and parents on the sexual needs of adults with mental handicaps.

SUMMARY

The field of mental handicap is changing rapidly as people move out of institutions into accommodation within the community. Increasing numbers of occupational therapists are choosing to work in the field, both in helping people to adapt to community living and in working with people who have always lived at home.

This chapter looked at ways in which mental handicap has been classified and at traditional ways of providing care in institutions. The traditional role of the occupational therapist was described in order to highlight how that role has changed. Changing attitudes to mental handicap were described, as well as changing patterns of care.

The current role of the occupational therapist was described in detail in three main areas of work: helping people to develop new skills for living, preparation for transferring from institutional to community living, and community-based occupational therapy.

CASE EXAMPLE 23.10 PROVIDING SUPPORT IN THE TRANSITION FROM COLLEGE TO OPEN EMPLOYMENT

Kathleen is 34 and lives in a group home with three of her friends. She had spent most of her life in institutional care since leaving the family home as a young child. She attended a 2-year course at the nearby college, 'Learning for Living', for people with a mental handicap.

A meeting was held to assist Kathleen to decide on what to do after leaving college, attended by her key worker, social worker, a representative of the college staff, an occupational therapist and a Pathways Employment Officer (Open Employment Opportunities).

Kathleen has communication difficulties and was unable to verbalise her needs and hopes. It had been observed that she had an interest in domestic tasks but there was no information as to her level of ability in this area of work. The Pathways Officer was not optimistic that he could secure paid employment for Kathleen on the basis of his brief assessment but suggested that she went on a work-experience placement in domestic work.

The therapist was involved in setting up a three mornings a week, 6 weeks' work

experience placement at an elderly persons' home. She worked alongside Kathleen, teaching her the specific duties of domestic staff, which involved working in the laundry and general cleaning. It was soon observed that Kathleen enjoyed her work and was always ready to leave for work on time. Her work was of a good standard and the speed of work was acceptable once she learned a routine that required her to work on her own initiative with little prompting.

The therapist reported back to the Pathways Employment Officer that Kathleen was now ready for a more permanent work-experience placement that would be converted into a paid position after a period of time for learning the job. A placement was found for her at another elderly persons' home where she worked alongside another domestic assistant, who supervised and supported her with advice from the therapist. She proved to be a very reliable worker, appeared to enjoy and take pride in her work and became much more sociable. Due to her learning difficulties she was unable to travel to her place of work independently and so required a taxi.

Following a 3-month period of training, Kathleen was offered employment by the local authority to work as a domestic assistant.

REFERENCES

Burke J P 1977 A clinical perspective on motivation: pawn versus origin, 31: 254–259

Chorley E 1948 Occupational therapy with the mentally defective. The Journal of the Association of Occupational Therapists 31: 14–16

Copeland M et al 1976 Occupational therapy for mentally retarded children. University Park, Baltimore

Creek J et al 1987 Building on basics. Therapy Weekly 14: 11

Creek J, Wells G 1988 Points of view on working together: qualified and unqualified staff in an occupational therapy department for adults with a mental handicap. British Journal of Occupational Therapy 51(6): 204–206

Erikson K T 1967 Notes on the sociology of deviance. In: Scheff T J (ed) Mental illness and social processes. Harper & Row, New York

Felce et al 1986 The Bereweeke skill-teaching system. NFER Nelson, Berkshire

Goffman E 1963 Stigma: notes on the management of spoiled identity. Penguin, Middlesex

Hall D M B 1984 The child with a handicap. Blackwell, Oxford, 193

Harvey F D 1986 A review of the assessment of people with a mental handicap: some important considerations, British Journal of Occupational Therapy 49(4): 119–121

Heaton-Ward W A 1975 Mental subnormality, 4th edn. Wright, Bristol

HMSO 1976 Better services for the mentally handicapped. HMSO, London

Hogg J, Raynes N V 1987 Assessment in mental handicap: a guide to assessment, practices, tests and checklists. Croom Helm, London

Kielhofner G 1988 The model of human occupation workbook. Workshops: London, Edinburgh, York

Kielhofner G, Burke J P 1980 A model of human occupation, part 1. Conceptual framework and content. American Journal of Occupational Therapy 34(9): 572–581

Mangen P 1982 Sociology and mental health: an introduction for nurses and other care-givers. Churchill Livingstone, Edinburgh

WHO 1980 International classification of impairments, disabilities and handicaps. WHO, Geneva

FURTHER READING

Bumphrey E (ed) 1987. Occupational therapy in the community. Woodhead Faulkener, New York

Cassidy N et al 1986. So then we will be outsiders: one resettlement team's experience of assessing and preparing people with mental handicap for life in the community. British Journal of Occupational Therapy 49(4): 103

Peck C, Hong C S 1988 Living skills for mentally handicapped people. London, Croom Helm

Issac D 1988 Adults with mental handicap: working with support staff to achieve occupational therapy aims. British Journal of Occupational Therapy. 51(4)

McGrowan C 1986 Moving on: an outline of group work with mentally handicapped people preparing to move out of hospital into a group home. British Journal of Occupational Therapy 49(4): 114

Sactuary G 1984 After I'm gone: what will happen to my handicapped child. Souvenir Press, London

Williams P, Shoultz B 1982 We can speak for ourselves. Souvenir Press, London

USEFUL ADDRESSES

The Campaign for people with mental handicaps (CMH)
12 Maddox Street
London WIR 9PL

The Royal National Society for Mentally Handicapped (MENCAP) Children and Adults
123 Golden Lane
London EC1Y ORT

British Institute of Mental Handicap (BIMH)
Wolverhampton Road

Kidderminster
Worcester DY11 3PP

Association of Professions for the Mentally Handicapped
126 Albert Street
London NW1 7NF

British Epilepsy Association
Crowthorne House
New Working Road
Wokingham
Berkshire RG11 3AY

24

Community

Penny Wheeler

INTRODUCTION

Community care is a comparatively new direction for mental health. Occupational therapists have begun to move from traditional settings to take part in providing a community service. This has led to therapists questioning and defining practice. The experience has served to strengthen an understanding of the principles behind the profession. Occupational therapy has had to address and resolve issues of role identification, the value of the occupational therapy process, and the management of therapists working in isolation. The solutions have been found to exist within the profession.

This chapter identifies the aspects of occupational therapy pertinent to community work:

- what is community care?
- beliefs of the profession
- settings and methods of delivering occupational therapy
- practising community occupational therapy
- resources available to the occupational therapist
- common problems related to community work
- management of the service
- summary.

Many of the methods used are the same as those used in institutional settings but the method of delivery and level of responsibility is different.

WHAT IS COMMUNITY CARE?

Community care involves the replacement of care previously delivered in large institutions by a wide range of services and facilities provided locally by collaboration between health, local authority and voluntary bodies.

Occupational therapists are trained to adapt to the resources available. Community care calls on the therapist to make full use of the resources existing in local areas and, if necessary, to create appropriate situations. Although the changes in services have forced occupational therapists to address many professional issues, they have extended practice rather than changed it dramatically.

'Most people who need long-term care can and should be looked after in the community. This is what most of them want for themselves and what those responsible for their care believe to be best' (DHSS 1983). Psychiatric services have been undergoing considerable change in style. There has been a gradual move away from institutional care since the 1960s but this move has accelerated following the government White Paper, 'Better Services for the Mentally Ill' (DHSS 1975). As a result of the paper there has been particular emphasis on developing community resources for the mentally ill in order to assist in the planned closure of local psychiatric hospitals.

There is evidence that if the movement away from inpatient care towards community care is to be successful, a range of rehabilitation and support services must be developed (McCreadie et al 1985). The 'Italian Experience' of the fast closure of mental hospitals was highly praised by some British observers but it highlighted that clients do not automatically become well when they are discharged from the institution. Clients and families need help from planned community services (Jones and Poletti 1985).

Vaughan (1983), in his discussion of brief care as current practice, says that day care, sheltered work, domiciliary support and other like options are essential in caring for the mentally ill in the community. Health Authorities throughout the country have been developing a range of services.

The demands on occupational therapy services have changed accordingly. This has provided an opportunity for therapists in mental health to review their practice and to improve the delivery of the service.

BELIEFS OF THE PROFESSION

Occupational therapists believe that a person can be seen as an open system (Kielhofner 1985), constantly relating with the external world. This is a two-way process, in which the person influences others and is also influenced. This is thought to be sequential although it may, at times, appear simultaneous.

INDEPENDENCE AND AUTONOMY

Powell-Lawton (1972) suggested that competence and functional ability have two components:

1. *autonomy:* the ability to function as an individual
2. *environmental control:* the ability to function within a particular situation.

Occupational therapists value the right of each person to act as an individual if they choose to do so. The therapist is concerned with the individual's belief in themselves, their motivation, and their belief in control over themselves and over external forces, in addition to developing, where necessary, the skills to carry out the planned action. In a community setting, the individual client has a great amount of responsibility in devising and implementing the treatment programme.

THE EXTERNAL WORLD

The external world consists of objects and people as well as space (Dunning 1972). The individual can use objects to impinge on the environment; for example, by painting with a brush, or the environment can impinge on the individual, for example, the steps up to a house force certain physical movements to be taken. In the same way, other people influence this process of interaction, for example, showing appreciation for a meal cooked or listening to a conversation.

A system can be defined as a set of parts interconnected and organised into a complex total, which works as a whole. The external world can be seen as a system. Society and the pattern of relationships experienced by the individual is a complex ever-changing picture. People with mental-health problems are interacting with three primary systems:

1. the health system, which may have one set of values
2. the family and informal support network, which could have another set of values and expectations
3. the wider system of society with its cultural norms.

Adaptation to function within these possibly contradicting groups calls for a high degree of skilled behaviour.

In institutional settings the occupational therapist enables the person to function within the sheltered environment of the hospital. In community work it is the normal everyday situation shared by the majority that is the milieu. This forces the therapist to consider more deeply the particular facets of the environment with which the individual has to cope. Interventions often have to take into account prejudice and poverty as well as the factors that enable integration with many different ideological groups (Etcheverry 1979).

THE INDIVIDUAL

An individual can be seen as a combination of values and beliefs, abilities (both motor and perceptual), emotions, and experience. Time also affects the individual; life is a continuing and developing process. Occupational therapists regard the person in the light of life stages as well as abilities and beliefs. Working with someone in the community results in assisting them to function in a wide range of life's roles as they actually occur.

In order to interact and function, the person must have the ability and desire to do so. Ability consists of movement, perception and thinking.

Cause of dysfunction	Example
Lack of opportunity	never leaving the house and therefore never meeting people
Adverse reaction when carrying out the behaviour	attempts at establishing relationships fail
Social pressure	pressure from the family to remain dependent
Physical dysfunction	a speech impediment
Perceptual difficulties	misperception of non-verbal communication shown by others
Low self-esteem	a fear of failure
Emotion and mood	depression

Fig. 24.1 Possible causes of dysfunction in interactional skills.

The desire to achieve function consists of motivation, beliefs and past experience of success.

Skills can be seen in patterns of behaviour that can be used to achieve a desired outcome. For example, riding a bike consists of motor and spatial performances. Once learnt, they become routines that can be produced with little effort and are then know as 'habits'. Dysfunction in interpersonal activities can be caused by a disruption in skills, see Figure 24.1.

OCCUPATION

The occupational therapist is primarily concerned with the interaction between the individual and the environment or system within which they live. This area of interaction is the area of occupation and function. There can be no interaction without some form of activity. It follows that activity and occupation are very broad concepts. Occupational therapists work with an enormous range of problems in functional ability.

Maslow's Hierarchy of Needs is often used to illustrate how areas of dysfunction are prioritised (see Ch. 6 p. 97). Using this framework, aspects such as personal activities of daily living are more essential than creativity and are addressed first. Once met it is possible to move on to the next driving force or need. Occupational therapists aim to enable people to meet their own needs and therefore to be independent. This is more possible in the community than in a hospital setting since the opportunities for choice and normal life-styles are increased.

The fundamental idea is that humans engage in activity and benefit both themselves and others by this active participation. The mores of society dictate which activities are acceptable. Occupational therapists remain within the standards of the relevant society and its cultural norms, the aim is to aid the person relate to and function with the immediate environment.

The pattern of occupation

Throughout the day and throughout one's life people engage in many different activities and occupations. These fall roughly into the following:

- personal- and self-maintenance
- social activities
- intellectual and creative activities
- work activities.

The occupational therapist looks at the whole pattern of the individual's day; the balance between work, leisure and play, taking into account subjective perception. One person may feel shopping is leisure, another that it is work. The pattern of occupation reflects the expectations of the individual (Parker 1976) and of the community. Working in the community gives the therapist the opportunity to use normal activity to reinforce the skills shown by the individual. It challenges and utilises the person's actual beliefs and expectations in a way that is difficult to simulate in the unnatural environment of a hospital.

Activity analysis

Not only does an occupational therapist study the combination of the individual and the system in which they interact, (both physical and human); but also the interaction and activity itself. An occupational therapist undertakes an analysis of the activity. This includes the required skills of the individual and the necessary physical and emotional environment (see Ch. 6 p. 92). Through this analysis, the therapist is able to identify suitable adaptations to the way the task is achieved so that the person is able to perform effectively.

In community settings adaptation and grading of activity is difficult to achieve because the therapist cannot control and alter all the experiences of normal life. An alternative approach is to identify whole activities that call for the desired outcome. It is the whole activity that is graded, not the components of the activity. These can be established to facilitate and utilise different abilities, for example, different levels of confidence and social behaviour are needed to attend a structured day centre and a local evening class.

SETTING ACHIEVABLE GOALS

The occupational therapist analyses the task and the skills necessary to accomplish it. The activity is then divided into achievable parts, taking into account the abilities and motivation of the individual. Great consideration will be given to establishing the correct goals for the individual. The person must feel able to complete it and yet it must not be so easy that it diminishes the importance of the task (Yerxa 1988). This area highlights occupational therapists' particular professional skills. It a matter of using the right activities at the right time and in the right way, for the right person.

Used by occupational therapists, activities are a prescribed treatment, offered with a remedial aim in mind. Within the context of the community, the activities are the actions of everyday life. The therapist will signify the importance of specific occupations and will reinforce achievement and functional ability.

The occupational therapist may not always use activity as a medium but it remains the aim of the intervention. Community work uses goal-directed activities, which form part of daily living, the individual plays a very large part in selecting the goal and medium.

The occupational therapist therefore works with an interconnected and dynamic combination of the person, the activity, and the environment. In institutional settings, emphasis is placed on adapting the interaction or activity to meet the needs of the individual. In community settings the emphasis of change is either with the individual or with the environment and system but the aim is always towards functional ability.

SETTINGS AND METHODS OF DELIVERING OCCUPATIONAL THERAPY

Occupational therapy services are delivered in a variety of settings:

- community teams
- day hospitals.

The types of occupational therapy services carried out include:

- sessional work
- independent treatment programmes
- use of structured leisure facilities.

COMMUNITY TEAMS

Occupational therapists may be members of community teams. It has become commonplace for therapists to be part of a multidisciplinary team but mental health teams are comparatively new. A typical team consists of:

- medical staff
- community psychiatric nurses
- psychologist
- social worker
- occupational therapist.

The development of teams has posed challenging questions about the role of the individual professions in community psychiatric services. There is a danger that occupational therapists in multidisciplinary teams are allowed to develop their identity as team members at the expense of their professional expertise. The roles of team members merge to produce mental-health workers who are multi-purpose practitioners, each carrying similar caseloads that do not necessarily reflect particular professional skills.

An occupational therapist working on a team must have a thorough and firm understanding of occupational therapy to ensure that the team has a valuable resource that can be appropriately used. This calls for professional maturity and a belief in the strengths of the profession. Once occupational therapists realise they belong to a group and once that group becomes cohesive in its statements and philosophy, the trauma of transition and definition of roles is reduced. This is achieved by clear, positive professional leadership and supervision.

At times a dilution of skills has been avoided by occupational therapists working as specialists rather than as key workers. This enables them to address specific referrals for occupational therapy and provide a service that can be used by key workers. Examples are: group work on various topics, contact clubs, functional assessment and treatment.

The therapist will assess and carry out treatment in a variety of places. Primarily this will be either the mental-health centre or the client's home. Other venues include leisure facilities, normal community facilities and health centres.

The clients seen reflect the expertise of the therapist and the needs of the team. In general occupational therapists are particularly skilled in assisting someone who is having difficulty in functioning, whether it is in the area of self-maintenance, work, or leisure. The broad training of occupational therapy allows staff to work with clients showing a range of problems and of varying degrees of severity.

DAY HOSPITALS

To have occupational therapists attached to individual units is a logical and well-accepted approach to service delivery. This method, however, does have the disadvantage that the therapist is often forced to work in isolation from occupational therapy colleagues. Support and good supervision are essential to avoid the reduction of specialist skills and to ease the role conflicts for the individual therapist. In such settings occupational therapists have often been trapped by the requirement to devise and implement programmes for groups of attenders rather than for individuals.

Whilst therapists have the necessary skills, it restricts their practice, and may result in professional stagnation.

SESSIONAL WORK AND INDEPENDENT TREATMENT PROGRAMMES

This is becoming a more-popular method of service delivery. Occupational therapists form teams to provide an occupational therapy service to a number of different units. This is one way of giving a viable service to the numerous small units resulting from the closure of the large hospitals. It enables professional support and supervision to be maintained. Therapists work together in carrying out appropriate treatment sessions in individual units and also in providing independent venues to which clients from many units may be referred. This method increases the autonomy of the occupational therapy service and enables greater flexibility in treatment programmes. One drawback is that it is harder for the therapist to bring about changes to the environment and approaches of the unit. The treatment and interventions are directed at the individual. It is easier to alter the approaches of other staff or the unit environment if the therapist is seen to belong to the group.

The venues used may be health premises or may be hired from other agencies, for example, the Arts Centre. Whilst the use of public facilities is very important, it should be noted that this complicates the treatment planning and implementation process. Time is taken to arrange facilities and transport resources, and arrangements are often cancelled without prior notice.

Delivering a service in this manner means that the occupational therapist has to relate to a large number of staff and clients. Clear communication channels are essential. It is vital to develop an effective method of participating in case management.

If these difficulties can be overcome, an efficient and effective occupational-therapy service can be provided. The individual therapist has professional support and supervision, professional role models, and a greater opportunity to mature professionally.

STRUCTURED LEISURE FACILITIES

One of the roles of traditional occupational therapy departments was to promote the constructive use of leisure time and to provide leisure or hobby activities for therapeutic purposes and for pleasure. Community care has provided the opportunity to develop a wide range of leisure facilities, day centres, drop-in centres and clubs. These may be run by occupational therapy helpers, volunteers, or the clients themselves. They may be part-time or full-time, in a variety of locations. If they are planned with care, clients can be given much greater choice in the type of day care they use.

PRACTISING COMMUNITY OCCUPATIONAL THERAPY

The trend towards community care has involved a move away from the pathological model of practice previously held by most health-care professions. This has resulted in the rejection for many of the label 'illness' in preference to the term 'mental health'. The individual or others still complain of feelings or behaviours which are perceived as not normal, however. Society is constantly moving the line between normality and abnormality.

The aims for the person are the same as in institutional settings.

TASKS AND ACTIVITIES

The occupational therapist in the community strives to use tasks and activities that are available to the public (for example, clubs, classes and sports centres) or to adapt and create activities that are as normal as possible. This has to take into account the priorities of individuals and the medium in which they prefer to express themselves.

The objective is to facilitate tasks that demand the right level of challenge for the person, are achievable, and contain no more than an acceptable level of risk. The freedom of choice carries with it the freedom to take risks. This requires informed choice. The therapist has to take some decisions on behalf of people whose cognitive

CASE EXAMPLE 24.1(a) MRS COLLIER

Mrs Collier, aged 52, is married with two sons both in their 20s, one still at home.

She came from a large family. She had always felt isolated and was the only one to go to the grammar school. Her parents were very strict and did not show affection or give praise. At the age of 13 she was raped by a man who worked for her father. She never told anyone about this but tried to commit suicide by drinking weedkiller.

Fifteen years ago Mrs Collier was admitted to the inpatient unit for 3 months when she was feeling depressed and suicidal. During this admission she told a doctor about the rape but couldn't bring herself to talk about it in depth. She continued to attend as a day patient for several years. Mrs Collier was employed as a cleaner in a shop during week-day evenings. This included the responsibility for securing the premises. She had been much better for the last 3 years until recently, when her feelings of agitation and depression returned.

The general practitioner referred her to the community mental-health team and she was allocated to the occupational therapist.

The long-term aims of treatment for Mrs Collier were:

- to help keep her out of hospital
- to give her an opportunity to talk about how she feels
- to try to help her feel more positive and to gain feelings of self-worth.

The short-term objectives were to:

1. meet on a regular (weekly then fortnightly) basis while she is feeling so depressed
2. encourage her to talk about her feelings of bereavement and loss
3. try to help her find a way to ask for what she wants, particularly from her family
4. encourage her to take up writing again which gives her great pleasure
5. try to increase her self-esteem by helping her to establish the positives of her character and aspects that give her satisfaction. Discuss the possibility of voluntary work in the future
6. identify strategies to help her sleep and relaxation techniques to still the mind
7. help her explore feelings about the rape (when she is ready).

abilities make it difficult to understand possible danger.

In community settings the occupational therapist has very little control over activities and tasks. This entails the individual client taking greater responsibility for the occupations performed.

THE ENVIRONMENT

The aim of treatment is to provide opportunities for the individual to interact with the environment. The service needs to create situations that

CASE EXAMPLE 24.2(a) MR BROWN

Mr Brown was 42. He had been diagnosed as suffering from schizophrenia since the age of 20. He had lived in hospital for the last 6 years and prior to that he had lived with his parents.

His father had been in the army, which necessitated much travelling. Mr Brown moved with the family and did not spend more than a year in any one school. He was a high achiever with good exam results.

At the time of referral he required 24-hour nursing supervision. He was living in a staffed hostel. He showed signs of paranoia, aggression, and delusions, although medication was keeping these under control. The symptoms became more apparent towards the end of the period of the neuroleptic depot medication.

He was thought to need remotivation and the opportunity to engage in constructive and useful activities. He was isolated and withdrawn. The long stay in a hospital setting had resulted in the loss of many previously learnt skills.

The long-term aim for Mr Brown was to enable him to move from a hostel to a supported satellite house. After the assessment the following aims of treatment were formed:

1. to increase motivation by facilitating the accomplishment of activities that he had defined as important, for example, gardening, darts, and swimming
2. to increase independence by providing the opportunity to develop skills, for example, social skills, work skills, and domestic activities.

enable this interaction, as well as utilising public facilities, for example, a coffee club that can tolerate the behaviour of the less socially skilled. The social support system may need to be adapted to understand and accommodate the needs of the person.

The approach of the occupational therapist does not just rely on the person to adapt to a fixed situation but also views the outside world and social system as adaptable. The focus of adaptation depends on the abilities and motivation to change of all concerned.

ASSESSMENT

The occupational-therapy process begins with a thorough assessment of the person and situation. The assessment procedures in the mental-health field are often difficult to identify and in community work become even more complicated. The content of the assessment varies from person to person and, to a certain degree, from therapist to therapist. On top of this there is the concept of the mental-health worker, which ostensibly negates the professional assessment.

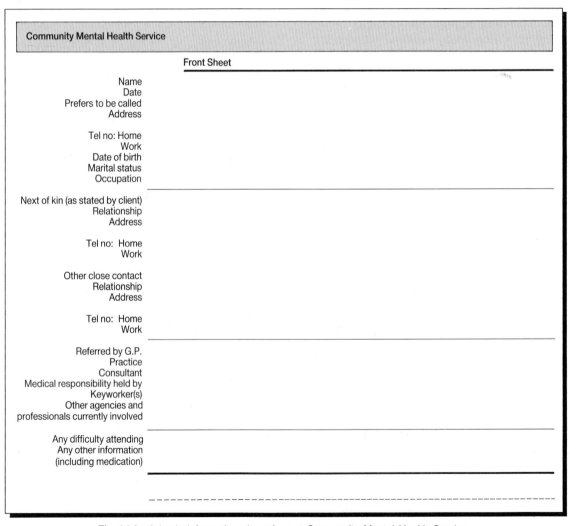

Fig. 24.2 A basic information sheet from a Community Mental Health Service.

Assessment is 'the process of collecting information systematically and organising it in a relevant and useful way' (Willson 1983). Many multidisciplinary teams advocate a common assessment procedure to be carried out by all members, particularly when members act as representatives of the whole team, for example, at an initial assessment, or when acting as a key worker. The concept of a common assessment undertaken by all members of the team enables the group to identify the crucial elements of information. The results are structured in a way that can be used by any of the members (see Fig. 24.2).

Since all health-care professions use interpersonal communication as a prime skill in working with clients, it follows that an assessment is conducted along fairly similar lines for the majority of the workers. Often a team will agree the manner of communicating any results, usually in a predetermined report form. The decision-making process involved in establishing a common approach enables members to explore issues of philosophy and policies, and of the values held by the individual professions. It may be important to the working of the team that this process is continually repeated, resulting in a reaffirmation of the common philosophy and an inauguration of new members, however, it may be at the expense of the professional contribution of individual members.

The dilemma of a common assessment procedure is whether or not to retain the specific professional approaches and techniques. Occupational therapy may have an advantage over many of the other disciplines as the ability to view the person, task, and the surrounding situation enables the therapist to undertake a comprehensive assessment without stepping outside the approaches commonly used by other occupational therapists.

The initial assessment

From the occupational-therapy perspective the initial assessment is very similar in method to those conducted in other settings. It usually consists of ascertaining the client or carer's view of the problem, introducing the service, and establishing a rapport (see Fig. 24.3).

It is necessary to gauge the severity of the prob-

CASE EXAMPLE 24.3(a) MR AND MRS ARNOTT

Mrs Arnott was 76 years old and suffered from Alzheimers Disease. She lived with her 78-year-old husband in their own bungalow. At the time of the referral they were experiencing a wide variety of functional, social, and financial problems.

Mr Arnott was very concerned about his wife's deterioration. He had to deal with all the daily problems alone, including personal and domestic activities, and dealing with his own feelings of bereavement, guilt and frustration. He was socially isolated. He was unable to leave his wife for more than 30 minutes, for brief shopping trips. He had no-one with whom to discuss his situation and did not know what help, if any, was available. Mrs Arnott had recently developed nocturnal incontinence and, in addition, the skin on her thighs had become inflamed.

The general practitioner referred Mrs Arnott to the local community mental-health team for the elderly. Mrs Arnott was allocated to the occupational therapist on the team. An initial assessment was carried out in the couple's own home. The problems were identified by Mr Arnott and the therapist helped him to place them in order of priority.

A day assessment was arranged at the local specialised unit for older confused people. During the day Mrs Arnott was examined by a doctor. She spent time in a variety of sessions in the unit's day care facility to observe her interactional and conversational skills. This was undertaken by the occupational therapist. With the assistance of Mr Arnott, the therapist administered the Clifton Assessment Procedures for the Elderly in order to establish both a behavioural and cognitive baseline.

The aims of treatment with Mrs Arnott covered two main areas:

1. To maintain her level of physical, mental and social function, and to slow down her rate of deterioration. To involve her more actively in her own self-care and to encourage her to be as mobile as possible.

2. To support Mr Arnott by offering advice and help over practical tasks, and the wide variety of resources available.

Community Mental Health Service	
	Assessment
Name	
Date	
Relevant personal history	
Social situation (including family, occupation, sources of support, etc.)	
Presenting problems (identified by client and/or worker)	
Goals or aims agreed with client	
Plans for interventions	
Review date	
Signed	

Fig. 24.3 A Community Mental Health Service assessment sheet.

lem, with particular reference to the safety of the individual and of others. This is an added responsibility for the therapist that does not arise in an institutional setting. The case may have to be passed on to another member of staff. The occupational therapist is representing the team and not only the profession. The therapist is acting as the first point of contact with the service and decides whether or not the referral to the service is appropriate. This aspect of the job also occurs only in community services.

The occupational therapist is well equipped to assess the global situation of the individual in the community; the abilities and difficulties, the task or activity causing concern, and the situation (both physical and social) within which the person functions. In addition to the more detailed assessments (the individual, tasks, and the environment and support system) described elsewhere, it is necessary to gather information about medication and financial circumstances. Although these areas have not been the responsibility of the profession, to date, they have always been important aspects that have been taken into account in assessment and treatment planning in the hospital.

The occupational therapist also carries out assessments of specific areas of dysfunction, for example, assertiveness, work skills, social interaction, and the daily pattern of activity.

Location

The location of the initial meeting will differ from professional to professional and from team to team. Economics may advocate that the person is seen at the mental-health centre but a much better picture of the situation is gained from an assessment conducted in the home.

CASE EXAMPLE 24.2(b)   MR BROWN

Mr Brown was assessed by the occupational
therapist on the community rehabilitation team.
His behaviour and performance was observed in
a variety of settings: in a group situation, in the
hostel, in community settings, and as an
individual. The activities performed varied from
leisure pursuits to domestic activities of daily
living.

An informal interview took place to exchange
information and to build up trust. A number of
self-assessment checklists were used to gain
further information and to ascertain Mr Brown's
response to his difficulties. These included
leisure and work interests; and life and social
skills. The self-assessment forms were also
completed by the nurse key worker in the hostel
to provide the means of developing an agreed
plan of action for all concerned.

The occupational therapist also undertook
formal assessments of Mr Brown's abilities in
the fields of personal and domestic activities of
daily living.

The ability to observe actual functional behaviour when carrying out an assessment in
someone's own home requires a mixture of
diplomacy, great sensitivity and opportunism, as
well as sophisticated observation and communication skills. The community setting reduces the
opportunity to use activities to assess function.
Great reliance is placed on self-reporting by the
individual or a description of behaviour by the
carer. This can provide the chance to identify
the perceptions of the individual and to examine
aspects such as motivation, beliefs, and autonomy.

The individual

The performance skills and abilities of the individual are assessed where necessary. Interactional dysfunction is the problem area for many
people who are functioning satisfactorily in self-
care and domestic activities. For others, such as
the confused or those showing behavioural disturbances, the ability to perform basic self-
maintenance tasks may be in question. Other
agencies or facilities may be used to assess precise
performance skills, for example, work skills
undertaken by government employment schemes.

The roles and expectations of the person are an
important part of the assessment and help to ascertain how they hope to interact with the outside
world. The traumatic phase of transition from one
role to another, with all the incumbent changes in
personal adjustment often cause the referral to the
service. The profession's view of life events assists
in identifying problem areas and possible remedial
action. Occupational therapy has always worked
within the individual's belief system and satisfaction with performance. A picture of the daily pattern of activity will be formed with reference to
the degree of fulfilment it gives. The concepts of
autonomy and choice are very important. Assessments include the locus of control and the perceived effectiveness, as reported by the person.

The occupational therapist also identifies the degree of motivation shown. This may relate to the
way the person needs to adapt or change or to the
desired outcome that will result in the environment changing. The difficulty stated by the individual is the primary problem assessed. This
allows the treatment process to progress at the appropriate rate and within the client's motivational
drive.

The task and activities

The exact situation in which the individual feels
dissatisfaction and dysfunction is identified and
examined. In addition, the occupational therapist
will detail circumstances in which the person feels
competent. This enables effective skills to be
recognised and utilised. The analysis of the activity requires the therapist to have a thorough
knowledge of all occupations and many fields of
employment. For example, many women referred
as showing depressive behaviour are going through
the ordeal of adjusting from being an autonomous
adult to being a partner and a parent or adjusting
to the reverse situation.

Tasks that may be identified as problems are
varied; they constitute many aspects of life for the
majority of society, and may cause the majority
degrees of difficulty. Common problems are adjustments to changes in role and the skills needed
to carry out the role, for example, child rearing,
or retirement. Another common problem is the

task of handling conflict, such as marital disharmony or a lack of assertiveness. A difficulty could
be in coping with the bureaucracy of the benefits
and welfare system. The assessment ascertains
what is required, whether it is information, skills
training; or emotional support.

The environment and support system

If relevant, the physical environment is assessed,
particularly when it is preventing autonomy. The
assessment may examine the physical attributes of
the situation or it may consider the whole environment, for example, assessing accommodation need
and deciding between a hostel, bed and breakfast,
and the family home.

The support system is an important component
of community work. Informal support is given by
family, friends, and colleagues. Formal support is
given by members of a service, including other
staff in the health service, social services, the
primary health-care team, voluntary workers, and
private care schemes.

Expectations of the support system greatly influence function. Just as the values and beliefs of
the individual are assessed, so it is part of the
therapist's task to assess the beliefs and motivation
of the support network. Gaps in the network are
identified, for example, periods of time without
help, a lack of emotional support, or little motivation for change.

RECORDING INFORMATION

The object of recording assessment and treatment
is to convey information about aims, process, and
progress. This is communicated internally, as a
memory jogger to the professional dealing with the
case, and to other members of the team should the
need arise. Information is also conveyed externally
to the primary health-care team, other sections of
the secondary health-care service, and to other
agencies.

One of the basic differences between traditional
practice and working in the community is in the
role of key worker. In this role staff are taking
responsibility for both case and all other notes,
whereas in hospital each profession formulates
their own records, resulting in duplication of information. In the community the onus is on the
key worker to keep notes that are up to date, comprehensive and truthful. The standards of practice
are those of occupational therapy but, in addition,
standards held by other mental-health workers
must be borne in mind since they influence team
policy. Areas of conflict should be discussed fully.
It is important to understand the values of different disciplines but the occupational therapist
must adhere to the standards set by the profession.

Records should be of a standard that can stand
up to scrutiny. They should be dated and signed.
They should document the process of intervention
as well as the progress. Occupational therapists are
familiar with using observable behaviour as the
basis of their records. In addition, care should be
taken to detail behaviour not seen as well as that
seen. Motivational drives should be noted since
these are frequently the reason for choosing one
treatment medium over another.

INTERNAL RECORDING

There are no hard and fast rules on how the
professional should record the information as it occurs. Some people make notes at the interview,
others prefer to wait until the session is completed,
and others record only changes observed. Actions that arise from the assessment should be
documented.

The team may devise a common structure to accommodate the information gathered. This usually
details contacts made, actions to be undertaken,
and a review date (see Fig. 24.4). There may also
be a common review format.

In general the standards of practice adhered to
by the occupational therapists are appropriate to
community work but the onus on the therapist
to keep accurate records is greater in the community than in a hospital setting. Most occupational therapists write notes on the basis that
they may be read by the client one day. Descrip-

```
┌─────────────────────────────────────────────────────────────────┐
│ ┌───────────────────────────────────────────────────────────┐   │
│ │ Community Mental Health Service                            │   │
│ └───────────────────────────────────────────────────────────┘   │
│                              Review _____      │
│                       Name  _____ │
│                       Date                                        │
│    New information since last review _____  │
│         Changes since last review                                 │
│       (as seen by client and by worker) _____   │
│    Present problems and goals/aims _____    │
│                             _____   │
│            Plan for interventions _____    │
│                             _____   │
│              Next review date _____    │
│                                                                   │
│            Signed _____ Date _____  │
└─────────────────────────────────────────────────────────────────┘
```

Fig. 24.4 A Community Mental Health Service review sheet.

tions tend to be of the situation from the individual's perspective and contain clear behavioural statements rather than speculation.

RECORDING INFORMATION FOR USE OUTSIDE THE TEAM

Ideally, general practitioners should regularly be kept informed about clients. This is usually done by means of a summary letter describing progress to date and the future plan of intervention. Other members of the primary health-care team, involved with the care, for example, district nurses, must also be advised of any changes to the intervention plans.

Information will usually be conveyed to other involved sections of the secondary health-care service by attendance at decision-making meetings, for example, ward rounds after the admission of a client. The decision about future care becomes a joint responsibility between the hospital and community, however, it is the community therapist who has to implement the decisions after discharge from the institution. When the responsibility for care moves from one part of the service to another, a summary of the situation and approaches used should accompany the individual. This may be an interim or a discharge summary (see Fig. 24.5).

Where other employing agencies and organisations are involved, thought should be given to the amount of information needed. There should be no breach of confidentiality, as there is no control over the way in which non-NHS agencies handle data. Files may be accessible to the client or carer in the future, if not now. Occupational therapists must conform to the guidelines set down by the service. Most occupational therapists would approach the problem of communicating information outside the NHS by encouraging the individual client or carer to give the relevant information personally.

CONFIDENTIALITY

It is essential that the service and professionals adhere to the standards of confidentiality laid down in the occupational therapy professional code of ethics and those detailed in service guidelines. Conflicts can arise from work in the community, for much of the time the therapist is assisting the client to interact within a social environment. Care has to be taken that in attempting to change the social network, no confidentiality is breached, for

Community Mental Health Service	

Discharge summary
_____

Name
Date of first contact
Date closed

Reason for closure (eg problems
resolved, failed to
attend, moved away)

_____

Address on closure

_____

Summary of interventions
made/type of contact

_____

Goals achieved/progress made
(related to the above)

_____

Agencies now involved/current
sources of support

_____

Signed_____Date_____

Fig. 24.5 A Community Mental Health Service discharge sheet.

example, when working with a wife and husband it would be important not to refer to information given in confidence.

Some disciplines advocate different levels of confidentiality and privacy, suggesting that people in 'socially sensitive' jobs (for example, police, teaching and the health service) require greater confidentiality than others. In general, occupational therapists would hope to apply the highest standards to all, regardless of their employment status. When information that does demand additional privacy is given, it should be kept in a manner that reduces the likelihood of its being unnecessarily or accidentally obtained, for example, in a sealed envelope in the notes. Some professional workers omit the information but this can lead to future difficulties for both the individual and any other professionals involved. Where there is doubt, the standards of the profession should be identified and followed.

Decisions have to be taken to identify the role and responsibilities of support staff, particularly in relation to access to information. This should include how the appointment system can be kept private.

Diaries are often used to record names and addresses, as well as events. It should be considered whether or not this can lead to potential breach of confidentiality. Diaries can be misplaced or read accidentally by others. The therapist should use a form of code to record appointments, etc. and should ensure the security of any information.

RESOURCES AVAILABLE TO THE OCCUPATIONAL THERAPIST

A resource can be defined as 'source or possibility of help'. The occupational therapist is concerned with shaping the actions performed by the client. Dysfunction may require help with learning new skills, in changing the task, or in creating a suitable environment and system within which to interact (physical and social). The resources available to an occupational therapist working in the community reflect these different approaches to intervention.

The support system around the client is often the most effective resource. This includes both informal and formal networks. The individual's perception of the adequacy and efficacy of the system is vital.

Occupational therapists work with an enormous range of resources and media, so the correct approach for any individual is available. This is no less true of community work than institutional settings, although it calls for great ingenuity and creativity. The activities used are not focused on single muscle movements or behavioural responses but rather on the sets of routine skills used by the majority of the population. The individual client may require skills practice and support, skills training, or the adaptation of the task to make the best use of remaining skills.

CASE EXAMPLE 24.1(b)   MRS COLLIER

Appropriate resources available to the occupational therapist working with Mrs Collier:

- individual sessions with key-worker occupational therapist
- support from family and two friends
- General Practitioner supportive
- Womens' Group
- Stress Management Group and individual relaxation instructions
- creative writing through the local Arts Centre
- volunteer bureau, occupational therapy support worker for those with special needs
- creative therapies, individual sessions offered in music, drama, dance, and art.

ACTIVITIES OF DAILY LIVING

- Community Living groups are run to identify the necessary skills and approaches that people have to take into account when planning to coexist with others. This includes topics such as personal hygiene and looking one's best. Peer-group pressure from others inside and outside the group

is a powerful shaper of behaviour. These are usually available to people with long-term mental-health problems.

- Various services can be brought into the home to assist with personal activities. These include community nursing, voluntary and private nursing schemes, mobile hairdressers and chiropodists. Assistance may be obtained when attending a day hospital, for example, help with bathing.

- Simple equipment such as toilet and bathing aids can be of great help to both the client and the carer. The use of Dycem can simplify a task to make it achievable. Labour-saving methods such as easy-care clothes or dry shampoo can drastically reduce the burden of care. Occupational therapists are skilled in the precise use of equipment to facilitate, but not eliminate, a task; to provide the just right challenge for the individual. As with all disciplines it is the ability to reject inappropriate treatments that marks a true professional. The provision of equipment depends entirely on the functional needs of the individual and not on the diagnostic label.

STRESS MANAGEMENT AND RELAXATION

Many occupational therapists in the community are teaching stress-management skills, either through groups or to individuals. Relaxation tapes are used to augment the treatment. The ability to cope with stress is crucial to coping with daily life; many people are prevented from gaining more out of life by their fears. The service sets up many different ways of meeting this need including the use of adult education classes.

MOBILITY

- Sports activities, fitness and swimming groups can be run in the community. Public facilities may be used or, if a more sheltered environment is needed, halls or pools can be hired. With enthusiasm from staff it is possible for people to join in organised events such as sponsored walks or marathons.

- Small pieces of equipment, such as chair

raisers and rails, can improve the quality of life for all concerned. Advice can be given to other disciplines on the appropriateness of certain items, for example, the effect of a self-lifting ejector seat on someone who is confused.

● Where necessary, wheelchairs may be provided, either on short-term loan from voluntary organisations or by prescribing the long-term use of a wheelchair for the individual. Care should be taken by staff to instruct on safe use and factors to monitor, such as tyre pressure.

Transport to facilities is a crucial consideration when planning a treatment programme.

CASE EXAMPLE 24.3(b)   MR AND MRS ARNOTT

The resources available to the occupational therapist as key worker for Mrs Arnott fall into a number of categories (not in priority order)
The NHS provision consists of:

● the community mental-health team for the elderly offering domiciliary assessment and support from a group of professionals – community psychiatric nurses, occupational therapist, and social worker
● the local specialised unit for the elderly confused has facilities including day-care services, night care, holiday relief and assessment
● the primary health-care team, including the general practitioner and district nurses.

Social Services provision including:

● specific rehabilitation equipment supplied by the occupational therapist
● home helps and additional facilities such as a laundry service.

The DHSS provide financial advice and benefits, particularly with regard to attendance allowance, and:

● Disability Service Centre for the provision of a wheelchair
● Local Carers' Group and Alzheimers Disease Society to support Mr Arnott
● Voluntary bodies, for example Age Concern who have a Sitter's Register and useful publications for information.

Availability, accessibility and financial cost to the individual and the service need to be identified. People with mental-health difficulties may find dealing with transport problems beyond their abilities. Facilities that specifically aim to help those with poor motivation need particular attention.

DOMESTIC ACTIVITIES

● Many people have domestic skills but are not able to put them into practice. The tasks seem overwhelming. In this case the occupational therapist assists with setting priorities. Aims are then broken down into small steps, which can be achieved. Depending on the need of the individual, there is either help with the task, or (preferably) success is reinforced when it occurs.

● Community Living groups are instrumental in teaching skills. The groups may be run in health-service property, hostels, colleges of further education, or community centres. The group provides knowledge and the opportunity to practise budgetting and cooking activities. Encouragement is towards healthy living.

● Assistance can be offered to those who find domestic tasks impossible or have placed them as a lower priority than other activities. Meals on Wheels may be provided, but provision at weekends needs to be considered. Home helps are a great boon, particularly when they are encouraged to take a wider view of their job to include, for example, shopping and the preparation of food. Laundry services and the use of easy-care fabrics reduce the burden of heavy washing.

SOCIAL ACTIVITIES

● Many people need help with joining a social group. A befriending scheme (run by the NHS or privately) can assist people over this initial hurdle. The occupational therapist needs to be familiar with the various facilities and organisations. This ensures the correct medium is chosen to provide the correct amount of challenge and satisfaction.

An Activation Team, consisting of unqualified occupational therapy staff, can support people in using facilities, offering help either in the home or in the local community.

- Skills training, both in interactional skills and in community living, can enable people to practise successful behaviour. Individual, as well as group, facilities need to be available. Feedback, often in the form of peer group response, is given on the behaviour seen. Consideration needs to be given to the venue used, as appropriate behaviour is most likely to be seen in appropriate settings.
- Environments that make best use of existing skills need to be created by the therapist. The interest and abilities of the clients dictate the exact nature of what is developed. The service needs to develop a range of different options, which cater for different groups of people with different abilities. The range should go from structured leisure facilities offering social contact without the label of illness to intensive input as in a day hospital, and to the use of ordinary social events open to all. Drop-in coffee clubs or contact clubs can offer a less structured but supportive atmosphere that suits the needs of many.

WORK ACTIVITIES

All occupational therapists will be aware of the many different motivating forces behind the drive for purposeful occupation, commonly called 'work'. This includes social acceptance and contact, a feeling of achievement, financial need, and intellectual and creative stimulation. Currently, employment is not available for all, particularly those with functional difficulties. The therapist needs to create and use opportunities to meet the need for work activities.

The assessment of work-related skills must be undertaken. The method is dependent on the individual and the nature of the work preferred. Government schemes at present in operation offer this facility. The Disablement Resettlement Officer is a useful ally for an occupational therapist. Occupational therapists need to ensure that a variety of work activities are established to meet the different needs of individuals. This should reflect the varied work pattern shown by the local community.

Schemes and projects offering suitable activities may involve gardening, decorating, printing, furniture restoration, cashier work and routine office work. The extent to which the occupational therapist is responsible for the establishment and running of these various facilities depends on the local resources. Wherever possible, the activities should be presented in as ordinary a manner as possible.

LEISURE ACTIVITIES

- As with social activities, some people require direction and support to undertake leisure activities. The therapist will attempt to find or organise activities that suit the individual needs of the client. Locally run classes abound and usually allow a reduction in fees for the unwaged.
- Projects and clubs can be set up for those who need more active assistance. Hobbies clubs enable crafts and creative activities to be undertaken in a sheltered environment, ensuring an appropriate task and social support. The venue should not be in hospital accommodation.

• While the specialist therapies (drama, music, art and dance) are not leisure activities, they do call on the creative ability common to many. Such therapies require equipment and space. They can be provided in specialised units accessible to people living in the community.

COMMON PROBLEMS IN COMMUNITY WORK

Whilst this is a challenging and exciting field of work, its comparative newness necessitates that occupational therapists review their philosophy and practice. The service and the profession have to work together to ensure that an efficient and effective pattern of care is offered to the client.

SETTING PRIORITIES

The service and professional managers must define the target client group, to ensure correct referrals and the identification of priorities. One role of the professional manager is to foster a special interest in the needs of the defined group. Ideally, personal interests and ambitions should enhance care in the service and not conflict with it.

Occupational therapists need to identify professional priorities. This requires an appreciation of the therapeutic process used and support in the decision reached.

Community work does not impose a structured framework onto the working week, so all team members must devise methods of managing time effectively. Cases and other duties have to be placed in order of priority.

IDENTIFYING THE APPROPRIATE USE OF SKILLS

In establishing priorities, the therapist has to define and describe the contributions of the profession. This may be to other team members, referrers or clients and, most importantly, to oneself. The therapist will need to gain confidence in the work and what can be offered under the name of occupational therapy. Occupational therapy does not have the advantages of some other disciplines whose skills and involvement have been defined by legislation (for example, medicine and social work). It is important for occupational-therapy staff to link together and identify a common code of practice.

The novelty of the community setting at first suggested that it called for a complete break with traditional practice. Experience has shown that this is quite incorrect. Community work in mental health has enabled a return to the basic beliefs and skills of the profession.

SUPPORT AND SUPERVISION

Occupational therapy is in its infancy in identifying the various methods of supervision. Traditionally, the final responsibility for a case was held by the doctor in charge but, as the pattern of health care changes, this changes, too.

There is a need for case supervision of an occupational therapist by an occupational therapist. Many managers have felt they do not have the knowledge of such a new field but they do have the knowledge and experience of occupational therapy. Case supervision requires an understanding of the system in which the therapist is working, and of the principles underpinning the profession, no matter what the field of work.

All singleton professionals require support in maintaining their approach and in dealing with being alone in a group setting. Occupational therapists have a particular need since the harmonising skills often shown may result in the lessening of the obvious differences between disciplines. New and established staff need support in their work. Any changes within the setting can result in transitional strain.

Occupational therapy requires a problem-solving ability to be effective. Contact with other occupational therapists can enhance the creativity. Unfortunately, some therapists find it difficult to resolve the conflict of long-term gain over short-term loss; for them time spent with colleagues is in opposition to that spent with clients. The role of the manager is to point out the consequences of this belief.

PROFESSIONAL ROLE MODELS

Traditional settings consisted of a department with a mixture of grades of staff. There were senior staff who could act as role models for junior staff. The move into the community and the dispersal of staff has altered this practice. New staff may use other disciplines as models, which results in a further blurring of roles. Professional networks need to be established to provide all staff with the ability to learn from others. Experienced staff need to be encouraged to take on a mentor role with colleagues and guide them through difficult situations.

EVALUATION

Occupational therapists are beginning to identify the need to question practice, to evaluate the work undertaken and to communicate this to others. To do this effectively, therapists should be encouraged to pursue specific topics and to learn the skills of evaluation and research. Research methodology, such as clinical trials, has limited value in community settings, however, sociological models of research and single case studies can be used to good effect.

MANAGEMENT OF THE SERVICE

The professional manager must be responsible for maintaining professional standards and ensuring effective methods of service delivery. The staff of a community occupational-therapy service are its most important resource. The manager must be able to motivate them and allow them to develop and mature as professionals. Effective management harnesses the creative and enthusiastic energy of staff.

Helpers and technical instructors can provide a flexible workforce to set up and run a variety of leisure-related facilities and groups. Good management and support of staff is vital. Staff should be appointed to one of the support services and not to a particular club or centre, to allow for greater flexibility.

Professional management can create a 'team spirit', which enables occupational therapists to share their expertise and skills and to work more confidently in the knowledge that they have their colleagues' support. This is increasingly important in community work where therapists are working in isolation and are having to respond to the changing needs of a new service.

SUMMARY

In conclusion, it will be seen from this chapter that the occupational therapists working in the community reflect the practice of their colleagues in hospitals but show a greater emphasis on the environment and system the client uses. Activities used to promote function are based on the normal activities performed by the majority of the population. Where it is not possible to use public facilities, effort is taken to present options as close to normal as possible. Community occupational therapists teach skills and routine sets of behaviour to allow people to make use of community resources.

The holistic malleable approach used by occupational therapists is ideally suited to community work in the field of mental health. Therapists already work in social services and other fields that are primarily set in the community. The philosophy of the profession fits well with the concepts and goals of community care. Occupational therapists need to build on the strong, wide foundation of the profession. This may be a new direction for mental health but it is familiar ground. It allows full use to be made of the comprehensive skills shown in occupational therapy. Individual practitioners need to be well supported, encouraged, and supervised in order to contribute to the community mental-health teams as occupational therapists. Community work calls for the creativity of occupational therapy. No doubt the pattern of health care will continue to change. Occupational therapists are more than able to develop their practice to meet the needs of the current and future situations.

REFERENCES

DHSS 1983 Care in the community: A consultative document on moving resources for care in England. DHSS, London

DHSS 1975 Better services for the mentally ill. DHSS, London

Dunning H 1972 Environmental occupational therapy. American Journal of Occupational Therapy 26: 292–298

Etcheverry E 1979 Curriculum planning for community occupational therapy. Canadian Journal of Occupational Therapy 46(5): 210–205

Jones K, Poleti A 1985 Understanding the Italian experience. British Journal of Psychiatry 146: 341–347

Kielhofner G 1985 A model of human occupation. Williams and Wilkins, London

Maslow A H 1970 Motivation and personality. Harper & Row, New York

McCreadie R G et al 1985 The Scottish survey of psychiatric rehabilitation and support services. British Journal of Psychiatry 147: 289–294

Parker S 1976 The sociology of leisure. Allen & Unwin, London

Powell-Lawton M 1972 Assessing the competence of older people in Kent, Action for the Elderly, Behavioural Publications, Kent

Vaughan P 1983 The disordered development of day care in psychiatry. Health Trends 15: 91–94

Willson M 1983 Occupational therapy in long-term psychiatry. Churchill Livingstone, Edinburgh

Yerxa E J 1988 Personal communication

25

Working in a transcultural context

Clephane A. Hume

INTRODUCTION

Many countries, such as the UK, USA and Australia, are now generally acknowledged to be multicultural societies. In day-to-day practice, occupational therapists in most areas of the country will encounter patients from a variety of national backgrounds in addition to the native population.

To rehabilitate a patient from the culture of a long-term ward into the community means reeducating him to cope with a range of new social demands, so the concept of working with patients from different cultures is one which most occupational therapists will readily understand. The purpose of this chapter is to provide some background information on transcultural problems, beginning with definitions of terms. A section on the nature of a multicultural society follows, covering the reasons for immigration and the main immigrant groups in Britain.

The chapter goes on to look at the many difficulties people have when forced to adapt to a new culture, some of which can aggravate existing psychiatric problems or create new ones. Attitudes to illness, and expectations of treatment vary widely in differing cultures, and the additional problems and misunderstandings that can occur are considered.

A section on occupational therapy with transcultural patients considers the need to provide an appropriate service, then discusses the assessment process, suitable skills, media and techniques, and common problems that arise. Finally, the multiracial team and problems with inter-staff relationships are examined.

DEFINING TERMS

An understanding of the processes of adapting to a new culture is required, so we look at what is meant by culture, immigration, acculturation and assimilation. For the sake of clarity, the following interpretations will be used here.

Culture

Culture is a concept that varies according to the context in which it is being used. For the purposes of this chapter, it may be regarded as comprising traditional beliefs and social practices that lead to accepted rules for social interaction within a particular locality or social group. Culture will be continually evolving in response to external influences such as changes in population structure, media and ideological influences. Specific information about the beliefs of the culture can be passed on from one generation to another.

Taft (1977) describes four aspects of adapting from one culture to another.

1. *Cognitive*—the beliefs and ideologies held by adherents of a culture, and the verbal and nonverbal structures used in thinking.

2. *Dynamic*—people's expectations and attitudes; social obligations recognised within a culture; and actual behaviour.

3. *The interrelationship between the cognitive and dynamic aspects*, for example, understanding why people behave in a particular way in a given situation, and knowing how to behave in order to comply with their expectations.

4. *Performance*—the skills, such as linguistic and technical, that are required for competent living in the new culture.

Immigration

Immigration means to enter a foreign country as a permanent resident. The immigrant is leaving his country of birth to establish a home and life in a new country.

Assimilation

Assimilation is a process of socialisation, the merging of the social networks of two ethnic groups. This means that both primary groups, such as friendship groups, and social institutions, such as local politics, are shared by the host country and the immigrant. One of the highest levels of assimilation is inter-racial marriage. Acceptance of this is a mark of real integration into the host community.

Acculturation

Acculturation signifies the adoption by one ethnic group of the cultural traits of another. It is a part of assimilation.

THE MULTICULTURAL SOCIETY

The benefits of a multicultural society should outweigh any disadvantages in that there is sharing of a rich variety of experiences and resources. Knowledge from several cultures can benefit the entire community.

For the average citizen, the most obvious evidence of a multicultural society is the variety of restaurants offering different styles of food, or a wider range of products in the supermarket. Benefits, however, go much deeper than this.

Opportunities for sharing different customs can lead to widening of horizons and broadening of experience. The arts and music can be enriched through greater appreciation of the work of others. Dialogues about religion can lead to deeper understanding, and sharing of religious practices, such as meditation, can also be extremely valuable.

Cultural differences may enrich society, but they may also create divisions within it. Some peoples retain a distinct identity within a discrete ethnic group, some integrate fully into the host society, and yet others become part of a mixed society where an amalgam of social practices prevails.

Broadly, differences will be evident in day-to-day lifestyle, including dress and personal habits. Other less-obvious differences are to be found in religious beliefs, values and attitudes. These will only be discovered on closer acquaintance, once mutual trust has been established. Some of these differences may create situations of conflict or lead to difficulties in settling in the host country.

This section looks at the reasons for which people migrate and at the main immigrant groups who have entered Britain.

REASONS FOR IMMIGRATION

Broadly, migrants can be divided into two groups: voluntary and involuntary.

Voluntary immigration

People may voluntarily decide to emigrate for the purposes of study, for better job prospects, improved quality of life, or for personal social reasons such as marriage.

Among some groups, a system evolved to facilitate immigration. One person saved enough money, possibly with help from his family, to come to work in Britain and then, in turn, gave financial assistance to someone else who could come to join him. This type of sponsorship led to chains of workers, and hence groups of people from the same area of origin may be found in a new locality. Recent legislation has curbed this type of immigration.

As modern travel makes international movement easier, more people are staying for short periods in other countries for career purposes, or for vacations. Occupational therapists are highly mobile professionals and may experience working in several different countries, especially in the early years of their career.

Involuntary immigration

Involuntary departure from one's homeland is usually the result of a natural disaster, a serious politically based disturbance such as war, or religious persecution. Even when a move in these circumstances is premeditated it cannot be regarded as voluntary.

Often, refugees will have the additional stress of a hasty departure, possibly having had to leave family and friends without knowing what has happened to them. Refugees or those in exile (long-term absence from country of origin) may find that their families have become split up, with members living in countries that are thousands of miles apart.

Resettlement via transit camps brings its own traumas, leaving lifelong psychological scars.

The circumstances behind the reasons for leaving can affect the composition of the groups of people who seek refuge in other countries. The displaced persons after the Second World War were mainly young men who had been in labour camps, whereas the Czechs who fled in 1967 were academics who found the regime incompatible with their beliefs. Many who left Cyprus during the troubles were able to join friends or relatives in the UK and, to some extent, the Asians who were forced to leave Uganda during the Amin regime were also able to find contacts and supports on arrival.

MAIN IMMIGRANT GROUPS

When people from one country move to a particular region and stay there for economic reasons, compatriots who follow may often stay near them. Groups of displaced persons may be settled in an area or dispersed according to current policies within the host country, causing certain ethnic groups to predominate in different areas. It is necessary for any therapist to be acquainted with the groups in the catchment area and to learn about their particular social rules and beliefs.

Space does not permit detailed consideration of different groups and their cultures, nor is this desirable lest stereotyping results. However, the reasons for immigration, date of immigration, main language and religion are included, followed by any significant general points. The reader is referred to Henley (1979) or Sampson (1982) for further reading.

Afro-Caribbeans

This group already had a multicultural heritage as the result of the slave trade from the west coast of Africa to the West Indies. Many people moved to Britain in response to a recruitment drive during the economic boom in post-war Britain.

Afro-Caribbeans speak English and often

Creole. Most are Christian, although many of the younger generation are Rastafarians.

There are differences between the islanders of the West Indies, so that someone who comes from Jamaica will not wish to be identified with Trinidad.

Asians

This is a very wide label, covering: citizens from all parts of the Indian subcontinent, Pakistanis, refugees from East Africa, residents of Southeast Asia and Chinese.

Indians

People from different parts of the subcontinent have come to the UK to seek work. Communities have become established as those already living in the UK have sponsored relatives or friends to come to join them. The main areas of origin are the Punjab and Gujerat.

The many languages spoken include local dialects such as Gujerati. Although many people have a knowledge of Hindi it cannot be assumed that this is understood and care should be taken to identify the correct language if the help of an interpreter is required.

There is a large number of cultures and religions within this overall group and people are often recognised as being Sikhs (from the Punjab) or Hindus (Gujerat) rather than members of a particular ethnic group. Inter-religious conflicts may cause stresses within a community. Hard work and family commitments are highly valued and customs in relation to dress and diet are respected. This may lead to children following an Indian lifestyle at home while adopting Western practices at school.

Pakistanis

Recruitment drives in Pakistan during the 1950s and 1960s sought people for the motor and textile industries.

People from Pakistan are likely to speak Urdu although some will use Mirpuri. Most are Muslims, followers of Islam.

In many instances men came alone and have been separated from their wives ever since, unless they have been able to return for holidays.

East-African Asians

During the time of oppression in Uganda in the 1970s Amin expelled Ugandan Asians and many sought refuge in different areas of the UK. Many were shopkeepers in the commercial class in Uganda and have been able to reestablish themselves here.

Their language depends upon the area of India from which they originally came but many speak English in addition to Swahili (the language of East Africa). They may be Hindus, Muslims or Sikhs. Their memories of persecution should be sensitively treated.

Southeast Asians, Vietnamese

From the 1970s onwards people fled from political oppression and are often referred to as the 'boat people' because of their escape by sea. They were settled from transit camps into different areas of the UK, though many have now moved to the south.

The principal religions of this region are Buddhism, Taoism and Confucianism. People speak the language of the country and may also have a knowledge of Cantonese.

As with other refugees, their experiences of refugee camps and extreme privations may leave indelible and painful memories.

Chinese

Chinese people have come from Hong Kong since the 1950s, generally in search of work. They represent a multiplicity of cultural groups so that generalisations are difficult. Chinese people are renowned for being a close-knit, hard-working community and the demands of their working day may set them apart from the host community.

Overseas Chinese usually speak Cantonese or Hakka, although the official language among the many in mainland China is Mandarin.

Some Chinese are Christian, some follow traditional religions or none at all.

Africans

Commonwealth citizens from different countries in Africa have come to study in the UK and some families have sent many generations here for education. In some instances students remain after completing their educational courses. Some will speak Swahili and local dialects will also be used. English will be familiar to many, although the intonation may not be immediately understood.

The predominant religions are Islam and Christianity, depending upon the country of origin.

Media reports of civil war and famine in certain African states can be worrying for those who have moved to the UK and can also present a false picture to the host community. The issue of apartheid also arouses strong emotions in people from the African continent.

East Europeans

After the Second World War refugees from states such as Poland, Lithuania and the Ukraine entered Britain. These people did not come from Russia, which now has jurisdiction over many of their homelands.

Each group has its own language, and most of the people are Christian. In general, people from Eastern Europe have adapted to life in the UK over the years, but although they may not immediately be thought of as immigrants, any more than citizens of the European Community, many have not learned to speak English and are experiencing problems in old age and widowhood.

South Americans

Political refugees from Chile and other South American states have sought asylum in Britain since 1973. Others have come as students at various times.

With the exception of Brazil, where people are of Portuguese origin, South Americans speak Spanish. Most countries within the continent are multicultural and this is reflected in the religions, although Christianity is widely recognised.

A host of emotional problems and uncertainties about family members who have been left behind pose extra stresses for this refugee group. Continuing problems in South America make it impossible for many people to return to their country of origin and the future remains uncertain.

Arabs, Iranians

Arab people in Britain may be students, wealthy businessmen or refugees from war-torn regions of Iran and Iraq. In the late 1970s Iranians were exiled following the overthrow of the Shah.

Arabic is spoken within all Arab states but the language of the Iranians is Farsi. The people are Muslim, and Islamic culture demands adherence to rigid sociocultural rules, particularly in regard to the status of women. Some of the behaviour accepted as the social norm in Britain is regarded with horror.

There are varying needs and problems according to different countries, for example, the Palestinian Arabs of the West Bank do not have the same civic status as Israeli Arabs and such differences should be sensitively approached.

ADAPTING TO A NEW COUNTRY

The normal process of socialisation is covered in Chapter 15. Additional obstacles must be overcome in becoming resocialised to another culture. Briefly, as the child grows and develops, he learns the social rules of the society in which he lives. First, he discovers what behaviour is acceptable within his family. This is then reinforced through the education system and the media and in interactions within the wider community. The adult has thus absorbed, and usually conforms to, a vast number of rules and complex sociocultural patterns of behaviour.

Someone moving to another culture has to compare the new behaviour patterns required with his previous experience and decide within himself the degree to which he wishes to modify his behaviour if he is to become resocialised and, therefore, more acceptable to the host community. This may be subconscious or a deliberate decision to adapt.

Learning everyday tasks, such as going shopping or travelling about in the local community, will require social skills that can be identified and learned relatively easily but other areas are more complex. Should diet or religious customs be modified? Can family and sexual roles be maintained? Should clothing styles be altered, other than for warmth? Many cultural rules are the result of closely interwoven social and religious practices, and to relinquish them can be painful and difficult.

Assuming that the individual wishes to change, he may do so at three different levels:

- adjustment, where there is no change in values but behaviour is modified to enable harmonious relationships
- adaptation, to modify his attitudes in line with those of the host culture
- integration into the social networks, becoming more like the native population. This implies a degree of change on both sides but to a greater extent on the part of the immigrant.

ACCULTURATION

Changes in cultural patterns take time to occur, according to the extent of differences between groups. Learning new social skills in adulthood is not an easy process and learning to cope in unfamiliar cultures may cause loss of confidence and identity.

The immigrant needs to develop competence in the social skills of the new culture before he is able to take on new roles but models to demonstrate such skills may not be available, particularly if an individual is not willing to admit to inadequacies in everyday behaviour, such as knowing how to turn on a tap or learning to use a knife and fork. These are small points but they add up to a feeling of incompetence that reduces self-confidence.

The culture shock experienced by new immigrants is stressful and the constant endeavour to do the correct thing and not cause offence is extremely tiring, as is speaking a foreign language.

ASSIMILATION

When a person has mastered the social processes and achieved acculturation, he has reached the stage at which he is accepted as an individual by the host society. He then has to become assimilated at a deeper level in order to be fully integrated. Someone who might be regarded as a nice chap but is not accepted as a town councillor or a potential son-in-law is not fully integrated.

The higher the level of assimilation reached, the more alike the native and the immigrant become. For the second-generation immigrant, who is socialised from birth into the host culture, the differences may be negligible. He may experience some clashes between parental behaviours and those which he learns at school but be able to cope with this.

If there is a visible difference, prejudice can make it virtually impossible for people to become fully assimilated. Colour can be a disadvantage in the same way as a disfiguring disability. Contemporary attitudes of resentment towards immigrants, who are seen as competing for resources such as jobs, may be reinforced by the media, creating problems with housing or employment and leading to general deprivation. Access to such resources is linked to assimilation.

FACTORS AFFECTING ASSIMILATION

Some of the main factors are:

- ability to learn new social skills
- availability of models to demonstrate new skills
- different appearance, such as skin colour
- language.

Other factors which affect assimilation are as follows.

● *Cultural distance* between immigrant and host community. This includes the history, culture and ideology of the host country. Scales for determining this distance in overseas students groups have been described by Cox (1986), who found that cultural distance had no relationship to academic success. Any problems recounted were related to difficulties experienced after arrival in Britain, such as language.

● *The length of time* for which an established group has lived in the community. A long-standing group such as the Jewish population is assimilated more easily than a more recent group such as the Vietnamese boat people. Existing cultural links and named contacts ease the transition.

• *Previous contact* with Western culture. Has it been possible for the person to talk with others who have visited the future host country prior to his departure? Has he met a host-country tourist in his own country and, if so, how realistic an impression did he gain? Has he had a briefing on arrival to explain some of the day-to-day differences? What are the communication problems: is there any common language?

• *Standard of living.* Someone may be materially better off by moving to, for example, Britain but may nevertheless be living in poor circumstances relative to the indigenous population. The person may have a loan to repay or may be sending money home to support his family.

• *Separate groupings* may develop in an attempt to preserve cultural identity and to feel 'at home' and these may create a barrier between the excluded host community and the immigrant group. The cultural distance thus perpetuated prevents integration and can lead to misunderstandings.

• *Racism and prejudice*, although often denied, cause the most obvious difficulties. Instances of victimisation may be denied by the host country and there is considerable reluctance in some areas to admit to any racial problems. The political and social systems may not come to terms with the problem.

• *Unavailability of familiar items*, such as foodstuffs, although apparently small problems in themselves, may accumulate to a sense of loss.

• *Adjustment from rural to urban life*, for example, from a village in Bangladesh to inner-city London, causes stress in some cases.

• *Pressure to succeed* often exists where there has been considerable financial outlay and sacrifice on the part of the family to enable the refugees to leave. This may heighten the feeling of responsibility towards the homeland, leaving little energy for focussing on the new surroundings. Any failure must be hidden from the family at home, creating additional stress.

Problems in assimilation

Difficulties described as occurring in multicultural societies are:

• need to preserve cultural identity
• racism and prejudice
• language and communication barriers
• sense of loss.

Other problems include:

• *Familiar cues* may be lacking in the environment, heightening the feeling of separateness. Street signs are in a foreign language. Styles of architecture may seem alien and familiar settings may not be available, for example, an outdoor meeting point where friends and neighbours can gather.

• *Segregation*, and efforts to retain cultural identity within groups.

• *Inability to communicate*, and therefore to understand at both conceptual and conversational levels, leads to retreat into the segregated group.

• *Cultural variations* may not be recognised. Failure to identify with those who have successfully managed to integrate weakens the ability to adapt to new social rules and roles. Subtle variations in temperament or attitudes may cause problems, for example, an individual who comes from a country where time is not important will not be popular in a culture where punctuality is highly valued.

• *Expected length of stay* may influence the reactions of people arriving in a country. Knowing that the stay is for a fixed period may enable someone to cope with quite severe difficulties.

• *A planned departure*, such as the desire to settle in Israel when circumstances permit, means that arrival in a new country represents the realisation of a dream or an ambition. The desire to assimilate is facilitated by motivation to settle.

• *Refugees*, in contrast, may have been exposed to torture and brutality, imprisonment or, at the least, fear of being caught escaping. Memories of the stress of living under threat, without freedom of speech, may scar the person for life and make adjustment to an alternative culture especially threatening. Family break-up may be an additional stress.

SECOND-GENERATION IMMIGRANTS

It must be noted that many apparent immigrants have been born in the host country. It is extremely upsetting for people to be asked where they have come from when they have spent all their lives in the UK and therefore feel British. However, as second-generation citizens, their expectations and experiences are different from those of their parents. Why should their rights and entitlements be different from those of any other British citizen?

The culture of their parents may lead children to a split identity between home and the wider society. The clash that may ensue between the cultures of the different generations can create considerable stress. Kolvin and Nicol (1979) have described some of the psychiatric problems affecting the children of immigrants.

An Asian girl, whose parents expect her to remain at home after school, may resent not being able to join her friends at the disco. She may also get into trouble if she speaks to male fellow pupils at the bus-stop. Many such teenagers can accept family life, watching Indian videos, and gain a sense of cultural identity from participating in worship at the local temple. They learn to switch from one culture to another and it is only when a major event occurs, such as an arranged marriage to someone still in India, that problems arise.

Expectations are gradually modifying so that a girl may now enter further education — where it is to be hoped that any restrictions on social participation will be sensitively accepted.

In later generations, the search for 'roots' may become stronger, with individuals returning to their country of origin to seek an understanding of their cultural heritage. Sadly, this may lead to a feeling of greater distance from both the original and the adopted culture.

ILLNESS AND THE IMMIGRANT

Living in a foreign country, or any unfamiliar society, may be an alienating experience but this is, of course, not always the case. Many people adapt over time and enjoy the variety of experiences and opportunities available without having any feeling of being set apart.

Others, however, feel that they do not fit in and this can aggravate existing problems. Depression may result, or hostility and anger towards the host community may be expressed both verbally and physically. It is only in rare circumstances that frank psychiatric symptoms emerge and these may be difficult to detect if the psychiatric staff involved represent the alien group in the eyes of the patient.

INCIDENCE OF ILLNESS

Are there real differences in presentation rates between races and if so, why? Is transcultural psychiatry a valid concept?

Cochrane (1977) in a study of mental illness among immigrants admitted to hospitals in England and Wales, identified relatively high admission rates for particular diagnoses among different ethnic groups. Irish and Scots people had the highest admission rate, compared to the native-born population, with high levels of alcohol and drug-related disorders. All immigrant groups had higher rates of admission for schizophrenia, due, perhaps, to differences in age structure between the groups.

The high incidence of admissions may be either a cause or an effect of migration. For example, social drift may be a consequence of schizophrenia, with people moving to seek a solution to their problems. On the other hand, the level of stress that results from immigration may precipitate psychiatric problems. Sometimes there is an acute reaction to immigration but, in other instances, years may elapse before psychiatric conditions manifest themselves.

Immigrants may be at variance with the existing groups within the country they join, for example, if the Scots and the Irish come from an area with higher incidence of alcohol problems in the first place, they will inevitably show a higher rate of incidence than other groups in their new locality.

More research is needed on the following questions. How many hidden cases of illness are there? Are patients known to their general practitioner or do they receive support from their own ethnic group? Is there considerable under-representation of certain groups among those who do get admitted? Does presentation affect diagnosis and are diagnoses accurate? Are there language or cultural blocks which prevent take-up of National Health Service resources, or does absence of alternative support actually precipitate admission?

Contributing factors

Particular symptoms may be linked to recognisable precipitating factors. Racism has an influence on depression. Fernando (1986) has detailed the incidence of depression in ethnic minorities and explains the implications of racist attitudes for minority groups. He suggests that racism is more than an added stress, it may actually damage self-esteem and create learned helplessness. To attempt to develop coping structures and to improve self-esteem for the individual is to deal with only one side of the problem. We should also try to treat the cause.

Antisocial acts by the indigenous population, such as setting fire to a group of Pakistanis in a car, or other harassment of immigrants, might lead to feelings of depression, paranoia, or anxiety.

Sometimes the death of a spouse precipitates referral, for example, a Polish man's Scottish wife dealt with day-to-day matters and shielded him from the difficulties resulting from his poor command of English. His reactions to bereavement were greatly magnified by his feelings of alienation.

CROSS-CULTURAL DIFFERENCES IN PRESENTATION

Concepts of illness obviously vary from one cultural background to another, from rural to urban settings and at different class levels within society, and also affect help-seeking behaviour.

Some cultures simply do not have words to describe a concept which is unfamiliar. 'My heart is heavy' may signify depression and is quite easy for others to understand but other descriptions and somatisation (physical presentation of psychological problems) of symptoms may be less obvious.

A client who presents with noisy, florid symptoms and is brought to hospital by the police may be diagnosed as experiencing hallucinations and delusional ideation. His resistance to hospitalisation may lead to compulsory detention and use of major tranquillisers to restore calm. Further investigation may reveal that such behaviour is the cultural norm in response to severe stress and that, far from being a religiously inclined schizophrenic, the person is doubly distressed at facing the extra difficulty of a non-comprehending host society. The problems surrounding this type of incident and misdiagnosis are further described by Littlewood and Lipsedge (1982).

The occupational therapist is less likely to be involved in crisis admission to hospital but may come across similar problems in the community. She will certainly encounter people who are not favourably disposed towards a health-care system that misjudges them through lack of understanding.

Occasionally, culture-bound syndromes may occur, with symptoms that seem bizarre to the Western mind but are familiar to patients (Littlewood and Lipsedge 1985). Conditions such as 'amok' (a Malay word for a state in which the person behaves in an uncharacteristic and very excited manner) are very rarely reported in the UK.

The concept of illness

In another culture, the concept of illness may be different from that of Western society. A headache may indicate a life-threatening illness rather than a relatively trivial reaction to the stresses of everyday life. The expression of symptoms may be in somatic terms; a headache or sore stomach may indicate depression.

The British attitude of maintaining a 'stiff upper lip' and being stoical in the face of pain is shared by some other cultures and may not always be helpful to the doctor who is endeavouring to ascertain the level of pain being experienced. In other countries, the appropriate reaction is to writhe or scream out in agony. These physical symptoms have parallels in psychiatry, where screams and tears may be deemed to be excessive expressions of distress.

The person's attitude towards illness is often reflected in his help-seeking behaviour.

Help-seeking behaviour

Each community has its own informal rules about how a sick person seeks help and from whom. Much care may be provided by lay people without any recourse to professional help; alternatively, a sick person may be encouraged to seek medical help fairly rapidly. The family may influence the decision, or other people in respected positions, such as teachers or priests, may suggest seeking help.

Help-seeking behaviour will also be governed by past experience and the ways in which the individual has learned to obtain help for an illness. It will also depend upon the level of social support available to the individual. If there is a family network and tried and tested family remedies, solutions may be sought through the advice of older or respected members rather than the NHS. People may accept illness as being the will of God, and outwith their control. This apparently passive reaction may be puzzling to hospital staff when the problem is one that is easily dealt with.

The sick person may not believe that Western medicine has the answer to a particular problem. Help may be sought from alternative forms of medicine, such as a herbalist or faith healer. This may be for language and communication reasons, as well as cultural factors. Knowledge of what medicine can provide is also relevant, as is an understanding of the nature of the illness itself. Fear of having a serious illness can often be a deterrent to seeking help, as is fear of stigma and shame on the family.

PROBLEMS IN DIAGNOSIS

Problems in making an accurate diagnosis, based on misunderstanding and lack of communication, will inevitably occur. Rack (1982) elaborates on cultural pitfalls in respect of different diagnoses. The occupational therapist is not primarily a diagnostician but obtaining information or observing behaviour that contributes to a diagnostic formulation is relevant and it is valuable to have some

understanding of common problems. The best way of learning how to obtain such information is by talking to an experienced practitioner and being as perceptive and sensitive as possible.

Lack of differentiation between words, and nuances in language, particularly in emotional descriptions, may create blocks to communications. Literal translations may be highly misleading.

CASE EXAMPLE 25.1

Soraya was an Iranian teenager, who had been living in Britain with her family for 4 years. She was admitted following parental concern about her withdrawal and lazy behaviour. In the ward, she appeared pleasant and responded to contact from others but did not initiate activity of her own volition. The staff felt that this lack of initiative might be a cultural behaviour, since the role of women was understood to be fairly subservient. However, Dr Khan, an Iranian, happened to visit the hospital and was asked if she would see Soraya. Dr Khan was very indignant at any suggestion that the problem might be cultural (she herself exemplified why it might not be) and was able to elicit that Soraya had delusional ideas about other people being endangered by her actions, explaining many of the presenting problems.

CASE EXAMPLE 25.2

Mr Chopra reported that his wife was not coping at home, failing to carry out normal household chores. Queries regarding her mood resulted in a reiteration of the above information, confirmed by the client. A few enquiries of a doctor familiar with the culture led to the discovery that neglect of social roles may indicate depression, although no understanding of the alteration in mood or ways of expressing this may be evident. Mrs Chopra received antidepressant medication and resumed her usual domestic round to the satisfaction of all concerned.

Loss of face

This is a concept that can only be partially understood by Western cultures. We know what it is like to feel a fool by making a social gaffe or a public mistake, we may feel embarrassed for an individual who is struggling to make a public speech, but loss of face is far deeper than this; the individual's self-esteem is ruined and his place in society may be lost, perhaps requiring a move elsewhere. His total existence is damaged; sometimes suicide is seen to be the only acceptable response. The slur and stigma extend to the family and may create considerable social difficulties.

Responses of individuals to questions may be coloured by attempts to avoid loss of face and this can be very exasperating for anyone who is unaware of the dynamics of the situation. It also has implications for psychiatry, as difficulties are masked and any probing is firmly resisted.

Somatisation

Probably the most well-documented example of how presentation of symptoms may vary from one culture to another is that of somatisation. Instead of the agitated, perhaps tearful, client who voices feelings of unhappiness, delusions of worthlessness or guilt, the doctor may be confronted by a person with a headache or sore stomach, for which no physical cause can be identified. Rather than pressing the individual, it may be possible to treat him for depression in the knowledge that this is a recognised presentation in people who have no language or concepts with which to describe it in other than physical symptoms.

Ongoing research in Bradford and Asia (Mumford 1989) indicates that the tendency towards somatisation may be less of a cultural difference than has previously been thought. British patients will describe similar symptoms if asked for this information in addition to verbalisation of mood.

Conceptual differences

A common language does not necessarily mean common conceptual patterns or symbolism and at this level communication becomes far more complex. For example, colours may have different meanings. Red is an auspicious colour for the Chinese and in Indian cultures white signifies mourning. Most people in the UK use an umbrella to give protection from rain, but someone from a warmer part of the world may think of it as a sunshade.

On a social basis, family relationships may be understood differently. Instead of the clearly defined relationships linked to the nuclear family, somebody from West Africa may talk about having many mothers, meaning his aunts and cousins. The extended family draws different distinctions.

Conceptual differences become integrated into value systems so that understanding and communication of illness behaviour may vary from group to group.

Mr Chopra (in Case example 25.2), who declared that his wife was ill because she would not cook his meals, would not find much sympathy for his attitude in some Western households.

Immigrants' ideas about Western society may be dependent upon television viewing rather than derived from direct experience, leading to some very distorted ideas.

Perceptual differences

These are complex. People growing up in rural or urban environments will learn to perceive their environment in different ways. The high-rise blocks of Hong Kong provide different sensory input to the villages of Bangladesh. There may even be different interpretations of round and straight; people who have been reared in a village with circular houses and an absence of straight-sided buildings will have a different sense of perspective (Gregory 1972).

If linked to conceptual differences, incidents may be interpreted completely differently and this may be relevant in psychiatric practice. A hearing from a spiritual healer, or seeing evidence that the evil eye has been cast upon one, may be readily understood by someone from West Africa. In the UK, to have second sight or communication with spirits may be regarded as a family gift. Neither of these is the same as hallucinations but both may be interpreted as such. Careful questioning is necessary to identify beliefs and the normality of the person's experience within the context of family values, even if it is at variance with that of the local community.

Obtaining information

There may be problems in gaining sufficient material upon which to base an assessment. Information is often contained within the family and rules of medical confidentiality do little to alter this. The social stigma of psychiatric illness may be seen as so damaging that help is not sought when it is required. The psychiatric team may therefore lack information that may be crucial to the management of the client.

There may be a reluctance on the part of a group to provide details about cultural norms. Fear of ridicule, resentment about prying, or a feeling of intrusion, together with doubts as to how the information may be used can all be problematic if mutual trust is not established.

SOCIAL FACTORS

Expectations

Doctors and other members of the treatment team may find themselves being expected to provide an instant solution, often when little information is being volunteered by the client. For the psychiatric practitioner this raises particular difficulties when the client is not willing to accept responsibility for his own progress.

A client may regard a cure through Western medicine as being impossible or, in contrast, a total cure may be expected from medication. Ideas as to what might happen to people in hospital may be based on the unfortunate experiences of others who have been misdiagnosed, or on the notion of bed rest as found in the general hospital setting. Television programmes may be responsible for influencing people's attitudes and psychiatric staff without uniforms do not conform to the expected image.

Family roles

Family structures may not consist of a nuclear family of husband, wife and two children but be an extended kinship system in the context of which all decisions are made. Having the family participating in the decision-making process may not be compatible with the team's goals of inde-pendence for the individual, even if there is no clash of opinions. It can be frustrating for the medical team to have to wait while overseas relations are consulted but to flout the convention will do nothing for the client's recovery or motivation.

The therapist should recognise that some of the attitudes found in the UK display shocking disregard for family values and responsibilities, and this may cause offence to others.

Social roles

These may be closely linked to religious and family customs. For example, they often include distinct divisions in sexual roles. A woman who has always maintained purdah may accompany her husband to Britain when he comes to study. Without her female relations her social network is non-existent, so how can she establish contacts in her new environment? She may not even be allowed to go to the shops alone.

Other women may find the freedom of their Western counterparts quite alien or, in some cases, despicable. Caring for her children may prove problematic and if they are of school age their experiences in the classroom may be totally alien to her.

The therapist must remember that topics such as assertiveness training for women may be quite unsuitable. It is not appropriate to impose one's own ideas of liberated behaviour on women who belong to male-dominated cultures.

Religion

For many people, religion may have a far greater significance in day-to-day life than that to which we in the West have become generally accustomed. Respect should be accorded to religious practices such as specific times for prayer, dietary rules and the need to have significant objects to hand. For example, in other countries it may be standard practice to cease work for prayer. Preferred foods may not be available and required dietary items be unobtainable. This will cause distress, the extent of which may not be fully understood.

Other problems may occur in the observance of religious obligations. One example is the difficulty of keeping Ramadan during the long hours of daylight in a British summer. The original requirement of fasting from dawn to sunset did not encompass such a long period.

PRACTICAL PROBLEMS

Access to resources

Difficulties in access to resources may prevent help-seeking. Time off work costs money that the person may not be able to afford. There may be an expensive or time-consuming journey to a health centre or appointments may not be available at a time when it is easy for the person to attend. There may be apprehension about attending 'mixed' clinics, the husband desiring to be present when his wife is examined. Fear of not being able to see a female doctor is a difficulty for many women and it should be possible to deal with this. Bad experiences, including those of friends, will affect future behaviour.

Communication

In the West we take our freedom of speech for granted. We may even question any apparent limitations put on it but our habit of talking frankly will not be shared by those from countries where censorship is the norm. People from all cultures will obviously show varying degrees of reticence in respect to revealing personal information and expressing feelings. For some, however, it is simply not socially acceptable to voice certain matters even within the family. To admit to problems is to disgrace the family as well as the individual.

Language

Ensuring that communication between two people is effective is always a problem in psychiatry. Use of jargon by client or therapist may prevent full understanding without either party being aware that the words have different meanings for each of them. Use of concise and straightforward language will help, even for clients with a good command of English. Being unable to communicate effectively is obviously frustrating and can lead to major loss of confidence and self-esteem.

Use of interpreters

If the patient's use of English is non-existent or poor and the therapist does not have a fluent command of the relevant language, then the help of an interpreter must be sought. This may sound straightforward, as most hospitals and social services have lists of competent linguists who are willing to help in this way and local community groups may also be able to assist, but the choice of interpreter is not as simple as it might seem. Use of a professional interpreter who is known to maintain confidentiality will result in greater understanding of particular groups and is the ideal situation. Other alternatives may, however, be necessary.

Clients' relatives may indicate their willingness to help but they may censor information. The husband may be more fluent than his wife, because of his work, and may therefore be asked to assist. However, the therapist does not know when he is providing a direct translation and when he is adding his own impressions of the situation. Finding out how the client sees the problem can be very difficult, particularly if marital difficulties exist.

Children may also be called upon to interpret for parents. Here, there is often a cultural, as well as generation gap. Parents may also feel inhibited about exposing their problems. Neither side should be expected to use this method of interpreting unless there is no other choice.

There may be a member of the staff from the client's country who could be called upon to help. Here, too, information may be adjusted to hide deficiencies or perceived unacceptable aspects that might reflect badly on the homeland. A common nationality does not, of course, mean a common language; there are many dialects and languages in the Indian subcontinent, for example. Even if there is a common language, there may be major social differences such as class, religion or politics. Any of these may prevent communication and possibly make the situation worse, if two opposing attitudes to a political regime come into conflict.

Special groups

In line with the general trend towards self-help, women's groups and other special groups are now beginning to be established. The latter are run by minority ethnic groups particularly for their own members and obviously have more credibility than a foreign professional.

Any service should include resources for interpretation and in some areas it is possible to recruit bilingual staff to assist in achieving this.

The elderly

A group with growing needs is the elderly. In addition to the general sociological problems associated with the elderly, members of minority groups may face particular disadvantages. Such problems may include deprivation, particularly separation from family as contact with the extended family is reduced or lost. Grandchildren may seem to be living in a totally strange world and the cultural distance may be distressing to the grandparents.

Communication difficulties may increase as elderly friends and relatives die, and those who speak the mother tongue become fewer. This, in turn, restricts social contact and the ability to participate in decision making about different aspects of life.

While local amenities may include a mosque or temple, the number of day centres that cater for special needs is small. There may be language barriers if people cannot converse easily in English. Someone who requires a halal diet (specially prepared meat) or kosher food will not feel able to attend. Equally, bland British food will not be appetising to people used to spicy Asian dishes.

Activities, too, may be culturally unacceptable and the person may thus feel alone, depressed and without a role or purpose in life. This should be combatted by involving consumers in planning resources and programmes. Amenities may also be established by community groups, such as the provision of a Chinese lunch club in a local church hall.

RACIST ATTITUDES

Psychiatric staff, regarding themselves as being sensitive to clients' need and behaviour, will resent any suggestion of racist attitudes but the problem does still arise.

Racism may occur in staff–staff or staff–client relationships, as well as in society as a whole. The consequences of each of these three areas have implications for client care. Racial stereotyping may affect choice of treatment as well as aggravating difficulties that may have led to the stresses which caused the client's admission in the first place.

When circumstances are such that the individual seeks psychiatric help, he may encounter racism within the hospital setting. This may take the form of racial stereotyping but it may also have implications for the methods of treatment selected. Limited experience may result in limited resources but may also lead to standardised responses. There may be greater use of electroconvulsive therapy (ECT) or attribution of a particular diagnosis at a higher frequency than that of the dominant culture. Such generalisations are obviously detrimental to client care.

Outright racism may occur, sometimes within the client group and sometimes between the client and staff. White clients may resist treatment from black or coloured staff. The reverse is unlikely. Covert prejudice is more difficult to deal with. Mimicking can be stopped but more subtle action may be less obvious.

Disregard for values and behavioural norms may not be regarded as racism but failure to provide the correct diet or to respect religious customs is both distressing and offensive to the individual.

In some parts of the country the person may be the only visibly different member of the client group, and this situation requires close monitoring to avoid scapegoating. Racial hostility, in addition to the stress of hospital admission, should be quickly countered and can, if circumstances are right, be put to educational use in breaking down existing barriers. Burke (1986) describes this issue in greater detail.

OCCUPATIONAL THERAPY WITH TRANSCULTURAL CLIENTS

Admission to hospital is a traumatic event for anyone but is much more so when the culture of the country itself is unfamiliar. Being ill in a foreign country can be a miserable experience. There are communication difficulties, lack of privacy and an expectation that you will disclose your personal problems within a group of strangers. Staff should recognise that what they regard as minimal self-disclosure or expression of feelings may represent a real effort on the part of the client, who may feel that he has already confided much.

This section first looks at the problems in providing a service to clients from another culture, then suggests how to conduct an assessment of such a client.

Appropriate culture-based skills, media and techniques, and common problems are then covered. Finally, staff–client and inter-staff relationships are discussed.

PROVIDING AN ADEQUATE SERVICE

Bavington and Majid (1986) indicate some of the problems in providing adequate services to different immigrant groups; a complex subject. Creating separate client groups implies continued segregation but an integrated service may not meet special needs. Occupational therapists will usually be required to treat clients within a multicultural setting and this can be very beneficial. It is worth considering, as in any treatment programme, how particular clients would benefit from selected activities. Specific groups may be indicated, the most obvious being separate male and female groups according to the conventions of purdah.

The question arises as to who should treat clients from various cultures. Someone from the same country would ensure language compatability but this ignores social and political differences and, likewise, differences in religion or dialect may be overlooked by well-intentioned staff.

Some black clients, for example, feel very strongly that they prefer a black therapist, others indicate no preference or may even attribute a higher level of expertise to a white therapist. In the UK the occupational therapist is unlikely to have options and will treat clients as they present, in accordance with the code of conduct of the College of Occupational Therapists.

INTRODUCING OCCUPATIONAL THERAPY TO CLIENTS

Since the aims of treatment are often not well understood by the general population, the therapist will have to find ways of overcoming both barriers to communication.

For many clients, occupational therapy is an alien concept and the need to achieve competence in skills may not seem relevant as the family will often assume the care of a mentally disabled relative.

As always, assessment is the first stage in the treatment process.

ASSESSMENT

In a transcultural situation the therapist has a greater than usual need to be aware of the client's social background, in order to put his problems into the correct context. Acceptable practice in one culture may not be suitable in another and every effort should be made to avoid undue stress caused by cultural misunderstanding. An awareness of underlying belief systems of different cultures will help to avoid this, although this knowledge takes time to acquire.

What to assess

As in any initial assessment, the therapist seeks to identify particular problems and general mental state, and to sort out immediate aims of treatment from those of a more long-term nature. In a transcultural environment some attempt should be made to assess the level of integration and ability to cope in the host society.

Assessing the level of integration

It is helpful to have some awareness of the extent to which any client is integrated into his new community. In addition to obtaining basic demographic data, some or all of the following questions could be considered:

- Which language/dialects are spoken?
- What is the country of origin and which region did the client live in?
- In the new country, what is his socio-economic background and does this represent a change in status?
- Are there clearly defined and rigidly enforced gender divisions or other social roles?
- Is there evidence of integration or is the person adhering rigidly to his social group?
- Which groups does the client identify with and what networks are being used?
- Is there a kinship system or is the person socially isolated?
- Is there contact between generations and is this an area of conflict?
- How far are the norms of the host country being adopted?

This material should enable the therapist to gain information about the individual's family life, including religion and diet. She will also gain an understanding of values and interactions and how these relate to the community in which the person is living.

Orque, Bloch and Monroy's ethnic/cultural system (1983) is designed as a framework for nursing care but also provides a useful guide for the therapist. Further information may be obtained by reference to Sampson (1982) or Mares, Henley and Baxter (1985) who describe considerations affecting multiracial Britain.

Standard occupational therapy assessment

Conventional occupational therapy assessment forms can also be completed, provided that the rater is aware of the relevance of the items for any individual. Additional points may be added for particular ethnic groups.

The occupational therapist should remember that assessment is a prerequisite for treatment planning and this is especially important in the transcultural context. Expecting a client to carry out a task that is unacceptable to his value system is of no benefit and many rehabilitation programmes have foundered on unrealistic expectations.

Areas which should be considered include:

- activities of daily living, with emphasis on social skills
- interpersonal relationships
- personal care
- leisure activities
- work, where relevant.

Attention must be given to:

- linguistic ability
- religion
- diet
- cultural norms and values
- place of birth
- length of residence in the UK, if the person was not born here
- contacts with the local community
- use of resources and available supports
- the extent to which contacts exist beyond the immediate family and ethnic group.

CULTURE-BASED SKILLS

As occupational therapy is essentially a practically based profession that aims to enhance clients' competence in daily living, many of the areas that transcultural work encompasses fall within this category. It is important to note that sexual division of labour may occur. The wife will carry out the domestic tasks and the husband will be the breadwinner. This division may be less clearly defined than in the past but it is not appropriate to ignore the boundaries that do exist.

A sensitive awareness of male–female relationships is also required. A man may not be able to discuss personal topics with a female therapist.

Rack (1982) suggests that occupational therapy is a meaningless concept to most Asians. What should the occupational therapist contribute in such a situation? Is activity really appropriate? The focus on 'doing' may well be alien, especially to the elderly, who are happy to sit and watch the world go by. Rack suggests cookery for women and physical activities for men, but what about programmes with a more psychotherapeutic basis? Bavington and Majid (1986) cite the example of group psychotherapy as practised with Asian clients in Bradford. One of the restrictions on this type of work is obviously communication, if the therapist does not speak the relevant language. It is the practitioner's responsibility to discover how appropriate particular techniques are in any locality but this section looks at the more appropriate skills and at problems that commonly arise.

Personal care

The therapist should be aware that in some Asian cultures the left hand is used for ablutions and the right for eating. It may be offensive to clients to see others eating with the left hand.

Personal hygiene may not be to an acceptable standard and the reasons behind this need to be investigated. It could be due to schizophrenic lack of motivation, to poor washing facilities, inadequate privacy, or simply to the fact that it is cold in the bathroom and washing is therefore unpleasant.

Choice of clothes may be an area for intervention and here finance may be a problem, as warm clothing is expensive. Sensitivity to clothing styles should be observed. An adolescent who wants to try all the modern styles may come into serious conflict with her parents.

Cooking and household management

For recent immigrants, this may be a major area for adjustment. If familiar foods are not available or if the dietary requirements of their religion cannot be met ways of overcoming these difficulties must be found. A trip to the supermarket may be necessary or the therapist may find herself becoming the learner in the local market. It may be the husband's role to do the shopping. The British habit of a weekly shopping trip is not shared by those who are used to fresh food from a local stall on a daily basis (see Fig. 25.1).

Longer residence does not necessarily mean good knowledge of resources, entitlements to benefits, or competence in practical skills that would be beneficial in daily life. The client's abilities and knowledge in these areas should still be assessed so that the educational aspects of treatment are not overlooked, or apparently simple everyday tasks ignored. Management of household tasks includes information about the socially acceptable ways of sharing communal responsibilities, for example, that you don't put out the rubbish every day. Methods of cleaning may be unfamiliar and may lead to unreasonable financial outlay. Operation of household appliances may require explanation. Many people may struggle for years, not wishing to appear inadequate at being unable to master a particular device.

Child rearing

This, together with household management, is usually one of the principal tasks for women. It may be necessary to advise on local practices in order to help to promote understanding of school and youth services, thereby reducing anxiety and conflict between generations. Discipline in the home may be more authoritarian than at school, or ideas about play can be at odds with the local norm. Discussion groups are a useful, and interesting, method of dealing with this.

Social skills

Much of the emphasis here needs to be on the social differences between different groups, for example, parents may be puzzled by their children's behaviour, feeling that it shows lack of respect for cultural traditions. A girl who is not allowed to go to the disco with her friends may still have assumed some of their social skills in dating behaviour, to the consternation of her parents.

Training groups may be needed to identify areas of faulty communication based on misunderstanding of non-verbal cues. A simple example is that nodding the head means 'No' to a Greek. Other

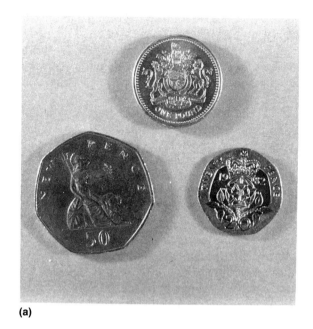

(a)

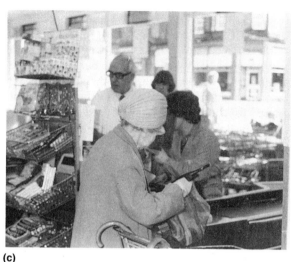

(c)

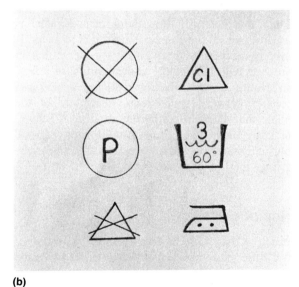

(d)

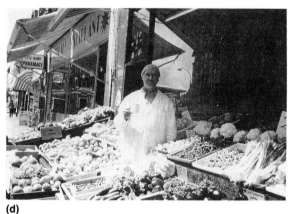

(b)

Fig. 25.1 Shopping is an area of great culture diversity, with the immigrant having to adapt in many ways.
(a) Local coinage is unfamiliar.
(b) Labels, such as laundry instructions, may not be understood.
(c) The checkout procedure at a supermarket is very different from shopping at a local market.
(d) A vegetable stall in a market may be more familiar but lack of language skills may cause problems.

gestures are more subtle and the rules for personal space are very variable between cultures.

Eye contact during conversation is complex. In South east Asia it is respectful to look down. A therapist who expects everyone to meet her direct gaze may find that people look away, apparently avoiding her.

Such examples may appear trivial but if allowed to persist may lead to serious misunderstandings.

Assertion skills may seem to be particularly

lacking in some cultures, according to the Western view. However, the acceptable standards of deference, as opposed to passive/aggressive behaviour, should be determined before any assertion training is suggested.

Work

Racial prejudice and general non-availability of jobs may already have caused clients considerable anxiety prior to their illness. Someone who has had a responsible job in his country of origin but is unable to obtain work of a similar status may feel very deskilled. Lack of fluency in technical language may be a problem here. A student who has failed his exams may have the added burden that he has failed to meet the family's expectations and finding an acceptable alternative may be extremely difficult. Longer-term residents in the UK, or people who were born here, may have considerable difficulty in finding work and, for the young, a lifetime of prospective unemployment will give rise to bitterness.

The occupational therapist should carry out work assessments and implement programmes as applicable for any rehabilitation programme. Prevocational assessment may be indicated or, if prospects are not good, preparation for unemployment may be the only alternative. The cultural implications of this are quite considerable in groups where most people have employment of some kind and loss of status and role are hard to bear.

Leisure

The Western concept of leisure is that it is time to be filled. For others, the time may be passed in conversation with family and friends and there is no concept of the need to be constructively occupied in creative activities, sports, or any of the other conventional occupational therapy recreational activities. Identifying opportunities for unstructured social contact in the community in order to combat a sense of isolation may be a more realistic course.

Crosscultural sharing of art or music may lead to enrichment and greater understanding and these and other arts can be beneficially utilised.

MEDIA AND TECHNIQUES

As in any treatment programme, activities should be selected to meet the needs of the individual. A variety of potentially applicable media and techniques is mentioned here in order to present some of the benefits and pitfalls of particular choices.

Practical activities

Focus on participation in domestic or practical activities, such as cooking, may be seen as a potential introduction both to therapy and to other clients. Multicultural cookery groups may appear to be a limited application of occupational therapy skills but nevertheless have a valuable educational role in fostering good international relations. Such sessions may improve social contact as well as increasing self-esteem.

There may, however, be designated male and female divisions that go deeper than some of the British opinions that kitchen activities are women's work. If a Muslim woman is in purdah, it will be the husband who does the shopping.

Craftwork

The 'occupational' aspect of activity may render it alien and unnecessary in the eyes of the client.

Traditional craft media may be relevant but the therapist should remember that what is a leisure pursuit for one may be a work activity for another. A tailoress may not appreciate being asked to join a patchwork group. Here again specific tasks may be traditionally male or female.

Yoga

Occupational therapists in psychiatric units have drawn extensively on Eastern techniques such as yoga and meditation. Relaxation and similar groups may not be as strange to immigrant clients as to the indigenous population. Sharing of techniques between clients and staff may be very helpful.

Groups

Sensitivity is needed in respect of exploratory

techniques, as self-revelation in a group context may be totally unacceptable to the client. It is certainly not possible if the linguistic skills of client or staff are not fluent. In settings such as drama groups the element of physical contact may be offensive and equally inappropriate.

Social activities may not be acceptable, for example, to take an Asian girl to a disco. A women-only swimming session would be much more suitable.

Individual work

Again, the focus on self-disclosure may be alien. The client–therapist relationship may be in conflict with the client's expectations of the curative powers of the staff. The notion of responsibility for self and the consequent problem-solving approach may be equally at variance with the individual's values and expectations.

As in any programme, individual and group activities require careful selection according to client needs at any particular time.

COMMON PROBLEMS

It is impossible to predict all the difficulties that the therapist may encounter, and it is the responsibility of the therapist to learn to recognise the needs in her own area. Some problems do commonly occur, however, and can be overcome.

Clients' names

Ensure that you are familiar with styles of address and pronunciation of names. There is nothing more demeaning than light-hearted attempts to use the correct name, or substituting an Anglicised version.

Names that are similar may be confusing to the therapist who finds that she has several clients who are referred to as 'Mr Singh'. This is because it is customary to use the Sikh title in everyday address. The family or personal name may not be given. Another potential pitfall is that the Chinese practice is to give the family name first, followed by personal names.

Unrealistic expectations on the part of the therapist

The therapist's idea of personal competence may be at variance with those of the patient and family. Independence and decision making without reference to the family may not be appropriate and the therapist should determine expectations before deciding goals. Individuality is not a valued trait in all cultures.

Overpromising

Clients may, in their attempts to do what the therapist wishes them to, promise to undertake tasks that are unlikely to be achieved. This may be to give the impression they do not need help to avoid loss of face, or simply as an attempt to please the therapist. A clear statement of expectations may help but some difficulties will have to be accepted.

Keeping appointments.

The therapist may feel frustrated by clients failing to keep appointments, being late, or dropping in unexpectedly. In a culture where time is valued differently from the West, none of these behaviours would be deemed unacceptable. It may cause problems in a busy department and here, too, explanations may help but remembering the differences might reduce staff's exasperation.

WORKING IN A MULTIRACIAL TEAM

Transcultural work obviously extends beyond that with clients. The occupational therapist will often find that she is a member of a multicultural team as well as a multidisciplinary one. Relationships are important and it should be remembered that transcultural colleagues may be facing considerable problems in adjusting to our practices. Friendly advice about ward routines and normal practices is usually welcomed by the newcomer. Interpretation of unfamiliar dialects and words may also be required.

It is important that the working relationship is clearly defined so that there is no possibility of friendly support between male and female staff being misconstrued as sexual interest.

Inter-staff relationships

Relationships between staff can lead to difficulties in any context (Pollock 1986) and the extra dimension of the multiracial team has already been discussed. Religious and racial prejudices run very deep and may be imported into the hospital to create unpleasant situations. In day-to-day teamwork there may be snide remarks, exclusion or behind-the-back comments.

In medical circles, psychiatry is sometimes regarded as one of the less attractive specialties, with continuing care and care of the elderly being the least highly regarded areas within the field. Staff from other cultures seeking work may therefore find it easier to obtain posts in these areas and feel devalued by their respective professions. The colour of one's skin may be a disability when facing an appointments committee. Alternatively, equal-opportunity employers may practise 'positive discrimination', a contradictory term that may make selecting the best applicant a difficult task.

Relationships within the team are usually on a hierarchical basis, with a team leader, normally the consultant. It is, however, common practice for much of the work to be delegated to other team members. Assumption of the authority inherent in this may be new to many and problems may occur if junior staff are reluctant to take on responsibility.

Different social roles can also cause problems, for example, a junior member of staff showing deference to a superior by walking along the corridor a few paces to the rear while trying to carry on a conversation. The converse problem arises if a staff member seems to be more dogmatic than the rest of the team would like.

Problems may arise when people come from the same country but do not share the same religious or political beliefs. Other team members cannot fully appreciate the differences and the atmosphere can be very strained. Even enquiring whether a visiting professional knows an individual from the same country may lead to a frosty answer, if they are allied to different political or religious groups.

This also extends to therapist–patient interaction and it is not easy for either if a foreign student is faced with an expatriate who does not support the existing regime.

A problem that sometimes occurs is that a team member will be asked to see and advise colleagues from other teams about the treatment of clients from her racial group. It is important not to make members of staff feel overloaded, nor to send them all the referrals of their own ethnic group. If the person chooses to specialise in working with her own group, then this is acceptable, but otherwise she may feel her career development is being restricted by not carrying a multicultural caseload.

Staff education

Given the diversity of backgrounds and needs, no one person can hope to be an expert on everything. It is, however, possible to build up a group of individuals who, together, can cope with most eventualities.

Education will be a continuous process but a few formal pointers at the outset are of benefit. Some disciplines pay more attention than others to the need for education for working in a multicultural society, but, even so, it is impossible to equip someone specifically for the needs of any particular area. The individual must take some responsibility.

If a particular racial group predominates in an area it may be feasible for the therapist to visit that country (Jopling 1979) in order to gain greater understanding of the original lifestyle. This is also helpful in terms of understanding the dilemmas of young second-generation immigrants being pressurised to return to their homeland.

If there is a team member with a particular ethnic background he or she will probably be willing to run educational sessions in which other staff can sort out queries and difficulties in that particular context. This has the benefit of dealing with real rather than hypothetical problems.

Locating potential sources of information within the local community should not prove too difficult once a few contacts have been established. Introductions can usually be provided, following some judicious questioning.

Consultation with local community relations councils, community associations and other organisations that may be involved, will be of value. Local community workers will have knowledge of problems and resources and can provide a wealth of valuable information.

SUMMARY

With a little judicious enquiry, sensitivity and willingness, the therapist can discover a wealth of knowledge and experience the rewards of this area of work. It is also possible to be an ambassador for one's clients by reducing the double stigma of mental illness and racial prejudice.

This chapter has considered some of the aspects of working in a multicultural society. Reasons why people have come to the UK are outlined, together with some of the problems encountered by people moving from one culture to another. Attention has been given to illness presentation and diagnoses and some of the special needs of clients have been indicated.

The role of the occupational therapist is outlined with reference to assessment, treatment media and some of the pitfalls that may be encountered. Teamwork in the context of the multiracial, multiprofessional team is also mentioned.

REFERENCES

Bavington J, Majid A 1986 Psychiatric services for ethnic minority groups. In: Cox J (ed) Transcultural psychiatry. Croom Helm, London

Burke A 1986 Racism, prejudice and mental illness. In: Cox J (ed) Transcultural Psychiatry. Croom Helm, London

Cochrane R 1977 Mental illness in immigrants to England and Wales: An analysis of hospital admissions. Social Psychiatry 12: 5

Cox J 1986 Overseas students and expatriates: sojourners or settlers. In: Cox J (ed) Transcultural psychiatry. Croom Helm, London

Fernando S 1986 Depression in ethnic minorities. In: Cox J (ed) Transcultural psychiatry. Croom Helm, London

Gregory R L 1972 Eye and brain, the psychology of seeing, 2nd edn. Weidenfeld and Nicolson, London

Henley A 1979 Asian patients and their families in hospital. Kings Fund, London

Jopling S 1979 A month in Pakistan, British Journal of Occupational Therapy. 42: 3

Kolvin I, Nicol 1979 In: Granville-Grossman K (ed) Recent advances in clinical psychiatry vol 3. Churchill Livingstone, Edinburgh

Littlewood R, Lipsedge M 1982 Aliens and alienists. Penguin, Harmondsworth

Littlewood R, Lipsedge M 1985 Culture bound syndromes. In: Granville-Grossman K (ed) Recent advances in clinical psychiatry, vol 5. Churchill Livingstone, Edinburgh

Mares P, Henley A, Baxter C 1985 Health care in multiracial Britain. Health Education Council and National Extension College Trust, Cambridge.

Mumford D 1989 Personal communication

Orque M, Bloch B, Monroy L 1983 Ethnic nursing care: a multicultural approach. C. V. Mosby, New York

Pollock L 1986 The multi-disciplinary team. In: Hume C, Pullen I (eds) Rehabilitation in psychiatry. Churchill Livingstone, Edinburgh

Rack P 1982 Race, culture and mental disorder. Tavistock, London

Sampson C 1982 The neglected ethic. McGraw Hill, London

Taft R 1977 Coping with unfamiliar cultures. In: Warren N (ed) Studies in crosscultural psychology, vol 1. Academic Press, London

FURTHER READING

Cox J L (ed) 1986 Transcultural psychiatry. Croom Helm, London

Eden S 1987 Ethnic groups. In: Bumphrey E (ed) Occupational therapy in the community. Woodhead Faulkener, London

Glendinning F 1979 The elders in ethnic minorities. Beth Johnson Foundation Publications, Department of Adult Education University of Keele and Commission for racial equality, Keele.

Hill C 1986 Towards a better understanding of elderly migrants. Australian Journal of Occupational Therapy 33: 2

Hume C 1984 Transcultural aspects of psychiatric rehabilitation. British Journal of Occupational Therapy 47: 12

Lipsedge M, Littlewood R 1979 Transcultural psychiatry. In: Granville-Grossman K (ed) Recent advances in clinical psychiatry 3, Churchill Livingstone, Edinburgh

Mares P, Henley A, Baxter C 1985 Health care in multiracial Britain. Health Education Council and National Extension College Trust, Cambridge

Taft R 1973 Migration: problems of adjustment and assimilation in immigrants. In: Watson P (ed) Psychology and race. Penguin, Harmondsworth

SECTION 7

Organisation, administration and management

26

Management

Sue Gore

INTRODUCTION

'The NHS exists to serve patients. The Government's main objective is therefore to establish a structure for the service which will enable health services to be planned and managed most effectively, and within which decisions can be taken quickly by those who are close to and responsive to the needs of patients. Changes in the structure alone will not be sufficient, the service must be managed in a way that enables those with prime responsibility for providing the services to patients to get on with the job.' (DHSS, 1979).

Some people fit more comfortably into managerial roles than others; it may be said that some are born managers. However, all occupational therapists, even the newly qualified, are required to manage people or resources. Most who enter the profession are drawn to the clinical aspect of the work and have an ambivalent attitude towards their managerial role but also demand the right to manage their own service, claiming that only an occupational therapist has the unique blend of skills required to understand their needs.

Shortage of resources is a continuing problem and the current emphasis on providing an efficient and cost-effective service to clients means that occupational therapists must carefully consider how best to prepare themselves for their role as managers.

WHAT IS A MANAGER?

The term 'manager' has now become established in the NHS. However, this has been associated with the mistaken assumptions that there is only one type of manager and that all people called managers operate in the same way. It is not easy to define the role of manager because the type of manager-role used must be based on the type of authority needed for the particular task assigned. Present-day management favours a more democratic style and this makes the role of the manager more difficult in attempting to consider the views of all people concerned rather than giving orders and using a more autocratic style.

Managers play a key role in the policy-making process, which determines the overall objectives of the service. Factors such as changes in population levels, socio-economic groupings or the number of elderly residents in a district affect the planning of the service. If the ultimate aim is to organise available resources to achieve objectives as efficiently as possible then the manager must encourage and support staff while constantly looking for improvements in performance.

In this chapter we will first look at how occupational therapy management has developed in Britain. The next section covers staff-development and staff-management issues, including training, performance review and industrial relations. Personal skills for the manager are discussed, including management of time, creative thinking and coping with stress. Communication is seen as a core management skill and is covered in detail. Finally, the management-control techniques of forecasting, manpower and planning are described.

A HISTORY OF OCCUPATIONAL THERAPY MANAGEMENT POSTS IN BRITAIN

Prior to the major reorganisation of the Health Service in 1974, occupational therapy services were mainly 'organised' on an individual hospital basis, with head occupational therapists relating managerially to the hospital administrator and in clinical matters working closely with the consultant medical staff.

In 1973 the Macmillan Report recommended the introduction of Managerial District Therapists and, in 1974, interim advice issued by the Department of Health and Social Services recommended that, while final arrangements were being agreed, senior occupational therapists should be designated as advisors to the District Management Team. The advisors had four principal responsibilities:

1. to advise the District Management Team on occupational therapy services
2. to help maintain professional standards
3. to participate in the development of rehabilitation services
4. to be the link with occupational therapists employed by Social Services.

No specific method of recruiting suitable candidates was laid down, but Districts were advised to ask all suitably qualified staff whether they wished to be considered. This interim arrangement was planned to last only a couple of years but it was not until late 1979 that is was finally decided to appoint district occupational therapists with managerial responsibility. These appointments were to differ from all previous arrangements in that the district occupational therapist would be the manager of all occupational therapy staff in the District and have a direct link to a member of the District Management Team.

'Patients First', a consultative paper on the structure and management of the National Health Service in England and Wales said, 'the first objective of the 1974 re-organization, the integration of services for patients in the hospital and in the community, has been substantially achieved. But there has been widespread criticism of the 1974 changes which the Royal Commission summed up as: too many tiers, too many administrators in all disciplines; failure to take quick decisions; and money wasted' (DHSS 1979).

As soon as 'Patients First' was issued, there was a growing concern that the DHSS recommendations on district occupational therapist posts had been made invalid. Had the government changed its mind? Was the emphasis now towards managerial authority at Unit level?

A circular, H. C.(80)8, was produced to provide the necessary guidance to Regional Health Authorities and the new District Health Authorities in implementing the changes in structure and management organisation that were needed to fulfil the aims of 'Patients First'. Paragraph 26 of H. C.(80)8 stated that District Health Authorities must consider management arrangements for many groups of staff, including the remedial professions. The criterion for establishing posts should be the anticipated workload and therefore full-time posts should be avoided unless it was certain that there was sufficient workload. The alternative was to combine an appointment at District level with one in a Unit. Districts made their own interpretation of the recommendations and so the number and grade of District appointments varied throughout the country.

In July 1984 the Government issued Health Circular (84)13, 'Implementation of the NHS Management Inquiry (Griffiths) Report'. This called for the appointment of general managers at Regional, District and Unit levels throughout the NHS but left the remainder of the management structure to be decided by each individual Health Authority.

The concept is said to be creative, positive, forward looking and, above all, about getting things done. We must therefore accept the challenges created by general management. The most important task is to identify, educate and develop potential managers for the future. In so doing we become a more managerially mature and respected profession and offer a greater contribution to improving the service to our clients.

STAFF DEVELOPMENT

The occupational therapy service includes both qualified staff and unqualified staff. The support services should not be forgotten as a department cannot function without them.

CAREER STRUCTURE FOR QUALIFIED STAFF

In order to recruit and retain qualified staff to a district it is essential to develop an appropriately managed service with an attractive career structure.

Students

Given adequate staffing levels, student placements are an essential component in a planned departmental structure, as the concept of clinical practice is to make a substantial contribution to the development of a 'competent and safe occupational therapist' (COT 1984). The benefits to students are well documented but a clinical department also benefits from taking students by building and maintaining strong links and good relationships with training schools. This enables a sharing of knowledge, information and professional expertise.

Participation in student training may be a daunting thought to a head of department with unfilled posts and a shortage of staff but a high percentage of students choose to seek employment in departments in which they received training. Therefore, the time and effort given to providing a good clinical placement now may be the solution to a recruitment problem in the future.

Further information about clinical training can be found in Chapter 29.

Clinical therapists

It is necessary to promote a staffing structure that will attract newly qualified staff who may choose to stay in the district and specialise in a particular field once they have gained experience.

Finalist students often choose a post that will offer them as much variety and experience as possible, since most are undecided about the area in which they wish to specialise. Thought must therefore be given to a rotational scheme for basic-grade therapists. The variety of clinical specialties and staffing establishments available will usually dictate the length and type of scheme feasible.

Senior staff

At the time of writing, it is not possible to progress very far professionally on the basis of clinical expertise alone, as promotion to a senior grade involves taking on a management role in some form, although this may change in future. Therapists may be reluctant to take the next step up the ladder of promotion as doing so can reduce their contact with clients. The development of clinical skills is, of course, crucial in establishing and maintaining an effective service but the functions of clinical specialist and manager cannot be separated from each other since effective management requires access to expert clinical knowledge.

Apprehension about promotion may also be due to a lack of training in management skills. Many therapists who lack adequate training assume managerial posts reluctantly and then have to struggle to fulfil their role.

A structured training programme for all grades of staff is essential in the development of any efficient and professional service. However, simply attending courses is not enough and senior staff need to encourage their Health Authorities to aid in further professional development.

Unqualified staff

The roles of the helper and technical instructor should never be underestimated. These staff can make a valuable contribution when there is a clear job specification and adequate support and supervision from qualified therapists. A variety of work is undertaken, from basic routine tasks to running specific groups and treatment programmes, necessitating four grades.

There is usually little difficulty in recruiting helpers and as a result there are few vacancies. In a profession that seems to have a fairly rapid turnover of qualified staff, helpers can provide the stability that every department needs for the sake of the clients being treated.

A problem that every department must have experienced is that of the newly qualified therapist having responsibility for supervising an experienced helper. In such a situation, there needs to be an honest and fair recognition of each other's skills, effective communication, mutual trust and diplomacy in arriving at decisions.

Back-up services

It should be noted that for an occupational therapy service to be efficient and cost effective in the use of clinical expertise it is essential to have access to back-up services, such as porters, receptionists, clerks and typists.

Domestic staff are also essential for the smooth running of a department, and there may need to be some negotiation about which aspects of cleaning are done by clients, as part of therapy, and which are done by the domestics.

It is helpful to have good working relationships with staff in the kitchens, in order to achieve cooperation with projects such as outings requiring packed lunches, and with the works department who can help with changes, such as alterations in the function of areas of the department.

PERFORMANCE REVIEW

Everyone working in the health services has made some sort of commitment to the provision of care for others. It is only possible for staff to concentrate fully on other people's needs and to care about them if they themselves feel secure, cared for and valued, and so employers should provide sufficient general support to staff.

Low morale, which can have a devastating effect on any service, is often caused by a lack of clear objectives or managerial appraisal of staff performance. Newly qualified and inexperienced staff risk being swamped by the unlimited needs and demands put upon them. Two questions in the minds of many employees are 'What is expected of me?' and 'How am I doing?' The answer to the first question lies in goal setting and planning, and to the second in monitoring and feedback. Confidence comes from being able to meet objectives and achieve valued goals. Lack of feedback can stifle a therapist who is striving to grow and develop her professional expertise. Training and encouragement to define and meet personal and departmental goals will produce confident therapists with no uncertainties about their role or performance. The capable managers of tomorrow must be confident in what they do today.

Effective managers are continuously assessing the performance of their staff informally but more formal methods could also be used. Managers could gain valuable insight into their own management style, the real effect of their policies and decisions, and could even learn more about those who work for them.

The subordinate would have the opportunity to influence the boss's thinking, express both positive and negative feelings about the work, and perhaps discuss opportunities for personal development. Some people genuinely want to be appraised because they desire to perform well. Constructive feedback, whether formal or informal, is an important way of measuring performance.

Individual performance review (IPR)

To be done well, this must be based on openness between reviewer and job holder. Regular formal reviews are required, as well as frequent informal discussions; IPR is not an annual exercise. Good performance management does not depend on periodic formal interviews, although they have their value. The real performance management consists of frequent meetings, at which performance is discussed, encouragement given and problems solved.

In a formal review, the manager and individual agree on key objectives for the coming period, usually a year. In producing this action plan, attention should be given to the individual's learning and development needs as they relate to the achievement of objectives. Objectives should be sufficiently challenging to ensure progress but not so difficult to achieve that failure and frustration are inevitable. The formal meeting should always end with a date being set for the next review meeting so that the monitoring process is continued.

An informal review provides a more frequent opportunity to check progress against the action plan. The more performance can be related to objectives and standards, the better idea employees have about what is expected of them, how they are performing and, if appropriate, what corrective action is needed. A positive environment that encourages open discussion can be created by beginning a review with acknowledgement of the employee's strength. Positive feedback is an important factor in increasing motivation and improving morale both as a reward and as a way of letting the employee know how to continue to behave.

When a manager has to give negative feedback there is sometimes a temptation to hesitate and not get quickly to the point. This can cause an atmosphere of suspicion and put the employee on the defensive. An ability to listen and engage in the give and take of two-way communication is necessary to overcome such barriers.

Feedback is a two-way process and can provide a sound basis for management development and career planning, which in turn contributes to a more effective use of staff resources.

TRAINING

Training is the responsibility of all grades of staff from District level through to the newly qualified; those responsible for the successful accomplishment of work are also responsible for maintaining the effectiveness of the employees undertaking that work. Managers are in a unique position to determine the training needs of those they manage. They are also in a position to measure the return on training investment, by monitoring the progress of their staff before and after training.

What is training?

Training can be defined as 'the systematic development of the attitudes, knowledge and skills pattern required by an individual in order to perform adequately a given task or job' (Craik 1986a).

To be effective, training must be systematic. The training process consists of four stages:

1. identify the training need
2. analyse the skills, knowledge and attitudes required for the job
3. plan and implement the training
4. evaluate the results.

Types of training

Many people think of training as taking courses that may lead to a qualification or at least a certificate of attendance. Courses are valuable for extending knowledge; and the main types are listed below.

- statutory
- essential
- refresher
- management
- DHSS
- day-release
- correspondence
- full-time
- part-time
- Open University
- trade union
- conference/seminar
- internal
- external.

Courses may be part-time, over a fairly long period, or they may be short and concentrated. There are other ways in which a manager can ensure that staff development takes place throughout the working life, rather than waiting for suitable courses.

External courses provide technical and professional qualifications and facilitate a broadening of the individual's experience. However, opportunities for self-development can also be found outside formal courses.

Many departments offer a rotation scheme for senior staff as well as newly qualified therapists. This is a way of gaining experience in the normal working situation and is aimed at developing existing knowledge and skills or acquiring new experiences.

Staff can also gain experience outside their normal duties by being assigned projects or special duties, for example, representing the department on working parties, joining a professional body or even organising a social event connected with work.

Group discussions can be used to give staff an opportunity to learn from the knowledge and experience of others. This can be as informal as a staff meeting or as formal as a case conference.

Every department has resources that can be used to extend our knowledge, including books to read, people to listen to and experiences to learn from.

Management training

Changes in the nature of the occupational therapy profession and of management in general now need to be reflected in a new style of management training. Formal classroom methods need to balanced by other approaches to stimulating and stretching management talent.

Managers tend to learn more effectively if theory is clearly connected with practice. This means firm links between:

- what a manager already knows through experience.
- the opportunity to learn new insights and skills
- the reinforcement of that learning through subsequent experience.

Management development involves maximum participation by the individual in selecting and specifying the approach to be applied in his or her case. Individuals should be encouraged to contribute their own values and experiences to any development experience rather than being expected to absorb information passively.

Training managers often means starting from the stage the manager is at in their personal development and preparing them for the next career move. Training should always use a manager's real-life issues and problems as the basis on which to build. In order to train effectively, it is necessary first to decide in some detail:

- what specific knowledge and skills a particular post involves
- what skills the individual already possesses
- what gaps in such knowledge and skills can be filled by training.

Time and money spent on training is only justified if the training contributes to the efficiency of the department and improves the performance and prospects of the employees. Evaluation of the total value of any training activity is therefore essential.

MANAGEMENT OF SELF

The occupational therapy manager often has a clinical caseload as well as her managerial duties but the two roles can be complementary. The first step towards being an effective manager is to manage one's own time and skills to best effect, which is as important for the clinician as for the manager.

MANAGEMENT OF TIME

As we go through our lives, feeling controlled by clocks, deadlines and schedules, we may have very mixed feelings about time and how we use it. Time is a scarce economic resource that many managers waste, mainly because they do not manage it. They reflect this when they say, 'Is it that time already? I don't know where today has gone' or 'I've worked so hard today yet I feel I haven't done anything'.

Common time management problems are:

- lack of objectives and clear priorities
- interruptions from people and telephone calls
- crises that upset planned activities
- meetings
- absence of long-term strategic plans.

Through careful analysis and a little effort most managers and clinicians can put a stop to trivial activities and redirect their time and effort to more important issues, thus saving at least 1 or 2 hours a day. The following four steps show how to manage time more effectively.

1. *Record how time is spent each day*
Keep a time log and record all activities at work for at least 5 days.

- describe in detail what happens, such as the *topic* of telephone calls, meetings and visits
- keep a note of the *duration* of each event
- note *who else* was involved.

Keeping a time log provides evidence of exactly where time is going and why, and clearly shows the difference between what the manager thought was happening and how exactly time is being spent. Keeping a time log will in itself be time consuming but the short-term nuisance will produce long-term rewards.

2. *Analyse how time is spent*
  a. *Outcome*: how successful were the various activities; were there any failures? A poor outcome can be caused by underestimating the amount of time needed to complete a certain task and this, in turn, can be the cause of unnecessary pressure. Be positive when estimating how long it will take to complete a task but, if anything, overestimate.
  b. *Type of work*: this can be subdivided into three distinct categories:

- the most important duties—things you *must* do
- the second most important duties—things you *should* do
- the least important duties—things you *like* to do.

Analyse how much time is spent on each set of activities and, in particular, the comparison between the most and least important duty. Also look at the amount of time spent on *managerial* work (that is, planning, organising) as opposed to *professional* skills (that is, exercising specialist clinical skills).
  c. *Delegation*: for each task undertaken, ask the questions:

- Could this have been delegated?
- If yes, to whom?
- If no, why not?

Are the reasons for not delegating valid? Management is about getting things done and delegating is about using others to carry out projects and tasks. It establishes the manager and subordinate as a team and often forces the manager to be more organised, requiring the art of good communication.

Despite the many advantages to appropriate delegation, many managers still avoid it, believing that to get a job done properly they have to do it themselves. Some managers feel they need to have total control, while others have a fear that they may be imposing on their subordinates if they ask them to do the work. Others also have the fear that their subordinates may do a better job, thus putting their own position under threat.

3. *Plan to succeed*
Decide how you can spend time in a more productive way by planning in order to succeed. Neglecting to set personal goals or write daily 'to do' lists may be a way of planning to fail.

a. Get into the habit of writing a 'to do' list every day, grading each task A-C, in order of importance. Be realistic and aware of time limitations, and avoid overscheduling, as only so many activities can be fitted into one day. It is far better to complete 10 out of 10 tasks than 10 out of 20. A sense of achievement produces energy and motivation, failure produces indifference.

b. Allow time for interruptions. Do not fill every minute with activity. Provide for the unexpected, such as clients being late for appointments or projects taking longer than estimated.

c. Review the list each day and refer to it throughout the day to keep objectives in mind.

d. If something is completed during the day that was not listed, add it to the list. Then at the end of the day it will be seen that more has been accomplished than was originally intended.

e. Build your day around the grade A, 'high pay-off' activities and leave the less important items for the time left over.

f. Plan to do something each day that will bring the achievement of personal goals a little closer.

4. *Review and assess the time-management process*
The time log exercise should be repeated at intervals to determine what, if any, progress has been made in managing time more successfully. Remember that time managed properly may also increase the effectiveness and capacity of others as well as yourself.

CREATIVE THINKING

In many situations managers could benefit from exercising creative thinking skills when dealing with difficult problems. Often, original and unusual ideas or solutions that have been suggested tend to be rejected or forgotten because they seem to be extreme or impracticable. There is also a tendency to keep on using well-tried ideas and solutions rather than spend time looking for genuine alternatives.

Brainstorming

Brainstorming is a technique that can be used to help overcome blocks to creative and innovative thinking, either individually or in a group.

When dealing with a difficult problem, an individual can brainstorm by writing down all the ideas and solutions that immediately come to mind. At this stage, do not stop to evaluate but concentrate on getting as long a list as possible. Setting a time limit (5–10 min) can help to force the pace and overcome any tendency to stop and evaluate what has been listed. When the list is finished take each in turn and consider all its aspects: strengths, weaknesses, implications, costs, acceptability, etc.

When brainstorming in a group:

- postpone evaluation and judgement
- encourage free thinking, record *all* ideas however extreme they appear
- encourage members to build on and expand ideas
- define the subject narrowly to avoid switching topics
- the more ideas collected the better
- encourage everyone to participate.

COPING WITH STRESS

The word 'stress' is used constantly in connection with emotional states and is usually associated with feelings we have about ourselves. However, stress is not necessarily a bad thing; what is unwelcome pressure to one person can be an exciting challenge to another. Life is most interesting and fulfilling when there is enough stress to give it interest but not so much as to cause distress.

The concept of stress, as taken from physical science, is force exerted on a structure or system which, if increased beyond a certain level, will cause deformity of the structure or system. Stress is also seen as a factor in disease.

Stress can be the cause of frequent absenteeism from work and repeated visits to the doctor with psychosomatic symptoms caused by prolonged reaction to stress, commonly digestive disorders, migraines or skin disorders.

The initial signs of too-high stress levels are easily detectable, for instance, the undesirable coping mechanisms of excess smoking, drinking and eating. High irritability, intolerance, poor concentration and unusual tiredness are all common stress indicators. It is normal to experience the physical results of increased adrenalin supply, such as headache, dry mouth; palpitations and muscle tension, at times of excitement or anxiety but an exaggeration of these symptoms may result in panic attacks that prevent the individual from performing the expected activities of daily living.

The first step in coping with stress is to acknowledge its existence. If a friend, relative or manager had the insight to recognise and point out stress indicators at an early stage, many of the long-term results might be countered.

Sharing worries can be constructive and helps to put life into perspective. People who habitually contain their anxiety, spending much of their time and thoughts alone, tend to produce negative and distorted views of events which increase tension. Close family members may be too subjectively involved with the situation to be able to offer positive support and understanding but a friend or colleague can be a valuable confidant.

It is possible for an individual to work out a plan to lessen the effects of stress and cope more productively with unavoidable life situations. This would involve:

- Planning ahead to reduce last minute hurrying and confusion.
- Enjoying meals in a relaxing atmosphere.
- Employing a regular pattern of exercise, which could lead to a satisfying involvement in a leisure pursuit and a fit body into the bargain.
- Developing a hobby which is relaxing and pleasurable to balance the stresses of a busy day.
- Resolving to master the techniques of muscular and mental relaxation, resulting in a more

peaceful state of mind and renewed energy. It must be emphasised that relaxation is an active pursuit, and cannot be achieved passively. It requires discipline and single-mindedness but is ultimately rewarding.

- Obtaining adequate rest and sleep. Ideally, at the end of a well-balanced day, which has included stimulus and rest, adequate nourishment, exercise and fresh air, the body and mind should be ready to enjoy sleep. It is wise to check practical points: comfort, warmth, ventilation and reduction of noise. Progressive muscular relaxation techniques may be employed.
- Being appropriately assertive and honest in a controlled manner. This removes the necessity to 'bottle up' and magnify negative feelings.
- Evaluating life goals to ensure that competive effort is going to produce the life-style that you really want. Setting realistic targets and giving self-congratulation on their achievement supplies the positive reinforcement required.

It has been said that the 'stress-proof' personality has a 'hardiness' that helps to protect against the effects of stress. This 'hardiness' comprises:

- *commitment* to one's work, family or other important areas of life
- *control* or the belief that one can influence what happens in one's world
- *challenge*, or an eagerness for change and a constant flow of new experiences.

A combination of these positive characteristics would indeed effect a productive and satisfying existence for all of us.

EFFECTIVE COMMUNICATION

Communication is the expression and exchange of thoughts and feelings. Managers tend not to invest enough time and effort in ensuring that their communication systems are effective (Stockport Health Authority 1985). They are sometimes guilty of being too optimistic about the successfulness of their communication systems.

Ineffective communications can lead to costly

errors in both financial and human terms. It can also lead to frustration and lack of commitment among staff. Effective communications are necessary to:

- ensure that work gets done correctly and that decisions are implemented
- minimise the effects of rumour and distortion
- let staff know what is happening in the organisation
- help give a better service to clients.

THE MANAGER'S ROLE IN COMMUNICATION

Talking to people is an important part of any manager's role: managers can spend up to 80% of their time in conversation with people. Effective communication depends on the means to, the capacity to and the will to communicate.

Managers have a responsibility to:

- tell their staff all they need to know to do their jobs to the best of their abilities
- keep staff informed of changes especially those that affect them directly
- ensure their communication systems are planned and work effectively
- check that all their communications are fully understood
- include communication as an integral part of their job.

Communication skills include informal face-to-face verbal interactions, both speaking and listening, telephone conversations, formal verbal instructions or presentations and written communications.

VERBAL COMMUNICATIONS SKILLS

Much day-to-day communication takes place verbally, either face to face or over the telephone, formally or informally.

Problems can arise from the fact that our expectations, needs and experiences greatly influence what we see and hear. Often the situation arises that the message received by the other person is not the message we intended to send.

In order to communicate effectively:

- know what you want to say
- adjust your message to the receiver
- be aware of any personal prejudices
- avoid jargon and unclear language
- set a time limit so that you get straight to the point
- put time and effort into listening
- devise a feedback channel, for example, paraphrase your understanding of what is being said and ask for confirmation
- reduce distraction and noise
- ask for feedback and *do not* assume anything.

Taking time in the beginning to make sure the message is clear can save hours of misunderstandings later.

How to improve your listening skills

The game of passing a whisper around a circle is a perfect example of how a message can be distorted. If messages can change so dramatically when everyone is concentrating on getting them correct, how much more jumbled can communications get in a busy office where there are countless distractions, interruptions and people coming and going?

Good listeners are rare but good listening skills are teachable. There are practical ways of improving these skills by following the simple rules devised by Davis (1977):

1. Stop talking! You cannot listen if you are talking.

2. Put the talker at ease. Help her to feel that she is free to talk.

3. Show the talker that you want to listen. Look and act interested. For example, do not open the post while someone is talking.

4. Remove distractions. Do not doodle, tap or shuffle papers.

5. Empathise with the talker. Try to put yourself in her place so you can see her point of view.

6. Be patient. Allow plenty of time and do not interrupt.

7. Hold your temper. An angry manager picks up the wrong meaning from what people say.

8. Try to keep argument and criticism to a minimum as it puts the talker on the defensive.

9. Ask questions. This encourages the talker and shows you are listening.

10. Stop talking! This is first and last because all other commandments depend on it.

Using the telephone

The telephone enables us to save enormous amounts of time; by communicating with people around the department, district and country without leaving the desk.

Telephone calls can also be very disruptive, for example, if carrying out an initial interview with a client. If privacy is desired, transfer calls to another extension or arrange for messages to be taken by the switchboard operator. Using the telephone is an integral part of the manager's job and it is important to remember the following points when making a call (Turla & Hawkins 1985).

- Plan what you want to say. Have a list of the topics you want to cover, any questions or information you want to convey or elicit so that you do not have to search your memory for what you want to say.
- State clearly who you are and be precise, avoiding non-words such as ahh! and ummm!
- Set a mental time limit on calls so you can get right to the point. If leaving a message, keep it short.
- If necessary, repeat or ask the receiver to repeat the message.
- Give important information clearly and spell out any difficult names or terminology.

When receiving a call:

- State clearly who you are.
- Take down the essential points; who is calling, their telephone number/extension, what they want, any special instructions.
- Repeat the message to check that you have all the details.
- Ask for any information that is not clear to be repeated.
- Keep a telephone message pad in a familiar place to write down messages and for other people to write down messages for you.

Verbal instruction

A great deal of time in any management or supervisory job is spent in instructing people. Whether you are teaching a client how to perform a task or telling someone how to get to the other side of the hospital, the principles remain the same.

The aim of instruction is to get something done:

- correctly
- safely
- quickly
- with minimum effort.

There are four main stages in giving verbal instruction:

- preparation
- presentation
- practice
- put to work

Preparation

1. Break down the information you wish to impart into simple parts or stages and note the key points that you will need to stress, such as safety.

2. Get ready any equipment or aids to instruction you may need but do not display them until required.

3. Ensure that all learners are in a good position to see and hear.

4. State the job or subject.

5. Create an interest in learning, for example, by using interesting visual display materials.

6. Check on existing knowledge.

7. Put the learner at ease.

Presentation

1. Tell, show or illustrate the job, the changes and the reasons, one stage at a time.

2. Stress the key points.

3. Instruct clearly, completely and patiently, and speak *to* the learner.

4. Proceed at a suitable pace.

5. Be pleasant, confident, alert and helpful—smile!

6. Avoid negative instructions, such as 'Don't ever do this'.

Practice

1. Have the job done or the instruction repeated back to you.

2. Correct any errors as they occur.

3. Continue to practise until you are satisfied with the learner's performance.

4. Identify any need for further training if this is appropriate.

Put to work

1. Indicate personal responsibilities.

2. Name the person who will help if difficulties arise.

3. Encourage questions: what, why, how, where, who?

4. Check performance, as necessary.

Making a verbal presentation

There are many occasions when the occupational therapist manager might need to make a verbal presentation, for example, when presenting an argument for increased staffing levels to the management board. There are several ways in which such a presentation can be made more succinct and attractive.

Decide the main message you want to get across and recognise that when making a verbal presentation you can only convey a limited amount of information in the time available.

Know your audience if possible and decide what their reactions are likely to be. Establish how much time you will need or have available for your presentation. Do not let the main thrust of your proposal get lost amongst irrelevant material.

Collect and sort out all the facts, opinions and ideas you will need and decide which can be used to best effect to back up your statements. Ensure your facts are accurate and up to date.

It is useful to have a framework to present your proposal/request, for example:

- *Introduction*: what your proposal/request is
- *Background*: essential facts about the situation
- *Interpretation*: what the facts/information mean
- *Conclusion*: what you think should be done
- *Summary*: the main points of what you have said.

Once you have prepared your proposal/request, think through any possible objections that might arise and look for any weak points.

- Is all the necessary information available?
- Have you checked out all the possible alternatives?
- Have you accurate details of actual costs/benefits/savings?
- Have you looked at all aspects?
- Can you provide answers to any possible questions that might arise?

Finally, it can be useful to draft out what you want to say and practise it beforehand.

EFFECTIVE WRITTEN COMMUNICATION

A great deal of written communication that is produced cannot be read by a large number of adults, either because they have difficulty reading or because the writing is too obscure. If written communication cannot easily be read and understand, then:

- people give up trying to read the information or misunderstand its contents
- time, money and effort are wasted
- lives may be lost as a result of badly written letters, notices and instructions.

Managers should pay special attention to written information given to staff and clients.

It is possible to improve written communication by:

- having a clear understanding of the purpose of the information being given
- having a clear idea of the readership and choosing an appropriate style of language

- sorting out essential points
- organising and presenting information in a logical sequence
- giving thought to an appropriate beginning to a letter/memo
- using words that the readership can understand
- avoiding long complicated sentences, jargon and gobbledegook
- using new paragraphs for new information or ideas
- providing accurate and complete information.

The importance of an ability to communicate is self-evident but needs to be emphasised. It is a skill in its own right which should be developed and perfected by all occupational therapists, not only managers.

MANAGEMENT CONTROL TECHNIQUES

Management control involves the measurement and correction of the performance of subordinates so that objectives, and the plans devised to attain them, are accomplished efficiently, effectively and economically. The control cycle consists of four elements (see Fig. 26.1):

1. *Planning*: determining policies and objectives, drawing up plans to achieve stated aims

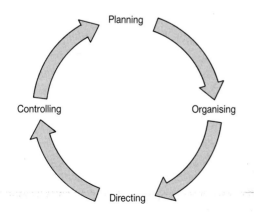

Fig. 26.1 The control cycle

2. *Organising*: converting plans into actions, for example, deciding who is responsible for each and when it should be completed

3. *Directing*: allocating work to staff, issuing instructions

4. *Controlling*: checking how work is progressing, setting standards, identifying problems, reviewing plans and evaluating actions.

AN INTRODUCTION TO PLANNING

Planning may be defined as the effective and efficient use of time and resources and involves:

a) establishing short, medium and long-term objectives
b) determining policies and procedures
c) developing operational plans.

The differences between efficiency and effectiveness are listed below.

Efficiency	*Effectiveness*
Do things correctly	Do what is really needed
Solve problems	Produce creative alternatives
Follow duties	Obtain results
Safeguard resources	Optimise the use of resources
Stay within budget	Reduce costs
Work within existing procedures	Update and develop procedures

Efficiency tends to be associated with day-to-day management, whereas effectiveness involves looking to the future in the medium and long term.

Planning is something we do every day of our lives. It is an essential component of the management process in controlling the resources of people, money and equipment. To exert control over people we need discipline and discipline can only be effective if we are clear about our aims and objectives.

Setting objectives

Management consists of achieving certain objectives by making the best use of resources, the most challenging and often most unused of which is the human resource.

In order to give our best to our work, each of us must know:

- what we are responsible for
- what is expected of us
- how we are performing.

Objective setting is a management tool that clarifies all these points for both workers and manager and allows performance to be measured objectively. It is concerned with:

- human resources
- productivity
- profitability
- telling people what is expected of them
- providing a regular check.

Setting clear objectives benefits the clinical therapist or unqualified member of staff by making appraisal of her performance more realistic, identifying her potential and defining training needs more clearly. The benefits to the manager are better results.

Forecasting

Forecasting is basic to planning and is concerned with probable events. Like other forms of prediction, it is a hazardous exercise. Nevertheless, it has to be carried out to assist in:

- making decisions about capital investment, for example, extending a hospital
- preparing plans, for example, manpower planning
- fixing staffing levels
- replenishing stocks, such as art materials.

The problem is not whether to forecast but how to do so. There are three methods of forecasting:

1. *Intuition*
2. *Statistical*: forecasting from historical figures
3. *Economic*: forecasting using a wide range of variables.

Forecasting techniques vary from the simple to the complex. It is sufficient here to concentrate on two of the more simple mathematical techniques for carrying out statistical forecasting.

Forecasting by past average

This method is used if the objective is to predict the quantity of an item required for the next time period.

$$\frac{\text{Forecasted quantity for}}{\text{the next time period}} = \frac{\text{Average quantity for}}{\text{previous time periods}}$$

For example, a hospital occupational therapy department has kept records over the last 6 months of the number of clients treated. The resulting figures are shown in Table 26.1.

Table 26.1

Month	No. of treatments
1	200
2	170
3	240
4	212
5	170
6	250

Forecasted treatments for month 7 = (200 + 170 + 240 + 212 + 170 + 250) ÷ 6 = 207. Using this technique, data may be obtained as in Table 26.2.

Table 26.2

Month	Actual treatments	Forecasted treatments	Error in forecast
1	200		
2	170		
3	240		
4	212		
5	170		
6	250		
7	200	207	−7

Table 26.3 shows that the forecast was very accurate for month 7 but in later months the accuracy decreased due to low treatment figures in months 1 to 5. This deficiency can be overcome by forecasting by moving average.

Table 26.3

Month	Actual treatments	Forecasted treatments	Error in forecast
1	200		
2	170		
3	240		
4	212		
5	170		
6	250		
7	200	207	−7
8	254	206	+48
9	229	212	+17
10	245	215	+30
11	283	217	+66
12	256	223	+33

Table 26.4

Month	Actual treatments	3-Month moving forecast	Error in forecast
1	200		
2	170		
3	240		
4	212	203	+9
5	170	207	−37
6	250	207	+43
7	200	211	−11
8	254	207	+47
9	229	235	−6
10	245	228	+17
11	283	243	+40
12	256	252	+4

Forecasting by moving average

This method recognises the shortcomings of forecasting by past average. A moving average is calculated simply by adding up the last 'n' number of observations and dividing by 'n'. When the next observation becomes available, the oldest observation in the earlier calculation is dropped, the new one is added on and a new average is calculated. The 3-month period is arrived at by inspection of the actual number of treatments, as shown in Table 26.4. This method has improved the forecast but further refinements can be made by making seasonal adjustments, noting staffing levels, etc.

ORGANISING

With the present emphasis on management budgetting and performance indicators, gathering information on workload, performance, outcomes, etc. has become increasingly important as part of the overall effort in deciding what a particular service requires in terms of amount of equipment and number of staff. The information gathered should help to show how the total workload is fluctuating or varying from past experience and, in more detailed form, to help predict future workloads.

Most hospital statistics are in the form of '*output*' data, that is, an historical account of what work has been accomplished, such as numbers of clients treated or new referrals received. These figures can be analysed to develop trend information and eventually to gain some measure of predictability of what may be expected for the future.

Another approach is to concentrate on looking at the work from the point of view of '*intake*,' that is, looking at referrals received to see if there is any possibility of adjusting the incoming workload. However, in many departments, which provide a mainly response service, there is little choice but to accept whatever workload is sent.

Analysing the data

1. *Output data*
   - Total annual figures are charted to show the rate of change from one year to the next. Use figures over a reasonable period of time, such as the last 5–10 years.
   - Total monthly figures are used to assess whether there are any recurring seasonal patterns and, by grouping the figures into half years, to show where increases/decreases of work exist.

● Total daily figures can be used to find out daily averages and the range between the lowest and highest days, and plotted to show weekly trends.

2. *Intake data*

These can be collected on an annual or monthly basis to show:

● Where the work comes from—which consultants/specialities are involved.

● Who the major users are —is there any possibility of smoothing out demands for the department services in order to iron out peaks and troughs.

● Changes in the balance of major users—have they changed and to what degree?

The data analysed above can help to provide answers to the following questions:

● How much work is currently undertaken by the department in 1 month and 1 year?

● Has the total volume of work changed appreciably during the past year, 2 years, 5 years?

● What variations are there from week to week?

● How predictable is the daily workload?

● How much does one day's workload differ from another?

● Have there been any significant changes in the balance of users and, if so, why?

● Who are the major users of the service? Is there any evidence of excessive use?

● Do departmental policies on priority and urgent cases need to be revised?

These techniques may seem crude but they are widely used and important management tools. However, therapy managers must remember that the 'quality' of treatment given is more important than the 'quantity'.

Analysing current manpower

The strengths and weaknesses of manpower currently employed will, to a large extent, determine future requirements. Managers should undertake regularly a number of analyses, such as the age distribution, absenteeism, wastage and qualifications of their staff. This will become easier

as more computerised personnel systems are introduced.

Age distribution

Looking at age distribution helps to determine the type of contribution staff make to a department, for example, increasing age may lead to higher sickness rates and decreased physical fitness but also to higher stability and increased maturity. It also helps to determine whether sufficient younger people are available to fill senior posts as they become vacant.

Managers should analyse the age distribution of their staff to determine:

● If any members of staff will be retiring in the next 12 months.

● What action needs to be taken to replace those staff, for example, restructuring jobs, reallocating work or recruiting and training new staff, especially if those retiring are long serving and experienced.

● What action, if any, needs to be taken to achieve a better balance in age structure, for example, through recruitment policies. Consideration should also be given to whether or not arbitrary age limits can be justified.

Sickness and absenteeism

Accurate information, although essential to a wellmanaged department, is not always available, nor is the significance fully recognised of the many factors that result in employees not attending work. Various causes of absenteeism are of course well known:

● holidays, with or without pay
● absence resulting from sickness
● maternity leave
● lateness and general bad timekeeping
● accidents.

Total losses due to all these causes can reach very high proportions in some departments.

Absenteeism should not be looked at in isolation but as one factor of many concerning both the individual employee and the department. Sickness, absence and lateness may be shown on a graph to highlight any trends. Often, the fact that staff know that a manager is keeping this information is enough in itself to bring about improvements in attendance.

Indicators of poor morale or low commitment to the job, such as low productivity and sub-standard work, are likely to be related to high levels of absence. This 'withdrawal from work' can vary from lateness to prolonged sickness. Managers should be aware of the various aspect of absence and see them as indicators of emerging problems, which are more easily dealt with in their early stages, perhaps through counselling.

Qualifications and training

Up-to-date information on qualifications and training undertaken by staff is important when planning current and future manpower resources. Professional qualifications, special skills, courses attended and training undertaken should all be recorded and used to identify any particular training needs, present or future, to be included in an annual training action plan.

The information should also be tied into any appraisal and career development scheme.

Computerised personnel information systems

An increasing amount of personnel information is, or soon will be, held on computer, therefore it is important to realise that this data is now subject to the Data Protection Act 1984 (see Ch. 17 p. 284)

Why have a computerised system?

It has become increasingly evident during recent years that existing methods of collection and analysis or manpower information do not meet the needs of either managers or operational and strategic planners. Recent developments in information technology have put within financial reach on-line computerised systems with the speed and capacity to deal with complex and rapidly changing organisations.

Data should be accurate, available to those managers who need it and, at the same time, be secure. Common records are held for all users of the data and available information is then drawn from the same source to:

- give managers on-line personnel records of the staff for whom they are responsible and provide up-to-date and accurate information about expenditure on staff
- give each authority the ability to control its establishment
- enable payroll information to be input directly from an appropriate district location through to the payroll computer
- provide accurate information for manpower planning.

Type of information held by computer

The data loaded into the system can be held in the following sections.

- *Management unit data*: information about each department built up through a hierarchical system to give an overall picture of the service across the district.
- *Establishment data*: information about a post, such as budgeted hours, location or salary scale.
- *Basic personal details*: information about an individual including name, sex, date of birth, address and nationality.
- *Post details*: information about the job itself, such as occupation code, contracted hours and grade.
- *Previous post details*: information about previous jobs held.
- *Education data*: Information on examinations passed and qualifications held.
- *Courses attended.*
- *Payroll*: information necessary for the calculation of pay, such as financial code, salary scale and salary point.
- *Non-attendance.*
- *Holiday information.*

- *Professional organisation*/trade union office held.
- *Specialist knowledge*, such as languages spoken.
- *Termination information*, such as reason for leaving and address of new post.

DIRECTING

In order to be efficient we have to maximise the use of available resources. The most important and difficult resource to manipulate is the human resource, maximisation of which is dependent upon good leadership.

Effective leadership depends on the ability to influence and be influenced by the team and its members in issuing instructions and allocating the work to be done in order to complete a given task.

The manager as leader has to have vision, set the direction, enable people to extend their capabilities, inspire loyalty and command respect. The ways in which instructions are accepted by people will depend on the ways in which they are given and on the ability, experience and motivation of the people receiving them.

As previously stated, present-day management favours a democratic style, using 'participative management', that is, involving people in the decision-making process so that they are more willing to accept and abide by decisions. It has traditionally been the manager's job to give orders and the employee's duty to do the job allocated. However, the more a manager can delegate authority, the more time there is to work on other tasks.

CONTROLLING

Controlling means checking how work is progressing and identifying deviations from the agreed objectives that are causing problems. Control includes setting standards, measuring performance against standards, obtaining feedback about results and correcting deviations from the standards.

To maintain effective control, certain fundamental principles must be complied with.

1. Controls must be set according to the job to be performed, that is, they must be flexible. There are many techniques available, which may or may not be relevant depending on the nature of the job.

2. Deviations from accepted standards must be reported immediately. Some control systems fail because the monitoring process provides information too late to be of immediate use.

3. Controls must relate to departmental and organisational procedures. It is simple to identify where deviations from objectives have occurred if the organisational structure of the department is well defined and responsibility for work done is clear.

4. Controls should be flexible and economical to operate. Any system should be sufficiently flexible to allow for alternative remedies when failures occur. Systems should be kept as simple as possible and must not cost more than they are worth.

5. Controls should be simple to understand and must indicate corrective action. Certain control techniques involve sophisticated mathematics and should therefore be summarised in a straightforward and easy to understand manner. It is essential that whatever technique is used for control purposes there must be a clear indication of the cause of any deviations and the possible remedies that might be applied.

SUMMARY

'The National Health Service is growing at a remarkable rate. A quality service which not only provides clinical excellence but also makes patients feel valued requires a quality management and organisation. To provide the best possible service from its resources, particularly as demands continue to grow, the NHS must always seek to make the best use of the resources available. Achieving this means giving managers more freedom to manage'.

Most managers learn by managing but in the changing role of management the biggest challenge lies not in the changes but in the people. People are looking for meaning in their work; because they are better educated and have higher expectations they want to be involved and contribute to the organisation in which they work.

This chapter has attempted to outline some of the skills required and techniques used in managing quality and productivity in occupational therapy today.

REFERENCES

Craik C 1986a Management training for occupational therapists, part 1. British Journal of Occupational Therapy 49(7): 220–223

Craik C 1986b Management training for occupational therapists, part 2. British Journal of Occupational Therapy 49(8): 253–256

COT 1984 Guidelines for clinical practice. COT, London

Davis K 1977 Behaviour at work, 5th edn. McGraw-Hill, New York

DHSS 1979 Patients first. HMSO, London

HMSO 1988 Working for patients. White Paper. HMSO, London

HMSO 1984 Implementation of the NHS management inquiry (Griffiths) report. HMSO, London

Stockport Health Authority 1985 First line management package: communication skills. SHA, Stockport

Turla P, Hawkins K 1985 Time management made easy. Panther, London

FURTHER READING

Stress management

Bailey R 1985 Coping with stress. Blackwell, London

Carnegie D 1977 How to stop worrying and start living. Cedar Books, Tadworth

Charlesworth E, Nathan R 1987 Stress management: a comprehensive guide to your wellbeing. Corgi, London

Kirsta A 1987 The book of stress survival: how to relax and live positively. Gaia, London

Livingstone, Booth A 1985 Stressmanship. Severn, London

Meichenbaum D 1983 Coping with stress. Century, London

Trauer T 1986 Coping with stress. Salamander, London

Appraisal

Long P 1986 Performance appraisal revisited. Institute of Personnel Management

Philip T 1983 Making performance appraisal work. McGraw-Hill, New York

Supervisor training

Honey P 1988 Improve your people skills. Institute of Personnel Management

Counselling

Megranahan M 1988 Counselling: a practical guide for employers. Institute of Personnel Management

General

Thomason G 1988 A textbook of human resource management. Institute of Personnel Management

Recruitment and selection

Courtis J 1988 Interviews: skills and strategy. Institute of Personnel Management

Fletcher J 1988 Effective interviewing. Institute of Personnel Management

Plumbley P 1988 Recruitment and selection, 4th edn. Institute of Personnel Management

27

Budgetting

Sue Gore

INTRODUCTION

Budgetary control has a fundamental role in the management process as it provides not only the financial resources that allow managers to implement plans and policies but also makes available the financial and statistical information necessary to control the use of resources. It is a strong management tool. Any budgetary system must be seen as an integral part of the managerial process and the people whose decisions affect the use of resources must be accountable for expenditure.

A budget may be defined as 'an estimate of income and expenditure for a stated period of account. A sum of money up to which a budget holder can spend.' (NAHA 1981, 2.1.4.) The 'stated period' is usually 1 year and the 'financial' year in the UK runs from April to March.

In understanding the budgetary process, the occupational therapist manager should be aware of the major financial issues affecting the service being managed and how these influence the day-to-day budget position. These issues are covered in the first section. Given this information and possessing an ability to understand the process of budgetting, the occupational therapist will be able to ask the right questions of treasurers, other budget holders, other managers and departmental staff. The budget process and budgetary management are described in the next two sections. The financial terms used in this chapter are defined in the Glossary at the end of this book.

NATIONAL HEALTH SERVICE (NHS) FUNDING

The National Health Service (NHS) is funded almost entirely by the Exchequer. Of that funding, 87.5% is raised through general taxation and a further 10.5% from national insurance contributions. The remaining 2% is raised from private patients, dental charges, prescription charges, etc.

BACKGROUND

The hospital service inherited by the NHS in 1948 was the result of initiatives taken by private benefactors and local authorities and funded solely by them. This meant that wealthier or more enterprising areas, or those blessed with particularly generous benefactors, acquired a better hospital service than other, less-fortunate areas (NAHA 1981, 2.2.1).

When the NHS came into being the intention was to provide a genuinely national service, and so it did. However, due to the existing imbalances the better-endowed parts of the country needed larger sums of money to fund their services than did less-fortunate areas. As money flowed in, the advantages of the better-off areas were consolidated.

As time went by it became increasingly clear that something had to be done to remove the old inequalities. This was not a simple task, as it could not be assumed that one need was the same as another and that a crude totalling of populations would effectively represent regional differences. The demand for health care generated by differing populations is influenced by the make-up of the population involved. The distribution of age and sex both make a difference; the increased demands on the health service by the elderly is an obvious example. The flow of patients between regions also varies, as some import patients from their neighbours and others export them. The extra cost of clinical teaching is another factor and so is the fact that, in general, it costs more to provide a comparable service in London than in the provinces.

Resource allocation

The Resource Allocation Working Party (RAWP) was appointed by the Department of Health and Social Security on 12th May 1975 in an attempt to plan something that previously had been largely determined by history.

This working party went further than anyone else had done in trying to assess the factors that influence the demand for health care and the cost of providing it. They considered resource allocation in three areas:

1. revenue
2. capital
3. allocations for teaching.

Using the size of populations as the main determinant of need, they considered seven different aspects of the health service:

1. non-psychiatric inpatient services
2. day and outpatient services
3. community services
4. ambulance services
5. family practitioner committee administration
6. inpatient services for the mentally ill
7. inpatient services for the mentally handicapped.

In each case, the population was weighted in the light of the criteria of need. Finally, these seven different weighted populations were combined into one figure, which gave a region's standing relative to other regions in the league table of need.

FINANCIAL PLANNING

A health authority is required by statutory provision made under Section 97 and 97a of the National Health Service Act 1977, as amended by the National Health Service Act 1986, to perform its functions within the total funds allocated by the Regional Health Authority. This means that each region within the NHS and, in turn, each District Health Authority is expected to provide its services within a given budget. The two principal financial responsibilities of health authorities are:

1. planning how to spend money
2. spending it efficiently.

The annual budgets prepared by health authorities are plans setting out in financial terms how the resources available to them are to be utilised in the course of the next financial year. In addition to these plans, health authorities are required to produce:

- operational plans, covering 1 to 3 years and revised every year
- strategic plans, offering a 5–10 year forecast and revised every three to four years.

However, this requirement changes with the implementation of the government's latest NHS reorganisation.

If plans are to be of use to health authorities, it is essential that they are costed and are capable of being implemented within the financial resources expected over the course of the planning cycle.

The whole process amounts to a set of compromises that attempt to relate what is desirable to what is practicable.

Spending of as much as 98% of NHS money is committed in advance by the pattern of established activity and the expectations of the public and staff about the sort of service that can and should be given. This means that only a small percentage of funds is available to cater for the unexpected and to accommodate future developments.

Strategic planning

Strategic plans are usually completed by the Regional Health Authority and District Health Authority on the basis of national and regional guidelines.

Operational planning

The operational or annual plan is a document that outlines the policies, priorities and strategies that the health authority intends to follow in providing services in the following years. This is of particular interest to occupational therapy managers as it is the principal channel through which service developments are identified and approved. Therefore, any changes required in the provision of a service and/or any additional resources required if approved, will appear in the annual programme.

This, then, is the mechanism for introducing change and, if appropriate, making the case for service developments. If a 'bid' secures a place in the annual plan, as agreed by the health authority, it then becomes a serious contender for funding when the annual revenue allocation is finally agreed.

Priorities are set at a number of levels in the health services, in national and local planning, in the clinical field and in commissioning research. Having to choose is a dilemma that confronts all managers involved in the health service.

It concerns not only how the services organises and manages itself but also the wider question of what it chooses to do with its limited resources.

In crude terms, this can be compared to people handling their own domestic budgets. Superficially, the NHS cannot provide a particular service or a particular improvement to the service because it has not got the money. The domestic equivalent is to say, perhaps, 'We can't have a continental holiday this year because we can't afford it'. The domestic budgetter might then go on to say, however, 'But if we delay buying a new car, cut down on cigarettes and economise on food we could manage a holiday abroad after all'. The question then is to decide whether the benefit of the holiday abroad is seen as outweighing the value attached to the things that have to be given up to make it possible. It is this sort of calculation, although of much greater sophistication, that has to be made by managers at all levels.

HEALTH ECONOMICS

Economics is about getting better value from the deployment of scarce resources.

The growing interest in health economics is not surprising. NHS funds have risen relatively slowly in real terms over the last few years. At the same time technological developments have conspired to increase costs, not only because they often require more expensive procedures but also because they increase the client population who would potentially benefit from treatment.

Economic appraisal is concerned with the ever-present need to make choices about how scarce resources are used. Resources are scarce in the sense that they will always be insufficient to enable individuals or society to pursue all the objectives they might desire. Accepting this means that choice is inevitable. It also means that using a resource in one way means foregoing the opportunity of having the benefits of its use in some alternative way.

Economics and financial management of health care are not ultimately about money. They are about choosing between the kinds of health service available to the public in order to achieve the best in human terms, as well as medical terms, that can be achieved with the resources available.

THE BUDGET PROCESS

Having received the cash limit for a given financial year, the treasurer, in consultation with the general manager and other senior officers, will compile financial estimates and make forecasts within the limits of the available funds and the planning policies of the health authority. Certain financial, statistical and other relevant information is required for the compilation of such estimates and forecasts and it is at this point that the district occupational therapist or occupational therapy manager should be involved.

These initial discussions usually take place towards the end of the calendar year and are the most appropriate means of providing the Treasurer with the necessary information on which the coming year's budget may be set.

Information relevant to these discussions would be, as in the following examples.

● The adequacy of the current year's budget, together with the identification of any particular problems that may have arisen, and possible solutions.

● Any identifiable shift in workload that may have a direct influence on the budgetary needs of the future. Where possible, this information should be supported by statistical evidence. It is at this point that the income element of the budget may need to be adjusted. An example of this would be if a particular department develops more

anxiety management groups, extends its relaxation teaching and reduces its income-producing activities.

The contents of these discussions will vary from district to district, for example, the draft budget may be calculated by the treasurer's department and agreed by the occupational therapy manager, or vice versa, but the outcome should always be an overall agreement that the budget is adequate in providing for the anticipated needs of the service.

Following the initial discussions and an agreed draft budget, approval from the health authority is required before a budget statement can be issued allowing the budget to become operational from 1 April, the first day of the new financial year.

DEPARTMENTAL BUDGETS

Traditionally departmental budgets are considered to be made up of two clearly defined components: pay and non-pay.

The pay budget

The staff establishment for a given department forms the basis of the pay budget and should allow for staff in post, vacancies, extra duty payments and employers on-costs. Employers on-costs are those costs over and above the salary payment incurred in employing staff, for example, the health authority has to contribute to the Government's National Insurance Fund for all employees and to the NHS Superannuation Fund for superannuable staff.

The figure for staff in post is the number of staff working on the day the budget was set, together with any staff that have replaced a leaver in the period between the budget setting exercise and the acceptance of it.

A cash allowance must be identified for known vacancies, to allow for recruitment expenses and, if appropriate, an allowance must be made to cover on-call, overtime, clinical supervisors' allowances and lecture fees.

In case of long-term sickness the cost will

generally have to be contained within the agreed budget and therefore any locum cover or overtime worked must be set against either an underspending or a negotiated additional allowance. Maternity leave is seldom allowed for and the general rule is that cover must be provided from within the overall total of the budget. It is always wise for a manager to seek financial advice regarding maternity leave.

The non-pay budget

The content of the non-pay part of the budget will vary very much from district to district, depending upon the agreement made at local level. However, the most common items under this heading are:

- travelling expenses
- staff uniforms
- clients' appliances
- materials
- equipment
- client entertainment
- occupational therapy aids
- occupational therapy sales (income).

As it is difficult to identify accurately the staff costs and materials used against the number of clients treated, it is often the case that a non-pay budget is based upon historical evidence of expenditure rather than on an assessment of need based upon quantified workload.

Budget adjustments

There are occasions when budgets need to be adjusted to take into account changes such as pay awards, changes in employers on-costs, new developments in the service and increased prices.

Pay awards are generally automatically fed into the budget by the treasurer, as are any changes to the employers on-costs. Increased prices due to the effects of inflation may or may not be allowed for in the budget. This needs to be identified when the budget is set because, if there is no allowance, the real value of the budget will diminish over the course of the year and expenditure must be planned to take account of this.

BUDGETARY MANAGEMENT

Budgetary controls are the systems set up to control and monitor expenditure. Budgetary management is the way in which these systems are operated. The process of managing the resources allocated to an occupational therapy service is little more than organising a domestic household budget but on a larger scale.

THE RELATIONSHIP BETWEEN THE BUDGET AND THE SERVICE

Full budgetary management means having full responsibility for the resources allocated to a particular service. Within the constraints of these resources, the manager is expected to provide the best possible service to the clients. The financial stability of a service depends on the ability to budget realistically for the expenditure it may be expected to incur in the following and subsequent years.

Virement

Virement is the ability to transfer funds from one financial account to another.

Each health authority, within its financial instructions, will make some reference to budget under- and over-spending.

Overspending should, of course, be avoided if at all possible. If it does occur then advice from the financial advisor should be sought and attempts made to correct the situation.

Underspending, although a happier state to be in, should never be excessive as this money could have been used by another service to provide client care. If the budget is underspent, perhaps because of an inability to recruit staff, then managers should be aware of the ability to transfer monies from one budget to another, perhaps from staffing into buying a new piece of equipment or from an underspent 'Materials and equipment' budget into providing some extra staff hours.

Virement and flexibility are the active means by which a manager and budget holder can fund changes in the pattern of client care.

Income

Income from sales is an everyday part of the budget process in most occupational therapy departments and will generally have been included as part of the overall department allocation. Income is credited against planned expenditure and the net sum allocated is the budget. It must be emphasised that therapy is not an income generator and any changes in treatment techniques used in a department that may affect income levels should be brought to the attention of the financial advisor so that any necessary adjustments can be made to the budget.

CONTROLLING EXPENDITURE

It is important when given the responsibility of managing a budget to recognise the sources of spending that can be charged to the budget and to understand how spending can be controlled.

All expenditure goes through the treasurer's ledger and is charged to the occupational therapy budget by a system of accounting codes. The coding of expenditure is therefore important if the correct budget is to be charged with the correct amount of expenditure. There are two systems available, centralised and department based.

A centralised coding system

This system dictates that all orders and invoices are passed on to the treasurer's department who, in processing them for payments, will allocate a code to each item of expenditure. This means that the treasurer's department determines exactly which budget holder is charged with the expenditure. A summary of all expenditures only becomes available when the monthly budget statement is produced.

Source coding

Source coding is a system whereby the occupational therapy manager or budget holder codes all orders or invoices before passing them on to the treasurer's department for payment. This system enables the manager to determine at source exactly which budget holder is charged with the expenditure. It also allows for the day-to-day control of expenditure as it arises. This applies equally to items purchased with petty cash, as these items are also charged to the budget.

BUDGET CONTROL REPORTS

Budgetary management depends upon the regular receipt of information on the state of the budget. This is invariably in the form of a monthly budget control report. Although these will differ in detail in different health authorities, the principles are generally similar. These reports should be available for every month of the year but it is not unusual for treasurers to begin producing them from the end of June onwards. The early part of the year is taken up with actually setting up budget reports on computer and checking their correctness before they are issued. Providing that establishments are not exceeded and non-pay budgets have been agreed at an adequate level, this delay should not cause any real concern.

Pay will inevitably form the greater cash component of the total budget. If the input hours are within the establishment and the establishment is correctly budgetted for then the pay budget should not cause concern. Non-pay budgets are often harder to analyse as the regular flow of payments is not so certain as that for salaries and wages.

The budgetary control report is simply a statement reflecting past activity. If the occupational therapy service is being efficiently and effectively managed they reflect a constant trend of reinforcing information showing that the service is under control.

AUDIT

Overseeing the financial management of the service are the auditors. The main function of an audit is to:

- check against fraud
- ensure that proper processes are being followed
- ensure that value for money is being obtained
- check that the authority's procedures are sound

- monitor whether the service is being provided economically and efficiently.

The auditors that most occupational therapy departments will have regular contact with are those employed permanently in the treasurer's department to undertake the internal audits. The audits that more directly affect health authorities are those carried out by the Department of Health auditors who visit an authority several times a year.

From time to time, departments may build up stocks of materials that are not for immediate use. If this is the case, then expenditure charged to the budget could be adjusted to take account of this unused stock and the expenditure spread over the months that the stocks are to be used in. The treasurer may offer advice about this if it is seen to be a problem. Stocktaking will be required at the end of the year, to enable statutory accounts to be completed as required by the DHSS.

SUMMARY

Good management is essential in occupational therapy and budgetary control has a fundamental role in the management process.

Budgetary management begins with an understanding of the factors that make up the budget and relies upon the regular receipt of information on the state of the budget. Given this information and understanding, the budget holder will be aware of the financial issues affecting the service and have sufficient knowledge, as a result, to ask the right questions of the treasurer and other managers.

Providing a quality service from scarce resources therefore requires a knowledge and understanding of the budgetary system and budget holders must be given responsibility for preparing their budgets and held responsible for and accountable to their line manager for their actual performance.

REFERENCES

The National Association of Health Authorities in England and Wales 1981 The National Health Service hand book. NAHA, Birmingham

FURTHER READING

College of Occupational Therapy 1984 Budgetary management package for district occupational therapists. COT, London
Drummond M 1984 Essentials of health economics. Research Unit, Aberdeen

National Health Service 1989 Working for patients. (White Paper) HMSO, London

28

Record keeping

Belinda Thompson

INTRODUCTION

Health-care services exist in order to identify people's health-related problems and needs, and to provide the best ways of solving the presenting problems, whether medical, physical or psychological.

Records made by each person involved in the client's treatment provide an essential communication network. In order that the occupational therapist's contribution is both effective and useful, it is necessary to examine carefully the whole concept of record keeping.

In this chapter, the types of records made by different professions are discussed. This is followed by detail of occupational therapy record keeping, including the effect of the Korner reports. Systems of record keeping are outlined, and the chapter ends with a discussion of effective report writing, an aspect of record keeping that concerns every occupational therapist.

KEEPING RECORDS

This section focuses on the types of records that make up the communication network and on the importance of confidentiality in record keeping.

WHAT ARE RECORDS?

Man has always recorded information that he needs to pass on to others or that he wishes to recall at a later date. Records then, whether in the form of cave drawings, writing or computerised data (Fig. 28.1) are means of communication and information storage. The records kept about a person and the treatment he receives are necessary both for information storage for the future and for communication between the professionals involved.

TYPES OF RECORD

Records differ in their content and style according to which member of the treatment team writes them. The following shows the difference between case notes, nurses' notes, occupational therapy notes and those made by community workers.

Case notes

As information about a client is collated by the medical records officer who processes the admission or referral, it is stored in the form of case notes. These are usually kept in a central base for ease of access by the different people who need to use them, for example, the ward to which admission has been made or the office of the centre or clinic.

Case notes contain all identification data about the client, usually on the front inside page, although the layout will vary between establishments. Figure 28.2 shows a form that came into use in a Health Authority in England on January 1987 as a result of the Korner recommendations (see page 491).

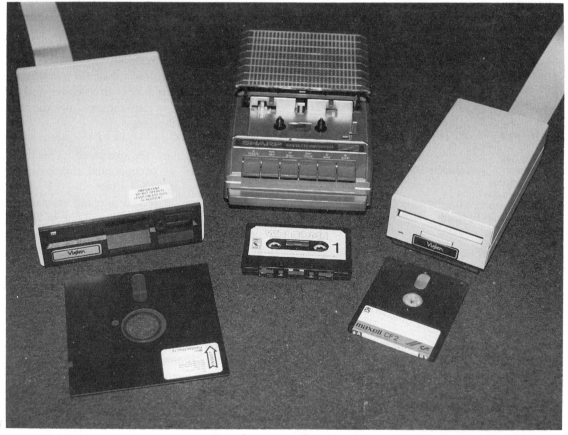

(a)

Fig. 28.1 There are many different types of records: paper, computer, microfiche, photographic, etc.
(a) Records can be stored on computer discs of various types (left and right), and on cassette (centre).
(b) An X-ray is a visual record form.

The case notes will also contain test, assessment or laboratory results and reports from any professionals involved, such as occupational therapists, art therapists or psychologists. Letters from social workers, doctors or relatives, and any other written communication, will also be included.

Nurses' notes

Within a hospital setting these are recorded on a daily basis, often in a system of easy-reference

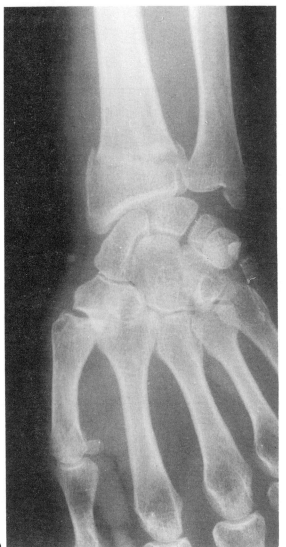

(b)

storage, such as a Kardex. On client discharge, or at periodic intervals during a lengthy stay in hospital, these notes are transferred, along with any drug charts, into the client's case notes. Nurses' notes detail a client's behaviour and any specific events or occurrences during the course of the day. They are also used by the nurse for reference during a doctor's ward round and during the changeover period when the next shift of nurses comes on duty.

Occupational therapy notes

The content of occupational therapy notes is covered on page 492, however, it is worth noting here how they fit into the client's case notes. The therapist's informal day-to-day notes are usually kept in the department office. The formal element of occupational therapy records, that is, reports and assessment results, are sent to the referring agent, usually the doctor, and eventually stored in the case notes.

Community workers' notes

Many health-care professionals, including occupational therapists, now work out of the hospital setting as part of community teams working with specific client groups, in general practice surgeries, health centres or clients' homes. The records they keep are as important as those kept in a hospital. In a community setting, however, communication between team members is made more difficult because they are not all based in one building.

The question of confidentiality is especially pertinent in this type of work as client records are carried around and stored only at the end of the day, or even every few days, at the central base or office.

CONFIDENTIALITY OF RECORDS

Records should only be accessible to people involved in the direct professional care of a client. It is imperative therefore that the system of keeping and storing records is not open to abuse and that those who do have access to records respect confidential ethics (see ch. 9).

Hospital	Casenote No.
District No.	
	G.P. Name
Surname Title	
	G.P. Address
Forename(s) Sex	
Date of Birth Age	G.P. Telephone No.
Address	
	Patients Tele. No. (Home)
	(Work)
Postcode LA Code	Address From which Admitted
Religion	Allergies
Place of Birth	Marital Status
Occupation/School (if child)	N.H.S. Number

NEXT OF KIN DATA

Name	N.O.K. Address
Relationship	
Telephone No. (Home)	
(Work)	Postcode

ADMISSION DATA

Consultant	Joint Consultant
Specialty	Joint Specialty
Admission Reason	Referred By
Operation	
Admission Date Admission Time	Need To Admit Date
Ward	Expected L.O.S. (days)
Method of Admission	Place Of Accident
Source Of Admission	Category of Admission
Intended Management	
Accompanying Healthy People Staying Overnight (Nos)	Has The Patient Been Resident In The Country For 12 Months Y / N
Is The Patient In Receipt Of A State Pension (State Type)	

Fig. 28.2 A sample identification data sheet.

(NB Continued on p. 489.)

Where records are kept

From the time an admission or referral has been made until the client is discharged from treatment, his records are kept on the ward or in the office concerned. They must always be kept in a lockable filing cabinet or trolley to prevent access by unauthorised personnel. Those who make the records or have access to them are responsible for respecting this rule.

In NHS hospitals or centres, a client's records

Fig. 28.2 continued

Medical records department

It is from here that the records were originally created on admission or referral and then sent to the ward or centre concerned. The medical records officer is the person who provides immediate custodial care of all medical records; legally, they belong to the government.

A visit to the medical records department is worthwhile in order to gain insight into its functions and purpose. Occupational therapy staff rarely have direct contact with the department and are consequently unaware of all its functions, which include:

- registering outpatient appointments
- receiving and registering general practitioners' letters
- maintaining a diagnostic index for research and statistical purposes
- recording all births, deaths, discharges and transfers to other hospitals
- storing case notes—the length of time the case notes are stored on return to the medical records department varies according to district policy. Many keep them for a specified number of years, for example, 20 years, while others keep them until the person's known death. Storage space is a determining factor, although many records are now transferred from paper to microfiche (see 'Systems of record keeping' on page 496).

Who reads records?

Any professional person involved in the care or treatment of a client is able to obtain access to that person's case notes. This includes nurses, doctors, therapists, psychologists, certain social-services officers and students of these disciplines. Some establishments do not permit access to case notes by unqualified personnel; this decision depends both upon management policy and on the staffing structure of a particular ward or department.

Should records that have been returned to the medical records department be required for research purposes, for example, as part of a case study by a member or student of the treatment team, then permission must be sought from the manager of the establishment via the medical records officer. If information is required by those not usually allowed access to records, or if more extensive information is required, then application is made to the Ethical Committee, which is based at the District Health Authority.

Traditionally, clients and their relatives have not had access to their own case notes. However, in certain establishments now, and in all occupational therapy programmes, the client is encouraged to become actively involved in decision making regarding his own treatment, so reports are written in a way that he can read and understand, that is, without technical jargon.

Disclosure of Information Act 1987

From April 1987 the DHSS brought into force the above act with the following effects:

- clients and/or relatives may have, upon request, access to client records kept by a social-services department
- all records must be written with this in mind, that is, their contents must be objective and without judgement or prejudice
- information that the team feels would prove to have a detrimental effect upon the client or relatives concerned should be marked 'Strictly confidential' and be kept seperately from the other records. Access to these records is given only to the professional team concerned.

Professional codes of conduct

Confidentiality is a fundamental part of the therapist's professional conduct, therefore it is important to understand and respect it.

All professionals with whom a client is likely to come into contact are required by their respective professional associations to acknowledge their understanding and acceptance of a professional code of ethics. In the case of the British Association of Occupational Therapists, it is stated, 'Occupational therapists shall respect confidential information available to them in the course of their professional duties.' (BAOT 1975) 'Confidential information' refers both to verbal and written material, including case notes and all client records. Allowing an unauthorised person access to written records is a breach of the ethic of confidentiality, as is talking about a client to anyone outside the treatment team or talking about a client in a public place.

It is for these reasons that pseudonyms and fictitious addresses should be used when using clients as Case studies for research or other purposes.

OCCUPATIONAL THERAPY RECORDS

The records made by occupational therapists fit into two broad categories:

- day-to-day notes
- formal reports.

The latter are used as a method of communicating the results of clients' participation in occupational therapy to other members of the team.

THE PURPOSE OF OCCUPATIONAL THERAPY RECORDS

We have identified what records are and who makes use of them. Next we examine what occupational therapy records are used for in the health-care services, including use in treatment, legal use and use in research.

Use in treatment

Assessment information and records of treatment

sessions are kept in written form for several purposes:

- to aid our memories, because to remember clearly all that we plan to do, and have done, with each client is impossible
- to provide a baseline to refer back to so that progress can be measured during treatment
- if a client is transferred from one therapist to another during treatment, written records will provide the second therapist with the information she needs to follow on
- records can provide a useful adjunct to verbal communication between two people who work with the same client and contribute to the same records
- if the client is readmitted or admitted to a different hospital the occupational therapist's report in the case notes will be available for future therapists.

Legal use

In the current climate of concern about the accountability of health-care staff, there is an increasing possibility of occupational therapists or other members of staff being accused of mismanaging a client who is in their care. In such cases, written records of actual treatment carried out by the therapist could provide essential information. If the case goes as far as the courts, records will be required for legal purposes.

All health-care establishments have a policy for the recording of any accidents or injury involving a member of staff and/or a client, usually on an accident report form, which demands specific, detailed information about the occurrence.

Research and statistics

In the long term occupational therapy records provide information that can be used for research and statistical purposes.

Statistics are needed in order to:

- justify the existing number of staff and facilities
- measure the effectiveness of the existing service

- plan for future needs
- justify proposed changes in the size or nature of the service, for example, creating a new post.

The way in which statistics from the professions allied to medicine are collected and used is currently undergoing radical change. Services are required to provide the DHSS with certain statistics but, as a result of the 'Korner Reports', the process and content of statistical collection are being revised.

THE KORNER REPORTS

Formerly, the statistics the DHSS has required from occupational therapists have been figures to represent how many treatment sessions take place within a department per therapist per year. These are collected at grass roots level by means of a daily register and are then converted into monthly figures, which are made available annually to the DHSS. Such records are used to justify the service given at present and to support recommendations for future changes, such as higher staffing levels and relocation of services.

However, occupational therapists and other professions allied to medicine have, for a long time, been concerned that their work has not been accurately reflected by this type of statistic, and the same concern was felt generally throughout the National Health Service. This led to the formation of the 'Steering Group on Health Services Information', chaired by Mrs Edith Korner, with the aims of:

- reviewing all health-services statistics
- studying how they are collected
- making subsequent recommendations.

Between 1982 and 1984, the steering group reviewed seven areas of major NHS activity and made their recommendations in what have become known as the 'Korner Reports'.

The fourth report, which concerned the paramedical professions, recommended compiling a basic minimum data set and recording additional information which is pertinent to each particular profession or geographical area.

Because this was a new system of record keeping and required all staff to be carefully trained to use it effectively, the DHSS gave the services staggered dates for implementing the different stages. Since 1 April 1988, all Health Authorities have been using the Korner system in its entirety. The method by which the required information is collected is at the discretion of the individual authority but an example is the computer software system, 'Comcare'.

Comcare data-collection system

The information recorded includes name and date of birth of the client, treatment given, location of contact and length of contact. Details are first entered in code form on paper and then programmed into a computer.

One problem that arose was the time required to complete the Korner forms with, for example, a department of eight staff taking a total of 2 hours per day to complete this task. Some health authorities are now replacing the forms with hand-held computers, making the task of collecting information easier and more accurate for both therapy staff and computer-processing staff.

To illustrate the way in which information is coded, assume that you need to record where initial contact with the client was made:

- inpatient at general hospital   code 328
- outpatient at general hospital   code 327
- inpatient at continuing care
  hospital   code 326
- home assessment/visit   code 325

The appropriate code would be indicated on the 'Comcare' record sheet and then fed into the computer (DHSS 1984).

CONTENTS OF OCCUPATIONAL THERAPY RECORDS

The occupational therapist keeps a set of records for each client she sees, the content of which is often of similar format to case notes but with specific details of treatment.

A sample set of records might include:

- a referral form
- an initial interview/assessment form
- continuation sheets
- occupational therapy reports
- results of any other tests or assessments
- any other written communication.

The referral form

Each department has a referral system that is suited to their particular needs and may or may not include a written form signed by a doctor. A referral to a community occupational therapist from a community source will often contain a lot of detail about the client, his social situation, problems, etc., as access by the therapist to more detailed information might be difficult and time-consuming if she has to travel to obtain it (see Fig. 28.3).

In a hospital setting, however, case notes and information are easier to obtain and so a referral form need not be as detailed. It is quite common in a hospital setting for the referral form to be completed by the person making the referral, for example the doctor, ward sister/charge nurse or social worker. In this case, it is preferable for the form to include only basic identification data about the client in order that:

- the referral form can be completed quickly so that the referral is not delayed
- the therapist can seek the precise information she requires after receiving the referral
- time is not wasted writing irrelevant information.

The most basic referral form might include the following:

- ward (where relevant)
- name of client's doctor
- client's name
- client's date of birth
- client's age
- reasons for the referral
- any precautions or contraindications
- signature, designation and date of the referring agent (see Fig. 28.4).

Social Services Department	Occupational Therapy Services

Referral to Occupational Therapy

Name of referring agent
Date

Name of client   Date of birth
Address and phone number   Age

Name of GP

Home situation

Family and social contacts

Occupation
Problems and/or reason for referral

Signed _____ Date _____

Fig. 28.3 A detailed referral form.

The referral form is often kept in the front of the client's notes, as it provides a quick way of identifying them. It is helpful to have the referral form in a different colour from the other notes.

Initial interview/assessment form

Like the referral form, this will vary according to the specific client group and establishment concerned. Initial interview/assessment forms can be broadly divided into two types:

- checklist
- open-ended

Checklist

This form is in more common use in settings where physical illness is the primary presenting problem, as it will contain factual information about a clients' abilities and problem areas. An extract may read:

Can the person transfer from: bed
                               chair
                               bath
                               toilet

a tick indicates independence.

Occupational Therapy Referral Form

Name
Date of birth
Age

Ward
Doctor

Precautions or contraindications

Reason for referral

Signed________________Designation________________Date______________

Fig. 28.4 A basic referral form.

Open-ended

For the majority of people with psychiatric problems, an open-ended system of information gathering is more suitable than a checklist because of the multifactorial nature of their problems. Such a form might include sections on:
'What is the clients' attitude to his/her job?'
'What social contacts does the client have?'

Figure 28.5 shows an example of an initial information sheet that is used in a community mental-health occupational therapy service and is a combination of the checklist and open-ended types.

These forms provide more detailed information than is generally presented on a referral form and, more importantly, it is information that the therapist has gleaned from her own contact with a client.

Continuation sheets

Notes, giving details of treatment sessions, the therapist's observations of the client, any other occupational therapy action that is relevant, and plans for further action, are recorded on sheets that are usually referred to as 'continuation sheets'.

Occupational therapy reports

Reports are usually written on a client after completion of the initial assessment, at discharge and at regular intervals in between. The frequency of reports depends on the type of client: long-stay clients may only be reviewed annually, whereas in an acute setting there may be weekly reviews. The occupational therapy report goes in the case notes but a copy must be kept in the department notes. Reports are discussed in more detail later on page 500.

Other written communication

This might include copies the occupational therapist receives of, for example, social-work reports, psychology reports or minutes of case reviews or other meetings where there has been occupational therapy involvement. For ease of reference these are best stored in date order, with the most recent to the front.

The rules of confidentiality must, of course, be applied to all occupational therapy records. This means that all occupational therapy staff, including helpers and instructors, should be aware of what the rules are, with the qualified staff ensuring that standards of confidentiality are maintained.

Community Occupational Therapy Service (Mental Health)

Initial Information Sheet

Name
Date of birth
Address
Tel

Referred by
Date of referral
Date of contact

Living alone/with

Main social/family contacts

Brief history of illness,
including diagnosis, hospital
admissions and present medication

Other professional contacts
Consultant
GP
CPN
SW
Hospital
DRO
Home help
Psychologist

Reason for referral

Convenient times to visit

Fig. 28.5 An initial information sheet.

SYSTEMS OF RECORD KEEPING

Until recent years all types of records were stored on paper but new technological advancements are changing the face of traditional systems of record keeping. We now have many alternative ways of recording and storing important information, which are safe for many years and make retrieval easy.

SYSTEMS ON PAPER

There are three main problems with records made on paper:

1 paper can decay, leaving the writing on it illegible and therefore worthless.
2 the frequent complaint that doctors' handwriting is illegible is often true and not all records are typed.
3 paper records are bulky to store and easily torn or badly creased.

However, medical records departments are gradually adopting more technological systems of keeping records. These will be covered in Chapter 17 and in 'Photographic records' on page 498.

The problem-orientated medical record

This is a system of 'paper' record keeping, originally developed in 1969 by Dr Lawrence Weed in response to the need indicated by many colleagues for a clearly defined and standardised method of recording client care, which could be used by the whole treatment team. The 'Weed' system of record keeping is in four sections:

1. identification and database
2. problem list
3. action plan
4. progress reports.

This brief summary of the problem-oriented medical record system is not intended to contain sufficient information to effect its implementation. However, this holistic approach to client care is one that occupational therapists will appreciate and which will merit further reading (Hayes-Roth et al 1972, Smith et al 1974, Kings Fund Centre 1988).

Identification and database

Information from case notes, initial client contact and any test or assessment results is included, providing a comprehensive picture of the client's medical, social and family history, and any other relevant facts or observations.

Problem list

A problem, or a factor that has a detrimental effect on the individual's performance in either his home, leisure or work life, can be identified in conjunction with the client and the team involved. As problems are identified they may be sub-divided into categories, as in the following examples.

1. psychological problems:
   a. experiences anxiety in social situations
   b. unable to fall asleep at night
2. social/family problems:
   a. not communicating well with spouse
   b. losing contact with friends
3. physical problems:
   a. poor mobility due to osteo-arthitis of right hip
   b. obesity.

New problems may be added as more information is obtained and problems need to be ranked in priority order so that an action plan can be made.

Action plan

In this section, a form of 'action' or treatment is suggested to correspond with each problem. As well as specific treatments, the plan may include further investigations to be carried out, client education or referral to other agencies.

Progress reports

Reports are written on the progress made with each problem and must be numbered and titled.

Should the form of treatment suggested not help towards solving the problem, then this should be noted and referral be made back to the 'action plan' stage.

COMPUTERS

Computers are increasingly being employed by occupational therapists in both the physical and psychiatric fields of practice, while interest in their use is becoming even more widespread, as evidenced by the formation of the National Special Interest Group in Microcomputers.

A computer and the required software can be one of the most expensive pieces of equipment bought from an occupational therapy budget. The cost in terms of time and finance to train staff in its use is also high and so it is likely that occupational therapy departments will also employ computers for work of a clinical nature, although this section only describes the value of computers as record keepers (Kings Fund 1988).

Computerised client records

There is great potential for the use of com-

Occupational Therapy	

Treatment Record

Name   Jo Barker   Date   11th Feb 1990

Date of birth

Treatment given   Group Relaxation - session 3 - Jacobson technique

Aims   Learn how to cope with anxiety in shops

Comments by client   Still doesn't feel fully comfortable in session, but feels improvement since last session — 60% relaxed

Comments by therapist   Making a good effort. Will try deep breathing next session, on an individual basis.

Name of therapist   A Person

Signature   A. Person

Fig. 28.6   A sample treatment record.

puterised client records, if staff are proficient in using the computer. Client-identification data, assessment results and reports can be programmed into the computer and further information added when required. For example, notes of each treatment session (see Fig. 28.6) can be entered into the computer rather than kept on paper, thus avoiding storage problems and the difficulty of interpreting the writing of another therapist. Reports can be produced more quickly than by conventional typing and photocopying methods.

Research

Computers make the process of researching stored client information quick, easy and accurate. Consider, for example, an occupational therapist who wants to evaluate the use of different relaxation methods with a person whose main problem is anxiety in social situations. Having entered daily notes, the therapist can then recall information from the whole treatment episode in the form of a spreadsheet (Fig. 28.7), a bar chart or a filled line graph. This form of presentation provides a summary for the therapist and for the client.

Data collection from treatment records:
J. Barker – use of relaxation techniques

Techniques	Session no.	Group (G) or individual (I)	Client assessment of state of relaxation
Jacobsen	1	G	50%
Jacobsen	2	G	50%
Jacobsen	3	G	55%
Deep breathing	4	I	60%
Autogenic training	5	I	60%
Autogenic training	6	G	50%
Taped music	7	G	45%
Jacobsen	8	G	55%

Fig. 28.7 A spreadsheet.

Other uses

Computers are used extensively for administrative purposes, as well as in the clinical setting, for example:

- word processing
- filing forms, charts and indexes
- monitoring supplies and equipment; what is in stock, awaiting delivery, due for payment or to be returned
- budgetting
- staff records
- patient administration statistics, for example, to monitor bed states.

Data protection

Personnel data, medical case-note data and other client information held on computer is protected by the 1984 Data Protection Act, its purpose being to protect information held about individuals, and to enforce a set of standards for the processing and disclosure of such information.

As computers have become standard systems for record keeping, it has been necessary to develop ways of maintaining confidentiality. For example, a District Health Authority can have a central computer terminal (based at the District General Hospital) that both receives and gives out information and that is strictly controlled by trained, authorised personnel. Secondary terminals might then be situated within departments throughout the district but these would be 'dumb' computers, that is, only information that has been programmed in at a particular terminal can be retrieved at that terminal. Records from these secondary terminals, and also from handheld computers used by community workers, could be fed into the central terminal on a regular basis. (see Fig. 28.8).

PHOTOGRAPHIC RECORDS

There is now a wide range of photographic methods of data storage available, although not all are used by occupational therapists.

Photographs, like paper systems of record keeping, have their limitations as long-term storage.

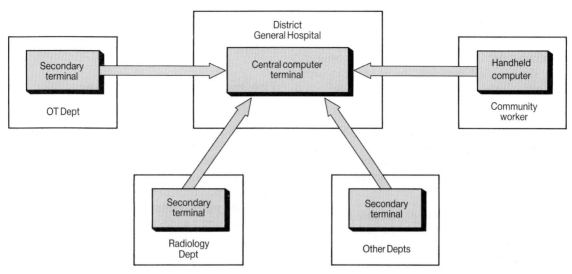

Fig. 28.8 A one-way system of computer terminals.

Any records that do require to be kept for a long period can be microcopied, which gives them the same advantages as records stored on microfiche (see page 500).

Videotapes

Like computers, video equipment provides the occupational therapist with another element of new technology to work with. Video equipment is widely used as a method of recording assessment and treatment sessions with people who have physical or psychiatric problems or a mental handicap and often proves to be very effective.

Video is a popular method of recording for several reasons.

● It is financially viable. The initial outlay for equipment (monitor, portable camera, battery and recorder) is not expensive in comparison to other items of equipment that might be bought for a department and it could easily be shared between departments. Operational costs include only blank cassettes plus electricity to run the equipment. Teaching staff to use the equipment need not be costly; one person with knowledge can teach others how to operate all the equipment within

half a day. As far as maintenence and repair are concerned, some large hospitals employ audio-visual technicians who will provide this service.

● Using videotaping, the client is able to participate actively in the process of recording his own treatment and in its evaluation.

● Viewing the videotape is often part of a client's treatment, giving him immediate feedback about how he is functioning. It is of value to both client and therapist that feedback following recorded therapy session is instant and objective (the camera never lies!).

● The tape provides a visual baseline from which to observe changes during treatment.

● The medium is appropriate for use with all age groups and is usually popular.

● Tapes can be analysed after a treatment session, particularly a group session, so that nothing is missed.

● They can be used to demonstrate a client's performance objectively to colleagues, for example, in a case conference.

● With the client's permission, recordings can also be used for student training, as they can be shown to large groups in order to give some idea of group or individual treatment without the intrusion of students into the treatment setting.

Microfiche

Microfiche is part of a process of recording written or diagrammatic information by photographing it. It is a system used especially by medical records departments, and has advantages over paper systems in that:

- it lasts longer
- it takes up far less storage space
- it is a safer way of storing information as it is less flammable than paper in comparable quantities.

The way the system works is that case notes and important statistical information are photographed using microfilm. Many individual photographs are then stored together on one presentation or 'slide' called a 'microfiche'. The microfiches are stored in envelopes called 'microjackets'.

Although this system of record keeping is not commonly found in occupational therapy departments, a medical records department could be approached, should the need arise, and might be willing both to photograph records and to lend their equipment for subsequent rereading.

Possible uses for microfiche in the occupational therapy department include:

- storage of client records for some time after discharge; it can be especially useful for therapists who have large case-loads and where storage space is limited
- storage of student records and reports
- storage of staff information, such as application forms and staff appraisal forms.

Microjackets must be used to ensure that records are protected from dust, light and extremes of temperature.

X-Rays

The X-ray is a photographic method of record keeping. X-rays are very short wavelengths that are capable of penetrating solid bodies and then printing, on photographic plate, shadow pictures of objects through which the rays have not passed. They are used in the diagnosis of physical abnormalities and to see the results or progress of treatment, such as surgery.

For the therapist, they are a useful addition to data collection about a client's condition, for example, the exact site of a fracture.

The medical photographer

Medical photographers are to be found in many hospitals, although not all. They are skilled in photography and take pictures of physical abnormalities and conditions that can best be demonstrated or recorded by the use of a photograph. Treatment methods are also illustrated by photographs and are used extensively in medical and surgical textbooks as teaching material for students of all disciplines.

REPORT WRITING

Written reports are an important way in which the occupational therapist communicates to other staff about her treatment of a client, although they are not a substitute for verbal communication.

Any reports will be kept in the client's case notes (with a copy in the occupational therapist's records) and so, when writing reports, it is worth remembering that all the team have access to case notes and therefore to occupational therapy reports.

WHAT IS A REPORT?

An occupational therapy report is a formal, written account of the therapist's work with a client.

There are usually many occasions during the working day when a therapist has need to communicate informally and verbally with other members of the team but the written report is an official channel through which to communicate ideas and information.

The occupational therapy report must initially identify the client by including personal data such as name, address and date of birth. It then aims to provide a brief and relevant picture of what occupational therapy has taken place, followed by an objective account of the results, relating them to the aims of treatment. The concluding section of the report will contain recommendations that must be based on fact and not on personal prejudice.

It is vital that all reports are signed and dated, otherwise they are invalid. It is also worth noting at the foot of the page to whom copies of the report should be sent.

Report formats

It is helpful when writing reports to have guidelines or a format to work to, so that nothing is missed out and the report is set out in a logical way. The format may be a series of general headings or it may consist of pre-set questions that require one- or two-word answers, or even ticks or crosses. The type of report written will depend upon the individual department; its policy, type of work, team preferences, etc.

At one hospital for adults with a mental handicap, the occupational therapy department uses a report format that matches its developmental frame of reference (see Fig. 28.9).

Occupational Therapy Department

Case Review

Name

Date of review

Occupational therapy programme
(to include timetable, performance,
attitude, motivation, punctuality, etc.)

Review of performance
Physical
Cognitive (intellectual)
Intrapersonal (emotional)
Interpersonal (social)
Performance

Needs (including all areas of need,
not just those the occupational
therapy department may treat)

Recommendations (including programme
changes, continuations, referrals to other
agencies and date of next review)

Signature_____Date_____

Fig. 28.9 A report format.

WRITING EFFECTIVE REPORTS

The people who read an occupational therapy report will want the information delivered to them quickly, comprehensibly and accurately. In writing an effective report, there are several important points to bear in mind.

- Appearance and legibility contribute greatly to the attention a report is given. A short, typewritten or neatly handwritten account that is set on the page in such a way that it does not give the appearance of a solid mass of grey is most likely to be read. A long report may contain more information but is of no value if no-one reads it. If there is no access to a typist and typewriter, handwriting must be neat and legible; interest is soon lost if a report is difficult to read. If photocopies of a report are to be distributed, they should be of good quality.
- The use of acceptable grammar, correct spelling and unambiguous words is important if the meaning of the report is to be clear.
- The content of the report must be succinct and include only pertinent details.

To summarise, if a report is to serve its purpose it must:

- be legible and generally well presented
- be factually accurate and objective
- be succinct and relevant

- not be out of date by the time it is written
- be seen and read by the appropriate people
- be signed and dated.

SUMMARY

All occupational therapists claim that their first priority in work is with the client. However, this chapter has tried to analyse the concept of record keeping and, in so doing, to identify its importance in occupational therapy. In summary, occupational therapists need to keep client records:

- to record treatment
- to communicate with other staff about treatment
- for legal purposes
- to justify our work
- as a basis for evaluating our work
- to support future changes/developments.

New technology is continually changing the way we store and retrieve information. It will be interesting to see what changes, if any, take place over the next few years. Maybe we shall all be equipped not only with diaries every year but with personal computers to replace the pen pushing and the piles of paperwork that everyone puts off until the last minute.

REFERENCES

British Association of Occupational Therapist 1975 Code of professional conduct for occupational therapists. BAOT, London
Department of Health and Social Security 1984 Steering group on health services information: 4th report to the Secretary of State. HMSO, London
Hayes-Roth F et al 1972 The POMR and psychiatry. British Journal of Psychiatry 121: 27–34

King's Fund Centre 1988. The problem orientated medical record (POMR): guidelines for therapists. King's Fund Centre, London
Smith L C et al 1974 Questions frequently asked about the POMR in psychiatry. Hospital and Community Psychiatry

FURTHER READING

COT 1987 Policy statement: access to patients' notes. COT, London
COT 1987 Statement on occupational therapy referral. COT, London

Hopkins H L, Smith H D 1988 Willard and Spackman's occupational therapy, 7th edn. Lippincott, Philadelphia

29

Clinical education

Sheena Blair

INTRODUCTION

WHAT IS CLINICAL EDUCATION?

Clinical education is a vital part of the educational process within a curriculum in occupational therapy. Pendergast (1971) considers that it is 'a continuum of integrated learning experiences directed towards maximizing the personal and professional growth of the student.' Booy and Lawson (1986) endorse such a view of integrated learning in their description of the progression throughout the training course from first year 'supervisor centred' aims and objectives towards 'student centred' learning in the third year. They also emphasise the necessity for a shared model of practice between clinicians and academics to clarify aims of clinical studies at all levels.

The minimum period of clinical practice suggested by the World Federation of Occupational Therapists is 1000 hours, spread throughout the whole course, at least 50% of which must be full time. The actual number of hours worked may vary in courses throughout the world and even within one country.

It is difficult to give a standard ratio of academic–clinical studies but one example is given in Figure 29.1. In this example, the alternating periods of theoretical and clinical studies allow for consolidation of knowledge and skill while providing a foundation of experience for the next block of college-based work.

Occupational therapy students will gain their clinical experience in a variety of settings, some of

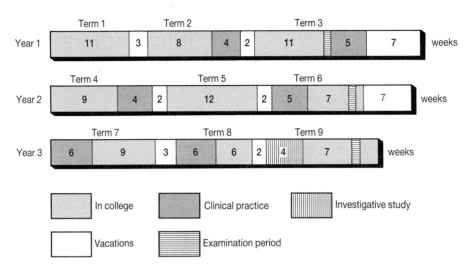

Fig. 29.1 Clinical placements within a course structure.

which are described in this book. Psychiatry offers a diversity of experience which is both challenging and bewildering for the learner, and it is not uncommon for students to feel overwhelmed by the multiplicity of problem areas, or to experience difficulty in transferring knowledge and adapting skills. Within this complex area, there is a need to establish firmly the identity of occupational therapy, outline the collaborative relationship with other disciplines and research the efficacy of our practice.

THE PURPOSE OF CLINICAL EDUCATION

'Education should separate individuals from a herd by means of an accentuation of their intrinsic difference; the manufacture of persons in regiments alike as peas is not its task.' (Molteno 1945)

The purpose of clinical studies is twofold:

- to offer an experience that allows the student to integrate theory with practice
- to cultivate behaviour and skills needed for effective practice.

The aims of each block of clinical education follow a carefully ordered sequence in which there is room for growing professional awareness and increasing clinical skill.

- The main function of the first-year placements is to give the student an understanding of the work of an occupational therapist within the clinical setting. The emphasis is on communication and handling skills, awareness of functional problems caused by illness or disability, and activity analysis.
- Clinical studies in the second year are concerned with understanding and applying the major frames of reference that underpin current clinical approaches. Opportunities are sought for developing an understanding of the many factors that influence the outcome of a rehabilitation programme.
- In the third year of training, students are expected to demonstrate increasing skill in treatment planning and evaluation. Emphasis is on management and use of resources, based on critical investigation and analysis.

Current courses of education have been designed to produce an enquiring, professionally confident student, with occupational therapy being the core topic of study. Staff involved in clinical studies must tailor their contributions accordingly, by employing appropriate teaching strategies and constructive feedback and by engaging the learner to seek out meaning. Booy and Lawson (1986) highlight the role of training schools in the continued education of clinical supervisors.

Recently, the difference between training and education has received considerable attention and the traditional emphasis on vocational instruction has been replaced by degree-level study. However, in a service profession, competency must be assured and that implies mastery of professional skills and techniques. According to Yager (1982), education can be defined as that which teaches process; how to think, how to transfer knowledge and how to analyse, rather than the syllabus outline and content. Successful education enables the student to live with uncertainty and, in psychiatry, this is an essential skill.

This chapter aims to consider aspects of clinical education concerning personal and professional growth, rather than to offer procedural or administrative guidelines.

General features of the supervision process are outlined, including the supervisor–student relationship, styles of supervision and the link between college and clinical setting. Common student problems are described in detail, followed by a section on counselling the student. The chapter then looks at factors influencing student development, such as establishing a learning climate, setting objectives and providing feedback. Examples of student placements are given. The final section covers the importance of assessment and suggests some strategies.

FEATURES OF SUPERVISION AND COMMUNICATION

Clinical supervision is most closely allied to what Bryne and Long (1973) call the 'attachment relationship', in which the novice is placed with an experienced practitioner. Within this situation, the novice is able to witness the direct application of specific knowledge and skill and the processes by which clinical judgements are reached and decisions made. The attachment relationship offers the possibility of mutual exploration of the student's and supervisor's respective roles. Rogers (1986) includes this exploration of roles in her concept of mentorship. Wallis (1977) also considers the negotiation of roles in the course of a learning

experience as intrinsic and necessary for learning.

The quality of experiential learning that occurs depends upon many factors, including the motivation of the learner, the teaching skill of the clinician and the strength of the supervisor–student relationship. Ultimately, the dream of education is to free, not control, and to nurture the desire to learn for life. Ekstein and Wallerstein (1972) urge that the natural scepticism of the student be used to fuel curiosity rather than be interpreted as doubt and criticism by the supervisor.

STYLES OF SUPERVISION

Styles of supervision vary according to the professional and personal confidence of the supervisor. Many clinicians are skilled in the procedures and administrative aspects of placements but may not necessarily inspire the wish to learn. Others are reluctant to set boundaries, preferring to allow the learner space to develop and relying on the effectiveness of dialogue as a teaching method.

Leonardelli and Gratz (1986) outline several teaching models that are relevant to clinical supervisors. They state that the responsibility of all teachers is to create the best possible learning situation for the student.

- The master–pupil model, which has been discredited as it tends to stifle enthusiasm and initiative, may reemerge in the authoritarian supervisor who 'talks at' and continually tests the student. Psychiatry can be clothed in mystery in order to suggest a superior and elusive knowledge that appears unattainable to the student.
- The apprenticeship model also has limitations in that it may encourage simple reproduction of the teacher's behaviour and overemphasise the importance of the skills component of professionalism. It is concerned with training and mastery of skill rather than with education and the fostering of self-directed learning.
- Mentorship is described by Rogers (1986) as a teaching behaviour that has many advantages. It is a nurturing process that extends role model possibilities for the learner. The distinguishing characteristic of a mentor is the

active involvement and acceptance of responsibility for shaping an individual career.

With each new learner, it is imperative to recognise individuality and to tailor objectives and teaching style accordingly. It has been said that to allow the student to 'learn the need to learn' may be the most useful contribution any teacher can make.

THE SUPERVISOR–STUDENT RELATIONSHIP

Occupational therapy in psychiatry carries intrinsic pressure that makes it necessary for staff to give each other support and encouragement. This support is also necessary for the student, to sustain belief in her own ability, therefore the supervisor–student relationship has a potent personal and professional effect.

Supervision is based upon effective communication, which includes what is heard, what is seen and the interplay between them. Staff regarded by students as helpful communicators are those who have a positive regard for the people they are endeavouring to teach, shown in enthusiasm, accessibility and willingness to share knowledge.

Yager (1982) suggests that a working alliance can be used to assist the learner to gain insight into her strengths and weaknesses. Many aspects of the student's ability to learn from experience are dependent upon the nature of this alliance, including:

- ability to integrate criticism without loss of integrity
- wish for progressive achievement
- professional confidence, based on the credibility of the supervisor.

Effective supervision

There is a need for the clinician to examine personal preferences and prejudices and attempt some self-understanding prior to assuming a supervisor role. It is easy to state that an atmosphere of openness should exist, where queries and criticisms are nonjudgementally heard, but it must be acknowledged that raw nerves are touched, insecurities

stirred and defensiveness aroused when our teaching, planning or practice is questioned. Recognising this is vital in order to prevent didactic or over-critical evaluations of students.

Entwistle (1983) suggests that teachers will often adopt methods of teaching that reflect their own preferences in learning. In clinical education, students sometimes comment that if they emulate their supervisor's style and practice they are given more positive feedback. Clearly, teaching style will affect attainment, therefore a repertoire of teaching behaviours is necessary to give the best opportunity for learning to the greatest number of students.

Methods vary from very structured programmes to ones that allow freedom to develop the student's own ideas and clinical approach. Teachers whose behaviour is considered enabling by students in psychiatry are those who:

- acknowledge individual learning styles
- accept responsibility for helping to integrate college learning with clinical skills
- appreciate that students learn best by doing
- permit enquiry, criticism and challenge without defensiveness
- offer remedial action for difficulties experienced.

Within the short time span of a clinical placement, the most likely role model for the student is the supervisor. Over the three or more years of occupational therapy training, a variety of role models will be presented to the student and the most comfortable or credible behaviours will be adopted.

Irby (1978) describes the need for clinical teachers to demonstrate high professional standards. Characteristics that attract imitation are:

- personal and professional confidence
- a capacity for self-criticism
- acceptance of responsibility
- recognition of personal limitations
- respect for others.

Students in the early stages of a placement feel it safer to directly replicate the clinical approach of their supervisor. This is noted particularly in specialty areas such as group psychotherapy, centres for the treatment of alcohol and drug abuse, or forensic work. As experience grows, personal style emerges. This pattern of initial compliance, leading to identification with the place or person and finally to internalisation of meaningful characteristics was outlined by Kelman (1963).

THE RELATIONSHIP BETWEEN COLLEGE AND CLINICAL PLACEMENT

Supervised clinical experience is an essential part of the educational programme, and provides the opportunity to synthesise theory with practice. A close relationship between college and clinical placement is imperative to ensure a shared frame of reference for teaching and learning. This relationship can be established by:

- regular meetings between clinical supervisors and college staff
- tutors' visits to placements
- a number of departments being the remit of one particular tutor
- mutual exchange of techniques or information, and shared teaching resources
- reciprocal teaching arrangements involving college staff in in-service training and clinical staff in course work
- mutual involvement in clinical supervisors' courses
- joint development of teaching aids such as videos, tape/slide presentations or static teaching displays.

Overlap between classroom and clinical situations

Within a period of clinical education it is possible to identify how a student learns and makes sense of occupational therapy. The setting emphasises 'doing' but this does not inevitably lead to understanding of the philosophical and theoretical bases or frame of reference that underpin practice. It is the joint responsibility of college and clinician to ensure that integration of knowledge, development of skills and growth of constructive attitudes to oc-

cupational therapy in psychiatry are taking place. Clinical practice offers a reality of involvement for the student that is both frightening and exciting. It has been stated that modelling is a useful teaching behaviour. Learners, however, rapidly sense a 'Do as I say and not as I do' approach. When such discrepancies occur, the supervisor's credibility suffers and the student's sense of professional identity is threatened.

The gap between the ideal situation that is often taught in colleges and the clinical reality can be illustrated by Case example 29.1. Treatment planning is a core skill of occupational therapy, however, much confusion may occur in the student's mind over where and when this takes place.

A transfer of focus occurs for students in clinical

CASE EXAMPLE 29.1

Anna was a friendly and adaptable student who found the weekly timetable on an acute psychiatric admission ward both stimulating and well-balanced in that it catered for a variety of emotional, interpersonal and practical needs. However, at her midway report it was considered by her supervisor that Anna could not analyse or articulate individual treatment aims within the programme of group activities.

In discussion with the visiting college tutor, Anna explained that, despite her having an awareness of individual needs and aims, at no time had she witnessed other staff or her supervisor formally record or definitely state clear goals within the programme for each individual client, apart from changes in medication. It appeared to the visiting tutor that the specifics of planning and judgement were not clearly outlined either in the course of daily events or in supervisory teaching sessions. Hence, Anna was confused about the insistence by college on specific analysis and sound treatment planning when she considered that what was occurring in the unit was proving therapeutic and useful without it. In turn, the supervisor considered that individual treatment planning was carried out continually 'in her head' but that there was insufficient time to formally record it.

Consequently, the problem for Anna's learning was that she was being criticised for lacking a skill that everyone agreed in theory was important but that could not be observed in practice.

practice. In college they are the central focus, whilst in the clinical area there is a shared focus of attention between patient care, management and countless other duties. This necessary juggling of priorities often causes anxiety and a feeling of dependency in the student, and creates a dilemma for the supervisor. The student may be concerned about not receiving sufficient attention, obtaining sparse feedback on performance and feeling that experiences are not tailored to her individual needs. The need for a mediator arises frequently, and this may be the head of department, the designated tutor or another college tutor who acts as an objective evaluator. This contact with college is vital and maintains the student's academic and personal link with the educational base. Visits from college staff usually occur following the midway report. This is also a time for reviewing the objectives and expectations of the placement.

COMMON PROBLEMS FOR OCCUPATIONAL THERAPY STUDENTS IN PSYCHIATRY

Working in the field of psychiatry is a daunting prospect to some, in that it demands a personal investment. Although this could be said of all areas in which occupational therapists are deployed, the therapeutic use of self is deemed to be an essential ingredient within psychiatry and the social sciences. Each area in psychiatry has inherent features that can complicate learning. These have to be allowed for in compiling objectives and in the assessment of performance.

Problems that may arise for the student include personal problems, professional role confusion and lack of clinical skills.

PERSONAL PROBLEMS

Overidentification

An anxious student may strongly identify with the supervisor in the hope that, by adopting the same style, she may achieve the same success. The danger of this behaviour is that individuality is lost and a personal style is not developed. Unconsciously or not, such imitation may be fostered by the supervisor and a frequently heard comment from students is that 'she only wants me to be like her.' Learners have to maintain their integrity and learn, with support, to value their own judgement.

Overidentification with clients can occur in practically every area, for example, with problems such as eating disorders, depression, anxiety and interpersonal difficulties. This shows in many ways, such as intense sympathy with the client, a desire to solve problems personally, wanting to become a valued and sought after carer, staying late at work or intervening passionately on the client's behalf. These may all be indicators that objectivity is being affected by personal needs. This is not to be confused with commitment, enthusiasm and individual styles of caring; the danger signals are shown when the student gives an excessive amount of time to one client for a variety of personal reasons. This needs discussion, either with a personal tutor, supervisor or some other objective person.

Sharf and Levinson (1964) outline the quest for omnipotence in professional training; occupational therapists, like other health professionals, may have flights of therapeutic zeal that meet our own needs rather than those of the people referred to our care.

High levels of anxiety

Occupational therapy is a service profession dependent upon doing and acquisition of skill but this may be rendered impossible by anxiety. Fear has a paralysing effect and can inhibit learning (Anderson and Graham 1980). Within occupational therapy in psychiatry, certain areas of performance are most likely to create anxiety, such as verbal reporting, leading groups or any situation where the student is heard by other health professionals. A progressive desensitisation has to occur by rehearsing the event and building upon small gains.

Certain client conditions, such as behavioural disturbance and aggressive behaviour, require special training procedures and considerable support from more experienced staff.

Feelings of therapeutic frustration

These may occur with those clients who appear to change very little during the allotted weeks of clinical practice. Such frustration is not, however, restricted to long-term or elderly clients but can also be experienced with the 'revolving door' syndrome of rapid discharge and equally rapid readmission. Students may encounter, for the first time, the impotence of clinical management with certain conditions and, in a pharmacologically dominated ward culture, may enquire 'Why occupational therapy?'. Problem solving, developing adaptive behaviour and change are events that the student may see only a tiny part of. The supervisor has the task of setting perspective to allow the student an understanding of the present situation and the sequence of events preceding it.

The effect on morale of seeing little result for therapeutic endeavours can eventually cause the student to attend only to the basic needs of clients and withdraw into administrative routines. Pitt (1984) describes three attitudes to the elderly that indicate frustration and ageist prejudice. These are defeatism, dominance and insularity. Elsewhere in psychiatry, similar protective devices against stress and a feeling a powerlessness are present and may be sensed by students.

Frustration may also be felt by students who feel they cannot emulate or match the skill of the staff. They feel therapeutically naive and are afraid of doing or saying the wrong thing. This fear may assume such proportion that it inhibits word and action and ultimately fuels feelings of failure.

Personal difficulties

Throughout the period of clinical placement, the supervisor needs to be sensitive to the emotional experience of the student. The first of ten elements of personal and professional growth listed by Fidler (1964) is change in self-concept and personal identity. Integrating criticism is hard for everyone and frequently dents self-esteem, therefore suggestions, comments and criticisms need to be made constructively and paced according to readiness for acceptance.

Working in someone's shadow is another feature of the clinical learning relationship that may cause either real or imagined problems.

PROBLEMS WITH PROFESSIONAL ROLE

Professional identity

The professional identity of the occupational therapy student is formed chiefly through identification with her supervisor. When the occupational therapist is seen to be integrated, at ease and accepted within the multidisciplinary team the student gains confidence in her professional role. Role blurring, which occurs in some treatment settings, can evoke insecurity unless the supervisor demonstrates that she is not worried by it.

The student's emerging professional self-image can also be buffeted by lack of appropriate referrals, by uncertainty about role or by other professionals using techniques previously considered to be the monopoly of the occupational therapist. One of two possible negative stances may be taken when this occurs:

- professional defensiveness, expressed as 'no-one understands occupational therapy'
- motivation to be accepted at all costs leading to denial of unique professional contribution and identity, for example, trying to become a behaviour therapist or group therapist.

Students need encouragement to drop their professional defensiveness and learn from other professionals. In order to help them do this, the clinical supervisor has to be prepared to acknowledge the potential difficulties of role blurring, provide learning situations that study collaborative working with other disciplines, and show the student how she can contribute professional expertise.

Team relationships

Occupational therapists frequently describe their role as 'integral' to the multidisciplinary team. Students are confused by this assertion if they do not observe the occupational therapist to be such an important member of the team. Frequently,

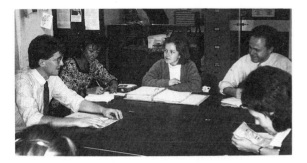

Fig. 29.2 A student taking part in a team conference.

they are caught between what the supervisor wishes would take place and the actual reality.

A treatment team must be viewed as any other group that requires time to work through certain developmental stages (Tuckman 1965). It is unrealistic to expect a student on placement for a month to take an active part in the team unless the climate and ethos of the unit is to welcome and use newcomers' impressions (Fig. 29.2).

Common difficulties for students include:

- unrealistically high expectations of the cohesiveness and effectiveness of the team; the student hopes for an ideal harmonious entity that values opinions from all sources
- disappointment when time in team meetings is taken up with discussion of pharmacological management, with less attention paid to social and interpersonal issues
- professional boundary problems and uncertainty about whether they can contribute to the assessment of clients in areas traditionally outwith the occupational therapist's role.

The supervisor needs to impart the attitudes and values of an integrative approach. Philosophies of teamwork are best taught within clinical education where the constraints can be witnessed alongside the strengths.

Coping with an eclectic approach in psychiatry

Appreciating an eclectic approach should not represent a major conceptual shift for occupational therapy students. The profession traditionally encompasses flexibility of thought, application and process, which are inherent qualities of eclectism. In patient admission wards increasingly demonstrate that a variety of approaches and treatment techniques can be used to meet client needs. Selection of the method of treatment that offers the greatest promise for alleviating problems and symptoms as quickly as possible is the core skill of an eclectic approach.

Problems exist, however, in learning how to choose from many possibilities, without becoming bewildered, in the very short time span of a clinical placement. Students will have learned the major models of treatment and can usually identify corresponding techniques. However, personal ideological preferences may exist to favour the psychodynamic, behavioural or humanistic model. The supervisor's task is to increase therapeutic and conceptual flexibility.

Active supervision is needed to help the student cope with the experience. This can include suggesting reading assignments, allowing ample discussion time for reflection and setting specific learning objectives.

PROBLEMS WITH SKILLS
Limited interpersonal skills

There will be students who, by personality and preference, are more suited to working with tools, machines or superficial interpersonal relationships than in the more intensive field of psychiatry. Psychiatry demands a measure of interpersonal skill, and the use of self is often thought of as the primary therapeutic factor. Certainly, it is necessary for any therapist to engage the motivation and participation of the client and this is partly engineered through the therapist–client relationship.

Within the study of occupational therapy, time is spent in the curriculum on social skills, interactional skills or interpersonal skills training. Despite this training, the reality of the event in clinical practice is often far removed from the role play in the classroom. Clinical practice provides opportunities for direct observation, practice of and feedback on a variety of interpersonal skills.

Objectives can be graded to allow progression from one-to-one encounters to small groups and ultimately to large groups. In this way, the student is able to develop increased self-awareness and security in interpersonal skills.

Interactional skills can be subdivided into listening skills, interviewing skills, counselling and group leadership skills. Students may be competent in one area but not in another. For example, they may demonstrate competent listening skills but lack group skills.

It would be a mistake to equate interpersonal effectiveness only with a vivacious outgoing personality. The steady reflective style of the gentler personality can be equally successful.

Problems in group situations

As Priestly and McQuire (1983) state, it is not unusual for experienced professionals to disclaim any interest in working with groups. Groups may be experienced as frightening, unpredictable and possibly damaging, therefore the newcomer understandably wishes to remain an onlooker.

In order to make the group experience less overwhelming, the model of treatment or approach must be first identified: is it geared to uncovering unconscious material, to supporting the client through a crisis or to self-help? The occupational therapy student faces a confusing array of approaches, techniques and milieus and the confidence to contribute can only follow identification of culture and observation of process.

Modelling plays an important part in learning how to work in groups, with cues taken from more experienced staff on what to say, how to phrase it and when to interject. Instruction, practice and feedback can be given on preparing for a group, introducing a session, facilitating interaction and ending a session. Difficulties arising with any one of these skills do not automatically imply that the student is unable to work in groups.

Confidence grows with success, allowing the student to attempt more complex interactions. Supervisors must hold a realistic view of what skill can be acquired in a short time and be accurate in diagnosis of areas of weakness, otherwise group work and a large section of psychiatry is 'written off' as not being within the individual's capabilities.

STUDENT COUNSELLING IN THE CLINICAL SETTING

Sometimes a problem may arise that requires particular assistance from either college staff or clinical staff. Such problems may include:

- difficulties with integration of criticism
- student–supervisor communication conflict
- finding it hard to bear the intense emotion of some psychiatric disorders
- feeling overwhelmed by role blurring, failure to grasp the rationale of occupational therapy in psychiatry or anxiety engendered when people appear not to improve
- lack of interpersonal skill highlighted by the length of 'settling-in time', inter-staff difficulties or poor group skills
- fear of failure, leading to compliancy and superficial understanding.

Counselling in the clinical practice arena is chiefly concerned with listening, exploring possibilities and mutually setting goals. Two types of counselling may be used with students on placement.

1. academic counselling, concerning problems with meaning and transfer of knowledge or difficulties in achieving clinical competency
2. personal counselling, concerning relationships or personal conflicts.

These are interlinked and combine to affect development.

Time puts a boundary on the amount of counselling possible, therefore it is always wise to involve the student's personal tutor and it is usually more useful if the student can take this initiative herself. Difficulties experienced in one placement may affect performance in the next, so it is imperative to maintain a consistent support system. The ultimate aim of all counselling is to enable the person to generate solutions for herself.

STUDENT DEVELOPMENT

One of the main goals of clinical education is to foster a deductive problem-solving approach. This requires the supervisor to have sound knowledge and to use an approach that integrates personal experience, relationships and meaning (Brown 1983). The following are some of the factors that can contribute to student development within clinical studies.

ESTABLISHING A LEARNING CLIMATE

Setting a learning climate is a feature of the work of Knowles (1972), who covered both the physical and psychological climate of the environment. The antennae of students are alert from the first few moments in a placement to the expectations, ethos and affective nature of the place. During the orientation period, familiarisation with people, places and timetables is taking place on one level while attitudes towards learning are more subtly communicated on another.

If the student perceives that active learning is the norm in a placement she will be influenced by it. This includes:

- the provision of books, journals and learning aids
- access to library facilities
- freedom of access to a variety of resource material, such as tape slides, directed reading material, learning packages, photographs and learning cassettes.

These provisions encourage experimentation and offer opportunities for students to find the alternative most applicable to individual learning styles or study habits. Numerous audio-visual aids which enrich learning are commercially available and can be used in tutorials, seminars and lectures. A balanced tutorial system including interdisciplinary teaching is most effective.

Fostering attitudes of enquiry

Encouraging a desire to learn in the student is the joint remit of clinical and academic staff. If a curriculum encourages intellectual curiosity, the student can rehearse presenting sound arguments. This ability to argue a theoretical point precedes problem solving with 'real' problems and gives confidence to apply theoretical knowledge. The teaching behaviour of the supervisor can keep alive a wish to investigate. Irby (1978) describes five positive aspects of the clinical teacher that foster the growth of the learner.

1. being accessible
2. observing, giving feedback on and evaluating student performance
3. guiding students, providing practice opportunities and developing skill in problem solving
4. giving case-specific comments
5. offering professional support and encouragement.

Value of peer group support

Whenever a number of students are on placement simultaneously a healthy cross-fertilisation of ideas can occur. Small group teaching, as described by Walton (1973), can be useful, particularly in understanding the feelings of students working in psychiatry. Tutorials are the most likely places for students to meet, identify and discuss issues common to the practice of occupational therapy. A number of teaching methods can be used on these occasions, including brainstorming sessions, buzz groups, workshops, seminars and case presentations.

Multidisciplinary learning

Occupational therapy in psychiatry cannot exist in isolation but requires collaborative input from other disciplines. Such interaction gives the student opportunities to learn sensitivity to the roles of others. This educational function of the multidisciplinary team is well recognised within the health service. Boufford (1978) believes that any health education must prepare the student to:

- be aware of the resources that other health professionals can provide for a client

● coordinate their care of the client with that of other involved professionals.

He suggests that the basic goals of the team are clear communication, goal setting, role negotiation and decision making. Defensiveness about professional boundaries can be lessened if education about the team is included in clinical studies.

PLANNING

Prior to the student's arrival, preliminary planning is essential to develop objectives, organise clinical experience and select teaching methods applicable to the student's stage of learning so that existing knowledge can be integrated with the new clinical experience.

Ambiguity is reduced by clear expectations, however, such expectations should be subject to a dialogue between student and supervisor and modified in areas where the student feels able to initiate personal objectives.

Objectives

The use of objectives is grounded in the assumption that the purpose of education is to help people change (Rowntree 1977). Objectives are statements of intent that can be an important teaching strategy and provide the main criteria for final assessment. They reflect the culture and constructs of each area. Yager (1982) considers that providing a student with a clearly defined list of goals and objectives may be the 'most important thing that can be done'.

A hierarchy of expectation is employed, increasing involvement and client contact as the placement progresses. (See Fig. 29.3 for sample objectives from the first clinical experience in a three-year BSc course.)

In psychiatry, a flexible attitude is required by each profession in order to be a part of the eclectic approach. The task of the supervisor is to assist assimilation of new information and to help integrate this without the student losing her sense of professional identity. We all vary in our method and depth of learning and it is necessary for teaching strategies to vary to accommodate each individual.

FEEDBACK

This is the means by which behaviour can be changed and skill increased. It is an active process akin to that described by Rogers (1986) as part of a mentor role. The nurturing process includes coaching, modelling, information giving and sharing clinical experience. Lack of feedback results in the student experiencing uncertainty, anxiety, lack of motivation and hostility. Barr (1980) postulates that inadequate feedback may be one of the reasons why students find clinical work stressful. Keuthe (1968) indicates that lack of feedback can be interpreted as a form of punishment. Most supervisors would agree in principle that continuous feedback should occur, thus enabling the learner to gain confidence and security.

For change to occur in knowledge, skills and attitude, feedback has to take place as soon after the event as possible. Also, feedback has to incorporate aspects of personal as well as professional change. Fidler (1964) states that the student must be helped to work towards an increased understanding of her own conscious and unconscious feelings and behaviour to provide assurance against their interference in the treatment process.

We all have our own information-processing systems, whereby we assimilate non-verbal cues and sift verbal communication before incorporating what is acceptable into our own frame of reference. The quality of communication and the student's interpretation of the feedback determine its effectiveness. Effective feedback requires effective listening before effective communication is possible! Non-specific comments about performance are as unhelpful as no feedback. Learners need coaching, acknowledgement of their strengths and remedies to overcome learning blocks. Judicious pacing is required to maintain readiness for accepting comments on personal development or skill; the individual's threshold for accepting praise and criticism needs to be shrewdly gauged. It is a complex task for the supervisor to match the amount of feedback she gives with the threshold of acceptance in the learner. Pacing is the greatest skill in feedback, ensuring that the wish to try again is continually encouraged.

However, it must be acknowledged that both parties have needs within this relationship.

Clinical practice no.1

Four weeks in duration

Placement: PSYCHOGERIATRIC DAY HOSPITAL

Description:

A busy hospital with up to 50 clients per day. The week is subdivided between 3 days for organically impaired elderly and 2 days for functional illnesses of the elderly. The multi-disciplinary approach to client care is well established, however, most of the staff with whom the student will be involved are helpers and nursing staff. A detailed weekly programme is run with individual treatment plans formulated after assessment. After 4 weeks the student should be able to give an informed account of:

- the size and complexity of the psychiatry of old age
- the contribution of day care
- the need for relatives' support
- the need for a multidisciplinary approach
- the specific contribution of occupational therapy

Week 1

At the end of the first week the student will have:

- identified staff members who liaise with the supervisor
- observed the daily organisational procedures of the hospital
- identified the main functional problems of those clients who attend on Monday, Wednesday and Friday
- approached and initiated conversation with a minimum of three clients who attend on Tuesday and Thursday
- attended and stated the purpose, in a written account, of the various review meetings held during the week
- discussed first impressions of the role of the therapist, functional difficulties of the elderly and day hospital organisation with the supervisor during the weekly feedback session
- revised notes on handling and interactional skills

Week 2

At the end of the second week the student will have:

- identified all staff members who are part of the multi-disciplinary team in the day hospital
- assisted the supervisor to plan an R.O. session, a baking session and a sensory stimulation group
- identified the main functional problems of those clients who attend on Tuesday and Thursday
- introduced self in a group session and encouraged and assisted one client within a session on Monday, Wednesday and Friday
- revised aspects of communication and written 200 words on constraints on communication with elderly confused clients

- reported informally to the supervisor the results of a dialogue between self and two clients, one male and one female, who attend on Tuesday and Thursday
- selected two clients, one with organic impairment and one with functional impairment, for the worksheet exercise
- taught one client one part of a procedure in the kitchen group or in an R.O. session
- recorded the organisation and preparation of one particular treatment session

Week 3

At the end of the third week the student will have:

- identified and listed the responsibilities of helpers in the hospital
- identified and recorded the role-specific skills of nursing staff in the hospital
- introduced the first two items in an R.O. session for clients moderately impaired by dementia
- analysed the therapeutic potential of one activity used with clients who have Alzheimer's disease and discussed this in the morning preparation session
- assisted in the pottery session and reported significant features to the supervisor
- reported verbally at the end-of-the-day review meeting on two clients' behaviour
- recorded the main interactional difficulties of confused elderly people
- identified what cognitive skills are assessed in occupational therapy and collected appropriate forms
- discussed with the supervisor, in a review session, support for relatives, demographic studies and a multidisciplinary approach to the problems of the elderly
- set one additional personal objective for the final week

Week 4

By the end of the final week the student will have:

- selected one article on the elderly from the file, read it and summarised it for the seminar
- prepared, organised, gathered clients for and conducted one R.O. session. Also run one communication session and one domestic session with supervision
- accompanied the therapist on one home visit and drafted an account of this visit, taking account of social and environmental factors
- taken part in planning one part of the reminiscence group and listed the therapeutic implications of this technique

Fig. 29.3 Sample objectives.

CASE EXAMPLE 29.2

Mary, a student on placement in an acute admission ward for 8 weeks in the final year of the traditional diploma course, was found at the midway assessment to have the following difficulties:

- inability to apply theoretical knowledge in the clinical setting
- difficulty in evaluating treatment sessions
- problems formulating written assessments.

Links clearly existed between the three problem areas. Strengths included sound interpersonal relationships with both clients and staff, clear verbal skill and sound management of self and resources.

Analysis of the difficulties with theory showed that the main problem was in relating what was happening clinically to the academic work that had been done some nine months earlier.

Action involved the student and supervisor selecting appropriate theoretical areas for review, including:

- the eclectic approach to treatment: an appropriate reading list and articles were offered
- work in activity groups: new objectives were set to offer practice in analysis, reporting and understanding the efficacy of group sessions
- psychotic illness was the main diagnostic group in the ward, therefore revision of associated functional difficulties was undertaken.

Specific analysis of the problems with evaluation showed that Mary could describe what happened in a group but not draw conclusions. Examples of group evaluations were given to Mary, showing conclusions drawn from the interaction, performance and non-verbal behaviour of the participants.

To aid written work, process recording of a selected group was suggested and carried out by both supervisor and Mary. The comparison highlighted areas that Mary could verbalise but not record. A guide was offered on how to structure reports and practice opportunities were increased.

CASE EXAMPLE 29.3

Alice was on a first-year 4-week observation block in a psychiatric day hospital. The main aim of this block was to gather information about the role of the occupational therapist.

Alice was overwhelmed by the new experience, the number of clients, the range of new procedures, the timetable and the attempt to retain information about the numerous community facilities involved.

Following discussion of objectives after the first week of orientation, it was decided that a range of learning aids could be used in Alice's own study time. Several packages of information on day care were given to Alice to work on at her own speed. These included:

- a series of overhead transparencies with information on the history, range and main advantages of day hospital facilities
- folder with details of community resources, self-help groups and advice centres. This was followed by a visit to the voluntary exchange centre to seek specific information on the possibility of clients becoming involved in voluntary work.

These were simple self-instruction aids that gave direction and reduced anxiety by providing a focus for study.

The student needs:

- coaching on a regular basis
- regular and planned supervision sessions
- scope to express individuality and not be compared with other students
- opportunities to practise clinical skills
- clarification of the purpose of clinical education.

The supervisor needs:

- feedback on teaching style

- frank evaluation of the placement by the student
- scope to apply individual style and not be compared with other supervisors
- confidence to relinquish authority and allow the student to develop skills
- continued opportunities to develop clinical teaching strategies, for example, regular short courses or other forms of study.

Case examples 29.2 and 29.3 are not intended as guides to follow in similar situations but rather as possibilities that were found to be useful in these particular instances. Analysis of the problem is often easier than finding solutions. It is necessary to identify accurately the learning block before offering further learning opportunities. Case example 29.2 looks at methods of tackling specific problems.

It can be difficult for the clinical supervisor to adapt to students at different levels or from different training schools. Careful examination of personal assumptions about what the student should be capable of at different stages is necessary. Case example 29.3 looks at gearing learning to the student's level.

ASSESSING CLINICAL COMPETENCE

THE PURPOSE OF ASSESSMENT

Every educational process requires assessment: the profession must be satisfied that competency is assured, the supervisor must discover whether objectives have been met and the student needs feedback on performance. Clinical education combines ongoing assessment designed for the benefit of the learner with regular formal grading designed to measure competence. Specific criteria for performance may be identified in the form of learning objectives.

Assessment should multidirectional (Pendergast 1971) and produce information that will benefit all involved. Although mutual assessment occurs naturally in any interchange, formal assessment is frequently a one-way event. This is regrettable in clinical education, which relies heavily upon continuous feedback and a learning alliance being maintained between supervisor and student. Assessment is a part of learning that is more usefully seen as a process than as an act of judgement.

ASSESSMENT STRATEGIES
Assessment formats

Clinical report forms cover the essential elements

of competency and provide a permanent record of performance. Most forms include a section for students to evaluate the learning experience, which provides a more complete account of the placement. The most useful feedback tool is the final appraisal section, which should humanise and individualise the report (Rowntree 1977).

Although there are many ways to design a clinical assessment form, some common features exist. The form will usually be subdivided into salient professional characteristics, for example:

- professional development
- interpersonal relationships
- communication
- assessment
- practice of occupational therapy
- treatment planning
- organisation and management.

Each of those sections will be further analysed for core skills and aptitudes that the student should attain a different stages of the course. Additionally, a method of differentiation may be required to indicate to the student the extent of success or failure. Some forms employ a clear visual aid such as a cross plotted on an X–Y axis (Fig. 29.4) whereas others note only pass or fail. Most clinicians would agree that the most vital formative assessment procedure occurs in the section where the clinician writes comments in support of the assessment decision.

It is important to ensure that the nature of the assessment form reflects the desired personal and professional changes throughout the period of education. Figures 29.5 to 29.7 show the progression required in the knowledge, skills and attitudes concerning the practice of occupational therapy from Year 1 to Year 3 of a BSc degree course in occupational therapy.

Finally, in any process of assessment the opportunity must be offered to the student to reflect upon the clinical experience and suggest to the clinician what the most and the least helpful aspects of the placement were. Again the design of such a form will vary according to the stage the student is at but it usually contains the following headings:

- level of supervision

X	CREDIT	PASS	FAIL	Y
Makes use of opportunities for learning	– – – – –	– ✕ – – – – – – – – – – –	– – – – –	Shows little motivation to learn
COMMENTS				

Fig. 29.4 An X-Y axis of professional development.

X	CREDIT	PASS	FAIL	Y
Shows understanding of the role of the occupational therapist				Unable to recognise the role of the occupational therapist
Can identify therapeutic potential in activities				Lacks the ability to perceive therapeutic potential in activities
Can handle clients safely				Is potentially hazardous in handling clients
Reacts calmly in difficult situations				Unable to cope with difficult situations
Teaches in a clear and logical manner				Teaching is disorganised and difficult to follow
COMMENTS				

Fig. 29.5 The practice of occupational therapy: aspects assessed in clinical placements 1 and 2.

- quality of feedback on performance
- special features of the placement
- assessment procedures
- links between college and academic work
- any recommendations or changes.

The report form is given to clinicians with an accompanying guide for completion. Each clinical supervisor is reminded of the main emphasis of the college work immediately preceding the placement and the aims of the assessment.

Student–supervisor evaluation

A report form that judges the performance of the student without an accompanying report from the consumer is incomplete. Irby (1978) includes a self-assessment form for teachers to gauge their own effectiveness. However, an honest exchange of views between teacher and student is the most potent way of giving feedback to the supervisor. Although it can be difficult for the student to write a report on her placement, such a report gives practice in realistic reporting.

It can be just as painful for supervisors to accept that they may be seen as authoritarian and difficult as it is for the student to accept negative appraisals. A period of clinical practice is just that for all concerned. We are all learning, practising and changing in this context.

X	CREDIT	PASS	FAIL	Y
Shows understanding of the role of occupational therapy with a variety of conditions				Unable to recognise the role of occupational therapy with a variety of conditions
Can apply theoretical knowledge to practice				Unable to apply theoretical knowledge to practice
Can identify therapeutic potential in activities				Lacks the ability to perceive therapeutic potential in activities
Can identify therapeutic potential of rehabilitation equipment				Unable to identify therapeutic potential of rehabilitation equipment
Actively participates in the selection and implementation of treatment programmes				Does not participate actively in selection and implementation of treatment programmes
Shows understanding of factors influencing treatment				Lacks awareness of factors influencing treatment
Teaches in a clear, concise and logical manner				Teaching is disorganised and difficult to follow
Can handle clients safely				Is potentially hazardous in handling clients
Reacts calmly in difficult situations				Unable to cope in difficult situations
COMMENTS				

Fig. 29.6 The practice of occupational therapy: aspects assessed in clinical placements 3 and 4.

Review of the learning experience

At the end of a placement it is wise for the supervisor and student to review the experience together. This has many advantages, including:

- giving the student time to wind down and put the experience into perspective
- highlighting areas of the placement that require rethinking by the supervisor
- offering the supervisor feedback on the learning environment and whether it is conducive to growth.

The review is a reflective process that can be conducted by questionnaire, interview or group activity. One method is to brainstorm, writing words, comments and thoughts about the placement on a blackboard until the surface is covered. Following this, the words are ranked into potentially positive or potentially negative phenomena. This offers a profile of the placement as seen through the eyes of each group. Over a year this can show if the students have been overloaded, if they are happy with the facilities, if more help is needed to make sense of theory and a host of other important information.

SUMMARY

This chapter has sought to highlight the specific characteristics of teaching in the clinical setting. It particularly stresses:

- the importance of the supervisor–student relationship and the need to achieve a constructive working alliance

X	CREDIT	PASS	FAIL	Y
Plans and implements treatment programmes to meet stated aims				Unable to plan and implement treatment programmes to meet stated aims
Realistically evaluates treatment procedures				Unable to evaluate treatment procedures
Modifies treatment in response to evaluation results				Unable to adapt treatment in response to evaluation results
Handles clients safely				Potentially hazardous in handling clients
Teaches clearly and effectively				Teaching is disorganised and difficult to follow
Reacts calmly in difficult situations				Unable to cope in difficult situations
Involves other agencies/professionals as appropriate				Does not involve other agencies/professionals
COMMENTS				

Fig. 29.7 The practice of occupational therapy: aspects assessed in clinical placements 5 and 6.

- the variety of supervision styles that a student may experience
- common difficulties encountered by students whilst on psychiatric placements
- ways in which a learning climate can be encouraged that allows all concerned to grow and develop skills.

The need for a better understanding of clinical education is recognised by all health professionals. This is especially so in occupational therapy when over 1000 hours is devoted to such studies. The following list suggests areas for further research:

- validity studies of existing clinical assessment procedures
- evaluation of the process of acquiring clinical competence
- application of recent research on students' learning styles in the clinical setting and investigation of the implications for clinical education
- design and trial of a system of continuing education for clinical supervisors.

REFERENCES

Anderson J, Graham A 1980 A problem in medical education: is there an information overload? Medical Education 14

Barr E M 1980 The relationship between student and clinical supervisor. British Journal of Occupational Therapy 43(10)

Booy M J, Lawson A 1986 Bridging the gap in clinical supervision. British Journal of Occupational Therapy 49(12)

Boufford J I 1978 In: Ford C W Clinical education for the allied health professionals. Mosby, St Louis

Brown G 1983 Studies of student learning: implications for medical teaching. Medical Teacher 5(2)

Bryne P S, Long B E L 1973 Learning to care. Churchill Livingstone, Edinburgh

Cracknell E 1977 Another view of students in the department. British Journal of Occupational Therapy 40(5)

Ekstein R E, Wallerstein R S 1972 The teaching and

learning of psychotherapy. International Universities Press, New York

Entwistle N 1983 Styles of learning and teaching. Wiley, London

Fidler G S 1964 A guide to planning and measuring growth and experiences in the clinical affiliation. American Journal of Occupational Therapy 23(6)

Ford C W 1978 Clinical education for the allied health professions. Mosby, St Louis

Gough H G 1957 Manual for the California psychological inventory. Consulting Psychologists' Press, California

Irby D M 1978 Clinical Faculty development. In: Ford C W Clinical education for the allied health professions. Mosby, St Louis

Kelman H C 1963 The role of the group in the induction of therapeutic change. International Journal of Group Psychotherapy 13(4)

Keuthe J L 1968 The teaching-learning process. Scott Foreman, Illinois

Knowles M S 1972 Innovations in teaching styles and approaches based upon adult learning. Education for Social Work (Spring)

Leonardelli C A, Gratz R R 1986 The relationship of purpose, objectives and teaching models. American Journal of Occupational Therapy 40(2)

Molteno E B F 1945 Beyond choices, chance or fate. Goodwood Press, South Africa

Pendergast N (ed) 1971 Principles of clinical education. Department of Medical Communications Health Sciences Center, Temple University, Pennsylvania

Pitt J 1984 Psychogeriatrics. Churchill Livingstone, Edinburgh

Priestley P, McQuire J 1983 Learning to help. Tavistock, London

Rogers J C 1986 Mentoring for career achievement and advancement. American Journal of Occupational Therapy 40(2)

Rowntree D 1977 Assessing students: how shall we know them? Harper & Row, London

Sharf M R, Levinson D J 1964 The quest for omnipotence in professional training. Psychiatry 27

Tuckman B W 1965 Developmental sequence in small groups. Psychological Bulletin 63

Willis M 1977 Aspects of management. British Journal of Occupational Therapy 40(11)

Walton H 1973 Small group methods in medical teaching. Medical education Book 1. Association for the Study of Medical Education, Dundee

Yager J 1982 Teaching psychiatry and behavioural science. Grune & Stratton. New York

30

Research

Averil Stewart

INTRODUCTION

This chapter aims to dispel some of the mystique surrounding the word 'research' by looking at what it is and why it is important to occupational therapy. It acknowledges the practical evaluative nature of most clinicians' work but aims to encourage research as being one of the primary means of documenting efficiency and effectiveness, and of validating techniques.

For the reader who is inexperienced in research, there is an introduction to different research methods, with examples of their application to occupational therapy and particular reference to psychiatric practice. Examples of the ethnographic method, survey and experimental methods are drawn from recent literature.

For the would-be researcher there is a section giving guidelines for the planning and implementation of research, with a very brief introduction to statistics. The references and bibliography are extensive in order to give the more serious-minded reader further opportunity to expand her knowledge and understanding.

In addition the importance of research for the development of the profession is discussed.

WHAT IS RESEARCH?

For many there is a certain perplexity surrounding the word 'research', stemming from uncertainty and ignorance, and yet this is something that every thinking practical person is doing as he goes about his daily tasks. In its simplest form it is the process of working out or explaining cause and effect or of showing the relationship between different factors. For example, it might be that, in seeking an explanation as to why a client has not arrived for an outpatient appointment, questions are raised in one's mind. Is this absence due to illness, to the breakdown of the ambulance or of communication, or has he had enough and decided to stay at home? For each of these questions possible answers might be surmised but would, in turn, need to be verified. If absences are frequent, do they reflect problems for the client, in the system or with therapy, and what action needs to be taken?

In another situation it might be that the therapist is planning a programme of activities for a group of clients. On the basis of previous experience she is able to predict with a degree of certainty which activities will be most effective, but can this conviction be elaborated and justified on the basis of concrete evidence of associations between the many variables? In some ways, a researcher is not unlike a detective seeking clues, asking questions and following up hunches in order to produce new information and possible explanations.

Such examples are simplistic and characterise intuitive behaviour but as the profession develops so there is pressure on individuals to quantify and to qualify what it is they do; to explain relationships between variables such as treatment and its effects, and to predict outcomes. Research may therefore be related to specific actions in order to understand them better or it may be to test out the theoretical framework or to provide evidence that will direct policies for the future.

DEFINITIONS

The Concise Oxford Dictionary defines research as 'a search or enquiry after; course of critical evaluation and endeavour to discover new facts by scientific study'. In the natural sciences, scientific method can be pursued more rigorously than in the social sciences. There can be greater precision

and experimental manipulation of the variables but people cannot be controlled so easily.

Scientific method in its purest sense is something that should be repeatable so that other researchers, undertaking similar observations of the same subject, under the same conditions, would get the same result. The personal opinions of an expert, no matter how much his professionalism may be respected, are not in themselves scientifically sound. Opinions need to be backed up by evidence, by data and by explanation. Relationships have been shown between stress and psychopathology (Lowe 1969). These relationships can be explained by a 'covering law', such as 'as stress factors increase so does the individual become more prone to psychopathology'; but such a law lacks the precision of those in the natural sciences, for example, Boyle's Law in physics. When dealing with people a multiplicity of factors may influence who does, or who does not, produce certain behaviours as a result of increasing stress. Laws in the physical sciences are precise statements or predictions of cause and effect but people do not respond like inanimate objects and therefore such a term is inappropriate. Regardless of laws of justice, of customary rules and social norms, much of human behaviour is prompted by a variety of motives.

Research in the field of occupational therapy must be directed towards assessing and evaluating all aspects of treatment in order that knowledge and understanding may be furthered. Therefore the client, the therapist's role, the nature of occupation, the environment and the theoretical basis for treatment from which the whole process stems are all issues for investigation.

Lest readers are inhibited from contemplating researching into something they wonder about, on the grounds that this is something for academics in ivory towers quite apart from the real world, this chapter aims to dispel some of those beliefs and to encourage therapists to embark on research of their own.

RESEARCH-MINDEDNESS

A questioning attitude should be a way of life for the problem-solving and imaginative therapist. If this is so then research need not be something that is superimposed but, by its very nature, is already part of the ethos of practice. Every record, routine statistic has the potential for contributing towards descriptive explanatory study. Of course, these data have their limitations. Collecting on its own, without reasons for so doing, without analysis and interpretation, is meaningless. However, it is often from cursory analysis of accumulated records that the gem of an idea worth following up emerges. Log and source books from student days, observational studies, first impressions, diaries and case studies can capture thoughts and ideas that on their own, or unrecorded, might have been lost but, once noted, may lead to more systematic pursuit. Diaries or even jottings help to keep the mind open to different perceptions and to develop a reflectiveness that is a critical component in a qualitative observational study. Mills (1970) in his classic article 'On Intellectual Craftsmanship' says 'you must learn to use your life experience in your intellectual work: continually to examine and interpret it . . . set up a file . . . keep a journal . . . of professional experience and professional activities, studies under way and studies planned'. Thus, early jottings can be the start of something bigger and the very effort of recording them increases critical awareness as well as developing fluency of style. Perhaps one of the most inhibiting aspects when research is being contemplated is possibly a secret desire to find the answer to life in the full knowledge that, in reality, little of great significance will emerge. Nevertheless, efforts to push forward the frontiers of knowledge, if not in themselves entirely successful, will have given the researcher greater appreciation of the process and enhanced professional development.

As notes accumulate, so may they be sorted, filed or even rejected. Rearrangements can act as a trigger for the unexpected, producing new ideas and stirring the imagination. 'Imagination is often successfully invited by putting together hitherto isolated items, by finding new connections' (Mills 1959). Alternatively conversations with stimulating colleagues can promote the debate, clarify the mind, prompt the search for evidence and so strengthen one's case.

Often the search for that evidence means repetition, thoroughness, persistency, frustration and boredom. Anyone who has done an activity sampling analysis of a client's or staff member's behaviour by recording their actions under specific categories at defined intervals of time, thus amassing hundreds of observations, must know of the tedium from personal experience. Similarly, those who have carried out surveys, perhaps knocking on doors, or worked out computer programs to test for significance amongst variables, will know of the frustrations generated by uncooperative clients or the insensitivities of modern technology. But, after all, the discovery of radium was not just a stroke of luck but the result of years of dedicated work.

There is a continuum of research-mindedness from the questioning, evaluative behaviour of competent therapists to the systematic accumulation of data in a search for explanations, and to life-saving discoveries after years of application, as shown in Figure 30.1.

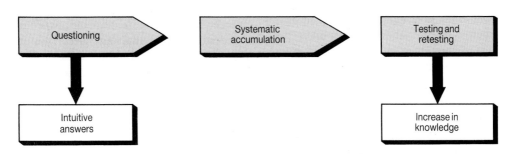

Fig. 30.1 The continuum of research-mindedness.

COMPLEXITIES AND LIMITATIONS

As one moves from the evaluative stance towards research methods, the complexities and limitations become apparent. Different methods produce different problems. For example, the correlations that might appear significant under experimental conditions may become distorted in the 'real' world.

Obtaining information

Whether there is only one observer or a number of different experimenters and interviewers, bias may creep in, threatening the validity of the study. Specially designed measuring tools, such as rating scales or questionnaires, may not meet operational definitions but instead be ambiguous and confusing. The simple questions, 'How would you rate your feelings today?' or 'When did you last cook a meal?' are open to a number of different interpretations. 'Today? Compared with when? Yesterday, or how I feel normally?' or 'Does a simple meal like beans on toast count, or do you mean a 'proper' three-course meal?' How many possible interpretations might there be to the question, 'When did you last go shopping?'

In interviews, open-ended questions such as 'How do you feel about . . . being in hospital?' give more scope for seeking out what is meant and clarifying ambiguities than is possible through more structured questions and rating scales in surveys. Thus the validity of unstructured interviews can be greater but such an interview is not so readily repeated by another interviewer and hence what is gained in understanding may be lost in replication and reliability.

In addition to the potential problems of measuring tools there is the variability in responses that different interviewees may give to the same interviewer, a response influenced by their perception of the characteristics of that person, such as age, warmth of personality or even social class. Labov (1969) found that black children in the United States were more at ease, and therefore gave more, when interviewed by casually dressed black experimenters who spoke the same dialect as the children. One might wonder to what extent professionalism could interfere in getting honest answers from clients.

Ethics

In dealing with people the question of ethics arises. The rights of the individual, privacy and confidentiality have to be respected. In addition, is it right to deceive subjects by, for example, giving them a placebo treatment? Is it justifiable to deprive some clients of treatment in order to have a control group? How far can subjects be exposed to detrimental conditions, such as sensory deprivation, or to simulated conditions that result in aggressive and uncharacteristic behaviour? (Milgram 1963, Zimbardo 1972). Much of the research in occupational therapy to date is of a descriptive nature and relatively free of ethical problems. Nevertheless, there is control through medical ethical committees thus ensuring, for example, that clients are not overexposed to surveys and interviewers and that the research proposal is of relevance. The frustrations and delays that are encountered in waiting for approval to begin cannot be overestimated (MacKintosh 1985).

Dealing with people

It is the 'people-aspect' of scientific methods in the social sciences that is probably the most problematic, yet without them there would be no research. People exhibit many variables, which can distort results. Variables include mood on a specific day; motivation and desire to cooperate, or not; previous experience, which may influence behaviour; personality, which may aim to please or to lie; age; comprehension; speech; prejudices and idiosyncrasies. Depending on the choice of research method, it is possible to control independent variables that may affect the outcome of the study but first they have to be identified in order that the research design may be valid.

WHY RESEARCH?

HISTORICAL DEVELOPMENTS

Occupational therapy as a profession is relatively young but with its origins rooted in history from before the days of Aesculapius (Macdonald 1970). Its development this century has been rapid, spurred on by the needs of victims of the Second World War. In 1987 over 9300 therapists were registered in the United Kingdom and, on the basis of earlier studies (Central Management Services 1980), approximately 35% were employed solely in the psychiatric field in the National Health Service. For many therapists their 'raison d'etre' is to treat clients, yet the changes in emphasis within the profession, from group work and the use of a wide range of therapeutic activities to activities of daily living and returning clients to the community, must raise many questions. Not least is, 'Could others have done this work just as, or even more, effectively?' and 'What would have been the consequences of not having done the work?' In these days of overlapping roles and increasing financial stringencies, there is an even greater need to monitor and evaluate existing services (Ellis 1981). Change comes about as knowledge expands and as new treatments affect outcomes. New treatments, such as depot drugs in the treatment of schizophrenia, influence policies thus redirecting staff from institutional care towards independent living in the community. Occupational therapists are inevitably part of the changing scene, sometimes being involved in a new initiative (Jeffrey 1985); sometimes being taken along on the wave of technological advances. The initiatives taken by the Department of Trade and Industry in installing microcomputers in 40 occupational therapy departments in 1983 and in setting up courses for therapists, thus alerting them to therapeutic potentials, is a case in point. It is not enough just to accept the inevitable changes which come with the introduction of new resources, however. The changes and their outcomes need to be studied systematically. As the profession develops there are increasing demands on practitioners to quantify and to evaluate the service.

The beliefs that are shared by the profession develop from tradition, prompted by events in history, influenced by contemporary values and nurtured jealously by its members. They can and should be challenged by these professionals, by colleagues and employers.

PHILOSOPHICAL ISSUES AND DILEMMAS

If a profession is to have greater autonomy and credibility it must monitor its practices and define the characteristics and functions that make it unique. Currently many models of practice are emanating from the United States (West 1959; King 1974; Mosey 1981; Kielhofner 1981). Emphasis on the concept of recovery of, and maintenance of, health through occupation is induced from observation and analysis of practice. Occupational therapists may believe that this model of 'health through occupation' is characteristic of the profession but it needs to be subjected to more detailed analysis and comparison with other professions. It could also be important to examine and analyse the concepts of work which are held by 'sick' people compared with those held by people who are healthy. The underlying beliefs of current theorists need to be tested in order that they can be falsified or proven, and so strengthened. Karl Popper (1957) says, 'tests should be attempts to weed out false theories—to find the weak points of a theory in order to reject it'. In addition he believes that research should not try to prove something for all time.

THE CYCLICAL NATURE OF RESEARCH

As indicated above, theories may be induced from professional practice. Observation of practice and intuitive explanations may lead to generalised statements and, thus, subsequent theories. Theories, in turn, can lead to establishing hypotheses and seeking ways of measuring factors to be observed. This probably seems more complicated than it really is; it is nothing more than a sequence of events making up a circle, as shown in Figure 30.2.

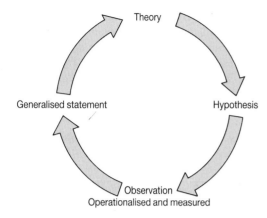

Fig. 30.2 The cyclical nature of research.

This simplified model shows how relationships stemming from observations might be explained on the one side, while established theories enable predictions to be made about behaviour on the other.

For example, reference was made earlier to a client failing to attend the department. Supposing absences were becoming increasingly frequent, it might be that, in this particular case, the therapist believed they could be explained on the basis of his having found the previous day's session very difficult and painful. If there was any relationship between these two variables then there are implications for the individual and for therapy. It would seem, therefore, that a systematic search for reasons for non-attendance would be highly desirable in order to refute the theory or, if there was any association thus leading to predictable negative behaviour, to examine policies and so determine action for the future.

Theories may be about attendance and participation or about more abstract concepts, often called constructs, such as 'personality', 'intelligence', 'obedience' and 'volition'. These constructs cannot be observed in themselves but they can be broken down into a number of components or factors deemed to make up that concept. Intelligence tests or personality inventories, for example, give observable measures or profiles that can then be systematically studied. This process of breaking down the construct into observable and measureable indicators is known as 'operationalisation'.

In Milgram's experiment (1963), designed to determine how far a subject would go in administering an electric shock to a 'victim' when so directed by an 'authority' figure, the construct of 'obedience to authority' was measured in terms of the voltage at which the subject desisted what seemed a bizarre and cruel activity. Thus, constructs in a theory once operationalised can produce data that can be used to demonstrate the correlation between two or more variables.

But how do we go about research in the first place? The following section will examine different methods.

METHODS OF RESEARCH

Different authors may categorise methods of research in different ways (COT 1985) but there are basically three different forms:

1. ethnographic or observational field studies
2. surveys
3. experiments.

The following brief descriptions and actual studies are intended to highlight differences and similarities between the different methods.

ETHNOGRAPHIC RESEARCH

In this style of research the investigator starts with an area of interest but without any clearly formulated questions or assumptions. Instead, it is his intention to find out through observation and/or participation in everyday events in the lives of the subjects what is important to them, how they see their world and what their values and beliefs are. Whether as participant or observer, or indeed in fulfilling a joint participant/observer's role, it is difficult in a complex society to study more than a relatively small number of people. Within the 'natural' setting the researcher will concentrate on the interactions between the participators, often examining covert behaviour and its meaning. Actors themselves may not be able to reflect on the full meaning of their actions for they are often inarticulate and the motives of much behaviour are subconscious. Thus the researcher infers meaning by understanding the context and the totality of the situation. Gradually, as questions and hypotheses are formulated, they are checked out and reformulated, leading to a theory on which future predictions can be made. Interviews in depth are one of the methods that may help confirm or reject impressions and interpretations.

Limitations

This method can lead to valid explanations and detailed understanding but it is most time consuming and laborious. Thousands of observations and quotations may be accumulated from transcripts and field notes written up after events. The categorisation of data can lead to different analyses and therefore emphasis. Another difficulty may stem from the role of the observer and whether he is there as a member of the group and accepted as such (Whyte 1955) or accepted as a researcher (Atkinson 1975). The 'secret' ethnographer has to be adept at adopting his membership role, ensuring that his cover is not blown, yet at the same time remembering and later recording details of interactions. Group rules have to be learnt and conformed with in order not to raise suspicion; dress, accent and inappropriate behaviour could all give the researcher away. An ethnographic study of drug addicts in society, for example, might involve 'going native'. However, it is doubtful that ethnographic studies that occupational therapists might undertake would have to go to such lengths.

Further problems with this form of research lie in the reliability of the observer's analysis. The question has to be asked: 'Would another researcher have selected out and recorded the same observations as being the most relevant?' The presence of a newcomer must have some effect on the interactions and the situation. 'To what extent would this be the same with another observer?' Thus, because of the danger of subjectivity, replication of this method is more difficult than with others. However, assessment of a particular

study's reliability and validity is usually made easier by the researcher giving an account of the methodology and detailed development of the process. In addition, triangulation, that is, comparing results from a variety of sources, helps to assure reliability. Triangulation also enables the typicality of the group under study to be assessed, thus allowing the findings to be generalised to other similar groups.

Advantages

Despite the disadvantages, this qualitative method has considerable relevance for occupational therapists in increasing their understanding of clients' or perhaps therapists' behaviour in different situations. While this method may lack the precision of research in the natural sciences it requires a certain artistry and intuitiveness in order to identify relevant material and make sensitive interpretations, as shown in Example 30.1, an ethnographic study of deinstitutionalised adults by Kielhofner (1981).

SURVEY METHOD

In contrast to the qualitative nature of ethnographic research, the survey method is more quantitative, produces 'harder' data and is more easily replicated. Questionnaires and structured interviews fit into this category.

This method requires a sample of people, randomly selected from the population being studied. Each person is given a set number of fixed questions under comparable conditions. This may take the form of a questionnaire or rating scale for self-completion, or for completion by a trained interviewer who should interact with the interviewee in a standard predetermined and consistent manner.

Limitations and advantages

Obviously a well-designed questionnaire can get a lot of information from a lot of people relatively cheaply and quickly but the structure of the questions is by no means easy, as was shown earlier in this chapter. If potential biases have been con-

EXAMPLE 30.1 FIELD STUDY OF
DEINSTITUTIONALISATION OF RETARDED
ADULTS (KIELHOFNER 1981)

Kielhofner and his fellow participant-observers
studied six residential settings and two activity
centres for retarded adults for periods of
between 10 and 35 months' duration. In the
early stages, residents were wary about giving
away information and inhibited in their behaviour
in the presence of the participant-observers.
However as the observers' presence became
accepted as part of the normal scene so did
residents' behaviour and conversation return to
their usual form and content.

Accounts of the methodology and quotations
reveal the richness of the qualitative approach.
The analysis brings to life some of the
theoretical constructs that influence behaviour
amongst owners and staff in these homes and
centres and helps the reader to understand and
predict some of the problems for mentally
handicapped adults trying to achieve

independence in the community. American
policies for deinstitutionalisation and their
implementation have resulted in owners and staff
being 'confronted with the monumental task of
social containment and control of human beings
who tend to demonstrate few of the culturally
valued characteristics.'

Owners therefore organise their businesses on
a profit-making basis in order to compensate for
doing the 'system's dirty work'. Residents were
therefore treated as commodities with caretakers
actively seeking to prevent training in areas that
would increase residents' independence or
disrupt daily routines. Understanding the
perspectives of the owners' of privately run
institutions alerts therapists to resistance to their
interventions.

This study demonstrates the obvious conflict
between economic realities and the process of
normalisation (Wolfensberger 1972). In addition
it provides a salutory warning for community
care in this country.

EXAMPLE 30.2 FIELD-OBSERVATION STUDY
OF THE ROLES OF OCCUPATIONAL
THERAPY STAFF (EDWARDS 1980).

This exploratory study of the roles of
occupational therapy staff sought information
about the profession for those planning
educational programmes for therapists.

During part of the field work Edwards
observed six therapists and three helpers on
alternate days over a period of 4 weeks, thus
leaving intervening days for sorting out the
previous day's observations. These had been
written up on cards, each covering an hour's
worth of each therapist's behaviour. Clinicians
were aware of her task and this awareness
minimised problems of role-pretending. Copious
notes were made and vast amounts of
qualitative information collected. According to
Edwards, 'The main problems associated with

observations are that the presence of the
observer alters what happens and/or that the
observer unintentionally selects what he sees,
records and reports according to his own biases.'

Varied as treatment was found to be, Edwards
observed that it was, at least in part, determined
by the social context in which it was given. It
also appeared that many therapists who had
been led to expect to spend the greater part of
their time in treating clients were in fact
spending about 75% of their time on secondary
tasks such as attending ward rounds,
communicating with other staff, checking
equipment and on administration.

This finding confirms results obtained in a
study of departments carried out by Central
Management Services (1980), using the survey
method, and has obvious implications for
occupational therapy education.

---

trolled through random selection then it can be
said to be representative of the population under
study, the findings therefore generalised to other
similar groups and descriptions of the population
produced. These may be superficial and lack the
qualitative depth of the ethnographic method but
their numerical or coded form can be taken further
to show where correlations exist between different
aspects. The correlations will not explain the

causation of variables but they can help in understanding social phenomena.

Many recent occupational therapy studies
(Beagen 1985; Chamove 1986; Durham 1982;
Hewitt et al 1981; Vaughan and Prechner 1986)
have made use of questionnaires and/or self-rating
forms and interviews in order to find out clients'
views and needs, amongst other things.

EXAMPLE 30.3 SURVEYING THE EFFECTS
OF A COMMUNITY LIVING SKILLS
PROGRAMME (DURHAM 1982)

Durham evaluated a Community Living Skills
(CLS) Programme for pre-discharge psychiatric
clients by comparing the data regarding skills
that daycare clients had found difficult with the
actual content of the CLS programme. The
results were used to modify and improve the
existing course so that it could meet the needs
of clients more effectively. Here, descriptive
information from a survey was used to predict
what might be of use to other people from a
similar population.

Durham concluded from her survey that 'many
patients need continuing assistance to use
existing skills and develop new ones, as they
move from hospital to the community and begin
to tackle unfamiliar situations'. However, while
identifying this need she has not been able in
this study, with the data available, to determine
the effectiveness of the course itself.

For this to be done a 'before and after'
experimental approach would need to be
adopted. Under these circumstances, perhaps
using questionnaires, interviews and
observations by other staff, a comparison of
people who follow the programme with those
who do not, might give evidence of change, for
better or worse, amongst those who have
participated in the course. However, this would
not necessarily prove that one had caused the
other. There are many variables involved and in
order to control these we need to look at the
experimental method in detail.

EXPERIMENTAL METHOD

The experimental method is the one most likely to
come to mind when thinking of research, conjur-
ing up images of rats in cages, laboratories with
sophisticated controls of variables, and impressive
statistical analyses. At a more practical, applied
and simple level, it may involve matching two
groups of people, subjecting one to the experimental method and measuring the performance of each
group before and after the experimental period.
Thus by starting off with scores for the two groups
and a statement 'that there is no difference between the groups', scores subsequent to the experimental period may be sufficiently different to
demonstrate that there has been a change and to
draw the conclusion that it has been affected by
the experimental condition. This change may or
may not be large enough to be considered as
significant.

The experimental method may go by a number
of different names such as 'pre-test–post-test' or
'laboratory' method. These names give a clue to
the design of the research, which sets out to show
the effect of one or more factors on a specific
situation, that is, it deals with the phenomenon of
cause and effect.

Variables

The experimental method requires careful structuring or designing in order to eliminate the possible effect of factors other than that, or those,
being studied. These factors are known as variables, literally 'things which vary'. Variables are
characteristics or properties such as age, weight
and stress tolerance, which differentiate one person from another and affect behaviour. Some variables can be grouped according to a category, for
example, male or female; others are ranked along
a scale, such as a rating scale, for levels of stress;
others, such as age and height, are very specific,
with precise measurement and exact intervals
whereby a person can be twice as old or half as
tall as another.

Independent and dependent variables

While talking about variables it is perhaps appropriate to distinguish between dependent and
independent variables. The independent variable
is the one that is thought to produce or to cause
change in the other, that is, in the dependent variable, or the one to be explained.

The independent variable is sometimes called
the explanatory variable since it can account for
change in the dependent variable. The independent or explanatory variable is the one the experimenter varies in order to investigate its effect
on behaviour.

The dependent variable is not under the
experimenter's control but will be affected by the
manipulation of the other variables. For example,

in studying relaxation techniques, the outcome, or behaviour, could be dependent upon the nature of the presentation, whether delivered by cassette or by live human voice; upon the environment, whether calm and comfortable or cold and distracting; on previous experience; on the preceding activity; or on personal levels of stress, to suggest but a few possible independent variables.

If it was the nature of the presentation that was under study and being manipulated by the researcher then all other possible explanatory variables should be systematically controlled. Control can be effected in a number of different ways:

- by ensuring that all groups receiving one or other treatment have the same extraneous variables, leaving only the independent variable to be changed from group to group
- by exposing each group to each of the possible explanatory factors
- by selecting members at random, thus ensuring that there is comparability between the groups without actually matching members across the whole range of possible characteristics.

Experimental design

A number of different experimental designs can be adopted, each with strengths and weaknesses. The simplest is perhaps the 'one group, pre-test–post-test method' (Fig. 30.3) but some would argue that this is more akin to a before-and-after survey approach and call it a 'quasi-experiment', similar to the study by Durham (1982) referred to above.

Let us suppose that a group of clients was introduced to a series of relaxation techniques using a recorded voice and that change was demonstrated through objective and subjective measurements of anxiety. In this situation it might be tempting to say that the relaxation had caused the change in behaviour. However there could be

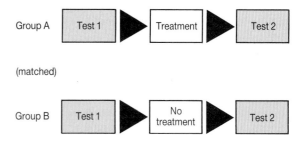

Fig. 30.4 The pre- post-test method for matched groups.

many other intervening variables to confound the outcome. Perhaps the change could have been attributed more to the approach of the therapist who introduced the relaxation period. For greater certainty about causal relationships a more sophisticated design is necessary (Fig. 30.4).

Under these conditions the only difference, for better or for worse, should be due to the experimental condition, or lack of it, and change therefore attributable to the factor which is different. However, life in the real world is not quite as simple as in the laboratory. If the nature of the experiment is known to staff then it could be possible for their biases to have an effect on one group or the other. For this reason, the experiment may be conducted as a double-blind, whereby only the experimenter knows which group is receiving the treatment and which the 'placebo'.

Under such circumstances, assessment of behaviour can be carried out by independent judges ignorant of who is getting what. This is a particularly common experimental procedure in drug trials, but occupational therapy cannot be compared exactly to treatments requiring passive acceptance as it involves the active participation of clients in their treatment programmes. A possible solution is therefore to expose each group to both the experimental and the control position but in reverse order (Fig. 30.5).

If both groups are identical there should be no difference in scores obtained in Test 1. If the treatment has an effect then differences will show between subsequent results for groups A and B. If however, the treatment has a lasting effect then one would expect to find a smaller difference in

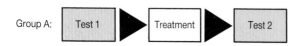

Fig. 30.3 The pre- post-test method.

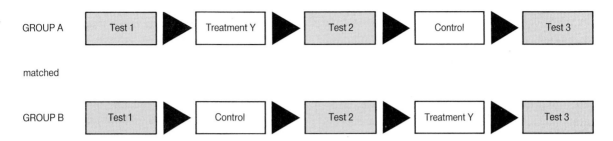

Fig. 30.5   Two runs with experimental and control conditions reversed.

EXAMPLE 30.4   A CONTROLLED STUDY OF A COMMUNITY LIVING SKILLS PROGRAMME (CAMPBELL AND MCCREADIE 1983)

An example of a small-scale controlled study of chronic schizophrenic day clients is given by Campbell and McCreadie (1983). Having identified 10 clients who fulfilled Feighner's criteria for 'definite' or 'probable' schizophrenia, these researchers assessed the clients using the Royal Edinburgh Occupational Therapy Assessment form, questionnaires, tests and discussion. The clients were then randomly allocated to one of two groups, one of which was to receive a 12-week graded programme of daily and community living skills. The numbers were small but nevertheless the post-test scores showed sufficient change for the conclusion to be drawn that 'change can be effected by occupational therapy even in a chronically handicapped group'.

Encouraging as conclusions like this may be to the enhancement and efficacy of the profession, they do raise questions regarding the long-term effects and whether in fact it was the treatment programme or the occupational therapist who contributed most to the improvement, and whether or not helpers or other staff could not have contributed equally as well. We should not be satisfied by one set of results but should continue to develop further tests of validity by investigating potential influencing variables.

Test 3 scores than in Test 2. If it is not possible to match subjects for all possible characteristics then a random selection divided between groups is assumed to distribute the variables equally between them and the groups are said to be matched. Any chance difference between the groups can be accounted for by probability theory and the use of statistical techniques.

Limitations

In a well-designed experiment it is easier to make connections between cause and effect. However, a number of problems are encountered with this method. Ethical issues come to the fore in the experimental method more than in any other. Is it right to withhold treatment or to deceive through the use of a placebo? When dealing with people there is a multiplicity of causes, many of which are difficult to control, such as previous experience and expectations. Furthermore, people may withdraw voluntarily or involuntarily through moving, or death, thus leading to a reduction in numbers and possible loss of reliability in findings. To obtain the cooperation of sufficiently large numbers over a sustained period of time can be a constraining factor on this method. Finally, as with other methods, the personal characteristics of the researcher can bias subjects' behaviour.

STAGES OF A RESEARCH PROJECT

The previous section has covered the three major research methods, ethnographic, survey and experimental, along with their limitations and advantages. This section now looks at how one might go about planning a research project, how data might be collected and later processed.

PLANNING

When a would-be researcher first starts thinking about a possible project or area of investigation there are several sources of information and help. Experienced colleagues, local colleges, libraries and literature are all worth drawing upon. Most researchers, even those with some experience, need advice on designing a study and how to collect and analyse data. Careful planning is necessary to ensure that faults are not built into the design for, once the field work is underway, it is often too late to compensate. When things do go wrong, or frustrations and boredom arise, then the moral support of a friend can be invaluable. Besides personal help from those whose commitment has been obtained, there are many texts that can assist and the College of Occupational Therapists, through its Research and Ethical Committee also provides useful documentation and advice (COT 1985).

Literature review

Having first got an idea, even if not clearly formulated, a review of the literature is essential in order to focus the attention and to highlight problems faced by other researchers within the same or similar field of study. Nowadays retrieval of possible relevant literature is speeded up by computer searches where cross-indexing of key words or phrases enables many articles to be scanned quickly. In addition, library searches may be performed by cooperative librarians or by personal reference to abstracts such as Index Medicus and Current Awareness Topic Searches (CATS). In September 1986 the first database in the UK to include a wide range of citations in therapy and related fields was produced. There is, in fact, a great richness of information available once one starts looking. An investigation of relevant literature can in itself be a fascinating and worthwhile experience, leading to useful accounts of the current state of knowledge.

The literature review will enable the potential researcher to discover if the gap in knowledge is purely personal, whether the topic of interest genuinely requires investigation, and whether previous studies have produced conflicting evidence

---

EXAMPLE 30.5   A LITERATURE REVIEW OF RELAXATION TRAINING TECHNIQUES (KEBBLE 1985)

Thorough 'reviews of relaxation training techniques' by Kebble (1985) contain descriptions of the techniques and their theoretical base, plus critical appraisals of some of the evaluative studies carried out by others. This might be described as armchair research but is nevertheless a vital starting point for future study and for encouraging greater critical awareness by occupational therapists and others in using the techniques. While 'results consistently conflict depending heavily on the quality of experimental design and methodology used ... relaxation training in general is a potentially effective and appropriate treatment in anxiety management ...'

---

or have not yet been replicated. There is nothing wrong in setting out to check out another's design, findings and interpretation.

When storing information from references, bibliographic cards can be invaluable if kept meticulously. If headed by the author's name, year and title of citation, and the publisher's name, they can be sorted readily for the reference and bibliographical section of the final report.

Aim of the project

From the review of the literature and thorough consideration of the information that is sought, it should be possible to formulate a brief statement of the aims of the project, questions to be answered and what it is intended to achieve. Having identified the problem to be investigated, a protocol will be needed if funds are to be sought. Formats may differ but essentially it should contain a title, brief background to the reasons for the study, its purpose, aims and value, the population or research subjects, methods to be followed for the collection and analysis of data, and the resources required. If the title is meaningful, containing key words to explain the nature of the study, then it will be more accessible to others once published and indexed in CATS or elsewhere.

Research design

The idea or problem to be investigated needs a framework and this is the research design, about which much has been written above. It would be naive and misleading to suggest that most research procedures progress smoothly from beginning to end like a chain, from stage to stage, from link to link. Alas the process may throw into relief some important factor overlooked at the planning stage; or another pertinent citation may be discovered in a bygone journal or appear unexpectedly in the current academic press; or subjects may disappear or die, leaving a less than satisfactory number for final analysis. Once data collection has been started there is little that can be done to stop the process, short of termination and admission of failure. It is probably better to continue, even if it means less reliable or negative results, than to have none at all. But let not such potential disasters dissuade the reader from beginning.

DATA COLLECTION

Major concerns with the collection of data lie with reliability and validity. These will be defined briefly before describing some of the different strategies for collecting data according to the research method being used.

Reliability

By reliability is meant whether or not the experiment can be repeated and similar results found, given the same conditions. In ethnographic studies it means the extent to which different observers would produce the same analysis and conclusions given detailed records for checking. Direct replication in this method is difficult.

Validity

Validity is the extent to which measures used are relevant to the variable being studied and measure the concepts that the researcher was aiming to operationalise. For example, it would be invalid to use scores from a biofeedback programme as a measure of the effectiveness of relaxation techniques when the subject's hands, while attached to the electrodes, were sweating profusely from previous exertion. This example would lack 'internal validity' because there would be an alternative explanation for the observable scores being produced.

'External validity' refers to the extent to which findings can be generalised to other similar groups. Validity can be defined further to have

- *predictive value* if the 'test' makes accurate predictions about future performance
- *concurrent validity* if it correlates well with other measures of the same concept
- *construct validity* if the test appears to conform to predictions about it based on theory.

Validity is checked and results from one method of data collection tested against another through the process of triangulation. This means using different research methods or sources of data to examine the same problem in order to refute or substantiate findings. In other words, if the same conclusions are reached using different methods then the confidence in validity increases, rather like using a triangulation point on a hill, or geographic features with a map, to give confidence in one's position.

Ethnographic approach

The ethnographic approach attempts to describe the nature of a complex issue, such as implementation of deinstitutionalisation policies and economic reality (Kielhofner 1981). Therefore the description and analysis of the role of the researcher and the process of the investigation is almost as important as the collection and interpretation of the data. Considerable information may be collected in the early stages before the variables have been operationalised. However, it does eventually require the researcher to focus attention onto specific interactions or events and to observe these systematically. This is known as progressive focusing, requiring greater selectivity and concern with detail. This detail may be extracted from field notes, checklists and audiovisual techniques, although it does depend to a large extent on memory and on records being made between sessions.

Observation

In order to focus on the necessary detail an observation schedule or checklist may be devised. Edwards (1980) completed time cards when observing therapists at work. These observations were structured as a result of predetermined categories arising from the early exploratory phase or initial pilot study.

Documentation

If access is possible, then reports such as case records, minutes of meetings, registers of attendance, records of accidents, and other forms of written material produced by others in the environment under investigation can add to the participant/observer's impressions and findings.

Interviews

Interviews may also be used for data collection with the nature of the interview depending on the stage the research is at and the significance of the person being interviewed. Those with some responsibility for the 'actors' might receive an exploratory interview at the beginning with in-depth and/or structured interviews being used during or after the field work. Interviews also play an important part in the survey method and will be discussed in greater detail below.

Survey method

The survey method tends to use interviews and questionnaires in various forms.

Exploratory interview

The exploratory interview is unstructured and requires considerable skill if the interviewer is to direct it in such a way as to gain information and insight from the respondent as to what he or she (the interviewee) finds important with regard to the issue under investigation. Essentially, its purpose is to establish ideas and possible research hypotheses. The interviewer has to establish a trusting and open relationship in which the respondent feels comfortable and cooperative. There needs to be an element of control without loss of freedom of expression. Such interviews should not be pressurised by a shortage of time.

The information gained will probably reveal feelings and attitudes, facts and fantasies, on a number of issues requiring subsequent follow-up. Hard facts and data are not expected at this stage. The interviewer must accept the respondent's views regardless of his own beliefs, and maintain a level of objectivity to the information given.

Pilot interview

Following on from an exploratory interview the researcher is able to identify potentially pertinent questions for the main survey. The wording and appropriateness would be tested out in a pilot interview given to a small but representative sample of the population being studied.

Standardised interview

The purpose and method of carrying out the standardised interview is quite different from the exploratory form. This should be the final version, with ambiguities eliminated. It will have been structured as a result of earlier investigations and tested rigorously during the pilot stage. Its purpose is to collect data. One of the disadvantages of the standardised interview, as with the standardised questionnaire, is that there is a degradation of data, and a loss of the refinements regarding individual differences, which would be available from in-depth interviews. Again interviewers require specific skills. In this case they need to ensure, as closely as possible, that there is 'sameness' with each respondent: the same questions and the same manner of asking.

Questionnaire

These are generally standardised in that they pose questions in a specific way. They may be self-administered or completed by a research worker.

An advantage of the latter approach is that it can ensure a higher response than from postal questionnaires and accurate identification of the respondent. After all, postal questionnaires can be passed on to another for completion, thereby possibly distorting the sample.

The response from postal questionnaires can be low and strategies should be sought to improve the return rate; by ensuring, for example, that questions are concise and explicit; that respondents appreciate the importance of the questionnaire and their contribution; and that the return postage is paid. However a low response need not be too great a concern if it remains a representative sample of the original population.

Pilot questionnaire

It is important to produce pilot questionnaires before launching the final version. When open-ended questions are set there can be many different responses. In order that these can be collated and the data programme prepared, pre-runs with a small representative sample are necessary.

Sampling

Apart from surveys such as the National Census, which includes everyone in the United Kingdom, the majority deal with only a sample of the population under study. If the sample is representative then statements made about it can be generalised for the population as a whole. This is obviously important for a variety of reasons, not the least being economic. However, in order to safeguard the sample's representativeness certain procedures have to be followed.

Probability or random sampling is the most common and infers that everyone in the population had an equal opportunity of being selected. This might be based on selecting every 'nth' person in order to obtain a sample 1/nth of the population; or by using a table of random numbers whereby each individual is given a number from 1 to n and then selected according to the distribution within the random table. A register of clients attending for treatment could be a sampling frame from which the random sample was selected.

Non-probability samples refer to those where only certain individuals may be selected, as in quota samples. If for example, a sample of clients attending the occupational therapy department was sought, and the percentage in different categories according to age was known, then the first to attend and make up the quota for each age group would form the sample. Later arrivals would not be included if their category was already complete, and hence do not have equal opportunities.

No matter how carefully the sample is drawn it cannot be totally representative of the total population. Lack of precision is known as sampling error and can be overcome through statistical techniques.

DATA PROCESSING

Depending on the research design, raw data may have been categorised and coded, or it may stand as individual scores that can be added together and subjected to various mathematical calculations. The questions of reliability and validity have been discussed. Now scales of measurement, descriptive statistics and tests of significance will be described.

While there are many texts that elaborate on statistical theory, in many instances a simple appreciation of statistical procedures is all that is required. An understanding in depth of statistical theory is certainly beyond the expectations of this chapter and of most colleagues. Indeed it might be said to be beyond the attainments of most behavioural scientists (Maxwell 1970). However, application of elementary statistical procedures should be within reach of most of those who have got this far in this chapter.

The nature of the data

Data may have been collected in a structured manner, by using stopwatches or standardised tests to measure learning speeds for example; or through less structured means of surveys, interviews and projective tests to measure levels of anxiety. Observation, per se, is completely unstructured until specific elements have been identified, operationalised and subsequently categorised. In the old days, data was transferred to punch cards. Now computers are used, resulting in much time being saved and processes being carried out more speedily. Whether by punch cards or computers, data must be coded and each code be mutually exclusive. Most survey questionnaires contain the opportunity for the respondent's answer to be fitted into an 'Other' category if those already listed are inappropriate. Alternatively the researcher may process the data by condensing all categories into two, for example, reducing social classes one to six into 'middle class' (1–3) and 'working class' (4–6). Obviously, such simplification into dichotomous variables has a degrading effect on the raw data but it may sometimes be considered more expedient for such a reduction to take place in order to simplify the analysis and so produce more general statements.

Scales of measurement

For practical purposes there are four scales, each lending itself to different statistical techniques. In order of complexity, they are

1. nominal
2. ordinal
3. interval
4. ratio.

The nominal scale places characteristics or attributes into different 'named' categories such as gender, male or female; marital status; or place of birth. The categories male/female are mutually exclusive and contain no order or level of importance. Subjects may come from Blackpool, Bognor or Ballingry, three towns on a nominal scale with no distinguishing characteristics identified, apart from the difference in names. However, if the place of birth was to be identified in terms of its proximity to London then they would fit into an ordinal scale as follows: Bognor, Blackpool, Ballingry. Taking this a step further, if the size of the town was the critical factor and subjects' place of birth was categorised according to the population being; less than 25 000; between 25 000 and 49 999; 50 000 to 74 999; and 75 000 or more; then we have a ratio scale since

the difference between each category is equal and there is a fixed zero point. On a ratio scale it is possible to show the mathematical relationship between items. However, not all scales with equal intervals start from zero. The Fahrenheit scale has equal intervals but it would not be true to say that 84° F was twice as hot as 42° F. Such a scale is known as an 'interval scale'.

The scale of measurement is important in determining which statistical procedures can be used. Obviously people falling into different categories in the nominal scales, for example, male or female, can be counted for their frequency and the 'mode' or category with the greatest number in it identified but these categories cannot be added together without losing their identity. On an interval scale, where intervals are of equal size, as in intelligence tests, scores from a number of individuals could be added together and divided by that number in order to find the 'mean' or average score.

Measures of central tendency

Measures of central tendency include the mean, mode, median and standard deviation. Reference has already been made to the mode as being the most frequently occurring number in a set of observations and to the mean as being the average score. The third measure of central tendency is the median, which is the middle score, with 50% of subjects having scores above it and 50% below. It can be found by placing all scores in rank order and then finding the one that is central.

Besides knowing the mode, median and mean scores it can be useful to know the range of scores about the central point, in other words how much spread or deviation there is from the central location. To know the range of scores, that is, the difference between the largest and the smallest score, adds to the description of the findings but it does not tell us how many might have very low or very high scores. The standard deviation is the statistic that gives us a measure of the dispersion. Given that the population of 100% fits into the bell-shaped curve of a normal distribution, then 34.1% of the population falls within one standard deviation below the mean and 34.1% falls above;

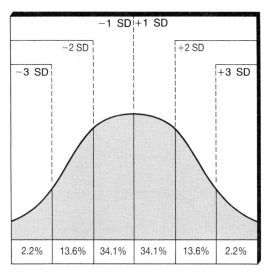

Fig. 30.6 A normal distribution curve, showing a fixed percentage of subjects falling into ranges measured by standard deviations.

13.6% of the population are contained between one and two standard deviations from the mean and 2.2% beyond two (Fig. 30.6).

Descriptive statistics

Measures of central location and dispersion have been described above. From these figures, patterns and relationships within the data can be seen and hence lead to inferences being made as the processed data are interpreted. In presenting the data, frequency histograms or bar charts can give a visual description with considerable impact, resulting in possible economy of words.

Taylor (1983), in his article describing the procedure for training agoraphobics in groups, demonstrates with the use of histograms the change after treatment in clients' involvement in activities, either accompanied or alone (Fig. 30.7).

Although the frequency measures shown in Figure 30.7 could not be subjected to statistical analysis since they were part of an ordinal scale of measurement, the anxiety measures arising from a self-report questionnaire, including rating scales, were appropriate for statistical analysis and showed a significant reduction. The graphs in Figure 30.8 demonstrate this very clearly.

The statistical calculation showed that the total anxiety score reduced significantly. Analysis of

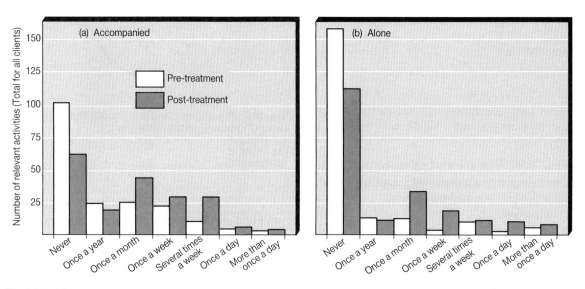

Fig. 30.7 Histograms showing frequency of relevant activities in a group of agoraphobics before and after treatment, accompanied and alone.
(a) Accompanied.
(b) Alone.

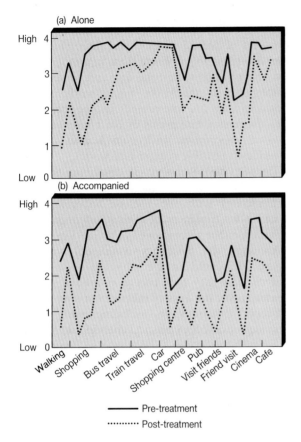

Fig. 30.8 Graphs showing anxiety levels before and after treatment.
(a) Alone.
(b) Accompanied.

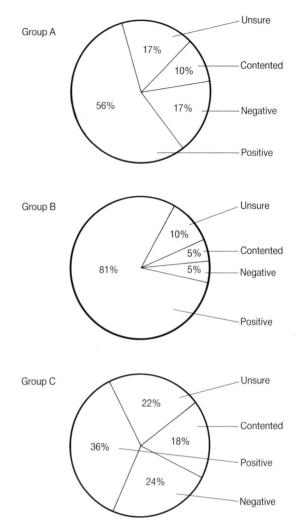

Fig. 30.9 Pie diagrams showing the attitudes of three different groups to occupational therapy.
(a) Group A.
(b) Group B.
(c) Group C.

pre- and post-treatment scores for different types of activity demonstrated a significant reduction in anxiety:

● at the 2.5% level for walking alone, shopping alone, shopping accompanied, shopping centre accompanied, bus and train travel accompanied
● at the 5% level for walking accompanied, visiting a friend alone and staying at home alone (Taylor 1983).

A number of the activities showed insignificant changes that would therefore suggest lines of action for future treatment.

Pie diagrams (Fig. 30.9) are another way of

quickly conveying information to the reader as shown in Burton's paper (1984) comparing the attitudes of three different groups of clients towards occupational therapy after their first week.

Burton's study highlights the need for further research into introductory procedures, education of other disciplines and how their attitudes can influence clients.

Tests of association and significance

Data can be presented to demonstrate patterns and relationships as above, or it can be used in a variety of tests designed to show the extent to which x is associated with y. Given knowledge of one, the other can be more easily estimated if there is an association.

The nature of the relationship can be seen if scores are plotted on graph paper, forming a scattergram. This is a way of showing the strength, or otherwise, of the relationship. The correlation may be:

- high and positive, for example, between children's age and height
- high and negative, for example between the age of cars and their value.

Or there may be no correlation between the two variables as, for example, between age and the consumption of alcohol (Fig. 30.10).

Even if such diagrams appear informative it must be remembered that correlation does not necessarily prove causation or that there is an association.

Statistical calculation of the correlation produces the 'correlation coefficient' (r). This score will lie between +1.0 and −1.0, that is, it can be between a perfect linear positive correlation or a perfect negative correlation. Zero correlation means that there is no relationship at all between the two variables.

The coefficient of correlation can be calculated by a variety of tests, each appropriate under different circumstances.

1. The Phi Coefficient (ϕ) may be used when both variables are dichotomous, for example, when one variable is pass/fail and the other male/female.

2. The Point Biserial Coefficient (r_{pb}) is a measure of association between one dichotomous variable and one interval or ratio variable.

3. Spearman's Rank Correlation Coefficient, as its name suggests, is the test to be used when the two variables are on ordinal scales.

4. Pearson's Product Moment Correlation Coefficient is used when both variables are measured on interval or ratio scales.

Formulae exist for each of these tests and statis-

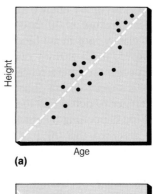

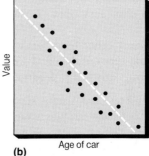

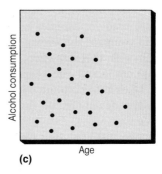

Fig. 30.10 Scattergrams.
(a) The relationship between children's age and height, showing high positive correlation.
(b) The relationship between the ages of cars and their value, showing high negative correlation.
(c) The relationship between age and alcohol consumption, showing no correlation.

tical tables will interpret the significance of r depending on the size of the sample.

Probability

Once r has been calculated using the appropriate measure it has to be determined whether or not this was likely to occur by chance alone. Suppose one is tossing a coin, out of 10 throws one would expect approximately half to be heads and half to be tails. However, if all throws produced heads you might suspect some interference and that the outcome was not simply due to chance alone. It is up to the researcher to determine the level of odds against something happening by chance. However, it is generally accepted that 20:1 or 95% level of certainty that something has not happened by chance alone is appropriate. Hence, Taylor's statement that probability of change happening by chance alone was less that 2.5% with some activities.

There are many other tests besides those listed above. Different types of data and sizes of samples require different statistical procedures.

1. Student's *t* test is a useful statistic for comparing means between samples which are usually smaller than 50. The measure will tell whether the samples have been drawn from the same population or whether there is a significant difference between them.

2. *z-scores* are used for samples larger than 50, for example, to compare the average age of marriage in Britain with that elsewhere. This makes certain assumptions about the shape of the distribution and takes into account both the means and the standard deviations of the populations being compared.

3. Chi square test (χ) is appropriate for nominal data and tests whether a particular pattern of frequencies in a table is likely to have occurred by chance. This test is one of a number of non-parametric tests and it is therefore worth making a final comment on the terms 'parametric' and 'non-parametric' which the reader may well come across.

Parametric tests are more likely to detect a significant difference or correlation at a particular probability level. They are used where the data has been measured on an interval scale at least, and the parameters of the population are known. They include z and t tests, and product moment correlation tests.

Non-parametric tests, on the other hand, do not make any assumptions about the shape of the distributions from which the samples have been selected. For example, the rankings of anxiety levels in two different groups may be compared using non-parametric tests, or the difference between men and women, before and after an anxiety-management programme. In the latter instance the chi square test would be used to test the hypothesis about the relationship between the different characteristics.

Advice

It will be appreciated from the above that the statistical component of research is far from simple and a little knowledge can lead the naive and uninitiated into a minefield of problems. Mathematical calculations and computer-assisted programs may be straightforward but advice from a statistician should be sought early on in the planning process in order to ensure that appropriate methods and tests are adopted, and all relevant questions asked. Good ideas cannot be incorporated half-way through a project.

For those who wish to develop their own knowledge and understanding of research and statistics, the references and bibliography at the end of this chapter could be a starting point. Alternatively the Open University course, 'Research Methods in Education and Social Science' is to be recommended.

TRENDS IN PRACTICE AND OPPORTUNITIES FOR RESEARCH

This final section takes us away from the serious side of statistics to considering the opportunities for and different functions of research.

The nature of the use of activity and its uniqueness to occupational therapy must inevitably be one reflecting changing atmospheres in departments and ratios of staff to clients. The value of different activities needs to be investigated. Also, to what extent is the relationship between client and professional of critical importance, and can other less well-qualified staff be equally therapeutic? In times of staff shortage this issue needs to be addressed.

Public awareness of issues regarding health leads to an emphasis on health education as a preventative measure and as part of the rehabilitation process. Occupational therapists are beginning to contribute to anxiety-management programmes from health centres and to run workshops for non-medical people who come into contact with disabled people. In the long term could a more extensive role as educator make more effective use of time and skills, rather than therapists expecting to have predominantly direct contact with clients and their treatment?

Occupational therapists are considerably involved in psycho-geriatric units and in the care of long-term clients. However, no matter how important the quality of life may be, resources are not infinite. Indeed as the old live longer and the young get fewer, compromise becomes necessary. What is the justification for highly skilled staff devoting their skills to this group of people? Should explanations for the deployment of staff be of an intuitive and subjective nature only?

As more psychiatric and mentally handicapped people are discharged into the community, the effectiveness of different pre-discharge assessments and training programmes needs to be examined and shared. Much time and energy can be wasted if individual teams of staff struggle to design their own schemes without either investigating what good practice already exists, or writing up their own experiences in order that others may benefit.

Other trends must include performance indicators and quality assurance: quantifiable measures resulting from systematic investigation. Whatever the research, it should produce useful answers to the many important questions confronting occupational therapists. In turn, results would have implications for clients, pay-masters and professional practice.

In thinking about current practice, trends and future opportunities as above, it is possible to identify three functions that research might fulfill.

1. It may be orientated towards developing policy, for example, to establishing, by objective means, what should be the minimum standards of staffing required for different categories of clients in units of different size in order to ensure effective practice.

2. Research could be described as 'action-research' where, for example, different approaches to assessment, or to treatment, are compared. Policy-orientated research and action-research are not always mutually exclusive, as will be seen below. In some instances policy may arise from the results of investigations into finding the most effective methods of working.

3. Yet another function of research can be to test out theory. This would seem particularly relevant today when occupational therapists are beset with many potential models and theories upon which practice can be based. Young (1984) says 'there seems, as yet, no defined limits to the depth to which the theoretical premise for occupational therapy may be plumbed. To date there is a scarcity of well-documented research pertinent to the theoretical constructs or the outcome of intervention by occupational therapy'.

The long-term value of each of these functions of research would be seen in greater efficiency and effectiveness, from improved quality of practice, and a strengthened and well-understood theoretical base. These functions in turn, could be carried out in different areas: education, management and clinical.

RESEARCH IN EDUCATION

Educational research has attracted considerable interest, with creative studies seeking to go beyond comparison and quantification of resources and outcomes. This author (Stewart 1979), in a comparison of occupational therapy education in schools in the United Kingdom, aimed to develop a greater awareness amongst educationists of the range of resources and approaches to education, which in turn led to a greater degree of sharing between schools and wider development of innovative practices. The field of education generally produces a cooperative and accessible population and there is scope for comparing, amongst other things, different teaching methods such as peer-teaching versus staff-teaching (Dunkin 1978), or the stages in students' intellectual development (Green 1980).

Moves towards degree-level education and the introduction of different routes to qualifying and so gaining entry to the profession, raise many questions worthy of serious investigation. Will changes in academic status have implications for costs and the quality of practice? Results from a comparison of competencies, that is, action-based research, could influence policy decisions, with obvious resulting effects on practice for the future.

RESEARCH IN MANAGEMENT

Within this growing profession there is a considerable shortfall of qualified personnel. Around 20% of funded posts are currently vacant (NAO 1986), and of these about 25% are in psychiatry as found by a cursory analysis of vacancies advertised in the British Journal of Occupational Therapy in 1986.

Occupational therapy is still a young profession in relation to others but, unless it can identify its unique contribution to rehabilitation, it faces the possibility of other health-care workers taking over some of its areas of practice. As knowledge expands and services are extended, so must there be continual appraisal in order to ensure that these limited resources are allocated appropriately and to effect.

The identification of the skills required for specific tasks in different areas of occupational therapy practice has important implications for manpower and training. Who does what best and why? The work of Edwards could form the basis for further analysis and differentiation of skills performed by helpers and other qualified staff, including occupational therapists in psychiatric settings. In evaluating occupational therapy helpers as behaviour therapists, Milne and Mason (1984) concluded that 'there was every indication from the objective measures that the six occupational therapy helpers who received the one-week course in behaviour therapy were able to become successful therapists'.

Management plans, when concerned, for example, with people with particular needs, are usually dependent on first identifying the popu-

lation, determining goals and the necessary requirements for their achievement. Bartlett, Gleeson and Young's (1985) rehabilitation survey of long-stay psychiatric patients at Park Prewett Hospital is an example of how data collected can lead to the implementation of appropriate programmes to the benefit of clients.

CLINICAL RESEARCH

It would seem that, over the years, occupational therapy has subsumed, and later rejected, a great variety of activities, as indeed has the world of psychiatry in general. Things come in and out of vogue. Computer software, whether in games, assessment, tests or wordprocessing, is claimed to have considerable potential (Roberts 1985), but how many occupational therapists have mastered this therapeutic medium? To what extent is it being used and by whom? Undoubtedly special interest groups stimulate the asking of questions and seeking of answers as well as giving support to individuals. Lone researchers may not have a viable population but, if working in conjunction with colleagues elsewhere, they may well be enabled to produce meaningful information that goes beyond the merely anecdotal. Hemphill's collection (1982) of evaluative processes actually gives further ideas for research and seeks collaboration between therapists.

SUMMARY

There are many questions waiting to be asked, thus giving potential for research projects.

This chapter has attempted to take away some of the mystique often associated with research, to introduce the reader to the different methods and stages of research, and to suggest some of the questions that are pertinent to the future.

It looked first at what research is and why it is carried out, followed by a detailed examination of three different research methods: the ethnographic, survey and experimental methods.

The different stages of a research project were

then covered, including planning, data collection and data processing. Finally, research trends and opportunities were considered, with questions pertinent to the future being suggested.

REFERENCES

Atkinson P 1975 In cold blood: bedside teaching in a medical school. In: Chanan G, Delamont S (eds) Frontiers of classroom research. NFER/Nelson, London

Bartlett S, Gleeson M, Young M 1985 Rehabilitation survey of long-stay patients at Park Prewett Hospital 1984, Final report. British Journal of Occupational Therapy 48(6): 179–180

Beagen D 1985 Spontaneity and creativity in the NHS: Starting a new group—psychodrama with adult day patients. British Journal of Occupational Therapy 48(12): 370–374

Burton L 1984 Introducing the concept of occupational therapy to patients in an acute psychiatric unit. British Journal of Occupational Therapy 47(6): 178–183

Campbell A, McCreadie R G 1983 Occupational therapy is effective for chronic schizophrenic day patients. British Journal of Occupational Therapy 46(11): 325–326

Central Management Services 1980 Report of a study of staffing in the remedial professions. DHSS, London

Chamove A S 1986 Exercise improves behaviour: a rationale for occupational therapy. British Journal of Occupational Therapy 49(3): 83–86

College of Occupational Therapists 1985 Research advice handbook for occupational therapists. COT, London

Dunkin N, Hook P 1978 Peer teaching: an alternative to lectures. British Journal of Occupational Therapy 41(8): 280–281

Durham T M 1982 Community living skills training. British Journal of Occupational Therapy 45(7): 233–235

Edwards J D 1980 Occupational therapy: role and education. MSc thesis submitted to University of Manchester

Ellis M 1981 Why bother to research? British Journal of Occupational Therapy 44(4): 115–116

Green M 1980 A study of the stages in the development of occupational therapy students in basic training. MSc Thesis, University of Southhampton

Hainey C et al 1973 A study of prisoners and guards in a simulated prison. Naval Research Review 30(9): 4–17. In: Potter D (ed) Society and the Social Sciences, Open . University Press, Milton Keynes

Hemphill B J 1982 The evaluative process in psychiatric occupational therapy. Slack, USA

Hewitt K, Wishart C, Lambert R 1981 Social skills training with chronic psychiatric patients. British Journal of Occupational Therapy 44(9): 284–285

Jeffrey L I H 1985 Newcastle play enrichment research programme. Paper presented at College of Occupational Therapists' European Congress, London

Kebble D 1985 Relaxation training techniques: a review, parts 1 and 2. British Journal of Occupational Therapy 48(4): 99–102; and (7): 201–204

Kielhofner G 1981 An ethnographic study of deinstitutionalised adults. Occupational Therapy Journal of Research 1(2): 125–142

King L J 1974 A sensory integrative approach to schizophrenia. American Journal of Occupational Therapy 28(10): 529–536

Labov W 1969 The logic of non-standard English. Georgetown monographs on language and linguistics, vol 22 excerpts. In: Giglioli P P (ed) 1972 Language and social context. Penguin, Harmondsworth

Lowe G R 1969 Personal relationships in psychological disorders. Penguin, Harmondsworth

Macdonald E M (ed) 1970 Occupational therapy in rehabilitation, 3rd edn. Balliere Tindall, London

MacKintosh D 1985 A comparison of carers of senile dementia sufferers in Dundee. Unpublished 3rd Year Student Project, Queen Margaret College, Edinburgh

Maxwell A E 1970 Basic statistics in behavioural research. Penguin, Harmondsworth

Milgram S 1963 Behavioural study of obedience. Journal of Abnormal and Social Psychology 67: 371–8. In: Wilson M (ed) 1978 Social and educational research in action. Longman, Harlow

Mills C W 1970 Appendix: on intellectual craftsmanship. In: The sociological imagination. Penguin, Harmondsworth. (First published in 1959 by Oxford University Press, Oxford)

Milne D, Mason H 1984 An evaluation of occupational therapy helpers as behaviour therapists. British Journal of Occupational Therapists 47(10): 311–314

Mosey A C 1981 Occupational therapy: configuration of a profession. Raven Press, New York

National Audit Office 1986 NHS: Control over professional and technical manpower. HMSO, London

Nicol M 1986 An evaluation of sensory integrative techniques with chronic schizophrenics. MPhil Thesis, Strathclyde University

Popper K R 1957 The unity of method from: The poverty of historicism. Routledge & Kegan Paul, London. In: Brymner J Stribley K M (eds) 1978 Social research: principles and procedures. Longman, Harlow

Roberts M 1985 The use of the BBC microcomputer with psychiatric conditions. British Journal of Occupational Therapy 48(6): 160–162

Stewart A M 1979 A study of occupational therapy education in the UK. Council for Professions Supplementary to Medicine, London

Taylor I 1983 Training agoraphobics in groups. British Journal of Occupational Therapy 46(2): 37–41

Vaughan P J, Prechner M 1986 A structured approach to psychiatric day care. British Journal of Occupational Therapy 46(1): 10–12

West W 1959 (ed) Changing concepts and practices in psychiatric occupational therapy. American Occupational Therapy Association, New York

Whyte W F 1955 Street corner society. University of Chicago Press, Chicago

Wolfensberger W 1972 The principle of normalisation in

human services. National Institute of Mental Retardation, Toronto

Young M 1984 Models of practice for occupational therapy.

British Journal of Occupational Therapy 47(12): 381–382
Zimbardo P G 1972 Pathology of imprisonment. Society 9: 4–8

FURTHER READING

Ackerman W B, Lohnes P R 1981 Research methods for nurses. McGraw Hill, USA

Calnan J 1984 Coping with research. Heinemann, London

Cox R C, West W L 1982 Fundamentals of research for health professionals. RAMSCO, Maryland

Evans K M 1968 Planning small scale research, revised edn. NFER, London

Greenstein L A 1980 Teaching research: an introduction to statistical concepts and research terminology. American Journal of Occupational Therapy 34(5): 320–327

Leedy P D 1980 Practical research. Macmillan, New York

Notter L E 1979 Essentials of nursing research. Tavistock, London

Open University 1979 Research in education and social science. Open University Press, Milton Keynes

Oppenheim A N 1979 Questionnaire design and attitude measurement. Open University Press, Milton Keynes

Partridge C, Barnitt R 1986 Research guidelines: A handbook for therapists. Heinemann, London

Reilly M 1962 Occupational therapy can be one of the great ideas of 20th century medicine. American Journal of Occupational Therapy 16(1): 1–9

Smith H W 1975 Strategies of social research. Prentice Hall, London

Glossaries

OCCUPATIONAL THERAPY TERMS

Activity: the state of being active, the exertion of energy.

Activity analysis: 'the process of examining an activity to distinguish its component parts' (Mosey 1986).

Activity synthesis: the process of combining different elements of activity and environment into an activity suitable for assessment or therapeutic intervention.

Adaptation: the process by which the individual adjusts to changes in his environment in a way that enables him to continue to function adequately.

Adaptive skill: a learned pattern of behaviour that assists the individual to function adequately within his environment.

Atomism: theory that all matter is made up of elementary units.

Belief: acceptance of fact, statement, object or theory as true or existing.

Client-centred therapy: a method of intervention in which the client is helped to become aware of his own potential and of ways in which he can work towards realising it.

Cognition: faculty of knowing, understanding, perceiving and conceiving.

Competence: the ability to perform skills to a level that allows satisfactory performance of life roles.

Dysfunction: inability to maintain the self within the environment at a satisfactory standard because of lack of skills necessary for coping with the current situation.

Environment: the human and non-human surroundings of the individual, including objects, people, events, cultural influences, social norms and expectations.

Frame of reference: the principles behind practice; the organisation of knowledge in a particular field to permit description of the relationships between facts and concepts.

Function: possession of the skills necessary for successful participation in the range of roles expected of the individual.

General systems theory: a way of thinking that combines holism and atomism. A way of studying the interrelationship between parts and wholes.

Health: the ability to function adequately in a balanced variety of roles, and achieve a sense of satisfaction from them.

Holism: the belief that the whole unit is qualitatively different from, and more than, the sum of its parts.

Human development: the gradual evolution of the individual through a series of predictable stages to full growth.

Humanism: a system of beliefs and a theoretical approach that is concerned with what it means to become fully human.

Identity: sense of self; knowledge of one's own individuality.

Intrinsic motivation: an innate drive to use one's capacity for action.

Model: a simplified representation of the structure and content of a phenomenon or system that describes or explains the complex relationships between concepts within the system.

Motivation: the force that causes people to act.

Multidisciplinary team: a unit made up of people of different professions who work autonomously but cooperatively to provide a direct client care service.

Occupation: any goal-directed activity that has meaning for the individual and is composed of skills and values.

Occupational form: the sociocultural and physical characteristics of an occupation that exist independent of the person engaging in the occupation.

Occupational performance: the actions of the individual elicited and guided by the occupational form.

Occupational role: the main social position held by an individual and the tasks performed in that position, for example, student, worker or volunteer.

Occupational therapy: the restoration or maintenance of optimal functional independence and life satisfaction through the analysis and use of selected occupations that enable the individual to develop the adaptive skills required to support his life roles.

Occupational therapy practice: the actions taken by the therapist to serve the need of the client for development of optimum function and independence.

Occupational therapy process: the series of steps by which professional philosophy, theory and content are translated into practice.

Paradigm: an agreed body of theory, explaining and rationalising professional unity and practice, that incorporates all the profession's concerns, concepts and expertise, and guides values and commitments.

Personal causation: the individual's capacity to initiate action with the intent to affect the environment.

Philosophical assumptions: basic suppositions about the nature of living beings, the nature of the universe and the relationships between them, upon which we build our knowledge.

Play: a variety of occupations that constitute a pleasurable way of passing time and are also the medium through which a wide range of skills can be learned and rehearsed.

Professional philosophy: shared beliefs, assumptions and values that provide the profession with its sense of identity and exert control over theory and practice.

Quality: degree or standard of excellence; characteristic trait or attribute.

Quality assurance: a method of ensuring that a service consistently achieves client satisfaction.

Reductionism: the belief that the structure and function of the whole can best be understood from a detailed study of its isolated parts.

Role: the set of expectations placed on an individual in a particular social context that become part of his identity and influence his behaviour. Each person plays a large number of roles, such as worker, parent, friend.

Self-care: occupation that enables the individual to survive and that promotes and maintains health, including mental health.

Skill: practised ability or facility in doing something.

Synthesis: combining separate elements together into an integrated whole.

Therapeutic medium: any activity which is used to develop competence in skills that the individual can use to sustain a satisfactory range of life roles.

Value: internal guidelines for assessing worth, desirability or utility, which allow the individual to set priorities for action.

Volition: the ability to choose between alternative actions; exercise of the will.

Work: any productive activity, whether paid or unpaid, that contributes to the maintenance or advancement of society as well as the individual. The work in which an individual spends most time usually becomes both an occupation and a major social role.

FINANCIAL TERMS

Accountability
Budgetary: responsibility and accountability for the control and utilisation of financial resources contained within a budget.
Management: accountable to named officer for all aspects of the service provided (including budget).

Accounting codes: a set of digits giving information about where expenditure is incurred, the budget it is costed to and the type of items the money has been used to produce.

Allocations
Capital: money made available to health authorities to enable them to build hospitals and clinics. Capital is also defined as goods to be used for more than 1 year, equipment costing over £7500, a works department scheme over £15 000 or any vehicle.
Revenue: money made available to health authorities to meet the running costs of the service. Running costs are the day-to-day expenses and include, for example, salaries and wages, food, drugs and the maintenance of premises.

Annual programme: sometimes called the operational plan, it is a document setting out the district's priorities and plans for a year or two years. It is reviewed annually.

Baseline: a starting point used in the budget setting process, based on the previous year's allocation and subsequent workload.

Baseline creep: changes in service that have an effect on costs but are not usually part of a defined development. For example, changes in treatment programmes may necessitate using more expensive materials or using new and more expensive, but more effective, equipment.

Budget: an estimate of income and expenditure for one year. A sum of money up to which a budget holder may spend.
Budget holder: manager responsible for a service or function. All costs for which she is responsible are brought together and compared with her budget. The budget holder does not necessarily need to be involved in the day-to-day running of the service but must have overall control of the service.
Budget manager: the day-to-day spender. This could include staff delegated down from the budget holder.
Budget statement: a paper issued annually, detailing the elements of funding for the year.
Budgetary control: the establishment of budgets, their maintenance and monitoring through the year.
Budget control reports (statements): produced monthly to show comparative information of expenditure against agreed budget.

Capital programme: a plan over a period of time, normally 10 years, showing costs, starting dates and final dates of schemes of work to be charged to the capital allocation.

Carry forward: an over or underspending by the authority that is taken into the next financial year. This does not necessarily apply to individual budget holders.

Cash limit: a limit imposed by the Government on the amount of cash a health authority may spend during a given financial year. This includes an estimated amount for the level of pay settlements and price rises. Separate cash limits are set for revenue and capital.

Consumables: anything that is not for resale and is not equipment, such as plastic aprons, rubber gloves, cleaning fluids, beverages.

Cost account: an off-shoot of the statutory accounts which produces information for individual units in terms of costs for inpatients, outpatients, etc.

Cost centre: any department, geographical area or activity that is identifiable by the individual code allocated to it for accounting purposes, usually a hospital or centre.

Development: schemes to change the level or type of service provided.

Enhancements: payments made for duties over and above the basic contracted hours and/or conditions of work.

Establishment: the total number and grades of staff in a particular department or branch of the service.

Expenditure
Non-recurring: one-off allocation or expenditure, such as a piece of equipment.
Recurring: continuous expenditure recurring each year and throughout the year, such as salaries.

Flexibility: the ability to move monies within budget headings.

Funding: allocation of monies to budget holders.

Gross pay: the total monies paid to employee before any deductions are made.

Incremental drift: cost associated with current staff receiving annual salary increments. These cause manpower costs to rise year by year with no distinct change in the service provided.

Index linking: automatic adjustment to baseline to take account of inflation.

Inflation rate: cash increase in cost not associated with a real increase in goods purchased. The rate is generally expressed as a percentage.

Manpower statistics: current analysis of staff contained within a budget.

Net pay: an employee's gross pay less deductions.

On-costs: the additional costs incurred over and above set salaries. The employer's contribution to employees' National Insurance and superannuation.

Operational planning: setting priorities and making plans for the year ahead.

Performance indicators: measurable items of workload set against established norms that enable relative performance to be measured.

Planned saving: certain actions, undertaken by a budget holder, which result in savings being made, for example, holding a post vacant for a set length of time.

Pump priming scheme: a scheme into which money is put in order to attract or save money, for example, money put into installing a computerised switchboard, which will eventually save money.

RAWP: an acronym for initials of the Resource Allocation Working Party, now used as a noun, verb and adjective.

Revenue consequences of capital schemes (RCCS): the annual running costs of a capital scheme.

Roll over: to take 1 year's budget as an agreed baseline for the following year's budget.

Slippage: the shortfall compared with planned spending, caused by delays in planning or execution of expenditure. It can be expressed in terms of money or time.

Source coding: budget holders' code documents originating spending on staff appointments, materials and equipment.

Stamp: Standard Manpower Planning; NHS computer-based system of manpower information.

Strategic planning: longer term plan, usually for 10 years, outlining general aims and directions based on Government's priorities for the health service.

Target allocation: money allocated through RAWP (see definition above) and in conjunction with the Health Authority's strategic plan.

Top slicing: money taken out of a Health Authority budget by the Department of Health for a particular project. For example, the Income Generation Department at the Department of Health may take money out of a region or group of regions budgets, before the money is allocated to them, in order to fund a national project.

Unit financial advisor (UFA): a representative of the treasurer's department who is designated to advise managers on any aspect of finance within their given function.

Uptake: utilising additional resources through increased service provision. Taking up monies offered.

Virement: the ability to switch funds within and between budgets, dependent on local policy.

Workload unit: a measure of workload performance in terms of a quantifiable indicator, for example, the number of clients seen in a department could be seen as the measure of output of that department.

WTE: Whole Time Equivalent. For example, a full-time occupational therapist works 36 hours per week. Someone working 18 hours per week is recorded as 0.5 WTE. Two people working 45 hours per week between them are recorded as 1.25 WTE.

Index